Textbook of

PLEURAL DISEASES

Textbook of PLEURAL DISEASES

Editors

Ashish Kumar Prakash
MBBS DTCD DNB EDRM FAPSR FNCCP MNAMS MICS MIACCAI
Senior Consultant
Department of Respiratory and Sleep Medicine
Respiratory Allergy Clinic
Medanta – The Medicity
Gurugram, Haryana, India

Anand Jaiswal
MBBS MAMC MD
Head and Senior Director
Department of Respiratory and Sleep Medicine
Medanta – The Medicity
Gurugram, Haryana, India

Randeep Guleria
MD (Medicine) DM (Pulmonary and Critical Care Medicine)
Chairman, Institute of Internal Medicine and Respiratory and Sleep Medicine
Director, Medical Education
Medanta (Global Health Ltd)
President, All India Institute of Medical Sciences
Bilaspur, Himachal Pradesh, India

Bornali Datta
MD MRCP (Edinburgh) CCST (UK)
Director
Department of Respiratory and Sleep Medicine
Project Lead, Mission TB-Free Haryana
Medanta – The Medicity
Gurugram, Haryana, India

Foreword

Randeep Guleria

JAYPEE BROTHERS MEDICAL PUBLISHERS
The Health Sciences Publisher
New Delhi | London

JAYPEE Jaypee Brothers Medical Publishers (P) Ltd

Headquarters
EMCA House
23/23-B, Ansari Road, Daryaganj
New Delhi 110 002, India
Landline: +91-11-23272143, +91-11-23272703
+91-11-23282021, +91-11-23245672
E-mail: jaypee@jaypeebrothers.com

Corporate Office
Jaypee Brothers Medical Publishers (P) Ltd.
4838/24, Ansari Road, Daryaganj
New Delhi 110 002, India
Phone: +91-11-43574357
Fax: +91-11-43574314
E-mail: jaypee@jaypeebrothers.com

Overseas Office
JP Medical Ltd.
83, Victoria Street, London
SW1H 0HW (UK)
Phone: +44-20 3170 8910
Fax: +44(0)20 3008 6180
E-mail: info@jpmedpub.com

Website: www.jaypeebrothers.com
Website: www.jaypeedigital.com

Inquiries for bulk sales may be solicited at: jaypee@jaypeebrothers.com

Textbook of Pleural Diseases / ***Ashish Kumar Prakash, Anand Jaiswal, Randeep Guleria, Bornali Datta***

First Edition: **2024**

Reprint 2025

ISBN: 978-93-5696-892-9

Printed at Replika Press Pvt. Ltd.

Dedicated to

This book is dedicated to

My Mother
Late Smt Renu Sinha,

My Father
Shri Vijay Kumar Sinha,

My Wife
Reena Verma Prakash,

My Son
Pratham Sinha,

My Daughter
Pankhudi Sinha,

and
the Whole Medanta Team.

CONTRIBUTORS

EDITORS

Ashish Kumar Prakash MBBS DTCD DNB EDRM FAPSR FNCCP MNAMS MICS MIACCAI
Senior Consultant
Department of Respiratory and Sleep Medicine
Respiratory Allergy Clinic
Medanta – The Medicity
Gurugram, Haryana, India

Anand Jaiswal MBBS MAMC MD
Head and Senior Director
Department of Respiratory and Sleep Medicine
Medanta – The Medicity
Gurugram, Haryana, India

Randeep Guleria MD (Medicine) DM (Pulmonary and Critical Care Medicine)
Chairman, Institute of Internal Medicine and Respiratory and Sleep Medicine
Director, Medical Education
Medanta (Global Health Ltd)
President, All India Institute of Medical Sciences
Bilaspur, Himachal Pradesh, India

Bornali Datta MD MRCP (Edinburgh) CCST (UK)
Director
Department of Respiratory and Sleep Medicine
Project Lead, Mission TB-Free Haryana
Medanta – The Medicity
Gurugram, Haryana, India

CONTRIBUTING AUTHORS

Abhijeet Khandelwal DNB (TB and Respiratory Diseases) Gold Medalist (Dr M Santhosham DNB-NBE Gold Medal) MBBS DTCD (Diploma in Chest and TB) FCCP (USA) EDARM (Europe)
Professor and Head
Department of Pulmonary and Sleep Medicine
Sri Aurobindo Institute of Medical Sciences
Indore, Madhya Pradesh, India

Abhishek Saini MBBS MD DM
Assistant Professor
Department of Gastroenterology
Sarvesh Health City
Hisar, Haryana, India

Aditi Singh MBBS DNB Fellow
Junior Resident, Department of Respiratory and Sleep Medicine
Medanta – The Medicity
Gurugram, Haryana, India

Ajay Kumar MBBS MD
Senior Consultant
Department of Pulmonology
Fortis Healthcare
Gurugram, Haryana, India

Amit Dhamija MBBS MD
Senior Consultant
Department of Chest Medicine
Sir Ganga Ram Hospital
Rajinder Nagar, New Delhi, India

Amit Kumar Mahapatra DM (Nephrology) MD (Medicine)
Senior Consultant, Nephrology and Kidney Transplant Medicine
Department of Nephrology
Medanta – The Medicity
Gurugram, Haryana, India

Anant Mohan MBBS MD
Professor and Head
Department of Pulmonary Medicine
All India Institute of Medical Sciences
New Delhi, India

Anuj K Bhatnagar MBBS MD
Professor and Head
Department of Pulmonary Medicine
Rajan Babu Institute of Pulmonary Medicine and Tuberculosis Hospital
New Delhi, India

Arvind Kumar MBBS MS (General Surgery) MNAMS FICS FACS FUICC
Chairman—Thoracic Surgery and Lung Transplantation
Institute of Chest Surgery, Chest Onco-Surgery and Lung Transplantation
Medanta – The Medicity
Gurugram, Haryana, India

Ashok Vaid MBBS MD
Chairman
Medical and Haemato Oncology
Cancer Institute
Medanta – The Medicity
Gurugram, Haryana, India

Ashwani Prakash MBBS MD (Anesthesiology) (Fellow)
Junior Resident
Department of Anesthesiology
Murshidabad Medical College and Hospital
Berhampore, West Bengal, India

Avi Kumar MBBS MD DNB EDRM
Senior Consultant
Department of Pulmonology
Fortis Escorts Heart Institute
New Delhi, India

Bhaumik J Kamdar MBBS MD (Respiratory Medicine)
Junior Resident
Department of Pulmonology
DY Patil Medical College and Research Centre
Navi Mumbai, Maharashtra, India

Bhavana Mastebhakti (Cardiology) Fellow (Pulmonology)
Consultant
Department of Pulmonology
Fortis Escorts Heart Institute
New Delhi, India

Bhawana Sharma MBBS DNB FCCM IDCCM
Consultant
Respiratory Medicine and Critical Care
Department of Critical Care
Medanta – The Medicity
Gurugram, Haryana, India

Deepak Govil MD EDIC FCCM
Vice Chairman—Critical Care Medicine
Medanta Institute of Critical Care and Anaesthesiology
Medanta – The Medicity
Gurugram, Haryana, India

Devireddy Madhava Reddy MBBS DNB FNB
Consultant—Critical Care Medicine
Medanta Institute of Critical Care and Anaesthesiology
Medanta – The Medicity
Gurugram, Haryana, India

Dhananjay Kumar Dubey MBBS MD (Anatomy) (Fellow)
Junior Resident
Department of Anatomy
Institute of Medical Sciences, Banaras Hindu University
Varanasi, Uttar Pradesh, India

Gargi Maitra MBBS MD
Consultant, Department of Pulmonology, Fortis Healthcare
Gurugram, Haryana, India

Hardeep Kaur Grewal MRCP (UK) FNIC FIAE
Senior Consultant—Clinical and Preventive Cardiology
Department of Cardiology
Medanta – The Medicity
Gurugram, Haryana, India

Harshvardhan Puri MBBS DNB (General Surgery) DNB (Thoracic Surgery)
Senior Consultant—Thoracic and Lung Transplant Surgeon
Institute of Chest Surgery, Chest Onco-Surgery and Lung Transplantation
Medanta – The Medicity
Gurugram, Haryana, India

JN Durga Rao Yadavalli MBBS MD DrNB
Consultant
Department of Rheumatology and Clinical Immunology
Medanta – The Medicity
Gurugram, Haryana, India

Kulbir Ahlawat MBBS MD
Vice Chairman—Diagnostic Radiology
Radiology and Imaging
Department of Radiology
Medanta – The Medicity
Gurugram, Haryana, India

Manan Bedi MBBS MD (Pulmonary Medicine)
Senior Resident
Department of Respiratory Medicine
Medanta – The Medicity
Gurugram, Haryana, India

Manish Bansal MD DNB (Cardiology) FACC FASE
Senior Director—Clinical and Preventive Cardiology
Department of Cardiology
Medanta – The Medicity
Gurugram, Haryana, India

Manoj K Goel MBBS MD
Director and Unit Head Pulmonology
Department of Pulmonology
Fortis Healthcare
Gurugram, Haryana, India

Mayank Pratap Singh DNB Fellow
Department of Respiratory and Sleep Medicine
Medanta – The Medicity
Gurugram, Haryana, India

Mohan Venkatesh Pulle MBBS DNB (General Surgery) DNB (Thoracic Surgery)
Consultant—Thoracic and Lung Transplant Surgeon
Institute of Chest Surgery, Chest Onco-Surgery and Lung Transplantation
Medanta – The Medicity
Gurugram, Haryana, India

Monika Madaan Gaur MD DNB FICOG FMAS
Specialist and Head
Department of Obstetrics and Gynaecology
ESIC Hospital, Manesar
Gurugram, Haryana, India

Mrinal Sircar MBBS DTCD MD (TB and Chest Diseases) DNB (Respiratory Diseases) EDIC EDRM
Senior Consultant and Head
Department of Critical Care
Fortis Hospital
Noida, Uttar Pradesh, India

Nafeesath PCP MBBS DNB
Junior Resident
Department of Respiratory Medicine
Lilavati Hospital
Mumbai, Maharashtra, India

Narendra S Choudhary MBBS MD DM
Senior Consultant
Department of Hepatology and Liver Transplantation
Medanta – The Medicity
Gurugram, Haryana, India

Nishant Gupta MBBS MD (Respiratory Medicine)
Consultant
Department of Respiratory Medicine
Medanta – The Medicity
Gurugram, Haryana, India

Pinky Goyal MBBS DTCD
Consultant
Department of Respiratory and Sleep Medicine
Medanta – The Medicity
Gurugram, Haryana, India

Pooja Tyagi MBBS MD FNB
Consultant—Critical Care Medicine
Medanta Institute of Critical Care and Anaesthesiology
Medanta – The Medicity
Gurugram, Haryana, India

Pralhad P Prabhudesai MD DNB FCCP (USA)
Consultant Chest Physician
Department of Respiratory Medicine
Lilavati Hospital and Research Centre
Mumbai, Maharashtra, India

Rahul Roshan DM MD DNB FCCP
Senior Consultant
Department of Chest and Allergy Disorders
BLK-Max Hospital
Noida, Uttar Pradesh, India

Rajiv Goyal DTCD MD MRCP (UK) (European Diploma in Adult Respiratory Medicine)
Senior Consultant and Director
Fellowship Program on Interventional Pulmonology and Thoracic Oncology
Rajiv Gandhi Cancer Institute and Research Centre
New Delhi, India

Rajiva Gupta MBBS MD MRCP
Head
Department of Rheumatology and Clinical Immunology
Medanta – The Medicity
Gurugram, Haryana, India

Rajkumar MBBS MD
Director, Professor and Head
Department of Respiratory Allergy and Applied Immunology
Vallabhbhai Patel Chest Institute (VPCI)
New Delhi, India

Reena Verma Prakash MBBS PGDMCH
Insurance Medical Office
CMO Department of Obstetrics and Gynaecology
ESIC Hospital, Manesar
Gurugram, Haryana, India

Roopanshi Jain MBBS DNB (Medanta – The Medicity, Gurugram)
Senior Resident
Respiratory and Sleep Medicine
Rajan Babu Institute of Pulmonary Medicine and Tuberculosis Hospital
New Delhi, India

Sandeep Katiyar DNB (European Diploma in Adult Respiratory Medicine) MNCCP FCCP (USA) MNAMS
Consultant Pulmonologist and Interventionist
Apollo Spectra Hospital
Director, Katiyar Chest Centre
Kanpur, Uttar Pradesh, India

Sandeep K Mittal MBBS DND IDCC
Senior Consultant, Department of Respiratory and Sleep Medicine
Medanta – The Medicity
Gurugram, Haryana, India

Sandeep Tilve DNB (Respiratory Diseases) FCCP
Consultant Pulmonologist
Department of Pulmonology
Green Lungs Clinic
Mumbai, Maharashtra, India

Sangeeta Basu Gupta MBBS MD (Paediatrics)
Consultant, Department of Paediatrics and Critical Care
Aarvy Hospital
Gurugram, Haryana, India

Saroj Meena MBBS DTCD DNB (Respiratory Medicine)
Specialist, Grade I
Department of Tuberculosis and Chest Diseases
National Institute of TB and Respiratory Diseases (NITRD)
New Delhi, India

Saurabh Mandilwar MBBS DNB (Pulmonary Medicine)
Speciality Medical Consultant
Department of Respiratory Medicine
Dr RN Cooper Hospital and HBT Medical College
Mumbai, Maharashtra, India

Shabd Prakash MBBS DTCD
Senior Specialist
Department of Pulmonary Medicine
ESIC Hospital
Gurugram, Haryana, India

Shubhi Singhal MBBS MD (Respiratory Medicine) DNB MNAMS
Attending Consultant
Internal Medicine, Respiratory and Sleep Medicine
Medanta – The Medicity
Gurugram, Haryana, India

Shweta Bansal MD DNB DM (AIIMS Delhi) EDARM MNAMS FAPSR (Fellowship Lung Transplant, Vienna Austria)
Senior Consultant
Department of Pulmonology and Sleep Medicine
Narayana Health
Gurugram, Haryana, India

Siddharth Chatterjee MBBS MD (Respiratory Medicine) EDRM (European Diploma in Adult Respiratory Medicine)
Senior Resident
Department of Respiratory and Sleep Medicine
Medanta – The Medicity
Ahmedabad, Gujarat, India

SK Chhabra MBBS MD
Department of Respiratory and Sleep Medicine
Ex-Director Professor
Pulmonary Medicine
Vallabhbhai Patel Chest Institute
Emeritus Consultant
Pulmonary Medicine
Primus Superspeciality Hospital
New Delhi, India

Sonam Singla MBBS DNB (Microbiology)
Attending Consultant
Department of Microbiology
Medanta – The Medicity
Ahmedabad, Gujarat, India

Sukhram Bishnoi MBBS DNB (General Surgery) DNB (Thoracic Surgery)
Consultant—Thoracic and Lung Transplant Surgeon
Institute of Chest Surgery, Chest Onco-Surgery and Lung Transplantation
Medanta – The Medicity
Gurugram, Haryana, India

Sumit K Pahariya MBBS DNB (Medanta – The Medicity, Gurugram)
Medical Officer
Department of Respiratory and Sleep Medicine
Rajan Babu Institute of Pulmonary Medicine and Tuberculosis Hospital
New Delhi, India

Surabhi Gupta MBBS DNB (Radiology) EDiR
Associate Consultant
Department of Radiology
Indraprastha Apollo Hospital
New Delhi, India

Vidhi Jobanputra MBBS MD (Respiratory Medicine)
Clinical Associate
Department of Respiratory Medicine
Lilavati Hospital and Research Centre
Om Clinic
Mumbai, Maharashtra, India

Vikas Deswal MBBS MD (Medicine) PDF (Infectious Diseases)
Senior Consultant
Department of Internal Medicine and Infectious Diseases
Medanta – The Medicity
Gurugram, Haryana, India

Vivek Singh MBBS MD (Pulmonary Medicine) Post-Doctoral Fellowship in Lung Transplantation (University of Toronto)
Director—Pulmonology and Transplant Pulmonology
Institute of Chest Surgery, Chest Onco-Surgery and Lung Transplantation
Medanta – The Medicity
Gurugram, Haryana, India

Yatin Mehta MD MNAMS FRCA FAMS FIACTA FICCM FTEE
Adjunct Professor—NBE
Past President—ISCCM
Chairman—Medanta Institute of Critical Care and Anesthesiology
Medanta – The Medicity
Gurugram, Haryana, India

PREFACE

ऊँ नमो देव्यै महादेव्यै शिवायै सततं नमः।
नमः प्रकृत्यै भद्रायै नियताः प्रणताः स्म ताम्।।

Pleural diseases are common in our day-to-day practice, yet there are not many textbooks which give an insight into pleural diseases, apart from Dr Richard W Light, which was originally published in 1983 and a new edition in 2007. Every year, millions of patients develop pleural effusion (or diseases) globally. Apart from pleural effusion, there are other pleural diseases, which are widely prevalent and need to be recognized, such as pneumothorax, hemothorax, chylothorax, and malignant pleural effusion. This textbook is intended to fill a perceived gap in this domain of a holistic approach to all pleural pathologies. All the chapters of this book are written by specialists, dealing with pleural pathology pertaining to specific diseases in their specialty.

The first two chapters describe *anatomy and physiology* of the pleura along with its development. The next few chapters discuss the *diagnostic aspects* of the pleura, such as chest X-ray and CT scan. One chapter is dedicated to chest USG, a common modality for management of pleural disease, and a bedside test used for point of care management in ICU.

Both the *common and rare entities* of pleural pathology are written about, using a wide angled lens and include all recent updates. In the wide remit of pulmonary science, the book zooms into the niche of pleural diseases with an individualized approach to each pleural pathology. There exists a plethora of textbooks on pulmonary medicine, critical care medicine, and internal medicine; this book is unique in being a textbook on pleural diseases written by *specialists* from multiple disciplines. We have ensured that a hepatologist has written about hepatic hydrothorax, a gynecologist has written about effusion due to gynecological issue, and so on and so forth. There are a few chapters on *topics which have not been addressed till date* (in any book?) like pleural disease in children and the pleura in lung transplant, which have been elaborated in this textbook.

Infection and its related complications, a common entity in pleural pathology, have been dealt with in separate chapters.

We have elaborated on *intercostal drainage (ICD) tubes*, their management, complications, and newer advances in two chapters. ICDs have evolved greatly in the last decade as have various drainage systems.

Along with substantial specialist input, we have attempted to pen down the vast experience of our whole team, both present and past, in this textbook.

I sincerely hope that those who read this book, both students and practitioners alike, will get a deep insight into the anatomy, physiology, and pathologies of the pleura. I hope this collection of expert writings will have a great impact in the management of pleural disease.

Ashish Kumar Prakash

ACKNOWLEDGMENTS

I extend my special thanks to Dr Naresh Trehan, the Chairman and Managing Director of Medanta – The Medicity. My gratitude also goes to Dr Vikram Sarabhai, whose inspiration led to the creation of this textbook on pleural diseases. Dr Anand Jaiswal's unwavering support has been the backbone of this book.

I am grateful for the consistent support from the entire Medanta Team, including Dr Bornali Datta, my DNB fellows, students, and the entire Respiratory Team. Their remarkable efforts have been instrumental in giving this book its complete shape.

We especially appreciate the constant support and encouragement of Shri Jitendar P Vij (Group Chairman) and Mr Ankit Vij (Managing Director) of M/s Jaypee Brothers Medical Publishers (P) Ltd, New Delhi, India, in publishing the book and also their associates, particularly Ms Chetna Malhotra (Senior Director—Professional Publishing, Marketing, and Business Development), and Ms Charu Lata (Development Editor), who have been prompt, efficient, and most helpful.

CONTENTS

CHAPTER

1 Pleural Anatomy

Dhananjay Kumar Dubey, Anant Mohan

INTRODUCTION

Vital organs like the heart and lungs constantly move and change volume in the cramped thoracic cavity in order to function. The pleura is an elastic serous membrane with a smooth, lubricating surface that covers the inner surface of the thoracic cage and the surface of the lung to create the pleural cavity **(Fig. 1)**. This resembles a sealed, damp, elastic plastic bag between the lung and the thoracic wall that helps to reduce friction. For the lung to function well, the pleura and pleural cavity are crucial, just as the pericardium and pericardial cavity are for the heart. Because of the significance of this arrangement, a bodily cavity surrounded by a serous membrane form in the embryo, and the actions required to keep the cavity open are taken before the development of the key organs. The pleura is a double-layered membrane, which are called visceral pleura and the parietal pleura.

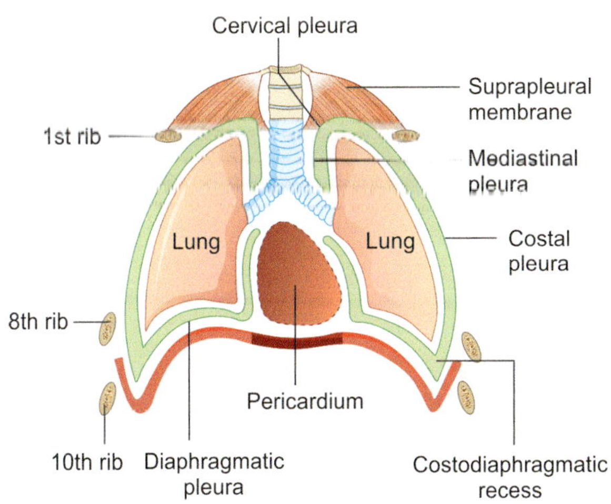

FIG. 1: Coronal Section in mid-axillary plane.

The innermost layer, which is in direct contact with the lung tissue, is the visceral pleura. It is a thin, translucent covering that closely approximates the lung's surface and contours. The lining of the thoracic cavity is made up of the parietal pleura, which is the thicker outer layer. This is anatomically divided into the costal, diaphragmatic, and mediastinal pleura. The mediastinal pleura covers the lateral aspect of the mediastinum, the diaphragmatic pleura covers the diaphragm, and the costal pleura lines the inner wall of the rib cage. The small area between the two layers of the pleura is known as the pleural cavity. This contains a small amount of fluid, called pleural fluid, which lubricates the pleural surfaces and allows them to slide over each other during breathing movements.

EMBRYOLOGY

The pleura develops from the mesoderm, one of the three germ layers during embryonic development. The somites and the lateral plate mesoderm are the two distinct sources from which the pleura originates. The pleural and peritoneal cavities, which will eventually be bordered by the pleura and peritoneum, are formed by the lateral plate mesoderm **(Figs. 2 and 3)**. The muscles of the thorax and abdomen are derived from the somites. The pleura separates into two layers, the visceral and parietal pleura, as the embryo grows and develops.

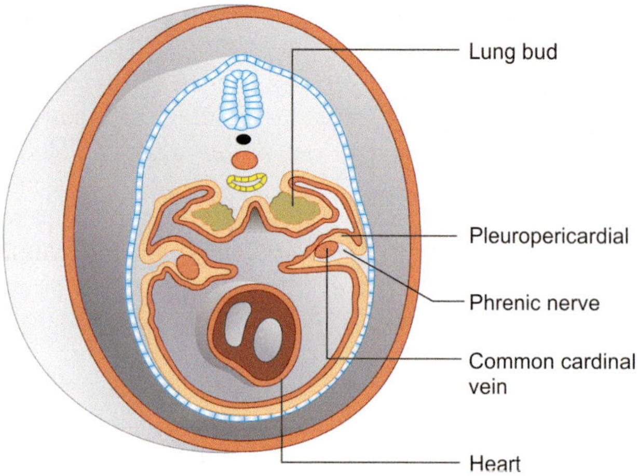

FIG. 2: Transverse section of developing embryo showing pleuropericardial fold, which divide thoracic cavity in to pleural and pericardial cavity.

The area between the two layers, which is known as the pleural cavity, is eventually formed by these layers. Initially connected to the peritoneal cavity, the pleural cavity separates from it as the septum transversum develops and eventually takes the form of the diaphragm. The coelomic cavity, a U-shaped cavity, separates into the pericardial, pleural, and peritoneal cavities in a systematic manner throughout development. This is achieved by the development of two membranes. The pleuroperitoneal membrane and septum transversum together produce the muscular diaphragm that divides the pleural cavity from the peritoneal cavity, while the pleuropericardial membrane does the same for the lungs and heart. Mesothelium[1] lines the interior of this recently developed pleural cavity. The trachea and main bronchi grow from the median mass of mesenchyme. These

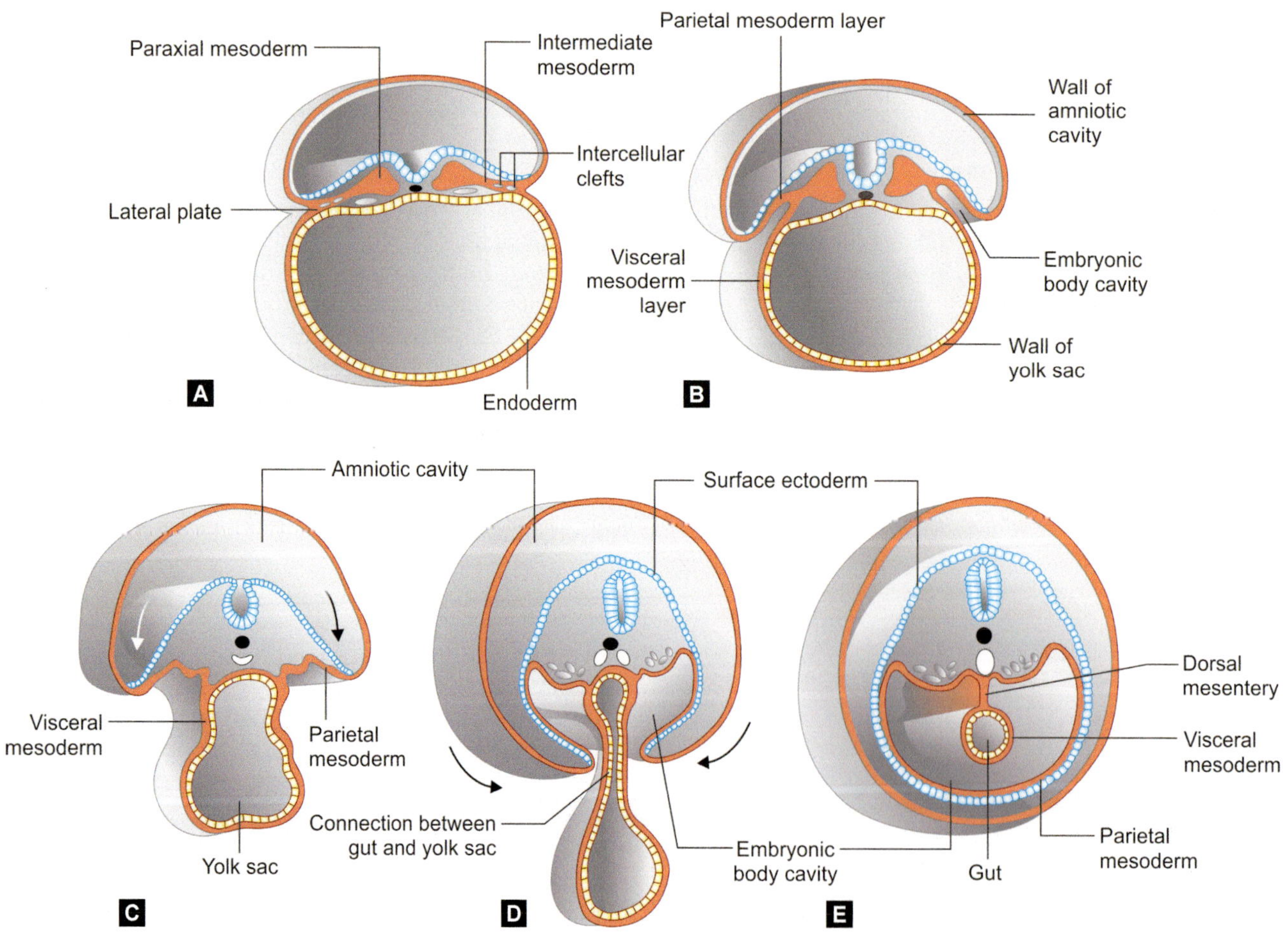

FIGS. 3A TO E: Transverse sections through embryos at various stages of closure of the gut tube and ventral body wall. (A) At approximately 19 days, intercellular clefts are visible in the lateral plate mesoderm; (B) At 20 days, the lateral plate is divided into somatic and visceral mesoderm layers that line the primitive body cavity (intraembryonic cavity); (C) By 21 days, the primitive body cavity (intraembryonic cavity) is still in open communication with the extraembryonic cavity; (D) By 24 days, the lateral body wall folds, consisting of the parietal layer of lateral plate mesoderm and overlying ectoderm, are approaching each other in the midline; (E) At the end of the fourth week, visceral mesoderm layers are continuous with parietal layers as a double-layered membrane, the dorsal mesentery. Dorsal mesentery extends from the caudal limit of the foregut to the end of the hindgut.

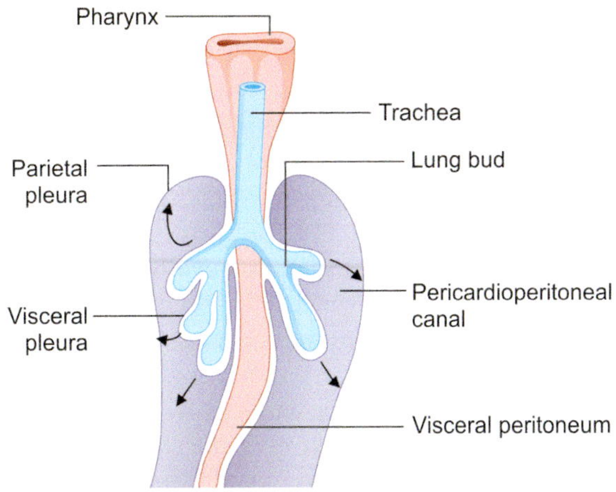

FIG. 4: Development of visceral and parietal pleura and invagination of lung buds into it.

growing bronchi buds grows outwards and while doing so it takes mesothelial layer along with it, which develops to become the visceral pleura **(Figs. 4 and 5)**.

HISTOLOGY

The connective tissue that makes up the pleura consists of fibroblasts, mesothelial cells, lymphocytes, and macrophages, among other cell types. The visceral pleura is a mesothelial cell-lined thin, delicate layer of connective tissue that covers the surface of the lung. Specialized epithelial cells, known as mesothelial cells **(Fig. 6)**, release a tiny amount of fluid that lubricates the pleural surfaces. The lining of the thoracic cavity is made up of a thicker layer of connective tissue called the parietal pleura.

Vascular supply, elastic fibers, and collagen fibers can all be found in the pleural tissue. While the elastic fibers enable the pleura to stretch and recoil in response to variations in lung volume while breathing, the collagen fibers give the pleural tissue tensile strength. The pleural arteries deliver oxygen and nutrients to the tissue's cells. Visceral pleura is made up of an acellular layer, which sits atop connective tissue, which is made up of blood, lymph, and nerve vessels. The thickness of the visceral pleura varies between species; it is thicker in humans, sheep, cows, pigs, and horses than in dogs, cats, and monkeys.[2] Since there are many microvilli on the inferior visceral pleura as well as the anterior and inferior mediastinal parietal pleura, their distribution is unequal. Additionally,

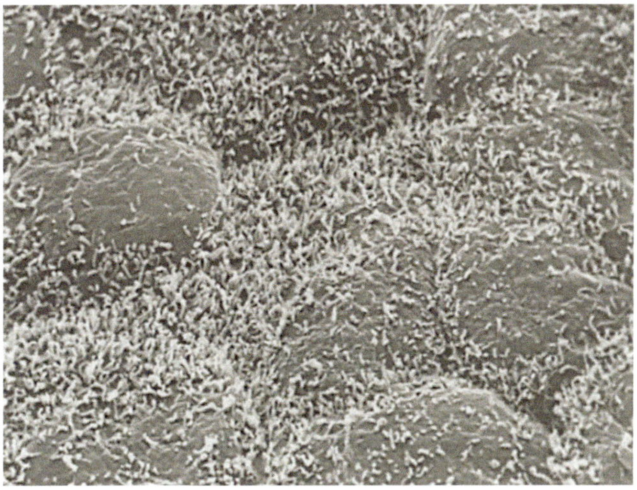

FIG. 6: Scanning electron micrograph showing parietal pleural mesothelial cells with a dense population of microvilli.

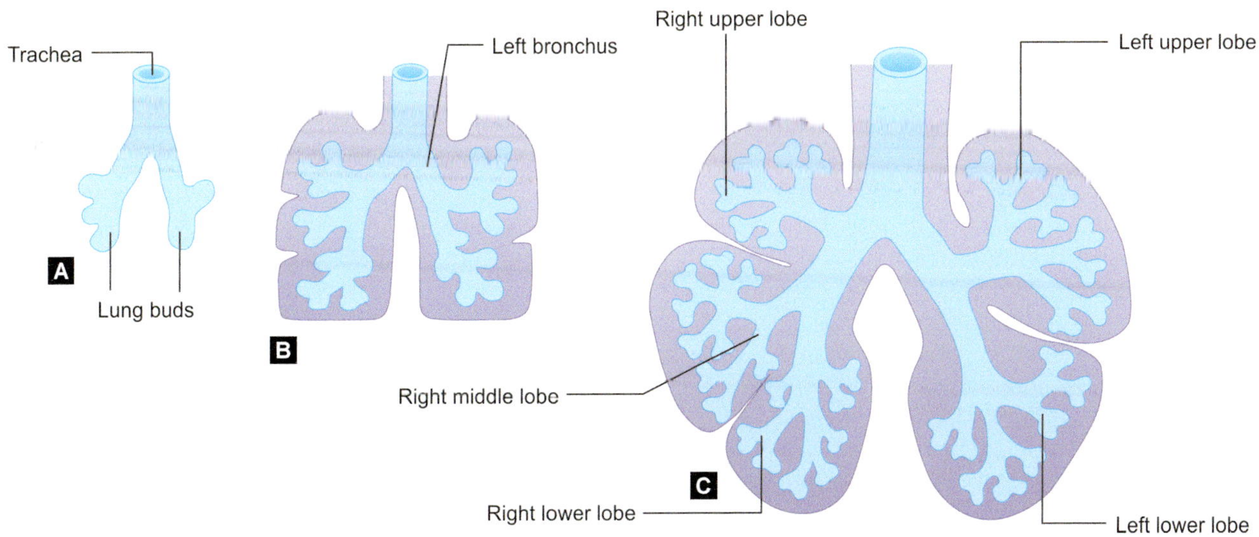

FIGS. 5A TO C: Stages in development of the trachea and lungs. (A) 5 weeks; (B) 6 weeks; (C) 8 weeks.

the comparable visceral pleura regions have more microvilli than the parietal pleura.[1,3]

Before, it was believed that the presence of microvilli assisted in the absorption of pleural fluid, but more recent research has revealed that they also play a role in minimizing lung–chest wall friction by generating a meshwork of glycoproteins high in hyaluronidase.[4]

The mesothelial cell layer is extremely brittle; frequently, mesothelial cells fall off the surface and are discovered floating freely in the pleural fluid.[5] The cells retract when the mesothelial layer is stimulated, yet they maintain their continuity by generating projections. When a layer of mesothelial cells is damaged, a defect results, which the mesothelial cells repair by mitosis and migration.[6] Mesothelial cells that are floating freely in the pleural fluid have the ability to transform into macrophages, which phagocyte various substances. Macrophages in pleural fluid can also be derived from alveolar macrophages and peripheral blood mononuclear cells.[7,8]

Over the pleura, mesothelial cells create a monolayer. They have the ability to develop into myofibroblasts in the presence of transforming growth factor beta (TGF-β).[9,10] This is a reason why TGF-β is used for pleurodesis because of the morphological alterations it causes. Furthermore, they release several substances, including nitric oxide, different cytokines, and fibronectin, different forms of collagen, elastin, and laminin.[11,12]

CELLULAR COMPONENT OF PLEURAL FLUID

Depending on the underlying cause of the pleural effusion, the cellular composition of the pleural fluid can change. Normal pleural fluid is sparsely cellular; however, cellularity increases in pathological states such infections, malignancies, or other inflammatory conditions. The kind and quantity of white blood cells (WBCs) might offer crucial diagnostic information. For example, a high concentration of neutrophils may be a sign of an infection, but a high number of lymphocytes may indicate inflammation or cancer. The presence of red blood cells (RBCs) in the pleural fluid can indicate a number of underlying health issues, such as cancer, trauma, or pulmonary embolism. Increase in shedding of mesothelial cells may occur in mesothelioma or asbestos exposure. Malignant pleural effusion can be identified by the presence of cancerous cells in the pleural fluid.

Normal pleural fluid distribution between the parietal and visceral pleura is equal. The friction between parietal pleura and chest wall is low, and visceral and parietal pleura always separate from each other as microvilli of mesothelial cells never interdigitate.[13,14]

In a study done by Noppen et al. pleural fluid volume in right lung is 8.4 mL ± 4.3 mL, and the volume of fluid is almost similar on both sides.[15] In animal studies, it is found that normal volume of pleural fluid varies from 0.04 to 0.2 mL/kg body weight.[16]

In a healthy adult, the amount of pleural fluid is normally quite tiny, between 0.1 and 0.2 mL/kg of body weight.[17] This trace amount of pleural fluid aids in the smooth movement of the lungs during breathing by lubricating the pleural surfaces. The amount of pleural fluid can grow in pathological diseases, such as infections, cancers, or congestive heart failure and result in pleural effusion. Depending on the underlying reason and length of the effusion, the volume of pleural fluid in these situations might range from a few milliliters to several liters.

Pleural fluids contain small amount of protein, which is mainly rich in low-molecular-weight protein, like albumin.

The ionic content and concentration in pleural fluid differs from serum. Compared to plasma, pleural fluid bicarbonate concentration is higher, sodium and chloride is lower, while potassium and glucose concentration is almost similar.[18]

BLOOD SUPPLY OF PLEURA

The pleura receives its oxygen and nutrition from a network of blood arteries that supply the pleural tissues. The intercostal arteries, internal thoracic arteries, and bronchial arteries are only a few of the blood vessels that supply the pleura. The parietal pleura is supplied by the intercostal arteries, which run along the underside of the ribs. The subclavian arteries give rise to the internal thoracic arteries, which supply the mediastinal pleura. These arteries also supply the pericardium and the anterior chest wall. The visceral pleura is perfused by the bronchial arteries, which emerge from the aorta. The bronchi and lung tissue are also supplied by these blood vessels. The pulmonary and bronchial veins, which empty into the left atrium of the heart, are responsible for the pleura's venous drainage. The blood is drained from the visceral pleura and lung tissue by the pulmonary veins. Four primary pulmonary veins emerge from the lungs and empty into the left atrium of the heart. They develop from the capillary beds around the alveoli. On the other side, the bronchial veins are responsible for removing blood from the parietal pleura and bronchi. The azygos vein, a significant vein that runs along the spine, is where the bronchial veins can drain directly, or they can drain into the pulmonary veins. The internal thoracic veins or the azygos vein, which in turn drain into the subclavian vein, are the final destinations of the intercostal veins, which run along the underside of the ribs. The pulmonary veins, bronchial veins, and intercostal veins are just a few of the venous blood sources that are involved in the complicated venous drainage of the pleura. Maintaining proper physiological function and minimizing fluid build-up in the pleural space depend on the efficient drainage of venous blood from the pleura.

PLEURAL LYMPHATICS

In order to maintain fluid balance and immunological function in the thoracic cavity, the lymphatic drainage of the pleura is crucial. The thoracic duct, the body's primary lymphatic channel, receives lymph from the pleura's extensive lymphatic network. Deep lymphatics and superficial lymphatics are the two basic classifications of lymphatic vessels in the pleura. The internal mammary, intercostal, and supraclavicular vessels run along the superficial lymphatics, which are found in the subpleural connective tissue and drain into the parietal pleural lymph nodes. The bronchopulmonary lymph nodes, which are close to the bronchi and pulmonary arteries, receive the deep lymphatics from the visceral pleura. Lymphatic vessels continue to drain into the tracheobronchial lymph nodes, which are situated close to the trachea and major bronchi, from the parietal pleural lymph nodes. Lymphatic veins pour into the pulmonary lymph nodes, which are found inside the lung tissue, from the bronchopulmonary lymph nodes. The thoracic duct, which empties into the left subclavian vein, receives lymphatic drainage from the pleura in the end. Before returning lymph fluid to the venous circulation, the thoracic duct also receives lymphatic drainage from other body areas, such as the lower limbs, abdomen, and left upper limb. Maintaining fluid balance in the thoracic cavity and moving immune cells and antigens between the pleura and lymphoid tissues both depend on the lymphatic drainage of the pleura. Pleural effusion, a disorder marked by an accumulation of fluid in the pleural space, can result from disruption of the pleural lymphatic drainage.

Red blood cells or carbon particles are reported to drain through stomas and the lymphatics surrounding them when injected into pleural spaces.[19,20]

While lymphatic vessels connected to the diaphragmatic pleura drain into the parasternal and phrenic group of lymph nodes, those connected to the mediastinal pleura flow into the mediastinal group of lymph nodes.

Lymphatic vessels of parietal pleura have many branches, and some vessels which are present under mesothelial layer have dilatation known as lacuna.[20,21]

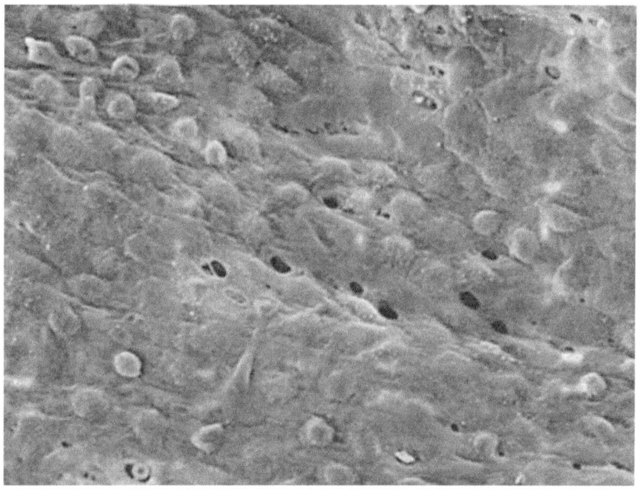

FIG. 7: A group of stomas is found at the anterior lower chest, caudal to a costochondral junction in a rat. The stomas show slight variation in sizes. (Scanning electron micrograph, original magnification × 1,500)

These lymphatic vessels are connected to pleural spaces through stomas of size 2–6 μm.[20,22]

Stomas are slit-like spaces where mesothelial cells which have microvilli are continuous with endothelial cells of lymphatic vessels **(Fig. 7)**.

Visceral pleura is rich in lymphatic vessels, which form interconnecting plexus over the surface of the lung and ultimately directed to hilum of the lung either by piercing the lung or crossing over the surface of the lung. Ultimately, all of these are directed to root of the lung. The large lymphatic vessels of visceral pleura have one-way valve through which lymph is directed to hilum of the lung.[5]

Visceral pleura is devoid of stoma, lymphatic vessels are separated from mesothelial cells by connective tissue layer; this is the reason why pleural fluid content is drained through parietal pleura lymphatic not through lymphatic vessels present over visceral pleura, as there is absence of stoma **(Fig. 8)**.[23]

In humans, milky spots are quite, invisible in the healthy pleura. However, thoracoscopy sometimes visualizes foci of parietal anthracosis near lymphatic vessels of the parietal pleura, which Boutin C[24] had called "black spots."

These "black spots" are aggregation of immune cells around lymphatic vessels.

According to Kampmeier (1928), Kampmeier foci are tiny milky patches that are collections of lymphocytes that are located on the surface of the lungs or pleura. Microscopically, these are collections of histiocytes, plasma cells, and other types of mononuclear cells that are clustered around the pleura's vasculature and

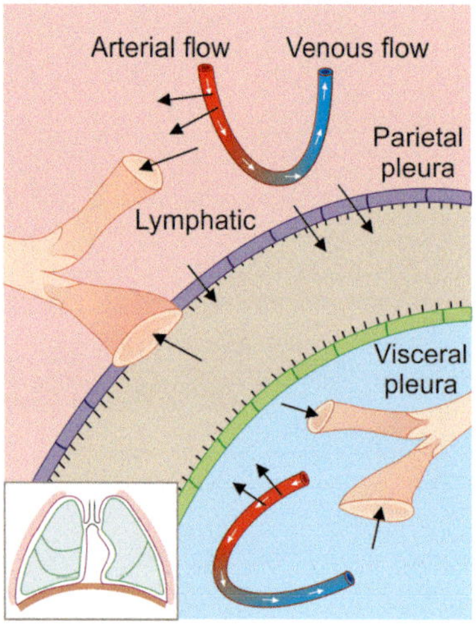

FIG. 8: Lymphatic drainage of pleura.

concentrate mostly in the mediastinal pleura. These small cellular aggregates are hypothesized to function as a defense mechanism in the pleura.

Asbestos fibers were discovered to be localized in these foci.[24] According to one view, these foci's high concentration of asbestos fibers causes the development of pleural plaques and mesothelioma.[24] However, it is not necessary that always black patches over lung are associated with pleural plaques.[25]

INNERVATION OF PLEURA

Sensory nerves that innervate the pleura transmit pain, touch, and temperature sensations from the pleural surface to the brain. These sensory nerves originate in the visceral and parietal pleura. The sensory nerves from the intercostal nerves, which are branches of the thoracic spinal nerves, richly innervate the parietal pleura, which lines the chest wall. The muscles and skin of the chest wall are likewise innervated by the intercostal nerves. Sensory nerves from the pulmonary plexus, a network of nerves derived from the sympathetic and parasympathetic nervous systems, innervate the visceral pleura, which surrounds the lungs, but their functional roles have not yet been determined.[26] The bronchi and arteries of the lungs are also innervated by the pulmonary plexus. Inflammation, infection, or damage to the pleural tissue can cause pain and other sensations, which are sensed by the sensory nerves of the pleura. Sharp chest pain that is frequently felt during breathing or coughing, for instance, can be brought on by irritation of the parietal pleura. On the other hand, inflammation of the visceral pleura can result in a deep-chest ache that is dull and painful. In order to diagnose and treat disorders that affect this tissue, such as pleurisy, pleural effusion, and pneumothorax, it is crucial to comprehend how the pleura is innervated.

Parietal pleura is innervated by intercostal nerves (T1–T11) and phrenic nerve (C3–C5), and sensitive to pain.

KEY POINTS

- Lung is covered by pleura, which is made up of two layers—visceral pleura and parietal pleura.
- Parietal pleura is thicker one and further divided into mediastinal, costal, and diaphragmatic pleura.
- Pleura develops from the lateral plate mesoderm after the formation of embryonic body cavity.
- Trachea and the lung buds develop from the adjacent mesenchyme after separation from the foregut, which invaginates into this developing pleura.
- Mesothelial cells are the lining cells of pleura containing numerous microvilli on their surface.
- In-between the two layers of pleura, there is very little amount of pleural fluid in healthy adults; it ranges from 0.1 to 0.2 mL/kg body weight.
- Costal pleura is supplied by intercostal arteries; mediastinal pleura is supplied by internal thoracic artery; and visceral pleura is supplied by bronchial artery.
- Pleura is richly supplied by lymphatics; parietal pleura drains into tracheobronchial and visceral pleura into bronchopulmonary lymph nodes.
- Stomas are slit-like spaces where mesothelial cells which have microvilli are continuous with endothelial cells of lymphatic vessels.
- Kampmeier foci are tiny milky spots, which are aggregation of lymphocytes present over the lung surface.
- Parietal pleura is innervated by intercostal nerve branches from thoracic spinal nerve and sensitive to pain, although visceral pleura is also innervated by pulmonary nerve plexus, but it is insensitive to pain.

REFERENCES

1. Wang NS. Anatomy of the pleura. Clin Chest Med. 1998;19(2):229-40.
2. Albertine KH, Wiener-Kronish JP, Roos PJ, Staub NC. Structure, blood supply, and lymphatic vessels of the sheep's visceral pleura. Am J Anat. 1982;165(3):277-94.
3. Yalcin NG, Choong CK, Eizenberg N. Anatomy and pathophysiology of the pleura and pleural space. Thorac Surg Clin. 2013;23(1):1-10, v.
4. Wang NS. The regional difference of pleural mesothelial cells in rabbits. Am Rev Respir Dis. 1974;110(5):623-33.

5. Peng MJ, Wang NS, Vargas FS, Light RW. Subclinical surface alterations of human pleura. A scanning electron microscopic study. Chest. 1994;106(2):351-3.
6. Efrati P, Nir E. Morphological and cytochemical investigation of human mesothelial cells from pleural and peritoneal effusions: a light and electron microscopy study. Isr J Med Sci. 1976;12(7): 662-73.
7. Bakalos D, Constantakis N, Tsicricas T. Distinction of mononuclear macrophages from mesothelial cells in pleural and peritoneal effusions. Acta Cytol. 1974;18(1):20-2.
8. Mutsaers SE. Mesothelial cells: their structure, function and role in serosal repair. Respirology. 2002;7(3):171-91.
9. Yang AH, Chen JY, Lin JK. Myofibroblastic conversion of mesothelial cells. Kidney Int. 2003;63(4):1530-9.
10. Owens MW, Milligan SA, Grisham MB. Nitric oxide synthesis by rat pleural mesothelial cells: induction by growth factors and lipopolysaccharide. Exp Lung Res. 1995;21(5):731-42.
11. Antony VB, Sahn SA, Mossman B, Gail DB, Kalica A. NHLBI workshop summaries. Pleural cell biology in health and disease. Am Rev Respir Dis. 1992;145(5):1236-9.
12. Lemos M, Pozo RM, Montes GS, Saldiva PH. Organization of collagen and elastic fibers studied in stretch preparations of whole mounts of human visceral pleura. Ann Anat. 1997;179(5):447-52.
13. Albertine KH, Wiener-Kronish JP, Bastacky J, Staub NC. No evidence for mesothelial cell contact across the costal pleural space of sheep. J Appl Physiol (1985). 1991;70(1):123-34.
14. Miserocchi G, Agostoni E. Pleural liquid and surface pressures at various lung volumes. Respir Physiol. 1980;39(3):315-26.
15. Noppen M, De Waele M, Li R, Gucht KV, D'Haese J, Gerlo E, et al. Volume and cellular content of normal pleural fluid in humans examined by pleural lavage. Am J Respir Crit Care Med. 2000;162(3 Pt 1):1023-6.
16. Noppen M. Normal volume and cellular contents of pleural fluid. Curr Opin Pulm Med. 2001;7(4):180-2.
17. Miserocchi G, Agostoni E. Contents of the pleural space. J Appl Physiol. 1971;30(2):208-13.
18. Rolf LL, Travis DM. Pleural fluid-plasma bicarbonate gradients in oxygen-toxic and normal rats. Am J Physiol. 1973;224(4): 857-61.
19. Albertine KH, Wiener-Kronish JP, Staub NC. The structure of the parietal pleura and its relationship to pleural liquid dynamics in sheep. Anat Rec. 1984;208(3):401-9.
20. Wang NS. The preformed stomas connecting the pleural cavity and the lymphatics in the parietal pleura. Am Rev Respir Dis. 1975;111(1):12-20.
21. Jones JS. The pleura in health and disease. Lung. 2001;179(6): 397-413.
22. Li YY, Li JC. Ultrastructure and three-dimensional study of the lymphatic stomata in the costal pleura of the rabbit. Microsc Res Tech. 2003;62(3):240-6.
23. Shinohara H. Distribution of lymphatic stomata on the pleural surface of the thoracic cavity and the surface topography of the pleural mesothelium in the golden hamster. Anat Rec. 1997;249(1):16-23.
24. Boutin C, Dumortier P, Rey F, Viallat JR, De Vuyst P. Black spots concentrate oncogenic asbestos fibers in the parietal pleura. Thoracoscopic and mineralogic study. Am J Respir Crit Care Med. 1996;153(1):444-9.
25. Mitchev K, Dumortier P, De Vuyst P. 'Black Spots' and hyaline pleural plaques on the parietal pleura of 150 urban necropsy cases. Am J Surg Pathol. 2002;26(9):1198-206.
26. Pintelon I, Brouns I, De Proost I, Van Meir F, Timmermans JP, Adriaensen D. Sensory receptors in the visceral pleura: neurochemical coding and live staining in whole mounts. Am J Respir Cell Mol Biol. 2007;36(5):541-51.

CHAPTER

2 Physiology of the Pleural Space

SK Chhabra

INTRODUCTION

The pleural space is a closed potential space between the visceral pleura, which lines the lung, including the fissures, and the parietal pleura, which lines the chest wall, diaphragm, and mediastinum. The two pleural membranes consist of a single layer of mesothelial cells, a layer of connective tissue, a superficial elastic layer, a loose connective tissue layer, and a deep fibroelastic layer. The two layers of the pleura are continuous at the lung hila, the visceral layer reflecting over itself lines the chest wall and the diaphragm to form the parietal pleura.

PLEURAL FLUID AND PLEURAL PRESSURE[1-5]

The two layers of the pleura are separated by a thin layer of fluid. The fluid provides lubrication and allows the visceral and parietal pleura to glide over each other without frictional resistance during respiratory movements. It has been suggested that the quantity of fluid is too small to provide adequate lubrication and surface-active phospholipids that have been identified in pleural fluid may be the actual lubricants. The fluid is also believed to facilitate lung expansion by mechanical coupling of the lung and the chest wall. The quantity of the fluid has to be minimal to allow these two mechanical functions during breathing.

The normal pleural space is filled with approximately 7–14 mL (0.26 mL of fluid per kilogram of body weight) of low-protein pleural fluid in a normal adult human. Approximately 0.15 mL/kg of fluid is produced hourly by the parietal pleura and quickly absorbed to keep the net fluid to a minimum. The pleural fluid is in a dynamic state with an hourly turnover of 30–75% of the water. This is accelerated by increased lung movements, such as during exercise. Protein and particles are turned over much less rapidly.

The pleural fluid normally has the following composition: glucose content similar to plasma, a protein concentration of 1–2 g%, low sodium content (1–2 g/dL), a low white cell count (<1,000 cells/mm^3), and a low lactate dehydrogenase (LDH) level (<50% that of plasma).

Any air that gains access to the pleural space is at atmospheric minus pleural pressure, whereas blood gases in parietal pleural capillaries are at a more negative pressure compared to atmospheric. Thus, air would quickly pass into parietal capillaries plasma and would not accumulate.

Generation and Importance of Pleural Pressure

At the functional residual capacity (FRC) of the lung, the elastic recoils of the lung (inward) and the chest wall (outward) are balanced but in opposite directions, creating a negative pressure inside the pleural cavity [pleural pressure (P_{pl})]. The P_{pl} is on an average about 5–6 cmH_2O at FRC, being more negative at lung apex and on deep inspiration. The inner surface of the thoracic cavity lined by the pleura as well as the outer surface of the lungs and the heart is exposed to this negative P_{pl}. The pleural negativity would tend to suck capillary fluid and gas from surrounding tissue into the space if it were not for other balancing factors.

The pleura transmits the force generated by the respiratory muscles to the lungs. As the chest wall expands during inspiration, due to the mechanical coupling provided by the thin amount of pleural fluid, the lung is pulled outward, thus decreasing the pressures inside the alveoli and drawing in air from the atmosphere.

The pleural pressure negativity also helps in cardiac filling due to the outward force on the heart. The P_{pl} thus plays an important role in regulation of volumes of the thoracic cage, lungs, and heart.

Interestingly, patients with obliterated pleural spaces appear to suffer no significant ill effects. Post pleurectomy, vital capacity remains nearly unchanged and so does the ventilation and oxygen uptake.

When the quantity of fluid is large, as in pleural effusions, or the fluid is replaced by air, the P_{pl} tends toward positive levels and the mechanical coupling between the chest wall and the lung becomes ineffective, and the lung becomes atelectatic. The chest wall moves outward due to its elastic recoil, thus occupying a bigger volume. The P_{pl} positivity in such cases also impairs cardiac filing. The cardiorespiratory and hemodynamic consequences depend on the magnitude of the pressure reversal as well the rapidity with which it develops in pathological conditions. In extreme cases, a decrease in arterial oxygenation and a fall in cardiac output would result.

Measurement of Pleural Pressure

Pleural pressure can be measured directly by inserting a sensor such as a needle or a balloon attached to a pressure transducer into the pleural cavity. The electrical signal from the transducer can be amplified and saved on a recorder or converted to a digital signal. However being invasive with attendant risks of a pneumothorax and infection, it is rarely required in clinical practice. Indirectly, an esophageal balloon in its middle part gives an approximation of the P_{pl}. Reliable measurements of esophageal pressures can be made with micromanometers.

Pleural Pressure Gradients

Due to the weight of the lungs and the effect of gravity, differences occur in the P_{pl} at different locations within the pleural cavity, with the pressure being lowest or most negative in the apical region and highest or least negative in the basal regions. It is estimated that the vertical gradient in P_{pl} is about 0.30 cmH_2O/cm on average.

As the alveolar pressures are constant throughout the lung, it follows that the distending pressure at different points in the vertical extent of the lungs varies with P_{pl} negativity, the alveoli at the apical regions being more distended than those at the bases. This also explains why pleural blebs occur almost exclusively in the lung apices. This also results in regional differences in the matching of perfusion and ventilation, with greater ventilation in the upper regions and greater perfusion in the basal regions.

FORMATION OF PLEURAL FLUID[1-5]

Starling Forces

Possible sources of fluid in the pleural space include pleural capillaries, the interstitial spaces of the lung, the intrathoracic lymphatics, the intrathoracic blood vessels, and the peritoneal cavity.

It was once believed that fluid formation occurs at the capillaries of the parietal pleura and the removal at the visceral pleura. More recent thinking is that both the formation and removal occur in health at the parietal pleura.

The volume and composition of the pleural liquid are regulated by several mechanisms, including the capillary hydrostatic pressures in the two pleural layers, pleural pressure and the oncotic pressures due to proteins in the capillaries as well as the pleural fluid, and the properties of the interface and the surface area available. The physical forces, called Starling forces, are the major regulatory mechanism in health.

The oncotic pressures in a compartment, which are due to proteins in the fluid, tend to hold the fluid within the compartment, while the hydrostatic pressures tend to push the fluid out of the compartment. The net movement of fluid from one compartment to another in health is governed by these pressures and described by the Starling equation:

$$Q_r = L_p.A[(P_{cap} - P_{pl}) - \sigma_d(\pi_{cap} - \pi_{pl})]$$

where, Q is the fluid movement, L_p is the filtration coefficient/unit area (or the hydraulic water conductivity of the membrane), A is the surface area of the membrane, P and π are the hydrostatic and oncotic pressures, respectively, of the capillary (cap) and pleural (pl) space; and σ_d is the solute reflection coefficient for protein, a measure of the membrane's ability to restrict the passage of large molecules. In health, the variables are the P and π, or the hydrostatic and oncotic pressures in the capillary and the pleural space fluid. Both the hydrostatic and the oncotic pressures are higher in the capillary plasma.

The hydrostatic pressure in the parietal pleura is approximately 30 cmH_2O, whereas the pleural pressure is approximately –5 cmH_2O. The net hydrostatic pressure favoring movement of fluid out of the capillary is therefore 30 – (–5) = 35 cmH_2O. Opposing this hydrostatic pressure gradient is the oncotic pressure gradient. The oncotic pressure in the plasma is approximately 34 cmH_2O, whereas the very small quantity of pleural fluid protein exerts an oncotic pressure of approximately 5 cmH_2O. Thus, the net oncotic pressure gradient of 34 – 5 = 29 cmH_2O tends to hold fluid in the capillaries. The net Starling force moving the fluid out of the capillaries and into the pleural space is 35 – 29 = 6 cmH_2O.

The hydrostatic pressure in the visceral pleura is approximately 24 cmH_2O. The net hydrostatic pressure-favoring movement of fluid out of the capillary in the visceral pleura is therefore 24 – (–5) = 29 cmH_2O. This is balanced by the net oncotic pressure gradient of 34 – 5 = 29 cmH_2O, tending to hold fluid in the visceral pleural capillaries. Thus, there is no movement of fluid in either direction in the visceral pleura. Moreover in humans, the visceral pleura is thicker; its blood supply is from the bronchial arteries and its capillaries are located deeper.

Animal studies have shown that there are local differences in pleural fluid formation and absorption. More fluid formation in the parietal pleura occurs over the ribs compared to that over the intercostal spaces and greater absorption occurs in the parietal pleura adjacent to the intercostal space rather than that overlying the ribs. There was also more fluid formation over the caudal ribs than over the cranial ribs. Further if the breathing frequency was increased, more fluid was formed.

There are other sources of pleural fluid formation in pathological conditions.

Interstitial Origin

The immediate source of pleural fluid in pathological effusions in most cases is the interstitial spaces of the lungs. Pulmonary edema due to volume overload or increased permeability is soon followed by the development of pleural effusion as the fluid from the lungs is cleared into the interstitial spaces and then into the pleural space. The amount of pleural fluid formed is directly related to the elevation in the wedge pressure.

The classic example is left heart failure. The occurrence of pleural effusion is related to the severity of pulmonary edema. It is more closely correlated with the pulmonary venous pressure than with the systemic venous pressure. However, patients with right heart failure due to precapillary pulmonary hypertension may have pleural effusions, although their wedge pressures are normal. This probably originates from the capillaries in the parietal pleura.

In pulmonary edema due to increased permeability of the alveolocapillary membrane (noncardiogenic edema), the amount of fluid that enters the pleural space is also increased as there is increased interstitial fluid. In both cardiogenic and noncardiogenic pulmonary edema, the effusion occurs without any morphologic evidence of pleural injury. Any lung injury can be associated with increased fluid in the interstitial spaces of the lung and this can result in pleural effusions. As the interstitial pressure increases within the lung, the fluid goes across the visceral pleura as the latter is a weak barrier to fluid movement.

Peritoneal Cavity

Pleural effusion is common when there is free fluid in the peritoneal cavity and if there are openings in the diaphragm. The flow occurs because the pressure in the pleural cavity is less than the pressure in the peritoneal cavity. The peritoneal cavity is the source of the pleural fluid in hepatic hydrothorax, Meigs syndrome, and peritoneal dialysis. There are no direct lymphatic connections between the peritoneal and pleural cavities.

Thoracic Duct or Blood Vessel Disruption

A disruption of the thoracic duct leads to accumulation of lymph in the pleural space, producing a chylothorax. This develops quickly and can be >1,000 mL/day. Similarly, a disruption of a large blood vessel in the thorax due to trauma or disease can result in accumulation of blood rapidly in the pleural space, producing a hemothorax.

Origin of Normal Pleural Fluid

The small amount of pleural fluid that is there normally enters the pleural space from the capillaries in the parietal pleura. Unlike pathological accumulations, the normal fluid has very less protein compared to normal interstitial fluid (1–1.5 g% compared to 4.5 g%, respectively) and therefore does not originate from the latter. The Starling forces discussed earlier also make visceral pleural very unlikely as the source and similarly, a lymphatic origin and a peritoneal cavity origin appear unlikely.

Normally, the rate of fluid formation at the parietal pleura is small (0.01 mL/kg/h) and almost all of this fluid is removed by the lymphatics in the parietal pleura.

PLEURAL FLUID ABSORPTION[1-5]

As fluid formation at the parietal pleura because of Starling forces is a continuous process and there is no gradient for fluid absorption through the visceral pleura, a removal mechanism is required to prevent accumulation of pleural fluid. This is accomplished by the parietal pleural lymphatics, where the fluid enters through the openings or stomas in the parietal pleura.

These stomas are in areas where the mesothelial cells are small and not flattened. Stoma diameter is not fixed but can increase when exposed to stimuli such as nitric oxide. No such stomas are present in the visceral pleura. Proteins, cells, and all other particulate matter are removed from the pleural space by these lymphatics. The lymphatic drainage may reach up to 500 mL/day. Interestingly, the capacity for lymphatic clearance is 28 times as high as the normal rate of pleural fluid formation.

While lymphatic removal is the major mechanism, there is some conflicting evidence on whether all fluid is removed by bulk flow through the lymphatics. Transcytosis contributes to the removal of protein from the pleural space and there may be a difference in the rate of removal of particles of different molecular sizes. Thus, aggressive diuresis may lead to an increase in protein concentration of the residual fluid.

PATHOGENESIS OF PLEURAL EFFUSIONS[1-6]

A pleural effusion is excess fluid that accumulates between the parietal and visceral pleura. Since the rate of formation of pleural fluid and the rate of its removal are balanced, resulting in minimal quantity of fluid in the pleural spaces, increased formation, decreased removal, or both should result in the development of increased fluid or pleural effusion. Since the absorptive capacity of the parietal pleura far exceeds the rate of fluid formation, both increased formation and decreased rate of removal are required for pleural fluid accumulation.

Changes in the balance of Starling forces or the rate of formation of interstitial fluid in the lungs will change the quantity of pleural fluid.

Increased Interstitial Fluid

The most common cause of increased pleural fluid in pathological conditions is increased interstitial fluid in the lung as discussed earlier. The increase in interstitial fluid may be due to heart failure, volume overload, or may be noncardiogenic due to lung injury. Examples are pleural effusions in patients with congestive heart failure, parapneumonic effusions, pulmonary embolism, acute respiratory distress syndrome, and in those who have undergone lung transplantation.

Increased Hydrostatic Pressure Gradient

As dictated by the Starling equation, increased intravascular pressure in the pleural capillaries increases the outward pressure gradient, increasing fluid formation. This occurs with right ventricular failure, left ventricular failure, pericardial effusions, or the superior vena cava syndrome.

A decrease in the pleural pressure (greater negativity) is much less common and can occur with bronchial obstruction, leading to atelectasis of the lower lobe or complete lung or when the visceral pleura becomes coated with a collagenous peel and the lung becomes trapped. Decreased pleural pressures also occur in diseases in which the elastic recoil of the lung is increased.

Increased capillary permeability can also lead to increased pleural fluid formation. In the Starling equation described earlier, this is reflected in an increase in L (hydraulic conductivity). Increased levels of vascular endothelial growth factor (VEGF) increase the permeability of the capillaries and contribute to accumulation of pleural fluid in certain instances. If the pleural surfaces become inflamed, the permeability of the capillaries may be increased.

Elevation of Systemic Venous Pressures

Patients with pulmonary hypertension and right heart failure commonly have pleural effusions due to the elevated systemic venous pressure, resulting in more pleural fluid formation.

Decreased Oncotic Pressure Gradient

It can be inferred from the Starling equation described earlier that changes in the oncotic pressure gradient can also affect the formation of pleural fluid. Normally, the higher protein concentration of the plasma holds back fluid in the capillaries. Increased pleural fluid protein levels that occur with increased permeability pulmonary edema, hemothorax, and with conditions in which the permeability of the pleural capillaries is increased changes the oncotic pressure gradient, favoring movement of fluid out of the capillaries in the pleura.

The effect of changes in oncotic pressure gradient is however not likely to be important because hypoproteinemia alone is thought to be a very uncommon cause of pleural effusion.

Other Contributory Mechanisms

In specific pathological conditions, other mechanisms play a role in the accumulation of pleural fluid. The presence of free peritoneal fluid in any cause of ascites leads to pleural fluid accumulation if there is a hole in the diaphragm. Fluid (chyle) will accumulate in the pleural space if there is a disruption in the thoracic duct and blood will accumulate in the pleural space if there is a disruption of a blood vessel in the thorax.

Decreased Pleural Fluid Absorption (Obstruction of Lymphatics)

An obstruction of the lymphatics draining the parietal pleura is the most common mechanism of decreased pleural fluid absorption. The lymphatic flow has a far greater capacity than what is used in health. Lymphatic blockade is an important factor that contributes to the development of a malignant pleural effusion but because of its great capacity to increase flow, it is not the main mechanism.

KEY POINTS

- Normally, a very thin layer of low protein fluid separates the two layers of the pleura.
- The pleural pressure is negative due to the elastic recoil of the lung and the chest wall acting in opposite directions, inward and outward, respectively.
- Pleural fluid formation and absorption occur at the parietal pleura in health.
- Balance of hydrostatic pressures in the parietal pleura capillaries and pleural space and oncotic pressure due to proteins in the two compartments determines the net fluid formation.
- The absorptive capacity of the lymphatics in the parietal pleura far exceeds the rate of formation.
- Development of pleural effusions in pathological conditions occurs due to one or more of the following mechanisms—increased hydrostatic pressure gradient, decreased oncotic pressure gradient, increased interstitial fluid, elevation of systemic venous pressures, decreased pleural fluid absorption (obstruction of lymphatics), and altered permeability of the pleura.

REFERENCES

1. Wang N. Anatomy and Physiology of the Pleural Space. Clin Chest Med. 1985;6:3-16.
2. Seaton A. Diseases of the pleura. In: Seaton A, et al. (Eds). Crofton and Douglas' Respiratory Diseases, 5th edition. Oxford, UK: Blackwell Science Ltd; 2000. pp. 1152-81.
3. Physiology of the pleural space. In: Light RW. Pleural Diseases, 6th edition. Philadelphia: Lippincott, Williams & Wilkins; 2013. pp. 8-18.
4. Zochhi L. Physiology and pathophysiology of pleural fluid turnover. Eur Respir J. 2002;20:1545-58.
5. Charalampidis C, Youroukou A, Lazaridis G, Baka S, Mpoukovinas I, Karavasilis V, et al. Physiology of the pleural space. J Thorac Dis. 2015;7(Suppl 1):S33-7.
6. Capp CM, Fellar Kopmn D. Non-malignant pleural effusions. In: Grippi, et al. Fishman's Pulmonary Diseases and Disorders, 6th edition. New York: McGraw Hill; 2022. pp. 1-36.

CHAPTER

3 Radiology in Pleura

Kulbir Ahlawat, Surabhi Gupta, Ashish Kumar Prakash

INTRODUCTION

To understand the radiology of pleura, it is very important to understand the various radiological modalities available for visualization of pleura. Imaging plays a pivotal role in identification, characterization, and management of pleural diseases. A basic chest radiograph often serves as the first imaging investigation in assessment of pleural pathologies. Since sir William Conrad Roentgen has discovered X-rays, there has been a significant advancement in the field of radiology, which now serves as a valuable tool in evaluation of pleura and its pathologies. Apart from the basic chest radiograph, other imaging modalities such as ultrasonography, computed tomography (CT), and magnetic resonance imaging (MRI) are also available. The initial and least expensive is the simple chest radiograph. The use of ultrasonography, a noninvasive modality with no radiation exposure, is an evolving concept in evaluation of pleural and lung pathologies; it is being discussed as a separate chapter in this textbook. In this chapter, we will be discussing the use of chest radiograph and other diagnostic modalities, apart from ultrasonography. Further, role of imaging using ultrasound (US), CT, or magnetic resonance (MR) depends on clinical context, initial imaging findings, and cost-effectiveness.

Different imaging modalities available are as follows:

- Chest radiograph
- CT, both high-resolution and contrast-enhanced (HRCT and CECT)
- US of chest
- MRI
- Positron emission tomography–CT (PET-CT)

CHEST X-RAY

Chest radiography till date is accepted as initial modality for the diagnosis of pleural disease. X-ray was discovered by *Willian Conard Roentgen*, revolutionizing the whole diagnostic armamentarium. Chest X-ray (CXR) is widely available nowadays and because of the digitalization, it has become more and more sensitive and specific. It is the first investigation of choice for any lung and pleural abnormality. The first step in evaluation of a chest radiograph before evaluating any pathology is to determine its technical adequacy, failing which one may overdiagnose or underdiagnose a disease entity. In an adequately positioned chest radiograph, the spinous processes should fall in line with an imaginary vertical line drawn midway between the clavicular heads. Scapulae should be rotated laterally to avoid superimposition on the upper lungs. There should be faint visualization of the vertebral bodies and disc spaces through the mediastinum. Motion blur can be assessed by noting the sharpness of the superior cortices of the ribs, vessel margins, and the diaphragmatic contours. Optimal inspiratory effort is assessed by noting the position of the right hemidiaphragm with respect to the ribs; this point should correspond to the sixth anterior rib or tenth posterior rib in the midclavicular line.[1] On a chest radiograph, the pleural pathologies can manifest as air (pneumothorax) or fluid (pleural effusion) in the pleural space or involve the pleural surfaces and present as thickening (ranging from benign pleural plaques to neoplasms) or calcification.[2]

PNEUMOTHORAX

The term pneumothorax describes the presence of air in the pleural space. A pneumothorax can be primary (with no underlying lung disease) or secondary (with underlying lung disease). An erect chest radiograph can easily demonstrate the pneumothorax **(Figs. 1 and 2)**. A pneumothorax is seen as an area of peripheral radiolucency (compared to adjacent lung), with a very thin but sharp line, representing the visible pleural edge. No lung markings can be appreciated lateral to the pleural edge. There may be complete or partial passive lung collapse. Other ancillary findings such as subcutaneous emphysema or pneumomediastinum can also be present. If there is tracheal or mediastinal shift toward the contralateral side of the pneumothorax, it is said to be a "tension pneumothorax." This is a medical emergency! It requires immediate management **(Fig. 3)**.

Various methods have been described in literature to estimate the volume of pneumothorax on a standard erect posteroanterior (PA) view radiograph.

Collins Method[3]

% of pneumothorax = 4.2 + 4.7 (A + B + C)

Distance between partially collapsed to **(Fig. 4)**:

- A—lung apex to apex of thoracic cavity (black color)
- B—midpoints of upper half of collapsed lung (red color)
- C—midpoints of lower half of collapsed lung (yellow color)

4.2—correction factor

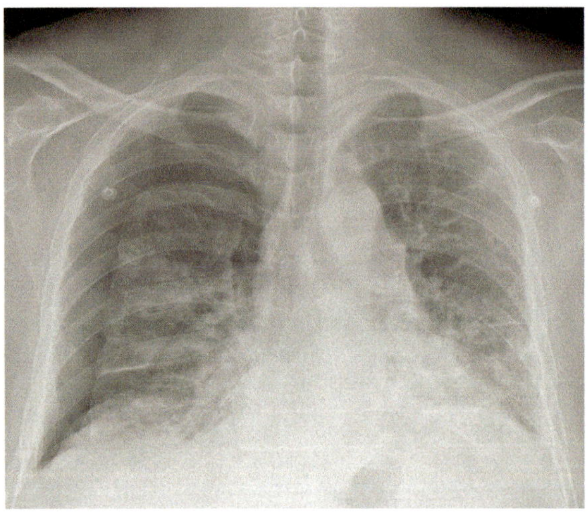

FIG. 1: Right-sided pneumothorax with lung margins clear.

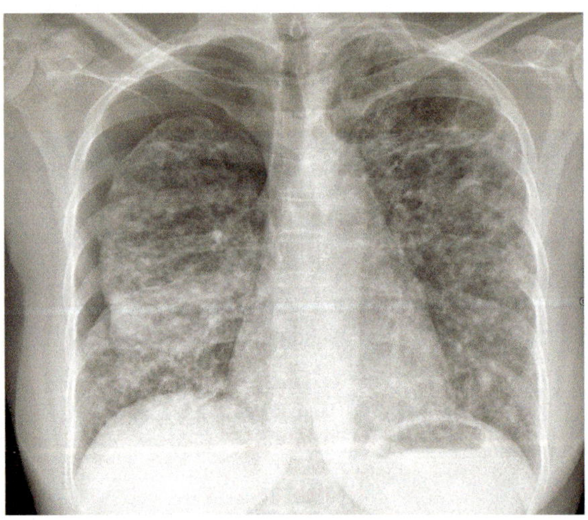

FIG. 2: Right-sided pneumothorax in a patient in underlying interstitial lung disease (ILD).

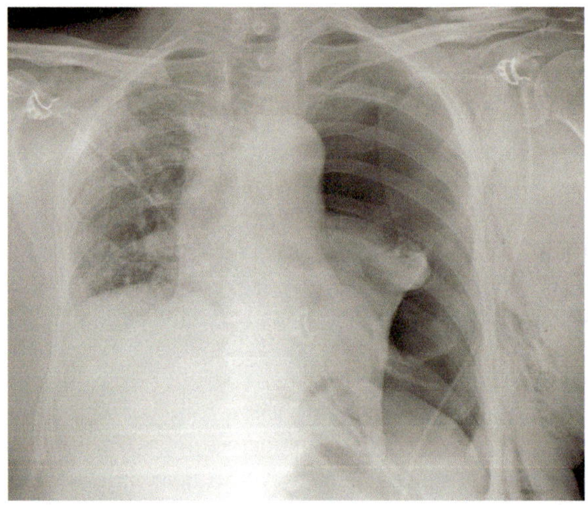

FIG. 3: Left-sided tension pneumothorax with mediastinal shift.

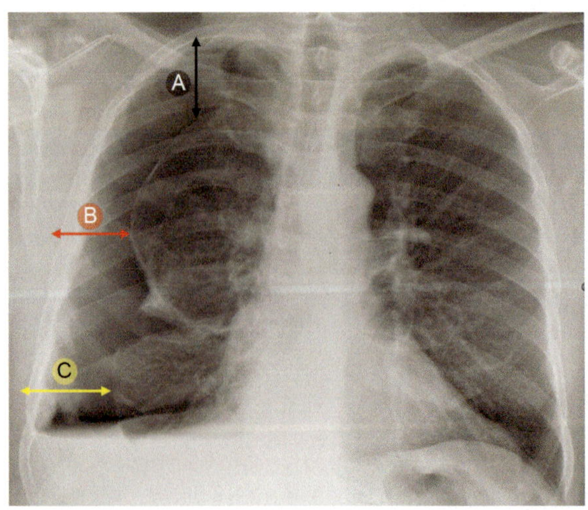

FIG. 4: Collins method to calculate size of pneumothorax: (A) Lung apex to apex of thoracic cavity (black color); (B) Midpoints of upper half of collapsed lung (red color); and (C) Midpoints of lower half of collapsed lung (yellow color).

Rhea Method[4]

The intrapleural distance is measured at the lung apex, lung base, and midpoint between the two and the average of these three is taken. The average pleural distance is marked on the nomogram, where *1 cm corresponds to 10% pneumothorax*. It is the easiest method to recall.

Light Index[5]

$$\% \text{ of pneumothorax} = 100 - (D_L^3/D_H^3 \times 100)$$

- D_L is the diameter of collapsed lung.
- D_H is the diameter of hemithorax on the collapsed side.

The simpler and more practical method involves measuring the distance between the lung margin and chest wall (at the level of pulmonary hilum), <2 cm is considered a small pneumothorax and >2 cm is considered a large pneumothorax. Quantification of pneumothorax is important to plan optimal management strategies, namely needle aspirations versus large-bore chest drains. Now as per the latest British Thoracic Society (BTS) guidelines, size of primary spontaneous pneumothorax (PSP) hardly matters for the conservative management.[6] In case of asymptomatic PSP if there is no significant pain or dyspnea or any hemodynamic compromise, conservative management can be tried regardless of size of the pneumothorax.

PLEURAL EFFUSION

Pleural effusion refers to the accumulation of fluid in the pleural space. The radiographic appearance of pleural effusion depends on the volume of fluid, position of the patient (erect vs. supine), and mobility of the effusion (free vs. constrained).

Distribution of Pleural Fluid in Erect Radiograph

The pleural fluid follows the gravity and is seen to initially accumulate in the most dependent region, i.e., between the lung base and dome of diaphragm on PA view, known as the subpulmonic region in the upright position. This is often difficult to pick on routine PA/lateral view radiographs as the upper edge of the effusion mimics the contour of the diaphragm, resulting in mild elevation of diaphragm, also referred to as the pseudodiaphragm appearance.

The posterior costophrenic sulcus being deeper than the lateral costophrenic sulcus is seen to accumulate significant pleural fluid, before being apparent on the erect PA radiographs. A lateral radiograph may prove beneficial in such cases, where obliteration of posterior costophrenic sulcus could represent pleural effusion not apparent on erect PA radiographs. At least 200–250 mL of fluid is required to cause obliteration of lateral costophrenic sulcus on erect PA view.[7] As the fluid quantity increases, the concave, upward slope of the fluid gives rise to the *"meniscus" sign* on erect frontal and lateral views. Sometimes this is also called *Ellis S* curve[7] **(Fig. 5)**, which is basically a radiological illusion. The radiological picture is not very easy to predict confidently about the height of fluid present in the pleural space. The exact upper limit is same throughout the hemithorax. The shape of meniscus is due to the layer of fluid which is of insufficient depth to create a noticeable shadow when viewed enface **(Fig. 6)**. Massive effusions can cause mass effect, demonstrated as contralateral tracheal and mediastinal shift.

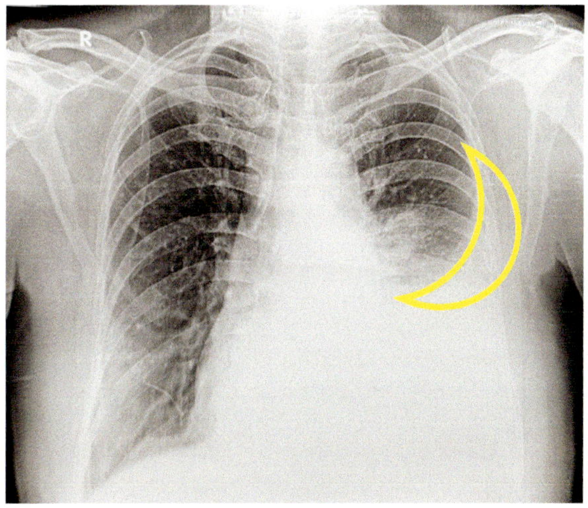

FIG. 5: Meniscus sign in the left side (pleural effusion).

Distribution of Pleural Fluid in Supine Radiograph

In the supine radiographs, the free pleural fluid layers posteriorly, resulting in a veil-like increased density of the hemithorax, which may often be difficult to detect. Other features include obscuration of the hemidiaphragm, reduced visibility of the pulmonary vessels below the level of the apparent dome of the diaphragm, increased opacity of the spleen in left-sided effusions, and thickening of the minor fissure.[8]

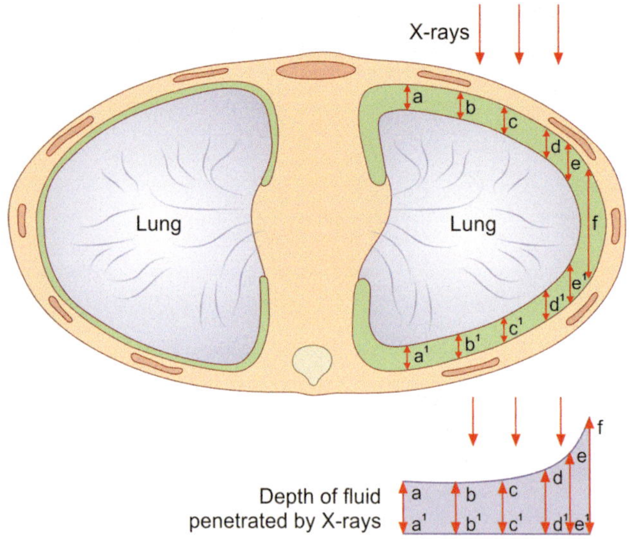

FIG. 6: Diagram explaining the meniscus sign. The distance between the chest wall and lung is same throughout the hemithorax. The fluid depth which is viewed enface a–a[1] and c–c[1] is not sufficient enough to cause radiodensity. If we move more laterally to d–d[1] and f–f[1], the beam of the X-ray passes through more and more pleural fluid, causing radiolucency which is a continuous phenomenon; hence, density gradually increases, causing meniscus sign.

Free pleural fluid can also cap the apex of the lung on supine radiographs, known as the *apical cap sign*.

Atypical Distribution and Loculation of Pleural Fluid

Loculated pleural effusions represent accumulation of fluid secondary to adhesions between contiguous pleural surfaces. The effusion typically produces biconvex mass-like opacities along the dependent costal pleural surfaces. When it occurs between two lobes, it can be misinterpreted as a pulmonary neoplasm on chest radiographs. However, fluid accumulations between two lobes **(Fig. 7A)** tend to resolve spontaneously or with diuretics **(Fig. 7B)**, and therefore have also been called *vanishing/pseudo-tumor/phantom tumor*.[9-11]

PLEURAL TUMORS AND TUMOR-LIKE CONDITIONS

Many neoplastic, both benign and malignant, and non-neoplastic pathologies can involve the pleura.

Basic Imaging Pearls (Table 1)

A peripherally placed opacity on chest radiograph can be localized in three different locations with respect to the pleura:

1. *Extrapleural opacity*: It originates from the chest wall and forms obtuse angles and a sharp medial margin in relation to the pleura.
2. *Pleural opacity*: It has partially or completely well-circumscribed margins and also forms obtuse angles with the pleura.
3. *Subpleural opacity*: It is localized to the lung parenchyma, has irregular margins, and forms acute angles with pleural reflections.

The general features on radiograph suggestive of pleural tumors include peripheral location abutting the chest wall, a sharp margin with the surrounding lung, and obtuse angle of contact with the chest wall/mediastinum. *If the angle of contact with the chest wall is acute, then it favors lesion to be of parenchymal origin* **(Fig. 8A)**, *and if the angle is obtuse (D shaped), then it suggests it to be of pleural origin* **(Fig. 8B)**.

PLEURAL THICKENING

Thickening of the pleura can be appreciated on chest radiographs. It can be focal or diffuse, benign or malignant. Diffuse pleural thickening is defined as thickening of pleura > 5 mm with total area of involvement >25% of chest wall if bilateral and 50% involvement if unilateral.[13] Apical pleural thickening is one of the most common findings seen on routine chest radiographs and is considered to be part of normal age-related changes; however, apical pleural thickening >2 cm requires further evaluation. On imaging, benign pleural thickening is seen as a diffuse involvement of pleura. Pleural thickening >5 cm in width, 8 cm in craniocaudal extent, and 3 mm in thickness usually points toward a benign etiology.[14] Furthermore, features such as volume loss, calcifications, and proliferation of extrapleural fat also support a diagnosis of diffuse benign pleural thickening. Nodular circumferential pleural thickening with involvement of mediastinal pleura suggests a malignant process.

COMPUTED TOMOGRAPHY—BOTH HIGH-RESOLUTION AND CONTRAST-ENHANCED

Computed tomography, formerly called *computed axial tomography scan* (*CAT scan*), is one of the latest imaging techniques, which plays a major role in medical imaging today. In CT, the patient is placed in a gantry, with an X-ray tube rotating around the patient, the X-ray beam used to radiate the patient can be pencil beam, fan beam, or cone beam in configuration. The multirow detectors simultaneously record the radiation that passes through the body, which is used to produce the image, available to us in its digitized format on our computer screens. Its

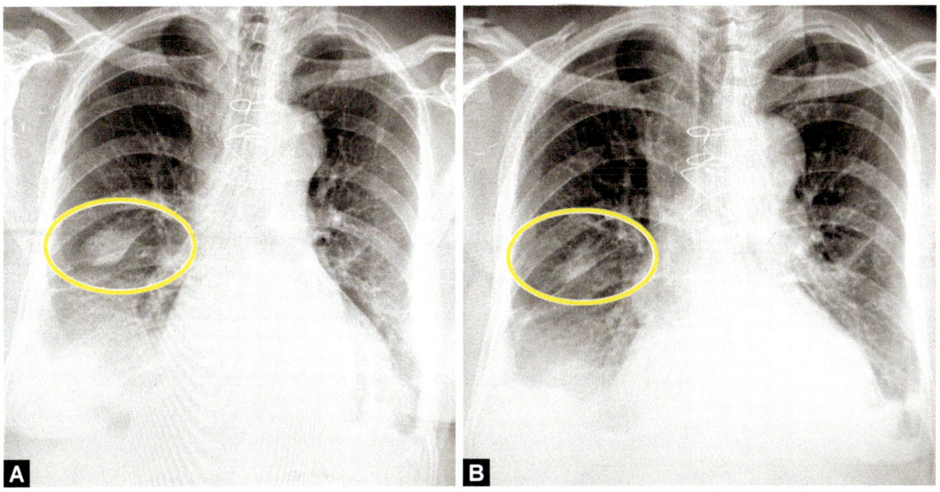

FIGS. 7A AND B: Fluid accumulation in fissure-vanishing/pseudo-tumor/phantom tumor. (A) Before and (B) after diuretics.

TABLE 1: Pleural versus pulmonary versus extrapleural lesions.[12]

Pleural	Extrapleural	Pulmonary
Obtuse angle	Obtuse angle	Acute angle
Displace pulmonary vasculature	Displace pulmonary vasculature	Engulf pulmonary vasculature
Centered along chest wall	Centered along chest wall	Centered in the lung
Tapered well-defined margins	Tapering margins	Nontapering, ill-defined margins
Changes location with respiration	–	–
Displace extrapleural fat outward	Displace extrapleural fat inward	–
Rib erosion unusual	Rib erosion common	Rib erosion unusual

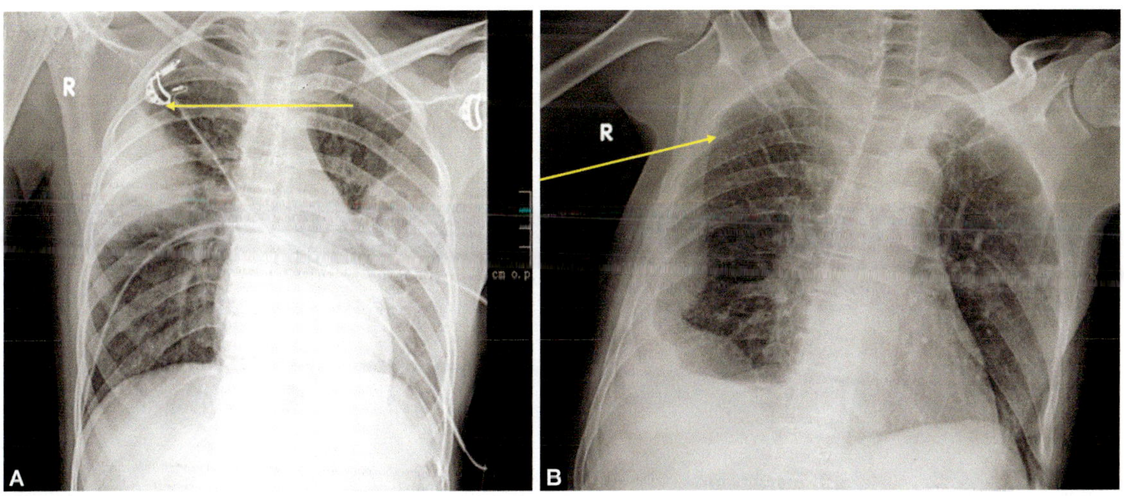

FIGS. 8A AND B: Difference between pulmonary and pleural lesions: (A) Acute angle favors—parenchymal origin and (B) obtuse (D-shaped) favors—pleural origin.

use in case of lung as well as mediastinal pathologies is well known.[15] Nowadays it is widely available, quick, and gives a detailed view of the internal organs.[16-18] In order to study the details of pleura, it should involve multislice thin sections (0.5–2.0 mm), which will enable subsequent multiplanar reconstruction[19-21] **(Fig. 9)**. The CT image generated is viewed on appropriate window settings to have a complete and detailed evaluation of lung parenchyma, mediastinal structures, and the bony structures of chest wall. The window width (W) refers to the range of CT numbers that a CT image contains, or in simpler terms the different shades of gray that it contains. The window level (L) refers to the center point or midpoint HU value in the window setting. Window setting for viewing lung parenchyma is W: 1,500, L: 500, for viewing mediastinum is W: 400, L: 40, and for viewing bone is W: 2,000, L: 500. Different organs of our body have different density through which the radiation beam passes. The linear attenuation coefficient for every material at the selected effective energy is converted to CT numbers known as *Hounsfield units* using the standard equation:

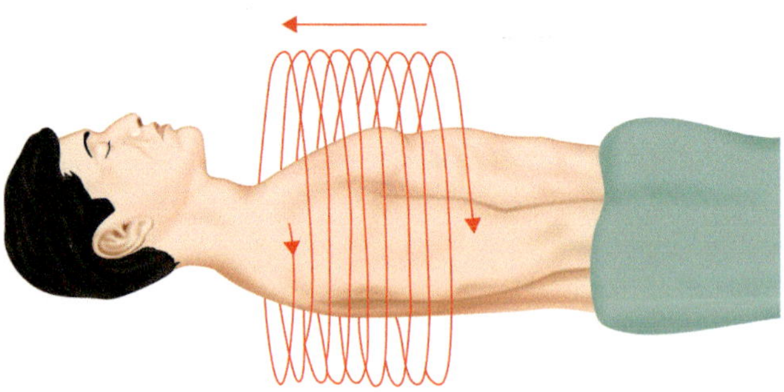

FIG. 9: Scanning geometry of a helical computed tomography (CT)—the schematic representations.

$$HU = (\mu_{material} - \mu_{water})/(\mu_{water}) \times 1{,}000$$

Contrast-enhanced CT is the best to view pleural abnormality and the image acquisition should be done after 60–90 seconds of intravenous contrast administration to allow maximum pleural enhancement called the *pleural phase*.[22] The pleural pathologies like fluid or blood or the masses obliterate the pleural space. It is very important to confirm the lesion obliterating pleural space that will be either pleural or parenchymal. In case of chest radiograph, the angle of contact between the opacity and chest wall helps us to determine if the lesion is pleural based or parenchymal in nature. CECT has good sensitivity and specificity to differentiate between the pleural and extrapleural lesions.[23,24] The free fluid looks like sickle-shaped fluid density in the gutter or the most dependent part of the chest posteriorly.[25] In case of loculated pleural effusions, there are fluid-attenuating lenticular densities showing fixed position[26] *(split pleura sign)* **(Figs. 10A and B)**. Rarely, the CT findings may be equivocal particularly when there is parenchymal abnormality like collapse/consolidation or loculated pleural collection, which form acute angles with the chest wall. When the lesions are in the posterior costophrenic recess, which is adjacent to the diaphragm, it is difficult to differentiate them from ascites. There are various CT findings to differentiate the pleural fluid from ascites,[25] as shown in **Figures 11A and B**. There are few important signs to be recalled as "**ABCD**" as shown in the diagrammatic representation **(Figs. 12A to D)**.

A. The *interface sign*: A hazy interface between the fluid and organs such as liver and spleen is indicative of pleural fluid, whereas a sharp interface between the

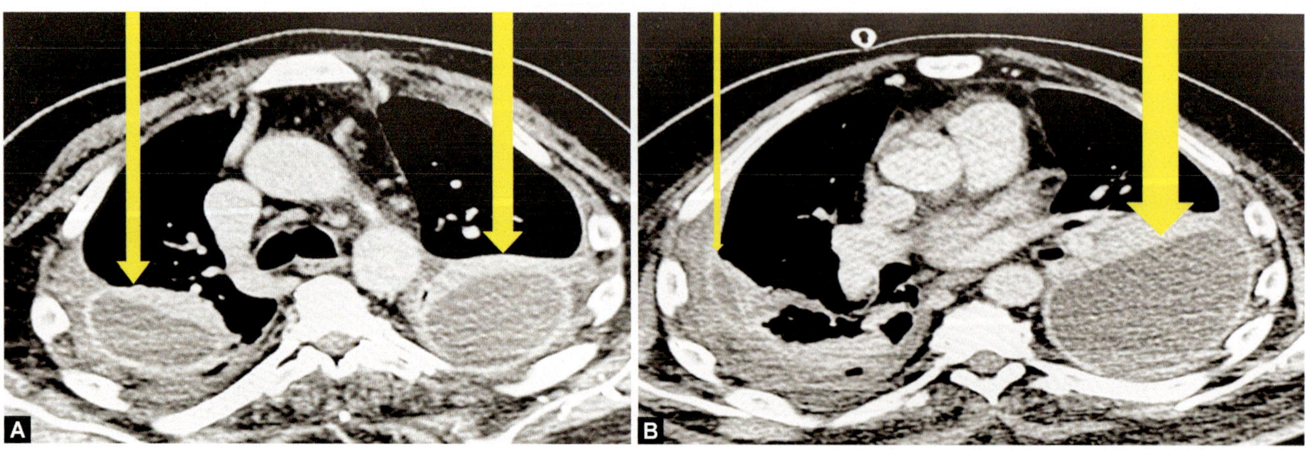

FIGS. 10A AND B: Computed tomography (CT) representing the bilateral split pleura sign (four yellow arrows). The width of the yellow arrow is representing the amount of loculated effusion.

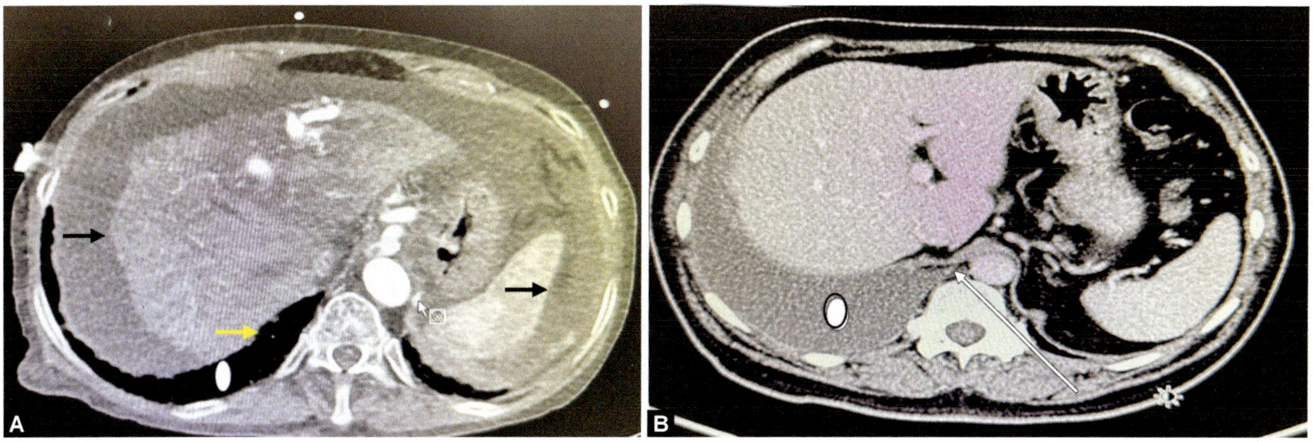

FIGS. 11A AND B: (A) 1-ascites showing interface sign (black arrows) and bare-area sign (yellow arrow) [bare area (white dot)—no fluid in case of ascites]. (B) Displaced crus sign—the right crus of the diaphragm is displaced (white arrow) laterally in case of pleural effusion [white dot (bare-area sign) in case of pleural effusion, unrestricted access to the posterior costophrenic sulcus].

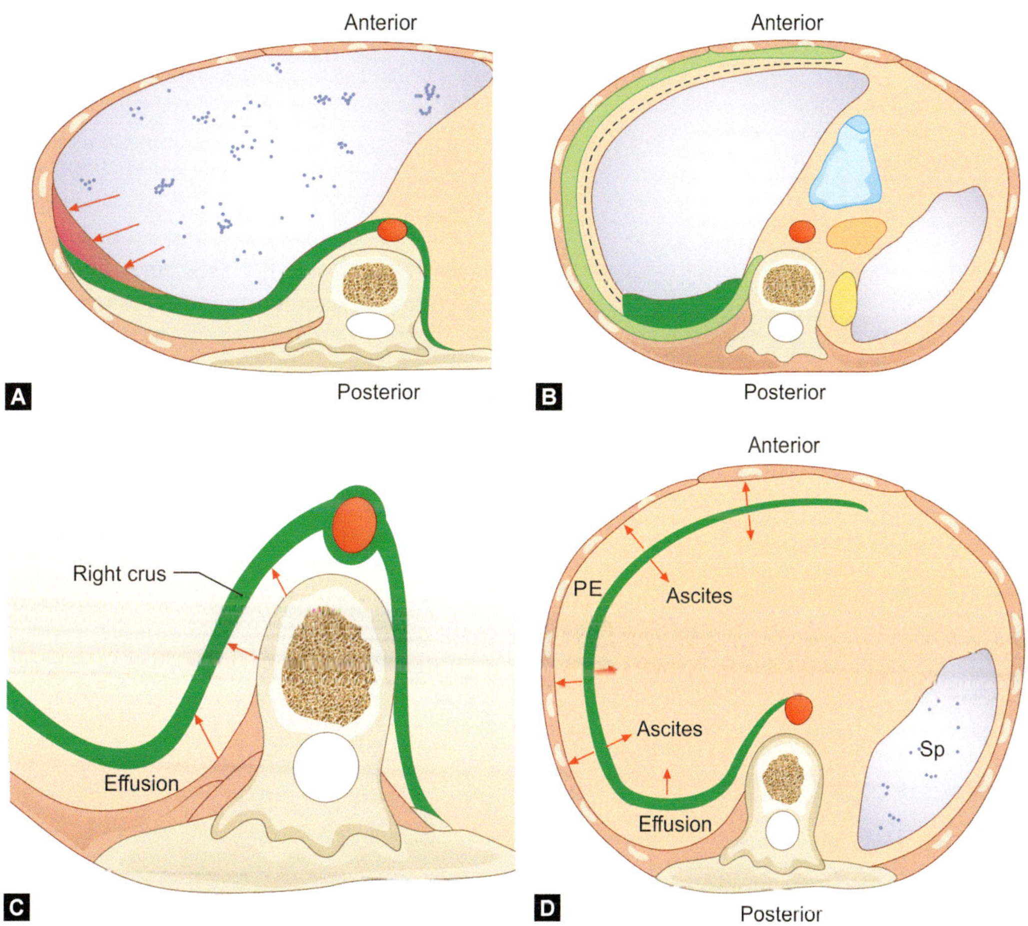

FIGS. 12A TO D: Diagrammatic representation of (A) interface sign, (B) bare-area sign, (C) crus-diaphragm sign, and (D) diaphragm sign.

fluid and abdominal organs is suggestive of ascites. Because diaphragm makes the interface, the organs such as spleen and liver are well delineated in case of ascites but not in pleural effusion.

B. The ***bare-area sign***: If there is restriction of fluid by the coronary ligaments from the bare area of the liver, it indicates that the patient has ascites. The pleural fluid has unrestricted access to the posterior costophrenic sulcus and is therefore also seen in relation to the bare area of liver.
C. The *displaced* ***crus*** *sign*: If the diaphragmatic crus is displayed away from the vertebral body by the fluid, it indicates that the fluid is in the pleural space, while ascites displaces the diaphragmatic crus toward the vertebral body.
D. The ***diaphragm*** *sign*: The fluid that lies outside the diaphragm is pleural fluid, whereas that lies inside the diaphragm is ascites.

Computed tomography is the most effective way for demonstrating abnormalities in the lung parenchyma and chest wall, which are not seen on the conventional chest radiograph. CT chest is very helpful in differentiating empyema with air-fluid levels from lung abscesses. Almost every disease of pleura has CT findings and are described in subsequent chapters of this book. CT is also helpful in differentiating benign versus malignant pleural effusion. A study done by Yilmaz et al.[27] in 146 patients suggested its sensitivity/specificity for pleural nodularity 37%/97%, pleural rind 22%/97%, mediastinal pleural involvement 31%/85%, and pleural thickening > 1 cm, 35%/87%, respectively. Another study done by Traill et al.[28] reported that 27 out of 32 patients with malignant pleural effusion had pleural nodularity or irregularity or pleural thickness > 1 cm. Chest CT is not indicated in all patients with suspected pleural disease. The coefficient density in CT is not very specific to distinguish among parenchymal lesions, solid pleural masses, or pleural fluids such as blood, serous fluid, or pus.[29] The coefficients of attenuation in CT scan cannot differentiate significantly between transudative and exudative pleural effusion.[30] Sometimes in case of hemothorax, there could be dual density **(Fig. 13)** inside the lesion in terms of HU units which may suggest the possibility of hemorrhage, but the gold standard is still the diagnostic tapping. In case of acute extravasated blood, the HU values tend to be high in comparison to chronic hemorrhage.[31] There is extensive literature regarding the HU units with respect to blood in pleural space.[32-33] One study done by Liu et al.[34] suggested a cutoff value of 15.6 HU or 30.0% of the perimeter/area (P/A) ratio to differentiate hemothorax from pleural effusion. In case of 15.9 HU cutoff or 56% of P/A ratio, better discrimination was obtained between hemothorax and empyema.

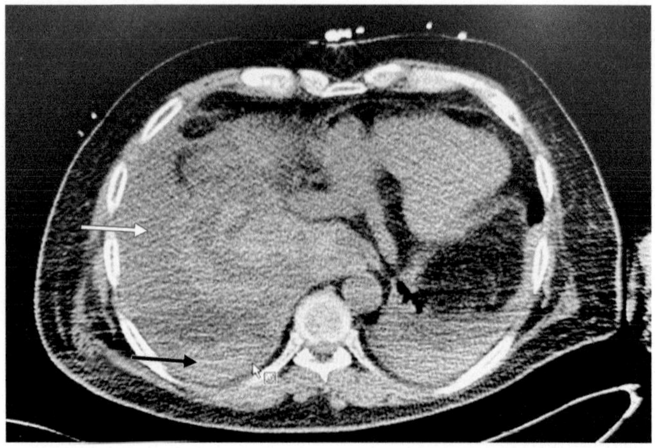

FIG. 13: Computed tomography (CT) showing double density in a post-traumatic patient (white arrow favoring fluid while black arrow favoring blood).

Computed tomography examinations of the chest can also give additional information regarding the effects of effusion on the underlying lung. Study done by Paling and Griffin[35] reviewed the chest CT of 46 cases in supine position with a moderate or large pleural effusion. The volume size of the underlying lung, especially lower lobe, was reduced in all patients, whereas atelectasis of the underlying lung was seen in 96% (44 of the 46) cases. Segmental collapse of the lower lobe was seen in 19 cases. Among 7 patients, the atelectatic segment was massive enough to cause complete collapse of the lower lobe. CT chest can also be used to evaluate the fissures (major and minor fissures).[36]

MAGNETIC RESONANCE IMAGING

Even today, CECT remains the most important radiological investigation in evaluation of pleural pathologies, but role of MRI in pleural pathologies can no longer be ignored. CT imaging has several limitations, including the use of iodinated contrast media, exposure to ionizing radiations, and restricted differentiation of pleural tumors from surrounding soft tissues. MRI provides superior contrast resolution and various MRI sequences can not only detect but also delineate pleural tumors more effectively than CT. It can be used to determine the invasion of surrounding tissues—chest wall, diaphragm, bone marrow, and endothoracic fascia, and in addition also provide functional information.[37] MRI is also serves as a radiation-free alternative in imaging, and therefore has huge potential in cases where repetitive imaging is required and in pediatric population. The choice of MR sequences is usually tailored to the clinical question and the individual case; however, the basic sequences that are acquired in almost all cases include multiplanar electrocardiogram-(ECG)-triggered T1 (T1-weighted), T2 (T2-weighted), and CE T1 (contrast-enhanced T1-weighted) with respiratory triggering and breath-holding techniques.[38] Additional sequences like short tau inversion recovery (STIR) sequences may be added to look for bone marrow involvement in malignant pleural pathologies. Dynamic contrast-enhanced MRI (DCE-MRI) DCE-MRI is used for functional imaging. It tracks signal changes after administration of contrast agents through sequential imaging. DCE-MRI can give information regarding vascularity and perfusion characteristics of a pleural tumors and monitor its response to chemotherapy. The diffusion-weighted MRI (DW-MRI) can help differentiate between benign and malignant pleural lesions. It is based on the mobility of protons in a given tissue; the malignant pathologies have restricted water movement and show higher signal intensity on DW-MRI compared to areas with free water movement. Despite its huge potential and diverse roles, thoracic MRI also comes with a set of limitations, namely the artifacts caused by respiratory and cardiac motion. Respiratory motion artifacts can be minimized by the use of breath-hold sequences and respiratory gating during acquisition.[39] Cardiac motion can be overcome by using techniques such as cardiac gating (gating using ECG) and using ultrashort sequences.

POSITRON EMISSION TOMOGRAPHY–COMPUTED TOMOGRAPHY

It is an increasingly utilized imaging modality in evaluation of malignant pleural conditions, especially mesothelioma and pleural metastasis. Fluorodeoxyglucose (FDG) PET-CT is a hybrid imaging technique, combining the benefits of FDG-PET, which provides metabolic parameters of a pleural tumor and CT, which has improved spatial resolution. It contributes to the diagnosis and staging of pleural malignancy, helps in planning of therapy, and also assessing response to the treatment. The procedure involves PET acquisition approximately 60 minutes after intravenous injection of 18F-FDG in conjunction with contrast-enhanced or unenhanced CT. To limit motion blur and reduce artifacts, use of respiratory-gated PET acquisition has been advocated; this improves the accuracy of standardized uptake value (SUV) and metabolic tumor volume measurements for intrathoracic neoplasms.[40] Integrated PET/CT has shown to be more accurate in the staging of thoracic malignancies than either modality alone. Like any other imaging modality, FDG PET-CT also comes with its own set of pitfalls and one must be aware of them before reporting a PET-CT. Inflammatory/infectious processes with increased metabolic activity can also show moderate-to-intense FDG avidity and may be wrongly interpreted as malignancy **(Figs. 14A and B)**; therefore, obtaining clinical history becomes absolutely essential before reading a FDG PET-CT scan.

Fluorodeoxyglucose Positron Emission Tomography–Computed Tomography in Malignant Pleural Mesothelioma

Fluorodeoxyglucose PET-CT is pivotal in imaging of malignant pleural mesothelioma. The typical findings in malignant pleural mesothelioma are unilateral circumferential or near-circumferential pleural and fissural thickening that shows FDG avidity and SUV

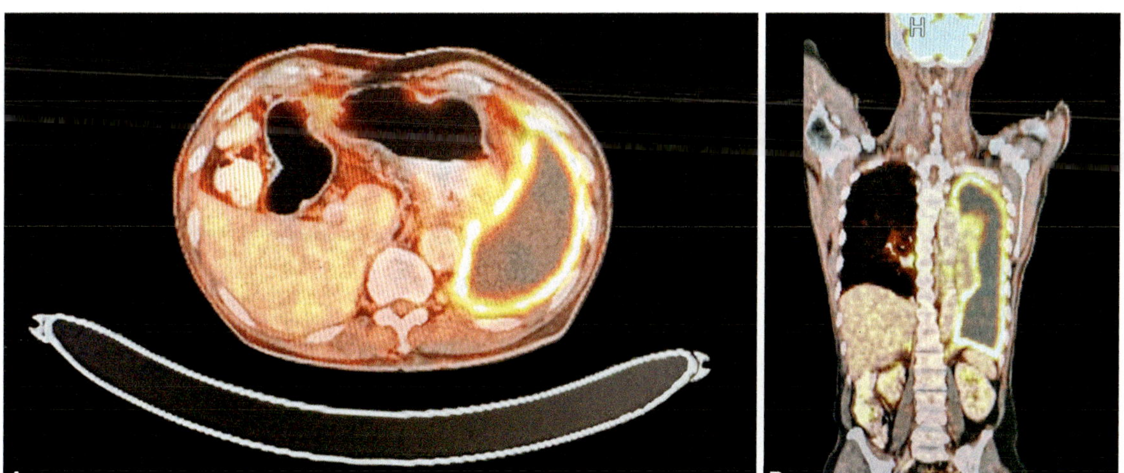

FIGS. 14A AND B: (A) Tubercular empyema patients with high uptake in PET in axial view. (B) Coronal section of PET–CT of tubercular empyema patients.

(PET–CT: positron emission tomography–computed tomography)

value > 2.0–2.2.[41] The tumor, node, metastasis (TNM) staging including the TNM system utilizes quantitative and qualitative parameters obtained from FDG PET-CT. An important role of imaging is to distinguish resectable tumor from unresectable tumor, preventing unnecessary thoracotomies and other morbid surgical procedures. This includes differentiation between T3 (resectable) and T4 (unresectable) disease and identifying involvement of N3 node and/or distant metastasis. FDG PET-CT has proven to be superior to other imaging modalities in this regard. The irregular and asymmetric morphology of malignant pleural mesothelioma poses difficulties in assessment of tumor burden; however, FDG-avid tumor volume values are an effective method to plan treatment and monitor response in patients undergoing radiation therapy. To overcome challenges in response assessment, owing to the asymmetric morphology of this tumor, Byrne and Nowak proposed a modified Response Evaluation Criteria for Solid Tumors (RECIST).[42] In this the tumor, burden is assessed by summing a total of six measurements of the tumor with maximum thickness perpendicular to the chest wall, with two measurements at reproducible landmarks carried out on three different slices, 1 cm apart.

KEY POINTS

- CXR is an initial modality for the diagnosis of pleural disease. CXR is widely available and is very sensitive.
- The ultrasonography of chest is noninvasive and no radiation exposure is very important for evaluation of pleural and lung pathologies. It can also be helpful for point-of-care management, emergency, and in intensive care unit.
- Other imaging modalities such as CT, MRI, and PET-CT are also available to evaluate for pleural diseases.
- CXR-PA view is the simplest, easiest, and quickest method to diagnose pneumothorax. There are various methods to quantify the pneumothorax (Collins, rhea, and light).
- The easier method is measuring the distance between the lung margin and chest wall, <2 cm is small and >2 cm is considered a large pneumothorax.
- In PSP, if patients are asymptomatic, conservative management can be tried regardless of the size of the pneumothorax.
- Meniscus' sign or Ellis S curve is a radiological illusion. The shape of meniscus is due to the layer of fluid which is of insufficient depth to create a noticeable shadow when viewed enface.
- When effusion occurs between two lobes (fissural). It tends to resolve spontaneously or with diuretics (vanishing/pseudo-tumor/phantom tumor).
- If the contact angle of the lesion with the chest wall gives a good clue regarding location, acute angle favors parenchymal while obtuse (D-shaped) suggests pleural origin.
- Pleural phase in CECT—when the image acquisition is done after 60–90 seconds of intravenous contrast administration.
- In loculated pleural effusions, there is split pleura sign.
- To differentiate between pleural effusion and ascites, there are few important signs to be recalled as A—interface, B—bare area, C—crus of diaphragm, and D—diaphragm sign.
- In case of hemothorax, there could be dual density inside the lesion in terms of HU units, which may suggest the possibility of hemorrhage, but the gold standard is still the diagnostic tapping.
- Inflammatory/infectious processes with increased metabolic activity can also show moderate-to-intense FDG avidity and may be wrongly interpreted as malignancy.

REFERENCES

1. Walz-Flannigan AI, Brossoit KJ, Magnuson DJ, Schueler BA. Pictorial review of digital radiography artifacts. Radiographics. 2018;38(3):833-46.
2. Qureshi NR, Gleeson FV. Imaging of pleural disease. Clin Chest Med. 2006;27(2):193-213.
3. Collins CD, Lopez A, Mathie A, Wood V, Jackson JE, Roddie ME. Quantification of pneumothorax size on chest radiographs using interpleural distances: regression analysis based on volume measurements from helical CT. AJR Am J Roentgenol. 1995;165(5):1127-30.
4. Rhea JT, DeLuca SA, Greene RE. Determining the size of pneumothorax in the upright patient. Radiology. 1982;144:733-6.
5. Light RW. Management of spontaneous pneumothorax. Am Rev Respir Dis. 1993;148(1):245-8.
6. Roberts ME, Rahman NM, Maskell NA, Bibby AC, Blyth KG, Corcoran JP, et al.; BTS Pleural Guideline Development Group. British Thoracic Society Guideline for pleural disease. Thorax. 2023;78(Suppl 3):1-42.

7. Davis S, Gardner F, Qvist G. The shape of a pleural effusion. Br Med J. 1963;1:436-7.
8. Woodring JH. Recognition of pleural effusion on supine radiographs: How much fluid is required? AJR Am J Roentgenol. 1984;142:59-64.
9. Oliveira E, Manuel P, Alexandre J, Girão F. Phantom tumour of the lung. Lancet. 2012;380(9858):2028.
10. Tesloianu DN, Chioarta M, Corduneanu D, Ignat AM, Petris AO, Tesloianu A. Does Phantom Tumor Really Exist? Maedica (Bucur). 2017;12(4):281-5.
11. Gefter WI, Boucot KR, Marshall EW. Localized interlobar effusion in congestive heart failure; vanishing tumor of the lung. Circ. 1950;3:336-43.
12. Sureka B, Thukral BB, Mittal MK, Mittal A, Sinha M. Radiological review of pleural tumors. Indian J Radiol Imaging. 2013;23(4): 313-20.
13. Downer NJ, Ali NJ, Au-Yong IT. Investigating pleural thickening. BMJ. 2013;346:e8376.
14. Jelen TH, Bankier AA, Eisenberg RL. Solid Pleural Lesions. Am J Roentgenol. 2012;198:W512-20.
15. Henschke CI, Yankelevitz OF, Davis SD. Pleural diseases: multimodality imaging and clinical management. Curr Probl Diagn Radio. 1991;20:155-81.
16. Kang MJ, Park CM, Lee CH, Goo JM, Lee HJ. Dual-energy CT: clinical applications in various pulmonary diseases. Radiographics. 2010;30:685.
17. Otrakji A, Digumarthy SR, Lo Gullo R, Flores EJ, Shepard JA, Kalra MK. Dual-Energy CT: Spectrum of Thoracic Abnormalities. Radiographics. 2016;36:38.
18. McCollough CH, Leng S, Yu L, Fletcher JG. Dual- and Multi-Energy CT: Principles, Technical Approaches, and Clinical Applications. Radiology. 2015;276:637.
19. Hallifax RJ, Talwar A, Wrightson JM, Edey A, Gleeson FV. State-of-the-art: Radiological investigation of pleural disease. Respir Med. 2017;124:88-99.
20. Hallifax RJ, Haris M, Corcoran JP, Leyakathalikhan S, Brown E, Srikantharaja D, et al. Role of CT in assessing pleural malignancy prior to thoracoscopy. Thorax. 2015;70:192-3.
21. Kalender WA, Sissler W, Klotz E, Vock P. Spiral volumetric CT with single-breath-hold technique, continuous transport, and continuous scanner rotation. Radiology. 1990;176:181-3.
22. Görg C, Bert T, Görg K. Contrast-enhanced sonography for differential diagnosis of pleurisy and focal pleural lesions of unknown cause. Chest. 2005;128(6):3894-9.
23. Leung AN, Müller NL, Miller RR. CT in differential diagnosis of diffuse pleural disease. AJR Am J Roentgenol. 1990;154:487-92.
24. Scott EM, Marshall TJ, Flower CD, Stewart S. Diffuse pleural thickening: percutaneous CT-guided cutting needle biopsy. Radiology. 1995;194:867-70.
25. McLoud TC, Flower CD. Imaging the pleura: sonography, CT, and MR imaging. AJR Am J Roentgenol. 1991;156:1145-53.
26. Aquino SL, Webb WR, Gushiken BJ. Pleural exudates and transudates: diagnosis with contrast-enhanced CT. Radiology. 1994;192:803-8.
27. Yilmaz U, Polar G, Sahin N, Soy O, Gülay U. CT in differential diagnosis of benign and malignant pleural disease. Monaldi Arch Chest Dis. 2005;63:17-22.
28. Traill ZC, Davies RJ, Gleeson FV. Thoracic computed romography in patients with suspected malignant pleural effusions. Clin Radiol. 2001;56(3):193-6.
29. Koh DM, Burke S, Davies N, Padley SP. Transthoracic US of the chest: clinical uses and applications. Radiographies. 2002;22(1):E1.
30. Abramowitz Y, Simanovsky N, Goldstein MS, et al. Pleural effusion: characterization with CT attenuation values and CT. AJR Am J Roentgenol. 2009;192:618-23.
31. Parizel PM, Makkat S, Van Miert E, Van Goethem JW, van den Hauwe L, De Schepper AM. Intracranial hemorrhage: principles of CT and MRI interpretation. Eur Radiol. 2001;11:1770-83.
32. Broderick SR. Hemothorax: etiology, diagnosis, and management. Thorac Surg Clin. 2013;23:89-96.
33. Kaewlai R, Avery LL, Asrani AV, Novelline RA. Multidetector CT of blunt thoracic trauma. Radiographics. 2008;28:1555-70.
34. Liu F, Huang YC, Ng Y-B, Liang JH. Differentiate pleural effusion from hemothorax after blunt chest trauma; comparison of computed tomography attenuation values. J Acute Med. 2016:1-6.
35. Paling MR, Griffin GK. Lower lobe collapse due co pleural effusion: a CT analysis. Comput Assist Tomogr. 1985;9:1079-83.
36. Proco AV, Ball JB Jr. Computed tomography of the major and minor fissures. AJR Am J Roentgenol. 1983;140:439-48.
37. Szczyrek M, Bitkowska P, Jutrzenka M, Szudy-Szczyrek A, Drelich-Zbroja A, Milanowski J. Pleural Neoplasms—What Could MRI Change? Cancers. 2023;15:3261.
38. Ohno Y. New Applications of Magnetic Resonance Imaging for Thoracic Oncology. Semin Respir Crit Care Med. 2014;35:27-40.
39. Puderbach M, Hintze C, Ley S, Eichinger M, Kauczor H, Biederer J. MR imaging of the chest: a practical approach at 1.5T. Eur J Radiol. 2007;64:345-55.
40. Feigen M, Lee ST, Lawford C, Churcher K, Zupan E, Scott AM, et al. Establishing locoregional control of malignant pleural mesothelioma using high-dose radiotherapy and (18) F-FDG PET/CT scan correlation. J Med Imaging Radiat Oncol. 2011;55:320-32.
41. Yildirim H, Metintas M, Entok E, Ak G, Ak I, Dundar E, et al. Clinical value of fluorodeoxyglucose-positron emission tomography/ computed tomography in differentiation of malignant mesothelioma from asbestos-related benign pleural disease: an observational pilot study. J Thorac Oncol. 2009;4:1480-4.
42. Byrne MJ, Nowak AK. Modified RECIST criteria for assessment of response in malignant pleural mesothelioma. Ann Oncol. 2004;15:257-60.

CHAPTER

4 Role of Ultrasound in Pleural Diseases

Pooja Tyagi, Devireddy Madhava Reddy, Deepak Govil

INTRODUCTION

Thoracic ultrasound is a bedside modality readily available to examine the chest wall, pulmonary parenchyma, and pleura. This noninvasive, radiation-free, repeatable, and real-time ultrasound examination is a powerful tool in the diagnosis of a multitude of disorders. We shall review the role of ultrasound in pleural diseases. The ultrasound examination of the thorax is limited by significant changes in impedance and access to deeper structures is affected by artifacts such as absorption, reflection, acoustic shadowing, mirroring, and ring-down artifacts. However, lung and pleural affections lead to changes in tissue composition and hence improved acoustic transmission leading to better ultrasound visualization. The ultrasound is an important clinical tool for point-of-care bedside evaluation.

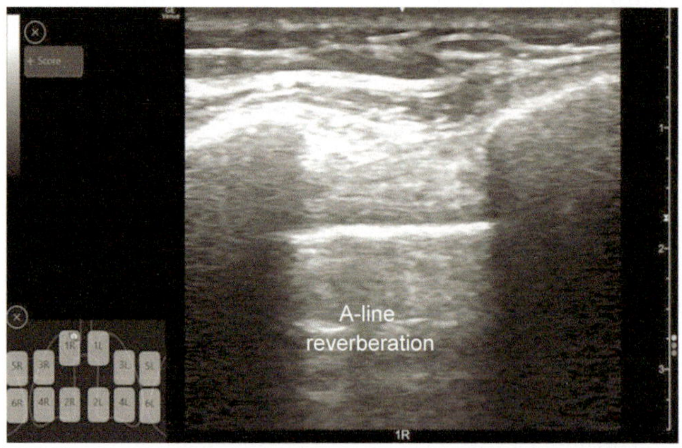

FIG. 1: Ultrasound image showing "A-line" artifact.

ULTRASOUND MODALITY

Pleural ultrasound can be easily carried out at the bedside, with low cost involved and serial examinations possible. Lung ultrasound is an exception, as it is based on varied artifacts while ultrasound of other organs is a direct visualization of the same. The acoustic impedance mismatch at the air and soft tissue interface results in a hyperechoic pleural line as most of the ultrasound beam is reflected at the pleura. Hence, an air-filled lung is not directly visualized instead an "A-line" artifact is seen on ultrasound as a reverberation artifact. Lung and pleural pathologies amounting to interstitium and pleural inflammation lead to "B-line" artifacts, which are hyperechoic vertical lines arising from the pleura and go down on scanned lung field replacing the "A-line" artifact, which is seen with normal aerated lungs **(Figs. 1 and 2)**.

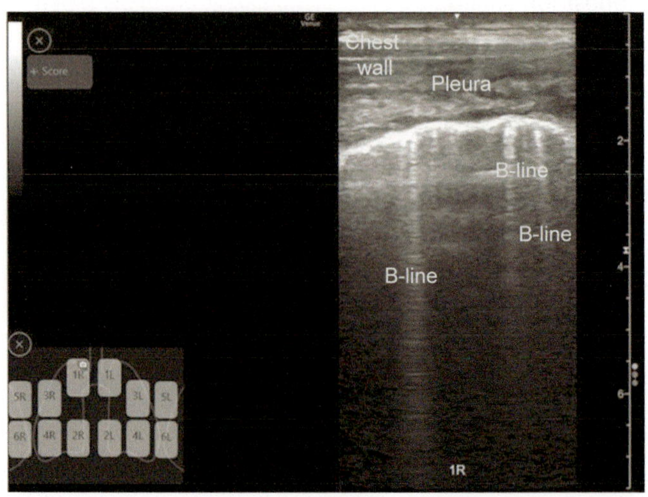

FIG. 2: Ultrasound image showing "B-line" artifact.

Lung consolidation and collapse lead to direct visualization of lung parenchyma, abolishing the "A-line" artifact. If a lung pathology does not involve pleura, it is not visualized due to air and soft tissue interface. Pleural effusions are directly seen.

Complete ultrasound examination involves looking at both right and left hemithorax in all anterior, lateral, and posterior lung fields. The patient can be examined in both supine and sitting upright positions. The probe is held perpendicular to the chest wall, and optimal resolution is achieved if the target structure is in the center of the screen.

The transducers used to examine the lung and pleura are curvilinear or phased array low-frequency probes of 5–9 MHz and for delineating superficial structures linear probe of 9–12 MHz is used. The probe orientation can be longitudinal or horizontal, placed in the intercostal space. By convention, the pointer is kept cephalad. The initial depth is kept at 18–20 cm and further gain and depth settings are adjusted to focus on target structures.

B mode is used for the visualization of pleural space, identifying pleural effusion, and delineating its etiology and characteristics while M mode enables observation of real-time dynamics of pleura.

NORMAL PLEURA ON ULTRASONOGRAPHY

In fully inflated lungs, apposed parietal and visceral pleura appear as pleural lines. It appears as a smooth hyperechoic structure with a subpleural hypoechoic line. The normal pleura is 0.2 mm in thickness and it lies 0.5 cm deep to periosteal reflection. The "lung sliding," which is a regular rhythmic movement with synchronized respiration, is a real-time ultrasound finding arising because the parietal and visceral pleura are in either direct apposition or separated by a small amount of intrapleural fluid. The pleura moves in respirophasic and cardiophasic fashion referred to as "lung sliding" and "lung pulse" in a normally aerated lung. The parietal pleura is better visualized than the visceral pleura as an echogenic line. This echogenic pleural line along with the adjacent ribs gives a characteristic appearance referred to as the "Bat sign." However, these two pleurae can be differentiated with high-resolution ultrasound. The visceral pleura can be seen with lung consolidation and deaeration of the lung; here it is then visible with the same echogenicity as the parietal pleura. Reverberation artifacts and reflection are primarily features of visceral pleura **(Fig. 3)**.

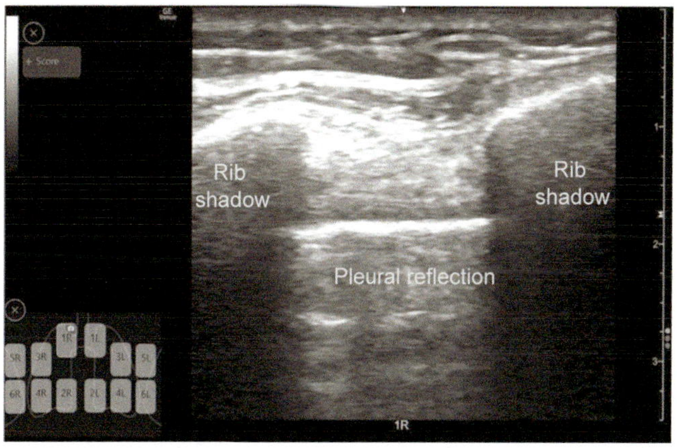

FIG. 3: Ultrasound image showing "Bat sign."

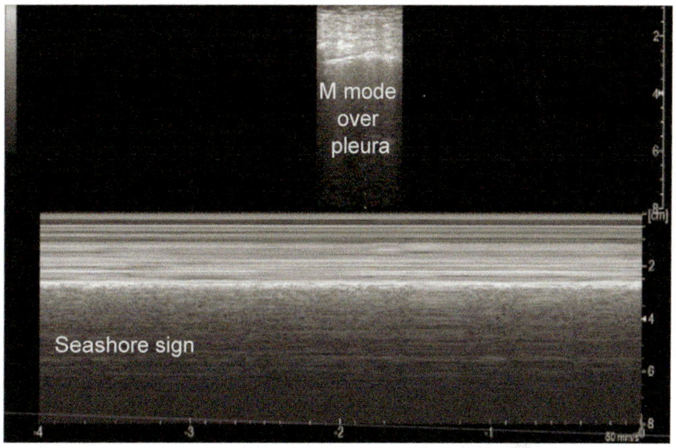

FIG. 4: Ultrasound image showing "Seashore sign."

The hyperechoic pleural line in between two ribs shimmering back and forth is a dynamic sign, seen on ultrasound as horizontal movement along the pleural line, at the lung apex in the supine position. The M mode, which detects motion over time, provides further evidence in lung sliding, especially helpful in elderly patients and in those with poor pulmonary reserve where appreciating lung sliding is otherwise difficult. The M-mode cursor is placed over the pleura, and two different patterns are seen on the ultrasound screen, motionless portion of the chest above the pleural line creates horizontal waves and sliding below the pleural line creates a granular pattern of the sand, the so-called "seashore sign" seen in normal lung **(Fig. 4)**.

PLEURAL EFFUSION

It can be diagnosed with physical examination, chest X-ray, computed tomography (CT), and ultrasound chest. With physical examination diagnostic accuracy depends largely on the size of the effusion and a minimum of 300 mL is required to be detected by physical examination alone. The factors, especially in critically critical care settings, such as body habitus, positioning, mechanical ventilation, subcutaneous emphysema, and noncooperation of the patient are all hindrances to proper physical examination. The sensitivity and specificity of physical examination for the diagnosis of pleural effusion is low compared to chest X-ray and CT of the chest.[1]

With a chest X-ray to diagnose pleural effusion minimum fluid required is 200 mL to blunt the costophrenic angle and 500 mL to obliterate the cardiophrenic angle, hence to be visible on chest X-ray.[2] Poor image quality, which is common in ICU settings, and the existence of lung mass may be misleading in interpreting the radiological image.

Computed tomography of the chest is the diagnostic modality for pleural effusion, but its limitation is the inability to distinguish between small pleural effusion and pleural thickening while exposing the patient to 7 mSv ionizing radiation, which is equivalent to 350 chest X-rays.[3] Moreover, it involves significant costs and transporting patients to radiological suites for imaging, which may not be always feasible in critically ill patients and lead to delays in diagnosis. Both chest X-ray and CT produce static images and do not consider the dynamic interplay between chest organs.

The pleural ultrasound gives us real-time dynamic information, which is radiation-free and can be performed bedside and repeated when needed. Even a small quantity of pleural fluid can be detected. Pleural ultrasound can be used to diagnose, asses the volume, and reveal characteristics of pleural fluid and plan further management. The amount of pleural fluid that can be detected by ultrasound is even 5 mL, although detection of 20 mL is more reliable and 100 mL can be detected with 100% sensitivity.[4,5]

Lichtenstein et al. in 2004 carried out a prospective study in acute respiratory distress syndrome (ARDS) patients comparing physical examination, chest and lung ultrasound with CT of the chest. They found that lung ultrasound had 92% sensitivity, 93% specificity, and a diagnostic accuracy of 93%.[5]

In 2008 Rocco et al. published a trial comparing bedside radiography and lung ultrasound in detecting pleural effusion in trauma patients. They showed lung ultrasound to be superior to chest X-ray in diagnosis of pleural effusion.[6]

In 2011 Xirouchaki et al. compared the diagnostic accuracy of lung ultrasound and bedside chest X-ray in ICU patients, which showed ultrasound to be 100% sensitive, 100% specificity, and 100% diagnostic accuracy in diagnosing pleural effusion while chest X-rays were 65, 81, and 69%, respectively.[7]

The pleural ultrasound is characterized by its high sensitivity and diagnostic accuracy in identifying and localizing pleural fluid. It is widely used as it is safe, easy to perform, small learning curve, and is highly acceptable to patients.[8] The International Consensus of Lung Ultrasound Experts states that for examination of pleura fluid, lung ultrasound is more accurate than supine chest X-ray and its diagnostic accuracy is consistent with CT of chest performed.[9] The pleural effusion is better visualized with low-frequency probe. The microconvex probe is the first choice to assess pleural fluid volume,[9] when not available a phased array or convex probe can be used. The probe should be small enough to fit into intercostal space with good spatial resolution.

In the absence of pleural effusion, on lung ultrasound, a "curtain sign" is seen during inspiration due to an air artifact generated from a causally moving aerated lung. In the presence of significant pleural effusion, a "jellyfish sign" or "flapping lung sign" is seen, which is seen due to mobile atelectatic lung as echogenic dense tissue within the pleural effusion **(Figs. 5 and 6)**.[10]

Characteristics of Pleural Effusion

Unless the effusion is loculated, it will be seen in the most dependent location in the thorax, depending on the position of the patient.

It has three important characteristics:

1. Pleural effusion appears as relatively hypoechoic to anechoic space.

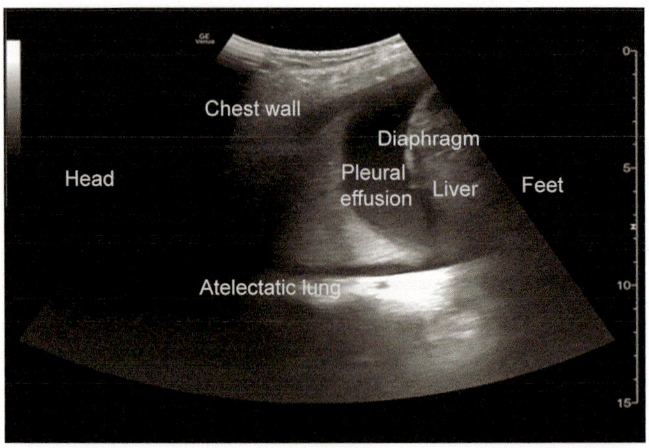

FIG. 5: Ultrasound image showing "Jellyfish sign."

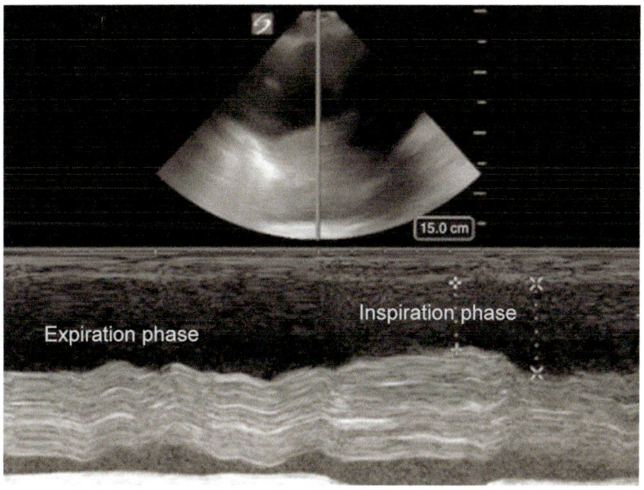

FIG. 6: Ultrasound image showing "Sinusoid sign" (dynamic sonographic sign showing the respiratory variation of distance between parietal and visceral pleura in the freely floating lung).
Source: Adapted from Patel KM, et al.[11]

2. Pleural effusion has anatomical boundaries within the thoracic cavity, surrounded by chest wall, compressed lung, diaphragm, and sometimes pericardium.
3. Pleural effusion has typical dynamic findings such as diaphragmatic movement, lung flapping, and plankton sign.

Dynamic Findings of Pleural Effusion

Dynamic findings include:

- Movement of compressed/atelectatic lung—commonly termed as "lung flapping" or "jellyfish sign", due to deaerated lung within the pleural effusion moving in respirophasic and cardiophasic manner.
- Movement of the diaphragm in a respirophasic manner—usually the diaphragm moves causally with inspiration, but in massive effusion paradoxical cephalad movement of the diaphragm is seen.
- Movement of elements within the effusion—cellular components, septations, or loculated walls move in respirophasic and cardiophasic manner.

Pleural Effusion versus Pleural Thickening

The "lung pulse" or "fluid color sign" is the most sensitive and specific sign to differentiate pleural fluid from pleural thickening, seen on color Doppler. It is the movement of effusion echoes synchronous with respiratory or cardiac cycle. The fluid color sign has sensitivity of 93% and specificity of 100% to detect even small pleural collection.[12]

Quantifying Pleural Fluid with Ultrasound

Assessment of pleural fluid along with clinical scenario wherein the respiratory distress is attributed to fluid accumulation, aids in decision making to drain the fluid.

There are many methods proposed to estimate the pleural fluid with aid of pleural ultrasound, but none is established best method. The accurate and reliable estimation of pleural fluid may not be feasible at all times, factors that might affect reliable estimation are:

- *Size of thoracic cavity*: Tall individuals have large thoracic cavity, leading to distribution of fluid over larger area, which may lead to over- or underestimation of fluid quantity.
- *Patient position*: Supine, upright, or lateral decubitus all influence fluid distribution.
- *Diaphragm position*: Phrenic nerve palsy, intra-abdominal hypertension, and diaphragmatic hernia all can influence pleural fluid estimation.
- *Associated condition*: Consolidation along with pleural fluid can impact correct fluid estimation.
- *Large effusions*: Entire section may not be visible in large pleural effusion.
- *Other factors*: Longitudinal or transverse scan, inter-observer variability, and operator expertise.

Vignon et al. measured distance between lung and posterior chest wall, which is also the distance between parietal and visceral pleura separated by the presence of fluid in pleural space, at lung apex and lung base, and compared maximum distance with amount of fluid drained. They concluded that a strong corelation existed between interpleural distance and fluid drained. They found that interpleural distance at lung base in right thoracic cavity, if >45 mm and >50 mm in left thoracic cavity, is suggestive of approximately 800 mL pleural fluid.[13]

Roch et al. assessed accuracy of lung ultrasound in predicting pleural fluid >500 mL in mechanically ventilated patients. They found that interpleural distance measured at lung base or fifth intercostal space (PLDbase or PLD5) by lung ultrasound correlated with the volume drained. To add more, PLDbase >5 estimated effusion >500 mL.[14]

Balik et al. measured maximum interpleural distance (Sep) at lung base at end expiration in mechanically ventilated patients and suggested that pleural effusion can be quantified as, V (mL) = 20 × Sep (mm). As per this study pleural fluid could be quantified and decision to proceed with thoracocentesis, if needed, can be made **(Tables 1 and 2; Figs. 7 and 8)**.[15]

TABLE 1: Assessment of pleural fluid volume.

Author	Study population	Formula	Results
Vignon et al.[13]	Mechanical ventilated vs. nonventilated	NA	Interpleural distance on right >45 mm (sensitivity 94%, specificity 76%), left >50 mm (sensitivity 100%, specificity 67%), predicted pleural effusion >800 mL. Positive linear correlation between distance and volume $r = 0.88$, $r^2 = 0.72$, $p < 0.0001$
Roch et al.[14]	Mechanical ventilated	NA	Interpleural distance at lung base >5 cm, predicted effusion volume >500 mL (sensitivity 83%, specificity 90%), PPV 91%, NPV 82%
Balik et al.[15]	Mechanical ventilated	V (mL) = 20 × Sep (mm)	Positive linear correlation between distance and volume $r = 0.72$, $r^2 = 0.52$, $p < 0.001$
Usta et al.[16]	Spontaneous breathing	V (mL) = 16 × D (mm)	Positive linear correlation between distance and volume $r = 0.89$, $r^2 = 0.79$, $p < 0.001$
Remerand et al.[17]	Critically ill patients	V (mL) = $L_{US} \times A_{US}$	Positive linear correlation between US volume and drained volume ($r = 0.84$, $p < 0.001$) and CT volume ($r = 0.90$, $p < 0.001$)

(A_{US}: cross-sectional area; CT: computed tomography; D: distance; L_{US}: paravertebral length; NA: not applicable; Sep: maximal distance between parietal and visceral pleura; US: ultrasound; V: pleural volume)

Source: Adapted from Brogi E, et al.[18]

TABLE 2: Measuring of pleural effusion by ultrasound.

Author	Probe position	Measuring method (end expiration)
Vignon et al.[13]	Along dorsolateral aspect of chest wall as posteriorly as possible, from base to apex in all intercostal spaces (ICS)	Measure maximal perpendicular interpleural distance from leading edge of dependent lung to posterior chest wall at apex and at base
Roch et al.[14]	Measure in posterior axillary line in 9th to 11th ICS, moving transducer cranially, in longitudinal scan	Measure mean of three different distances—lung and diaphragm, lung and posterior chest wall at base, lung and posterior chest wall at fifth ICS
Balik et al.[15]	Along posterior axillary line, moving cranially	Measure maximal distance between parietal and visceral pleura at lung base
Usta et al.[16]	Along midscapular line, moving cranially	Measure maximal distance between visceral pleura and mid diaphragm
Remerand et al.[17]	Along paravertebral ICS	Measure the distance between ICS where fluid is visualized L-us and at half point of L-us, area is manually measured

Source: Adapted from Brogi E, et al.[18]

Compression atelectasis, an important ultrasound finding, suggestive of lung collapse also correlates with the degree of pleural fluid accumulated [ultrasound image **(Fig. 5)**].

Assessment of Pleural Fluid Nature with Ultrasound

The sonographic appearance of pleural fluid depends on nature, cause, and chronicity of pleural fluid accumulated. The pleural fluid can be characterized as exudative or transudative broadly, depending on the different pathological process involved. Further pleural fluid could be an empyema, hemothorax, or a malignant effusion. Ultrasound findings based on analysis of pleural fluid echogenicity, changes in pleura thickness, and lung parenchyma, all aid in diagnosis of etiology of fluid accumulated.

In a prospective study, Yang et al., studying possible use of ultrasound in delineating etiology of pleural effusion, found that the internal echogenicity could be anechoic, complex nonseptate, and complex septate. The echogenicity of fluid could be homogeneous or nonhomogeneous.

1. Effusion is anechoic when it is echo free.
2. Complex nonseptate when echogenic material is seen inside accumulated effusion.
3. Complex septate when fibrin strands or septa are seen floating inside pleural fluid.

Usually, anechoic fluid is transudative in nature while internal echogenicity or septae are suggestive of exudative fluid, additionally pleural thickening and lung

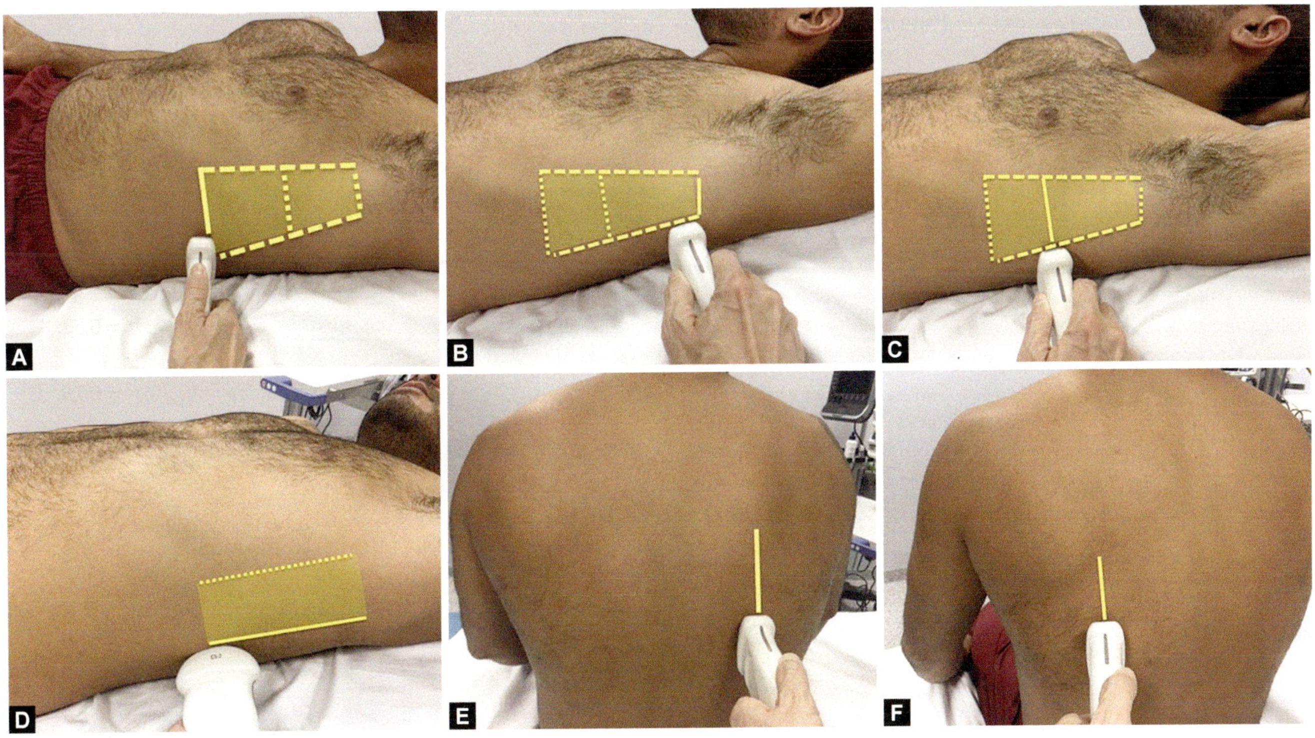

FIGS. 7A TO F: Position of the probe and the marker on the chest wall.
Source: Adapted from Brogi E, et al.[18]

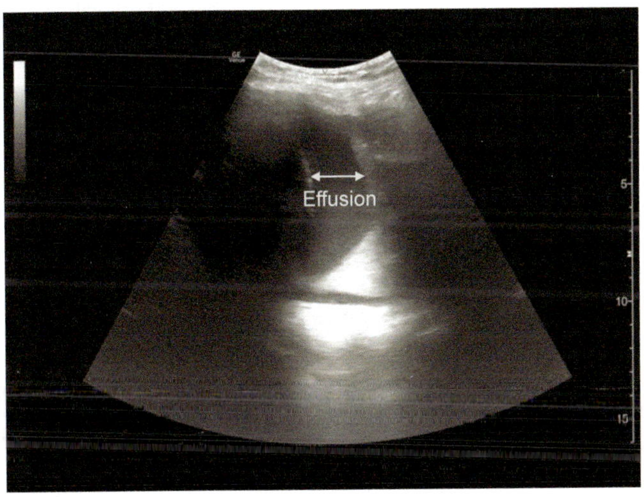

FIG. 8: Ultrasound image showing how to quantify the pleural fluid volume.

parenchyma changes are also indicative of exudative fluid. However, two-thirds of exudative fluid is anechoic in nature **(Table 3)**.

Empyema

A parapneumonic effusion eventually can lead to empyema. The lung ultrasound has 69% sensitivity and 90% specificity to detect parapneumonic effusion. While CT of chest has 77% sensitivity and 65% specificity, on the other hand chest X-ray has 62% and 60%, respectively. This suggests that lung ultrasound is superior to other modalities regarding specificity to detect parapneumonic effusions.[19] Three stages recognized in the course of an empyema as exudative, fibrinopurulent, and organizing stage. These stages with their characteristic findings are distinctly seen with lung ultrasound.[20] The ultrasound findings in an empyema can predict clinical outcome to an extent. Chen and colleagues found that a subset of patients with septations had increased length of hospital stay, had fewer chest tube free days, and were more likely to require fibrinolytic therapy or undergo surgical interventions.[21]

Hemothorax

Bleeding into pleural space could be a result of chest trauma or any inflammatory process like tuberculosis or malignancy. A hemothorax appears echogenic on ultrasound due to its cellularity, which creates extensive acoustic reflections.[22]

A layering effect seen due to cellular accumulation in gravity-dependent fashion results in a "hematocrit sign", appearing highly echogenic in dependent areas. Hemothorax with or without pneumothorax can be reliably detected with ultrasound, and ultrasound chest to

TABLE 3: Differentiating nature of pleural fluid.

	Exudate	Transudate	Hemothorax	Empyema	Malignant effusion
Internal echogenicity: Anechoic/ complex nonseptate/complex septate	Can be septate/ nonseptate/anechoic	Anechoic	Hyperechogenic	Septate	Can be complex septate or nonseptate
Echogenicity: Homogeneous/ nonhomogeneous	Can be homogeneous or nonhomogeneous	Nonhomogeneous	Homogeneous	Homogeneous	Homogeneous
Pleural thickness	Thickened	No	Thickened	Thickened	Irregular pleural thickness

Source: Adapted from Brogi E, et al.[18]

detect or rule out hemothorax—pneumothorax is essential part of extended focused assessment with sonography in trauma (eFAST) algorithm. The sensitivity of ultrasound to detect hemothorax after trauma was equivalent to chest X-ray, but ultrasound was found to be faster, taking 1 minute versus 15 minutes needed for an chest X-ray.[23] A meta-analysis of 12 studies of ultrasound for pleural effusion in trauma settings showed sensitivity 67% and specificity 99% for ultrasound to detect hemothorax[24] **(Fig. 9)**.

Fresh blood collected is echo free or poor, while old or collected blood has echogenic shadows or visible clot[25] **(Figs. 10 and 11)**.

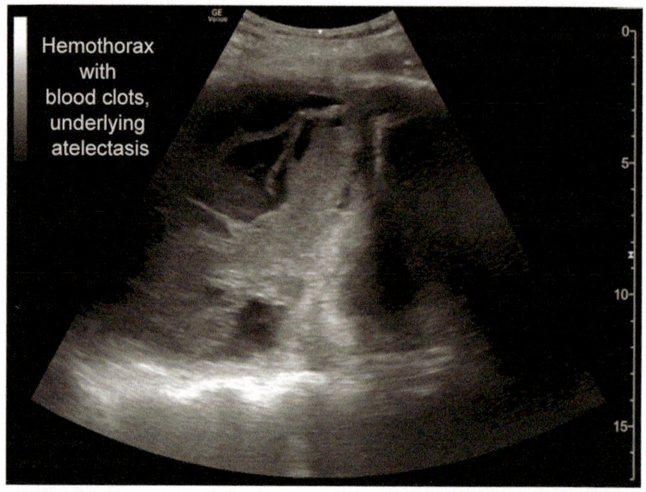

FIG. 10: Ultrasound image showing hemothorax with underlying atelectasis.

Malignant Pleural Effusion

The ultrasound findings of malignant effusion depend on chronicity and degree of inflammation in pleural space.

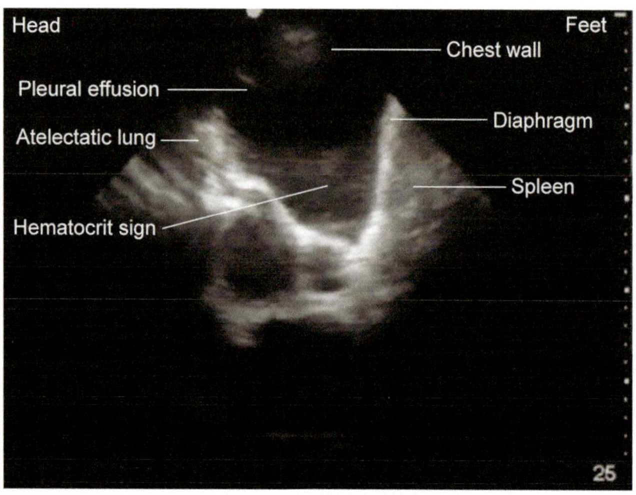

FIG. 9: Ultrasound image showing "Hematocrit sign."
Source: Adapted from Jose Cardenas-Garcia J, et al.[26]

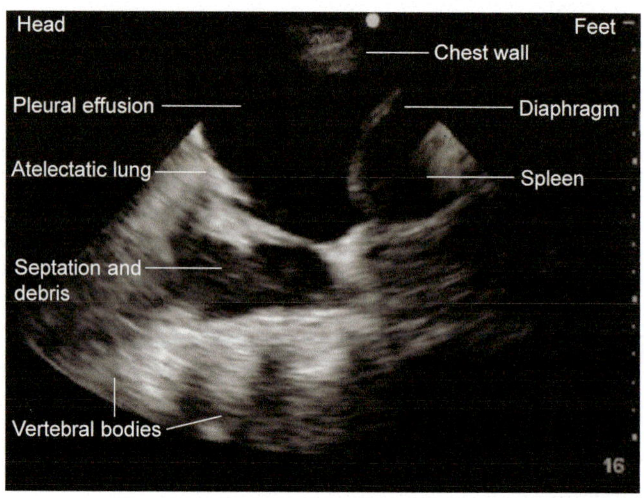

FIG. 11: Ultrasound image showing "Plankton sign."
Source: Adapted from Jose Cardenas-Garcia J, et al.[26]

A prospective study by Qureshi et al. in patients suspected of malignant effusion included pleural thickening >1 cm, pleural nodularity, and diaphragm thickness >0.7 cm as findings suggestive of malignant effusion.[27] Pleural thickness of >1 cm alone has 88% sensitivity and 48% specificity for malignant effusion.[28] The positive predictive value increases to 100% if pleural thickness is accompanied by pleural nodularity and increased diaphragm thickness.[27]

PNEUMOTHORAX

It is the accumulation of air between parietal and visceral pleura. A pneumothorax can be broadly classified as traumatic or nontraumatic, further nontraumatic pneumothorax can be primary spontaneous or secondary spontaneous in nature. Traumatic pneumothorax is the most common life-threatening condition, seen in over 20% of patients with blunt chest trauma and nearly 40% with penetrating chest trauma.[29] Small (nearly 10%) and medium pneumothorax (11–40%) are generally not life-threatening and their management varies.[30] A delay in diagnosis and its management, especially when patient is on mechanical ventilation, can lead to progressively increase in pneumothorax and hemodynamic instability.[31] In these situations a quick bedside ultrasound examination can rapidly detect the pneumothorax and expedite treatment options. The lung ultrasound has an established role in diagnosis of traumatic pneumothorax; hence, it is also an important part of eFAST. In one prospective study wherein lung ultrasound for diagnosing pneumothorax was compared to chest X-ray alone, a composite standard (chest X-ray, CT chest, clinical course, and invasive interventions) and to gold standard CT scan only.[23] The result showed eFAST examination had a sensitivity of 58.9% with positive likelihood ratio of 69.7 and specificity of 99.1% when compared to composite standard. The sensitivity of ultrasound and chest X-ray were 48.8% and 20.9%, respectively and specificity of 99.6% and 98.7%, respectively.

Another prospective study by Ball et al. noted that up to 76% of all traumatic pneumothorax were missed by supine anteroposterior (AP) view interpreted by trauma team in emergency.[32] This reveals poor sensitivity of chest X-ray to detect pneumothorax in rushed emergency scenarios and utility of rapid bedside ultrasound to aid in diagnosis.

Lichtenstein et al. have shown that ultrasound has sensitivity of 95.3% and specificity of 91.1% for detecting pneumothorax in intensive care unit (ICU) patients.[33]

Sonographic Signs of Pneumothorax

The ultrasound findings suggestive of pneumothorax are absence of lung sliding, absence of lung pulse, absence of B lines, and presence of lung point. Lung sliding, which is the movement of pleural line with respiration, is a strong negative predictor of pneumothorax.

- *Absence of lung sliding*: The air in between pleural and visceral layers seen in pneumothorax prevents visualization of visceral pleura leading to absent lung sliding that is to and fro movement or shimmering of pleural line is not present. When an M mode is placed on examined area leads to "barcode" or a "stratosphere sign", which is a pattern of parallel horizontal line above and below pleural lines representing lack of movement. The negative predictive value for lung sliding is reported as 99.2–100%, indicating that the presence of lung sliding effectively rules out pneumothorax.[33,34] Lung sliding may not be present in other conditions such as ARDS, pulmonary fibrosis, large consolidation, pleural adhesions, atelectasis, right mainstem intubation, and phrenic nerve palsy.[35,36] Specificity ranges from 60% to 90% depending on studied patient population.[33,34] The combination of lung sliding with other signs improves accuracy of diagnosing pneumothorax despite variable specificity. Another way to detect lung sliding is use of power Doppler eliciting subtle lung sliding in patients where it may be difficult to visualize otherwise. The power Doppler being very sensitive detects subtle flow and movement of pleural line. With presence of lung sliding, the power Doppler lights up the pleural line with color flow. The requisite being the probe needs to be held steady and avoid patient movement so as to prevent artifacts and erroneous color flow at pleural line as power Doppler is very sensitive **(Fig. 12)**.
- *Comet tail artifacts or B lines*: These are reverberation artifacts, which appears as hyperechoic vertical lines extending from pleura to lower screen edge without fading, they move with lung sliding and respiratory movements. These comet tail artifacts appear due to acoustic impedance difference between air and water. The loss of these comet tail artifacts is seen in pneumothorax due to presence of air in pleural space, which hinders propagation of sound waves, eliminating acoustic impedance gradient. Also, as visceral pleura is not visible due to presence of air. The negative predictive value of this artifact is high 98–100%, essentially presence of even a single B line rules out presence of pneumothorax.[35,37] If lung sliding is absent along with presence of A lines sensitivity and specificity for a occult pneumothorax is high as 95% and 94%, respectively.[37]

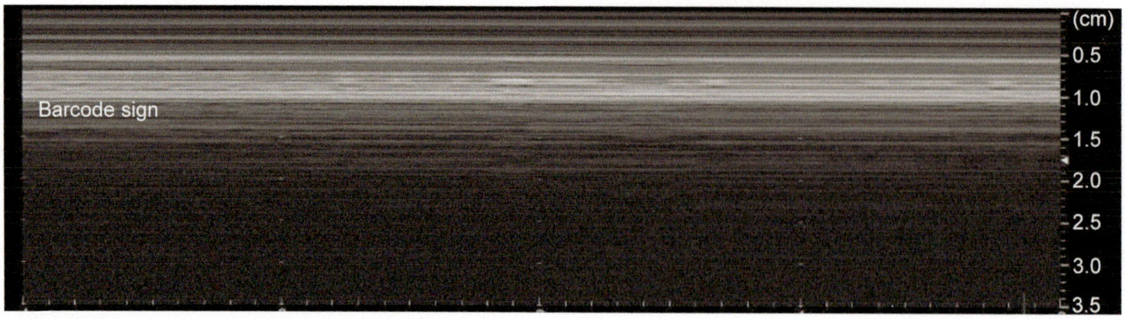

FIG. 12: Ultrasound image showing "Barcode sign."

- *Lung point sign*: This sign is confirmatory of pneumothorax, 100% specific. The lung point is useful in determining the size of pneumothorax, as it occurs at the border of pneumothorax. It is basically due to lung sliding intermittently coming into contact with chest wall during inspiration. The more lateral or posterior the lung point is, larger is the pneumothorax. Though the specificity is 100%, sensitivity of lung point sign is low around 66% and lung point is not seen in large pneumothorax leading to total lung collapse.[37,38] Anterior location of lung point in midclavicular line is suggestive of small pneumothorax. Studies suggest concordance between pneumothorax size on ultrasound and CT chest being within 1.9–2.3 cm.[39] The determination of size of pneumothorax is important in decision making for management of pneumothorax based on clinical scenarios. Further on M mode, alternatively seashore and stratosphere patterns are seen.
- *Lung pulse*: It is the rhythmic movement of pleural line synchronous with cardiac oscillation. The lung pulse is essentially seen when the cardiac oscillations or vibrations are transmitted to lung pleura in poorly aerated lungs. Normally, it is not seen in a well-aerated lung, as the lung sliding is dominant and resistant to cardiac oscillations.[35]
- *Other signs* relevant in diagnosis of complex pneumothorax are:
  - *Double lung point*: At times two lung points are visualized, alternating patterns of sliding and nonsliding intermittently appearing at two opposite sides of scan, two lung point representing two ends of air trapped in pleural space. Pneumothorax with air trapped is seen in chronic pulmonary pleural diseases, acute lung contusions. When this is strongly suspected clinically, patient chest should be examined more laterally in supine position.
  - *Septate pneumothorax*: Here the absence of lung sliding may be associated with B lines and presence of lung pulse in the same scan where parietal and visceral pleura may still be touching due to presence of septa, likely seen in failed pleurodesis. Presence of lung point is confirmatory in such cases.
  - *Hydropneumothorax*: Normally aerated lung and pneumothorax (air–air interface) are seen as lung point with ultrasound; however, air–fluid interface is seen differently on ultrasound. In hydropneumothorax, pleural effusion appears anechoic while pneumothorax gives a reverberation artifacts as A pattern seen below pleural line, absence of lung sliding or pulse, and absence of B lines. Opposition between these two points is known as "hydro point". It shares the same diagnostic power as lung point in diagnosis of pneumothorax.[40]

OTHER PLEURAL DISEASES

Pleural Inflammation

On ultrasound, irregularities of pleural margin, thickened pleura, subpleural consolidation, pleural effusion with or without fibrinous bands, and septa can be identified. Pleural fibrosis is differentiated from pleural effusions by its mixed echogenic or hypoechoic appearance, with or without calcification.

Pleural Neoplasm

Benign tumors of pleura are relatively rare, seen on ultrasound as round or oval shaped, well demarcated, hypoechoic, or moderately echogenic.

Malignant pleural neoplasms being mesothelioma, metastasis, and transpleural growth of lung tumors. The signs of malignancy being irregular thickened pleura with heterogeneous echo patterns, associated pleural effusion and infiltration of adjacent structures.

USE OF ULTRASOUND IN THORACOCENTESIS

The British Thoracic Society pleural disease guidelines 2010 concluded that site selection for all pleural aspiration should be ultrasound guided.[41] Pleural ultrasound to drain pleural fluid reduces morbidity, by preventing postprocedure pneumothorax or inadvertent organ puncture.[42,43]

Ultrasound-guided thoracocentesis can be done in two ways either as site marking or direct needle guidance.[44] In former, the appropriate site for pleural fluid aspiration is marked on skin with aid of ultrasound and fluid is removed without use of ultrasound. Here however patient repositioning can lead to fluid redistribution, as a result fluid aspiration should be done immediately after site marking. While in latter is the direct needle guidance technique, which is the preferred technique, the needle is visible in real-time and constantly monitored. This can be technically challenging but is safer in comparison to the site marking technique. The "V" point demarcates the maximal thickness pleural effusion, formed by the edge of the collapsed lung and diaphragm creating a "V" shape, wherein thoracocentesis can be safely performed. It is recommended that 1–1.5 cm pleural fluid be present between the chest wall and the lung, measured during inspiration to avoid complications. The needle is inserted at the superior margin of the rib to avoid injuring the neurovascular bundle. The PLAPS point (intersection of vertical posterior axillary line and horizontal line at lower blue point) is where all fluid accumulates in the supine position; hence, scanning this area is a must **(Fig. 13)**.

A few important steps in performing safe pleural ultrasound-guided thoracocentesis include:

1. Identify the pleural effusion.
2. Identify a safe trajectory for needle insertion.
3. Identify the depth for safe needle insertion.
4. Identify the safe angulation of needle insertion.
5. Identify the correct guide wire or catheter placement.

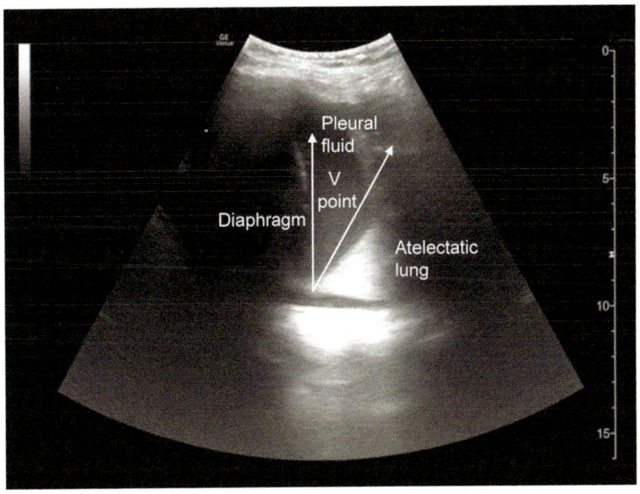

FIG. 13: Ultrasound image showing "V" point.

FUTURE DIRECTIONS

Bedside point-of-care portable ultrasound is the advanced stethoscope in the care of the critically ill and has nearly replaced the stethoscope at the bedside with high diagnostic accuracy. In rural and remote areas where radiology imaging facilities are far-fetched, ultrasound is a boon, especially with tele ultrasound and remote reading, where images are read from a distance, providing accurate diagnosis in a short time. The clinicians and radiologists are often at the crossroads where lung ultrasound is concerned, the best solution is, where point of care ultrasound is needed in acute and critical conditions, it is performed at the clinician bedside, while in complex cases where a more detailed formal diagnosis is needed, ultrasound is performed by radiologist.

CONCLUSION

The utility of pleural ultrasound cannot be underestimated, taking into consideration the ease to perform, fast learning curve, quick interpretation, radiation-free, repeatability, and accessibility. Pleural ultrasound has surpassed physical examination and chest radiography in a big way. The high sensitivity and specificity in diagnosing the pleural disease nearly equals the CT, without the transport to the radiological suite. All this indicates more pleural ultrasound needs to be used by clinicians to get quick results and better diagnostic accuracy.

KEY POINTS

- Ultrasound is an important clinical tool for point-of-care bedside evaluation.
- Bedside ultrasound is a useful instrument for the assessment of chest pathology, specifically in pleural diseases.
- Pleural ultrasound plays important role in evaluation of pneumothorax, pleural effusions, trapped lung, pleural based masses, and parenchymal masses abutting the pleura and in direct vision placement of needles for thoracocentesis.
- The portability and cost-effectiveness in comparison with other imaging modalities give ultrasound an upper hand in diagnostic evaluation.
- Pleural ultrasound can be easily learned and applied with acceptable diagnostic accuracy.

REFERENCES

1. Tasci O, Hatipoglu ON, Cagli B, Ermis V. Sonography of chest using linear array versus sector transducer: correlation with auscultation, chest X-ray and computed tomography. J Clin Ultrasound. 2016;44(6):383-9.
2. Blackmore CC, Black WC, Dallas RV, Crow HC. Pleural fluid estimation: A chest X-ray prediction rule. Acad Radiol. 1996;3(2):103-9.
3. Fazel R, Krumholz HM, Wang Y, Ross JS, Chen J, Ting HH, et al. Exposure to low-dose ionising radiation from medical imaging procedures. N Eng J Med. 2009;361:849-57.
4. Röthlin MA, Näf R, Amgwerd M, Candinas D, Frick T, Trentz O. Ultrasound in blunt abdomen and thoracic trauma. J Trauma. 1993;34(4):488-95.
5. Lichtenstein D, Goldstein I, Mourgeon E, Cluzel P, Grenier P, Rouby JJ. Comparative diagnostic performance of auscultation, chest X-ray, and lung ultrasound in ARDS. Anaesthesiology. 2004;100:9-15.
6. Rocco M, Carbone I, Morelli A, Bertoletti L, Rossi S, Vitale M, et al. Diagnostic accuracy of bedside ultrasound in ICU. Feasibility of detecting pleural effusion and lung contusion in patients on respiratory support after blunt thoracic trauma. Acta Anaesthesiol Scand. 2008;52(6):776-84.
7. Xirouchaki N, Magkanas E, Vaporidi K, Kondili E, Plataki M, Patrianakos A, et al. Lung ultrasound in critically ill patients, comparison with bedside chest X-ray. Intensive Care Med. 2011;37(9);1488-93.
8. Walden AP, Jones QC, Matsa R, Wise MP. Pleural effusion in ICU; hidden morbidity with therapeutic potential. Respirology. 2013;18(2):246-54.
9. Volpicelli G, Elbarbary M, Blaivas M, Lichtenstein DA, Mathis G, Kirkpatrick AW, et al. International evidence-based recommendations for point-of-care lung ultrasound. Intensive Care Med. 2012;38(4):577-91.
10. Lichtenstein DA. Lung ultrasound in the critically ill. Ann Intensive Care. 2014;4:1.
11. Patel KM, Ullah K, Patail H, Ahmad S. Ultrasound for Pleural Disease. Beyond a Pocket of Pleural Fluid. Ann Am Thorac Soc. 2021;18(5):749-56.
12. Wu RG, Yang PC, Kuo SH, Luh KT. Fluid colour sign; A useful indicator for discrimination between pleural thickening and pleural effusion. J Ultrasound Med. 1985;14(10):767-9.
13. Vignon P, Chastagner C, Berkane V, Chardac E, François B, Normand S, et al. Quantitative assessment of pleural effusion in critically ill patients by means of ultrasound. Crit Care Med. 2005;33(8):1757-63.
14. Roch A, Bojan M, Michelet P, Romain F, Bregeon F, Papazian L, Auffray JP, et al. Usefulness of lung ultrasonography in predicting pleural effusion >500 mL in mechanically ventilated patients. Chest. 2005;127(1):224-32.
15. Balik M, Plasil P, Waldauf P, Pazout J, Fric M, Otahal M, et al. Ultrasound estimation of volume of pleural fluid in mechanical ventilated patients. Intensive Care Med. 2006;32(2):318-21.
16. Usta E, Mustafi M, Ziemer G. Ultrasound estimation of the volume of pleural fluid in postoperative cardiac surgery patients. Interact Cardiovasc Thorac Surg. 2010;10(2):204-7.
17. Remérand F, Dellamonica J, Mao Z, Ferrari F, Bouhemad B, Jianxin Y, et al. Ultrasound approach to quantify pleural effusion at the bedside. Intensive Care Med. 2010;36(4):656-4.
18. Brogi E, Gargani L, Bignami E, Barbariol F, Marra A, Forfori F, et al. Thoracic ultrasound for pleural effusion in the intensive care unit: a narrative review from diagnosis to treatment. Crit Care. 2017;21:325.
19. Svigals PZ, Chopra A, Ravenel JG, Nietert PJ, Huggins JT, et al. The accuracy of pleural ultrasonography in diagnosing complicated parapneumonic pleural effusion. Thorax. 2017;72:94-5.
20. Patail H, Patail H, Ahmad S. A man in his 30s presents with shortness of breath and productive cough after recent pneumonia. Chest. 2020;157(3):e91-e93.
21. Chen KY, Liaws YS, Wang HC, Luh KT, Yang PC. Sonographic septations: a useful prognostic indicator of acute thorax empyema. J Ultrasound Med. 2000;19:837-43.
22. Dietrich CF, Mathis G, Cui XW, Ignee A, Hocke M, Hirche TO. Ultrasound of pleura and lungs. Ultrasound Lung Biol. 2015;41:351-65.
23. Kirkpatrick AW, Sirois M, Laupland KB, Liu D, Rowan K, Ball CG, et al. Hand held thoracic ultrasound for detecting post traumatic pneumothorax. The Extended Focused Assessment with Sonography for Trauma (eFAST). J Thanatol. 2004;57(2): 288-95.
24. Rahimi-Movaghar M, Yousefifard M, Ghelichkhani P, Baikpour M, Tafakhori A, Asady H, et al. Application of ultrasound and radiography in detection for hemothorax. A systematic review and meta-analysis. Emergency (Tehran). 2016 summer;4(3): 116-26.
25. Reuses J. Sonography of the pleura. Ultraschall Med. 2010;31: 8-22.
26. Jose Cardenas-Garcia J, Mayo PH, Folch E. Ultrasonographic Evaluation of the Pleura. PLEURA. 2015;2.
27. Qureshi NR, Rahman NM, Gleeson FV. Thoracic ultrasound in diagnosis of malignant pleural effusion. Thorax. 2008;64:139-43.
28. Hassan WA, Alkarn AF, Kamel M. Can chest ultrasound differentiate between benign and malignant effusion. Egypt J Bronchol. 2015;9:165-9.
29. Di Bartolomeo S, Sanson G, Nardi G, Scian F, Michelutto V, Lattuada L. A population-based study of pneumothorax in severely traumatised patients. J Trauma. 2001;51:677-82.
30. Baumann MH, Strange C, Heffner JE, Light R, Kirby TJ, Klein J, et al. Management of spontaneous pneumothorax. An American college of chest physician Delphi consensus statement. Chest. 2001;119:590-602.
31. Enderson BL, Abdalla R, Frame SB, Casey MT, Gould H, Maull KI. Tube thoracotomy for occult pneumothorax. A randomised study for its use. J Trauma. 1993;35:725-30.
32. Ball CG, Ranson K, Dente CJ, Feliciano DV, Laupland KB, Dyer D, et al. Clinical predictor for occult pneumothorax in severely injured blunt poly trauma patients. A prospective observational study. Injury. 2009;40(1):44-7.
33. Lichtenstein DA, Menu Y. A bedside ultrasound sign ruling out pneumothorax in critically ill. Lung sliding. Chest. 1995;108(5):1334-8.
34. Blavais M, Lyon M, Duggal S. A prospective comparison of supine chest radiography and bedside ultrasound for diagnosis of traumatic pneumothorax. Acad Emerg Med. 2005;12(9):844-9.
35. De Luca C, Valentino M, Rimondi MR, Branchini M, Baleni MC, Barozzi L. Use of chest ultrasound in acute care radiology. J Ultrasound. 2008;11(4):125-34.

36. Murphy M, Nagdev A, Sisson C. Lack of lung sliding on ultrasound does not always indicate a pneumothorax. Resuscitation. 2008;77(2):270.
37. Lichtenstein DA, Meziere G, Lascols N, Biderman P, Courret JP, Gepner A, et al. Ultrasound diagnosis of occult pneumothorax. Crit Care Med. 2005;33(6):1231-8.
38. Lichtenstein D, Mezière G, Biderman P, Gepner A. The lung point: A ultrasound sign specific to pneumothorax. Intensive Care Med. 2000;26(10):1434-40.
39. Ball CG, Kirkpatrick AW, Feliciano DV. The occult pneumothorax, what have we learned? Can J Surg. 2009;52:E173-9.
40. Volpicelli G, Lamorte A, Tullio M, Boero E, Stefanone V. Worsening cough and dyspnea following thoracocentesis. Chest. 2013;144(2):e1-e3.
41. Havelock T, Teoh R, Laws D, Gleeson F; BTS Pleural Disease Guideline Group. Pleural procedures and thoracic ultrasound: British Thoracic Society Pleural disease guidelines 2010. Thorax. 2010;65 (Suppl 2):ii61-76.
42. Zanforlin A, Gavelli G, Oboldi D, Galletti S. Ultrasound guided thoracocentesis: the V point as a site for optimal drainage position. Eur Rev Med Pharmacol Sci. 2013;17(1):25-8.
43. Canty EP, Walter JM, Corbridge T, Barsuk JH. Complications of thoracocentesis: incidence, risk factors, and strategies for prevention. Curr Opin Pulmonary Med. 2016;22(4):378-85.
44. Wrightson JM, Fysh E, Maskell NA, Lee YC. Risk reduction in pleural procedures: sonography: simulation and supervision. Curr Opin Pulmonary Med. 2010;16(4):340-50.

CHAPTER

5 Approach to Pleural Effusion

Randeep Guleria, Shubhi Singhal

INTRODUCTION

Pleural effusion is the most common disease among all pleural diseases and affects 1.5 million patients per year in the United States.[1] The accumulation of the pleural fluid may present as a manifestation of over 50 recognized pleuropulmonary and systemic causes. Among 5,625 patients who were subjected to a diagnostic thoracentesis over 25 years in a university hospital in Lleida (Spain), the most common diagnoses were heart failure (HF) (28.7%), cancer (26.3%), pneumonia (15.9%), tuberculosis (TB) (6.3%), postsurgery (4.4%), pericardial diseases (3.6%), and cirrhosis (2.6%).[2] However, these figures may not represent the common causes in the low and middle-income countries and emerging markets. Infections, especially TB are a relatively common cause of pleural effusion in these countries. According to a small study conducted in a tertiary care hospital in West Bengal, India, the most common cause of pleural effusion was TB (64.67%), followed by malignancy (14.67%), parapneumonic effusion (7.33%), cardiac failure (5.33%), and other minor causes.[3]

Therefore, keeping local causes in mind, a systematic approach is required for the analysis of pleural fluid, to narrow down the differentials and guide-specific treatment.

This chapter will provide a broad and individualized approach to patients with pleural effusion.

ETIOLOGY

Pleural effusions may develop due to transudative causes, which result due to rise in hydrostatic pressure, i.e., HF or decrease in oncotic pressure, i.e., hypoproteinemia, with a normal capillary permeability[4] or due to exudative causes, which arise due to increased capillary permeability and lymphatic obstruction.[5]

They can be widely classified as exudative and transudative **(Box 1)** based on the Light's criteria (described further).

BOX 1 Classification of pleural effusion.

- Exudative:
    - Malignancy
    - Parapneumonic effusion and empyema
    - Tuberculosis
    - Pulmonary embolism
    - Rheumatoid arthritis
    - Other connective tissue disorders
    - Benign asbestos effusion
    - Pancreatitis
    - Post myocardial infarction
    - Post coronary artery bypass graft
    - Yellow nail syndrome
    - Drugs (nitrofurantoin, amiodarone, ovarian stimulation therapy, immunotherapy, etc.)
- Transudative:
    - Left ventricular failure
    - Liver cirrhosis
    - Hypoalbuminemia
    - Peritoneal dialysis
    - Hypothyroidism
    - Nephrotic syndrome
    - Mitral stenosis
    - Constrictive pericarditis
    - Urinothorax
    - Meigs syndrome

INITIAL STEPWISE APPROACH IN A PATIENT WITH PLEURAL EFFUSION

History and Examination

This is an important step that helps narrow the differentials to the etiology and gives us a better idea about the further investigations that need to be ordered to arrive at a diagnosis.

Symptoms

Dyspnea is a common and nonspecific symptom. It may be caused due to a plethora of causes in a patient of pleural effusion, such as diaphragmatic dysfunction, reduced chest compliance, and passive lung collapse.

Cough, another nonspecific symptom is also common with the pleural involvement. Cough is usually dry and irritating; however, in case of a productive cough, an alternate infective etiology or parenchymal involvement should be ruled out.

Chest pain is usually pleuritic in nature and is attributed to the presence of pain receptors in the parietal pleura, which get irritated due to pleural inflammation, mostly in exudative pleural effusions. It is described as a sharp, stabbing pain, usually localized to the inflamed part of pleura that gets aggravated on deep inspiration, coughing, yawning, sneezing, etc., due to friction in the inflamed pleural surfaces as depicted in **Figures 1A to C**. This pain usually gets resolved or becomes dull aching as the effusion increases, as the apposition between the pleura and hence the friction reduces.

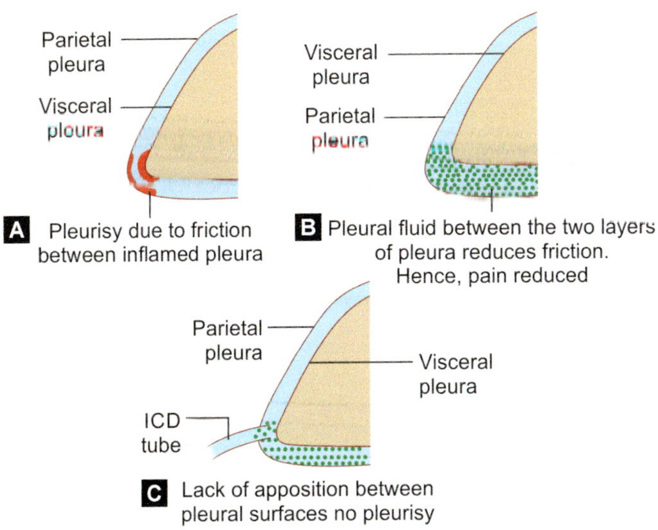

FIGS. 1A TO C: Figure eliciting nature of change of pleuritic chest pain in case of pleural effusion.

Fever, weight loss, and loss of appetite may also occur, and are usually associated with tuberculous pleurisy, infections, or malignancy. Presence of hemoptysis would suggest an associated underlying parenchymal or airway pathology.

Skin, joint, and eye symptoms may be associated with a connective tissue disorder, which are known to cause pleural effusions.

Comorbidities

Comorbidities such as HF, renal disorders, and liver disease may lead us to a transudative cause of effusion secondary to the fluid overload and should be looked upon for.

History of a connective tissue disorder, hypothyroidism, pancreatitis, lymphangioleiomyomatosis, and immunoglobulin G4 (IgG4) disease should always be ruled out if the initial diagnosis is not made, as these may give rise to pleural effusions.

Occupational History

A detailed history should be elicited to rule out history of exposures such as that of asbestos even if it is years prior to the presentation (for associated mesothelioma or benign effusions).

Drug History

A thorough history of drug intake such as nitrofurantoin, amiodarone, immunotherapy, phenytoin, and methotrexate is important and should not be missed.

Miscellaneous

History of recent coronary artery bypass grafting (CABG), central line placement, biliary intervention, cerebrospinal fluid (CSF) shunt placement, peritoneal dialysis, and trauma should always be ruled out if the diagnosis is unclear, before approaching to the next step.

Examination may indicate systemic features of connective tissue disorders or malignancy. A large effusion without mediastinal shift may indicate an endobronchial mass, mesothelioma, or associated pleural fibrosis.

Thoracic Imaging

Chest Radiograph

The posteroanterior (PA) chest radiographs become abnormal when ≥200 mL pleural fluid is present. However, accumulation of as less as 50 mL fluid can produce a costophrenic angle blunting on lateral chest radiographs.[6] Chest X-ray (CXR) in PA view can appear normal with up to 500 mL.[6] Most radiographs in intensive care unit (ICU) settings are in anteroposterior, supine view, which cause accumulation of pleural fluid in the dependent chest and can therefore cause one to underestimate an effusion or even miss it as it causes a uniform haze.

Bedside Ultrasound

Thoracic ultrasonography has now become a routine investigation in evaluation of pleural effusions. It not only tells us about the size of the effusion, but also provides information on presence of septations and loculations with a better sensitivity than a chest computed tomography(CT) scanning.[7] Ultrasound-guided thoracocentesis also reduces the incidence of iatrogenic pneumothorax and other complications. It also helps in diagnosing pleural thickening, especially when used in conjunction with color Doppler.[8-11] Ultrasound can detect pleural masses and can also at times help differentiate malignant from benign effusions.

Computed Tomography of Chest

Although, this is not a necessary investigation in all cases of pleural effusion, it might be useful in certain cases such as where etiology is not obvious, loculated effusions, when a mass is suspected or a detailed visualization of lung parenchyma, mediastinum, and when pleura is required. Contrast scans may reveal irregular or nodular pleura which is suggestive of a malignancy and it also helps in guiding for an appropriate site for sampling through needle aspiration or biopsies. CTs may sometimes direct us toward pulmonary and extrapulmonary clues that may lead us to the diagnoses, such as lung mass, mediastinal lymphadenopathy, cysts, consolidation, fractured ribs, and esophageal mass.

Pleural Fluid Aspiration

Indications

All patients with newly detected, radiologically confirmed pleural effusions of unclear etiology should undergo diagnostic thoracocentesis. Aspiration should not be performed for bilateral pleural effusions in a clinical setting strongly suggestive of a transudate unless there are atypical features[12] such as significant disparity in the size of the effusions, fever, pleurisy, septations and loculations, and disproportionate hypoxemia, which warrant diagnostic sampling.

Contraindications

- Insufficient pleural fluid (<1 cm fluid depth, adjacent to the parietal pleura)
- Coagulopathies
- Skin infection at the needle insertion sites

Once the indications of pleural aspiration have been ensured and the contraindications ruled out, thoracocentesis must be performed in all cases of radiologically confirmed pleural effusion (except for in cases where a transudative cause is obvious).

It is recommended to use a 21 G, 50 mL needle for diagnostic aspiration. In case a parapneumonic effusion is suspected and pH needs to be measured, fluid should be directly drawn into a heparinized blood gas syringe and processed. Rest of the sample should be divided into separate containers for microbiology (5 mL), biochemistry (2–5 mL) and cytology (remaining sample, at least 20–40 mL). Sample should also be sent for other investigations depending upon clinical suspicion such as adenosine deaminase (ADA), triglycerides, and amylase. In case of suspicion of infection, fluid should additionally be inoculated in blood culture bottles to increase diagnostic yield, especially for anaerobic organisms.[13]

Once the fluid is aspirated, a step-by-step algorithm helps to narrow down the differentials and have a more focused approach toward a patient.

Appearance and Odor (Table 1)

Fluid may appear straw-colored, serous, bloody, frank blood, turbid or frankly purulent. Centrifugation of turbid fluid helps differentiate empyema from chylothorax and pseudochylothorax. In the case of a clear supernatant, empyema is likely, whereas in a supernatant that remains turbid, a chylous or pseudochylous effusion is more likely. Hemorrhagic pleural effusions, maybe due to traumatic aspiration, pulmonary embolism with infarction, postcardiac injury syndrome, or benign asbestosis. A grossly bloody aspirate may suggest the presence of a hemothorax, which is confirmed by a pleural fluid hematocrit > 50% of serum hematocrit. Rarely, food particles in the fluid may be due to an esophageal rupture, bile-stained fluid may be seen in biliary fistula and an anchovy sauce-like fluid may be noted in a ruptured amoebic liver abscess.

Putrid odor in turbid fluids may indicate anaerobic infection or empyemas. In rare circumstances, an ammonical odor may be suggestive of urinothorax.

TABLE 1: Appearance of fluid and its possible diagnosis.

Appearance of fluid	Possible diagnosis
Turbid	Empyema, chylothorax, pseudochylothorax
Hemorrhagic	Traumatic aspiration, pulmonary embolism, post-cardiac injury, benign asbestosis
Milky	Chylothorax and pseudochylothorax
Food particles	Esophageal rupture
Bilious	Biliary fistula
Anchovy brown	Ruptured amoebic liver abscess

Differentiating Exudative and Transudative Effusions

Light's criteria should be used to differentiate between exudative and transudative effusions:

- Pleural fluid protein/serum protein > 0.5
- Pleural fluid lactate dehydrogenase (LDH)/serum LDH > 0.6
- Pleural fluid LDH more than two-thirds of the upper limit of normal serum LDH

Pleural fluid is classified as exudate if one or more of the aforementioned criteria are met.

However, due to the compulsory requirement of simultaneous blood samples and the pleural fluid LDH being included in 2 out of 3 criteria, its diagnostic accuracy is reduced and it is, therefore, often criticized.[14-16] Light's criteria have a high sensitivity but a moderate specificity for exudative pleural effusions; therefore, 25–30% of transudates are misclassified as exudates, especially the ones due to HF patients on diuretics as they increase the concentration of protein, LDH, and lipids in the effusion. For such patients, the following single-test criteria may be applied to reclassify the effusion as transudative:[17,18]

- Serum-to-pleural fluid albumin gradient > 1.2 g/dL
- Serum-to-pleural fluid protein gradient > 2.5 g/dL

Pleural fluid levels of N-terminal pro-B-type natriuretic peptide (NT-proBNP) > 1,500 pg/mL corroborate well with transudative effusions due to HF. However, routine measurements are not of much utility due to a good correlation with the serum values so it is almost equally as effective.[19-21]

pH

Normal pH of pleural fluid is approximately 7.60 with the transudates having a usual normal range of 7.40–7.55 and exudates having a normal range of around 7.30–7.45.

pH may get reduced due to excessive lactic acid and carbon dioxide production as a result of an increase in local metabolism in conditions with high cellular load such as infections (bacteria) and pleural malignancies (tumor cells) and due to a fall in hydrogen ion reflux across abnormal pleural membranes.

The main utility of pH is in differentiating simple from complicated parapneumonic effusion or empyema, as complicated effusions indicate a high likelihood for intercostal drainage. pH levels of <7.2 usually indicate a complicated parapneumonic effusion and, hence warrant drainage. Pleural fluid should be drawn directly from the pleural space and pH should be measured within 1 hour. Air, lidocaine, or excessive heparin may alter the measured pH.

Glucose

In most cases, pleural fluid glucose level is similar to blood glucose. A low pleural fluid glucose (<60 mg/dL) may result due to impaired diffusion across diseased pleura or increased utilization and may be found in cases of complicated parapneumonic effusions or empyema, rheumatoid arthritis, esophageal rupture, malignancy, urinothorax, and tubercular pleural effusions.[22] It usually falls with the pH but is a less accurate indicator of a need for intercostal drainage than pH.[23]

Cell Count (Table 2)

In normal circumstances, the pleural fluid white cell count is <2,000/µL, with macrophage predominance (75%), followed by lymphocytes (23%) and 2% constituted by the rest of the cells (mesothelial, neutrophils, and eosinophils).

Differential cell counts serve as an important test to narrow the differential diagnosis. A polymorphonuclear predominance is noted in acute processes such as parapneumonic effusion or empyema, early tubercular pleurisy most commonly, followed by relatively uncommon causes, such as acute pancreatitis, lupus pleuritis, and pulmonary thromboembolism. A lymphocyte predominance (>50% lymphocytes) is most commonly noted in malignancies and TB. Other less common causes include sarcoidosis, chronic rheumatoid pleuritis, chylothorax, yellow nail syndrome, and drug-induced effusions. Eosinophilic predominant (>10%) effusions are mostly seen in the presence of air or blood in pleural space. It may also be seen in case of malignancies, EGPA, pulmonary infarction, parasitic infections, and benign asbestos effusion.

TABLE 2: Differential count predominance and its possible diagnosis.

Differential count predominance	Possible diagnosis
Polymorphonuclear cells	Parapneumonic effusions, empyema, early tubercular effusions, acute pancreatitis, lupus pleuritis, and pulmonary embolism
Lymphocytes	Malignancies, tuberculosis, sarcoidosis, chronic rheumatoid pleuritis, chylothorax, and drug-induced
Eosinophils	Pneumothorax, hemothorax, malignancies, eosinophilic granulomatosis with polyangiitis (EGPA), parasitic infections, and benign asbestos effusions

Mesothelial cells are normally found in small numbers in pleural fluid. *If mesothelial cells are >50%, TB is usually unlikely and other causes should be ruled out.*[24]

Lactate Dehydrogenase

Pleural fluid LDH forms two of the three Light's criteria and is a marker of pleural inflammation. Very high LDH levels (>1,000 IU/L) may be seen in case of empyema, rheumatoid pleurisy paragonimiasis, and malignancy.[25-28]

Lactate dehydrogenase levels are usually raised in the case of TB also; however, it is much lower compared to that in empyemas.

Protein

Pleural fluid protein levels are measured in order to categorize it as either exudative or transudative as per Light's criteria. It is also used as part of a few newly defined calculators for pleural fluid classification. Pleural fluid protein > 3.0 g/dL favors an exudative effusion in most cases.[15,29]

Cytology

This is a quick and minimally invasive test to diagnose malignancies. More than one sample should be sent and analyzed as early as possible so as to increase the yield. Studies have found a yield of 65, 27, and 5% respectively from the first, second, and third samples.[30] Sensitivity also depends on the type of malignancy, with ovarian cancer having the highest sensitivity of up to 85%, followed by adenocarcinoma (78–83%), breast cancer (65%), small cell (53%), mesothelioma (29%), and squamous cell (25%).[31] A higher volume of sample (at least 75 mL) is recommended for cytological examination for a better yield and a possible molecular profiling.[32]

Specific Tests

These are the tests that may be done for patients with specific clinical suspicion, to reach a definitive diagnosis.

Adenosine Deaminase

The diagnosis of TB is mostly established based on a lymphocyte-predominant exudative effusion with ADA > 40 U/L. ADA may also be raised in case of empyema, rheumatoid pleuritic, and malignancies. In view of the higher incidence of TB in India, this should be sent as a routine investigation in India and other TB endemic areas. Interferon-γ levels are found to be equally diagnostic but ADA is preferred due to cost effectiveness.

Amylase

It may be useful in suspected cases of esophageal rupture, pancreatic disease-associated pleural effusions, and malignancies. Isoenzyme analysis may be used for further differentiation.

Triglyceride and Cholesterol Levels

These may be ordered when suspecting chylothorax or pseudochylothorax.

Others

Tumor markers in suspected malignancies, creatinine levels in cases of suspected urinothorax, β-2-transferrin in suspected ventriculoperitoneal (VP) shunt-related effusions, bilirubin levels in suspected bilothorax, etc.

This is not an exhaustive list and a detailed discussion on such ancillary investigations is done in subsequent chapters.

Additional Evaluation in Case of Inconclusive Reports

In certain cases, despite revisiting the history, examination, and pleural fluid analysis, a definite conclusion cannot be made and further evaluation may be required.

- *Repeat pleural fluid analysis*—such as a second cytology sample, in cases where previous reports do not correlate with the clinical picture
- *Additional biomarkers*—when initial reports raise a suspicion, additional investigations such as ADA, amylase, triglycerides, cholesterol, etc., should be sent
- *Additional imaging*: CT pulmonary angiography in case of suspected pulmonary thromboembolism, not only aids in the diagnosis of thromboembolism but also gives an idea about any pulmonary infiltrates, masses, or mediastinal lymphadenopathy. Magnetic resonance imaging (MRI) may be done to distinguish benign from malignant effusions by different signal intensities on T2-weighed images. Positron emission tomography (PET)/CT may be done to look at the uptake or to guide an appropriate biopsy site in case of suspected malignancy.
- *Pleural biopsy*: This may be closed, image-guided, thoracoscopy-guided, or video-assisted thoracoscopic surgery (VATS) guided. A closed pleural biopsy, usually done by Abram's needle is useful in case of diseases causing diffuse pleural involvement, such as tuberculous or rheumatoid pleuritis. With the advent of thoracoscopy, closed pleural biopsy is less often done nowadays. The yield is likely to be lower in case of patchy pleural involvement, such as in malignancies. An image-guided pleural biopsy is preferred in cases with pleural involvement, such as pleural masses, nodules, and thickening.

  Thoracoscopic pleural biopsy is preferred when a closed biopsy is inconclusive and no obvious mass or pleural abnormality can be found. It has an added advantage of direct visualization of pleura, a more targeted sampling, and an option of doing pleurodesis in the same sitting whenever desired. The diagnostic yield for malignancy is 80–95% and in one study, 66% of the patients who had a negative blind biopsy result got diagnosed on thoracoscopy.[33]

- *Bronchoscopy*: It is not indicated unless an endobronchial process (such as hemoptysis and bronchial obstruction) is suspected clinically or on CT.

APPROACH TO A PATIENT WITH PLEURAL EFFUSION (FLOWCHART 1)

Below is a flowchart, depicting a systematic approach to a patient with pleural effusion.

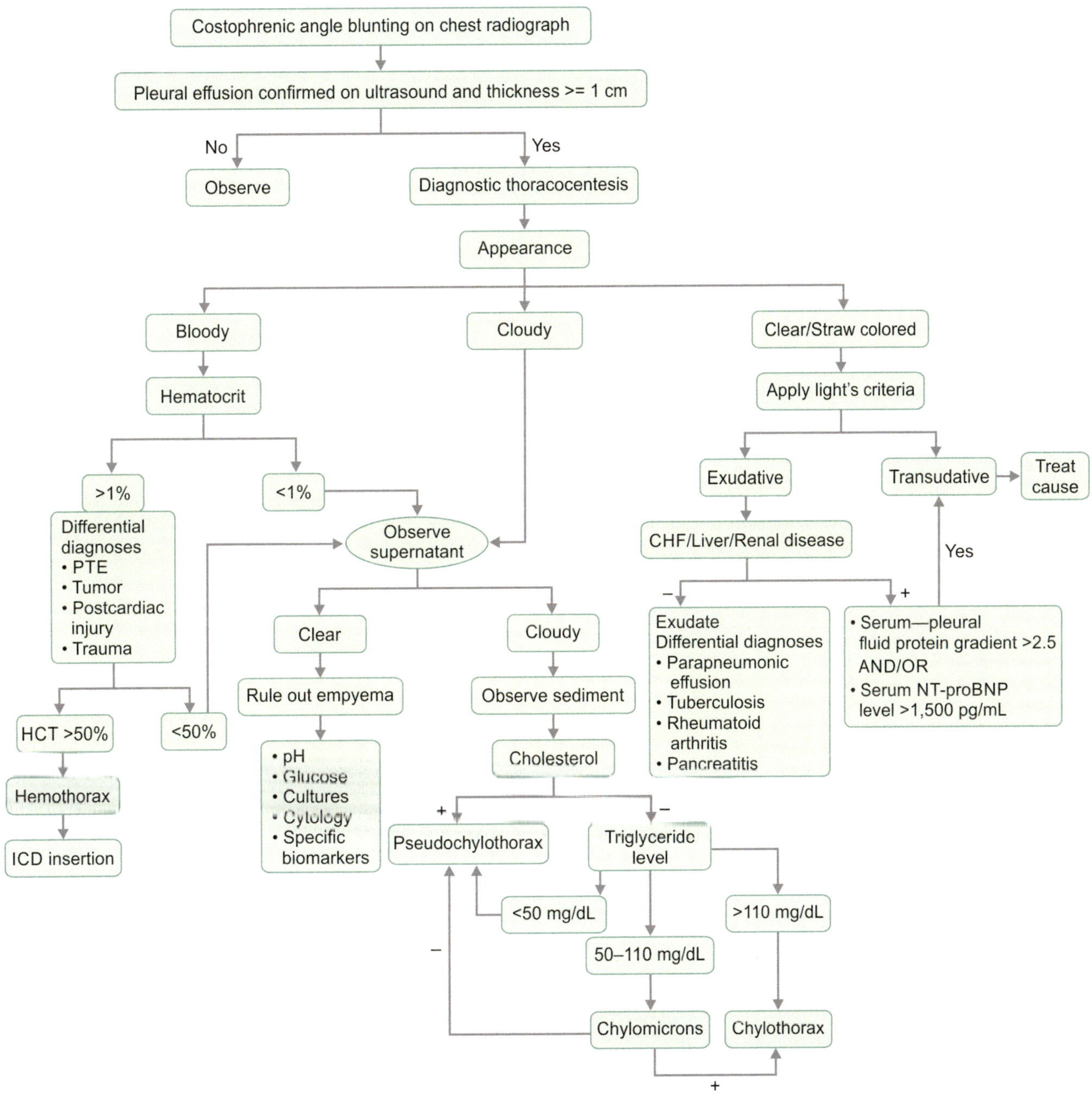

FLOWCHART 1: Approach to a patient with pleural effusion.

(CHF: congestive heart failure; HCT: hematocrit; ICD: intercostal drainage tube; PTE: pulmonary thromboembolism)

KEY POINTS

- Pleural effusion is the most common disease among all pleural diseases.
- Pleural effusions maybe classified as transudative and exudative based on Light's criteria.
- Transudative effusions are caused due to increased hydrostatic pressures or reduced oncotic pressures with normal capillary permeability.
- Exudative effusions are caused due to increased capillary permeability and lymphatic obstruction.
- A thorough stepwise approach is necessary to evaluate all the cases of pleural effusion in order to make a correct diagnosis and treat accordingly.
- Evaluation includes a detailed history, examination, thoracic imaging, and a comprehensive pleural fluid analysis.
- Pleural fluid should be routinely analyzed for appearance, odor, glucose, protein, cell counts, LDH, and cytology.
- Based on the clinical suspicion, additional pleural fluid investigations may be sent accordingly.
- Additional investigations such as computed tomography pulmonary angiogram (CTPA), PET/CT, and pleural biopsy may be required in certain undiagnosed pleural effusions.

REFERENCES

1. Kugasia IAR, Kumar A, Khatri A, Saeed F, Islam H, Epelbaum O. Primary effusion lymphoma of the pleural space: Report of a rare complication of cardiac transplant with review of the literature. Transpl Infect Dis. 2019;21(1):e13005.
2. Porcel JM, Light RW. Diagnostic approach to pleural effusion in adults. Am Fam Physician. 2006;73(7):1211-20.
3. Bar PK, Mandal S, Banik T, Barman R, Mandal A. A clinicopathological study of pleural effusion with special reference to malignant aetiology in a tertiary care hospital in West Bengal. Transudative pleural effusions. 2019;7(4):266-72.
4. Chetty KG. Transudative pleural effusions. Clin Chest Med. 1985;6(1):49-54.
5. Light RW. Diagnostic principles in pleural disease. Eur Respir J. 1997;10(2):476-81.
6. Blackmore CC, Black WC, Dallas RV, Crow HC. Pleural fluid volume estimation: a chest radiograph prediction rule. Acad Radiol. 1996;3(2):103-9.
7. Kearney SE, Davies CWH, Davies RJO. Computed tomography and ultrasound in parapneumonic effusions and empyema. Clin Radiol 2000;55(7):542e7.
8. Lipscomb DJ, Flower CDR, Hadfield JW. Ultrasound of the pleura: an assessment of its clinical value. Clin Radiol. 1981;32(3):289e90.
9. Wu RG, Yuan A, Liaw YS, Chang DB, Yu CJ, Wu HD, et al. Image comparison of real-time gray-scale ultrasound and color Doppler ultrasound for use in diagnosis of minimal pleural effusion. Am J Respir Crit Care Med. 1994;150(2):510-4.
10. Roch A, Bojan M, Michelet P, Romain F, Bregeon F, Papazian L, et al. Usefulness of ultrasonography in predicting pleural effusions > 500 ml in patients receiving mechanical ventilation. Chest. 2005;127(1):224-32.
11. Eibenberger KL, Dock WI, Ammann ME, Dorffner R, Hörmann MF, Grabenwöger F. Quantification of pleural effusions: sonography versus radiography. Radiology. 1994;191(3):681e4.
12. Hooper C, Lee YG, Maskell N; BTS Pleural Guideline Group. Investigation of a unilateral pleural effusion in adults: British Thoracic Society pleural disease guideline 2010. Thorax. 2010;65(Suppl 2):ii4-17.
13. Ferrer A, Osset J, Alegre J, Suriñach JM, Crespo E, Fernández de Sevilla T, et al. Prospective clinical and microbiological study of pleural effusions. Eur J Clin Microbiol Infect Dis. 1999;18(4):237-41.
14. Heffner JE, Brown LK, Barbieri CA. Diagnostic value of tests that discriminate between exudative and transudative pleural effusions. Primary Study Investigators. Chest. 1997;111(4):970-80.
15. Porcel JM, Peña JM, Vicente de Vera C, Esquerda A, Vives M, Light RW. Bayesian analysis using continuous likelihood ratios for identifying pleural exudates. Respir Med. 2006;100(11):1960-5.
16. Babyak MA. What you see may not be what you get: a brief, nontechnical introduction to overfitting in regression-type models. Psychosom Med. 2004;66(3):411-21.
17. Porcel JM, Ferreiro L, Civit C, Valdés L, Esquerda A, Light RW, et al. Development and validation of a scoring system for the identification of pleural exudates of cardiac origin. Eur J Intern Med. 2018;50:60.
18. Porcel JM. Identifying transudates misclassified by Light's criteria. Curr Opin Pulm Med. 2013;19(4):362-7.
19. Porcel JM. Utilization of B-type natriuretic peptide and NT-proBNP in the diagnosis of pleural effusions due to heart failure. Curr Opin Pulm Med. 2011;17(4):215-9.
20. Han ZJ, Wu XD, Cheng JJ, Zhao SD, Gao MZ, Huang HY, et al. Diagnostic Accuracy of Natriuretic Peptides for Heart Failure in Patients with Pleural Effusion: A Systematic Review and Updated Meta-Analysis. PLoS One. 2015;10(8):e0134376.
21. Han CH, Choi JE, Chung JH. Clinical utility of pleural fluid NT-pro brain natriuretic peptide (NT-proBNP) in patients with pleural effusions. Intern Med. 2008;47(19):1669-74.
22. Light RW, Ball WC. Glucose and amylase in pleural effusions. JAMA. 1973;225(3):257-60.
23. Heffner JE, Brown LK, Barbieri C, DeLeo JM. Pleural fluid chemical analysis in parapneumonic effusions. A meta-analysis. Am J Respir Crit Care Med. 1995;151(6):1700e8.
24. Lo Cascio CM, Kaul V, Dhooria S, Agrawal A, Chaddha U. Diagnosis of tuberculous pleural effusions: A review. Respir Med. 2021;188:106607.
25. Light RW, Girard WM, Jenkinson SG, George RB. Parapneumonic effusions. Am J Med. 1980;69(4):507-12.

26. Arnold DT, Hamilton FW, Elvers KT, Frankland SW, Zahan-Evans N, Patole S, et al. Pleural Fluid suPAR Levels Predict the Need for Invasive Management in Parapneumonic Effusions. Am J Respir Crit Care Med. 2020;201(12):1545-53.
27. Balbir-Gurman A, Yigla M, Nahir AM, Braun-Moscovici Y. Rheumatoid pleural effusion. Semin Arthritis Rheum. 2006;35(6):368-78.
28. Ahn CS, Shin JW, Kim JG, Lee WY, Kang I, Im JG, et al. Spectrum of pleuropulmonary paragonimiasis: An analysis of 685 cases diagnosed over 22 years. J Infect. 2021;82(1):150-8.
29. Porcel JM, Light RW. Pleural Fluid Analysis: Are Light's Criteria Still Relevant After Half a Century? Clin Chest Med. 2021;42(4):599-609.
30. Garcia L, Ducatman BS, Wang HH. The value of multiple fluid specimens in the cytological diagnosis of malignancy. Mod Pathol. 1994;7(6):665-8.
31. Kassirian S, Hinton SN, Cuninghame S, Chaudhary R, Iansavitchene A, Amjadi K, et al. Diagnostic sensitivity of pleural fluid cytology in malignant pleural effusions: systematic review and meta-analysis. Thorax. 2023;78(1):32-40.
32. Xu Y, Hu AY, Wang SM, Wang Q, Pan YC, Zhang SH. A retrospective analysis of pleural effusion specimens based on the newly proposed International System for Reporting Serous Fluid Cytopathology. Diagn Cytopathol. 2021;49(9):997-1007.
33. Harris RJ, Kavuru MS, Rice TW, Kirby TJ. The diagnostic and therapeutic utility of thoracoscopy. A review. Chest. 1995;108:828-41.

CHAPTER

6 Transudative Pleural Effusion

Sandeep Tilve, Sumit K Pahariya

INTRODUCTION

Once the basic analysis of the pleural fluid is done, we classify them into two broad groups, namely exudative pleural effusions and transudative pleural effusions. The diagnostic and prognostic implications of transudative effusions differ completely from exudative ones. Unlike exudative pleural effusion, which is characterized by an inflammatory response and increased permeability of the pleura, transudative effusion is typically caused by imbalances in hydrostatic or oncotic pressures. This imbalance leads to the accumulation of a clear, protein-poor fluid in the pleural cavity.

PATHOPHYSIOLOGY (FIGS. 1A TO C)[1]

An imbalance in pleural fluid dynamics either increased hydrostatic pressure or reduced oncotic pressure or both leads to accumulation of fluid in the pleural cavity. If the rate of fluid drainage is less than the rate of fluid accumulation, the pleural fluid level increases in the pleural cavity leading to pleural effusion. Increased interstitial fluid can also cause pleural fluid accumulation. This happens more or less in all the etiologies of transudative pleural effusion.

CAUSES OF TRANSUDATIVE PLEURAL EFFUSION

Congestive Cardiac Failure

Congestive cardiac failure (CCF) is the most common cause of pleural effusion. About 45–50% of all pleural effusions are because of CCF. CCF is also the most common cause of transudative pleural effusion. Around 80% of transudative effusions are due to CCF.[2] Patients of decompensated heart failure (HF) who need diuretic therapy during their admission, around 87% of them show pleural effusion radiologically.[3] Pleural effusion in CCF is due to increased interstitial fluid in the lung due to elevated pulmonary capillary pressure. Rarely, pleural effusions may occur in association with isolated right heart failure. CCF-associated effusions are typically bilateral, but if unilateral, they are more commonly seen on the right side; however, unilateral pleural effusion does not exclude CCF. In a review of six series, 783 patients with pleural effusion because of CCF, among them 125 (16%) patients had right-sided pleural effusion, and 55 (7%) patients had left-sided pleural effusion.[4]

Diagnosis

The diagnosis of CCF-related pleural effusion is usually made by history, symptoms, physical examination, and radiological investigation. Thoracocentesis is not routinely advised in every patient to make a diagnosis.[5] Clinically, patients of CCF with pleural effusion presented with classic signs and symptoms of CCF. The patient usually complains of increasing shortness of breath (especially on exertion), pedal edema, and orthopnea or paroxysmal nocturnal dyspnea. Rarely, do patients come with complaints of chest pain.

On physical examination, signs of cardiac failure such as jugular venous pulse, bilateral pitting pedal edema, abdominal distention, ascites, and hepatojugular reflux are present, along with rattle and left-sided S3 gallop. In respiratory system examination, decreased tactile vocal fremitus was noted during palpation, dull node

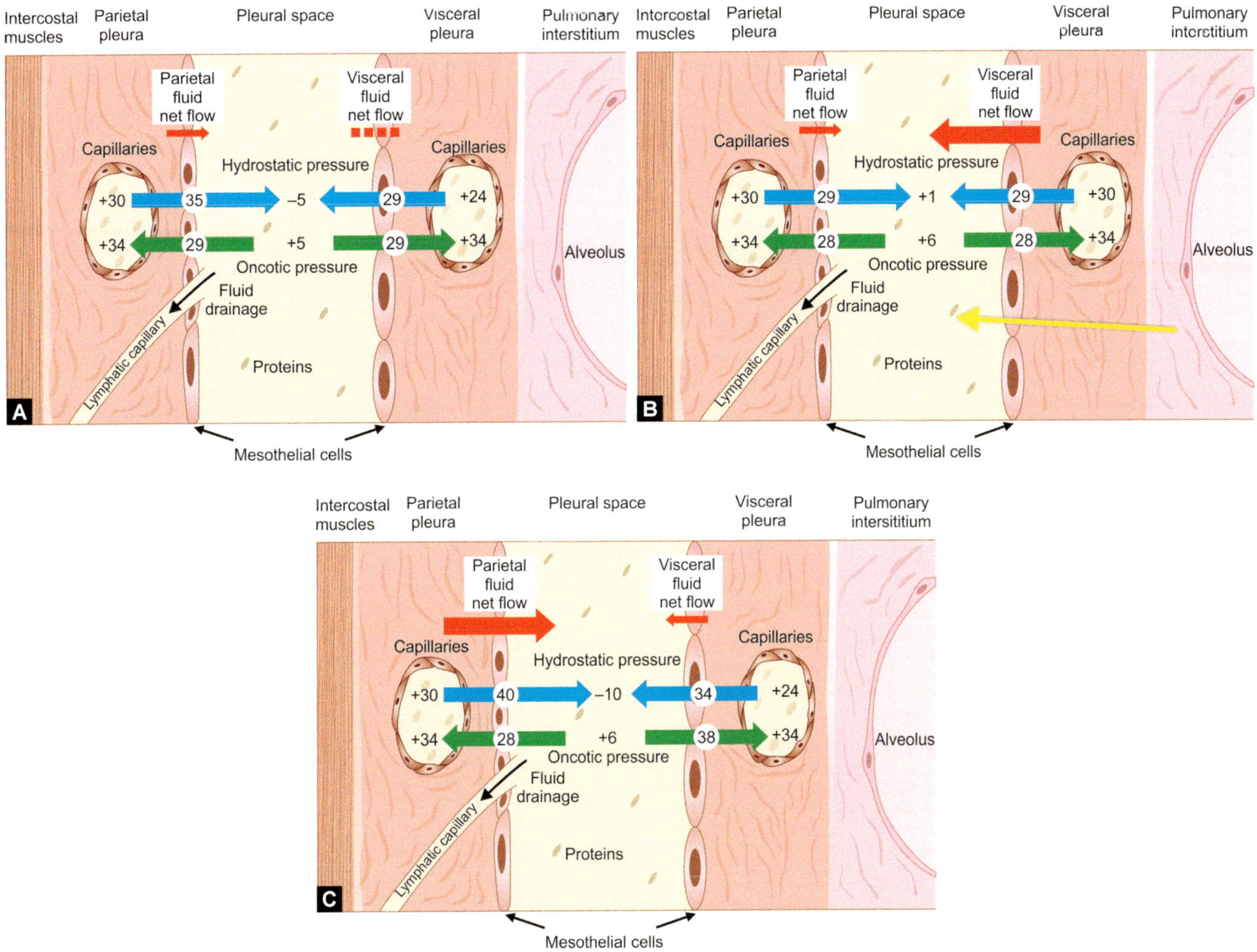

FIGS. 1A TO C: Schematic representation of the movement of fluid: (A) In the pleural space in normal conditions; (B) In heart failure; and (C) In trapped lung. (A) In normal lung and pleura, the balance of hydrostatic and oncotic pressures promotes the formation of pleural fluid. Pressure gradients show a net flow of fluid from the parietal pleura and that balance is maintained in the visceral pleura (pressures in cmH_2O); (B) In heart failure, fluid in the pulmonary interstitium increases due to increased pulmonary capillary pressures. A fluid that enters the pleural space exceeds the drainage capacity of the pleural lymphatic capillaries; and (C) In the trapped lung, a previous inflammatory process has produced a thick, fibrous visceral pleura. The inability of the lung to expand leads to a negative hydrostatic pleural pressure and this alteration of Starling's forces lead to the formation of a pleural transudate. Pleural effusion may be verging on exudate, depending on how recent the active inflammation was.

on percussion, and decreased breath sound elicited on auscultation. All these findings confirm the presence of pleural effusion.[6] In cases where clinical findings are not conclusive, thoracentesis and analysis of fluid is mandatory.

Pleural Fluid Analysis

The fluid typically meets the biochemical characteristics of a transudate by Light's criteria.[7] However the ability of Light's criteria to exclude transudative pleural effusion is low.[8] Due to this fallacy, pleural effusions associated with heart failure can be misclassified as exudates, especially when patients are on diuretic therapy. One study showed that 28% (5 of 18) patients with pleural effusions due to congestive heart failure (CHF) were misclassified as exudative effusions when Light's criteria were applied. In these cases, serum-pleural fluid albumin or total protein gradient can be used to distinguish a transudative effusion from an exudative effusion. Gradient (or gap) > 1.2 g/dL indicates that the pleural effusion is transudative in nature, regardless of whether it meets Light's criteria or not.[9]

The level of N terminal-pro-brain natriuretic peptide (NT-pro-BNP) in pleural fluid can also be used to make the diagnosis of pleural effusions due to cardiac origin. If the pretest probability of pleural effusion due to heart failure is high and alternative diagnoses are less likely, then an invasive procedure thoracentesis can be avoided and an elevated serum NT-pro-BNP level will be diagnostic for pleural effusion due to CCF. If the pretest probability is low or alternative diagnoses are considered in addition to heart failure, then a thoracentesis should be performed. If the NT-pro-BNP levels in pleural fluid are high then this would be more diagnostic of heart failure as one potential cause for the pleural effusion. Furthermore, if the pretest probability is equivocal for CCF and lights criteria also misclassify transudative CCF effusion as exudate, a high pleural fluid NT-pro-BNP level would also be diagnostic. In a recent meta-analysis, the diagnostic yield of NT-pro-BNP in CCF-induced pleural fluid showed a sensitivity of 94%, specificity of 91%.[10] A meta-analysis was done by Zhou et al.[11] which included 8 studies, found out that level of NT-pro-BNP in the pleural fluid has high diagnostic accuracy and, on that basis, the cardiac and noncardiac origin of pleural effusion can be differentiated.[12]

Management

The main aim in the management of transudative pleural effusion is to treat the underlying cause. So, treatment of pleural effusion due to CCF consists of diuretics, *Digitalis*, and/or afterload reduction (decongestive management and removal of excess amount of fluid from the body by diuresis). Generally, most of the patients have improved after optimization of cardiac failure treatment (medical or surgical).[13] Medical management of CCF includes the use of diuretics, angiotensin-converting enzyme (ACE) inhibitors, and β-blockers, sometimes the patient needs a pacemaker insertion or surgical correction of cardiac valvular abnormalities. Sometimes, massive effusions may produce severe dyspnea or respiratory distress, in such cases therapeutic thoracocentesis should be performed, in which around 500–1,500 mL fluid is removed from the pleural cavity, providing symptomatic relief to the patients.

A prospective study of 60 patients with pleural effusion secondary to CCF showed that in 89% of cases pleural effusion resolved after 2 weeks of treatment with diuretics.[3]

Occasionally, clinician encounters a patient with massive effusions and refractory heart failure. Initially, therapeutic pleural tapping improves the symptoms but the effusion cannot be controlled with medical therapy, chemical pleurodesis with doxycycline, tetracycline, betadine, or talc should be considered in this situation. Some theory suggests that chemical pleurodesis interferes with fluid movement from the alveoli to the pleural cavity and might increase the severity of alveolar edema, but fortunately, there is no clinical evidence in support of these theories. Unilateral pleurodesis sometimes causes an increased fluid accumulation in the opposite pleural cavity.[14]

Hepatic Hydrothorax

It is a clinical entity that refers to the presence of pleural effusion in a liver cirrhosis patient and also patients do not have any other reason for pleural effusion (cardiac, lung, or pleural disease). Prevalence of this condition varies from 5 to 10%.[15] Pleural effusions due to liver disease are usually unilateral and commonly seen on the right side, but it is not always true as it can be seen on the left side only (16%), or can be present as a bilateral accumulation of fluid (16%).[15] Respiratory symptoms depend upon the size of the effusion, in small effusion, patients may be asymptomatic while dyspnea and chest pain are suggestive of submassive or massive effusion. In chronic liver disease patients, low serum albumin level is frequently present, which leads to decreased plasma oncotic pressure, which is responsible for excess pleural fluid formation. Initially, fluid get accumulated in peritoneal cavity from there it goes in pleural cavity, so ascites is present in almost every patient who presented with pleural effusion. Even in the presence of mild ascites, which do not show clinical symptoms, effusion can be detected with the help of ultrasonography.[6,16] There are two mechanisms that are responsible for the movement of ascitic fluid into the pleural cavity. First, the presence of diaphragmatic pores, and second is presence of intraperitoneal and intrapleural pressure gradient. During inspiration, intrathoracic pressure becomes negative which further facilitates movement of fluid from abdominal space to pleural cavity.

An experiment conducted by Lieberman et al.,[17] in which they introduced labeled albumin into the peritoneal cavity, later they found out that the concentration of the labeled protein in the pleural fluid was higher in comparison to plasma or thoracic duct lymph. It confirms that fluid in the pleural cavity came from the peritoneal cavity. However, when tracers are injected into the pleural cavity, they are not detected in the ascitic fluid, indicating unidirectional flow.[18]

Ongoing studies also suggested that excess pleural fluid in these patients came from the peritoneal cavity. As discussed earlier there are some diaphragmatic defects that are present, fluid passes from these pores and is responsible for effusion. Due to ascites and increased intra-abdominal pressure, the diaphragmatic muscles get stretched and microscopic defects are formed. Another reason is the pressure gradient difference; hydrostatic pressure is higher in the peritoneal cavity in comparison to the pleural cavity, due to the accumulation of fluid in the peritoneal cavity first. This is responsible for the unidirectional flow of fluids. Hepatic hydrothorax is more commonly seen on the right side because diaphragm developmental defects are more common on that side and the left hemidiaphragm is more muscular and thicker.[19]

Diagnosis

Patients may be asymptomatic in whom pleural effusion is an incidental finding on chest imaging performed for other reasons or they may have pulmonary symptoms of shortness of breath, cough, hypoxemia, or respiratory failure associated with large pleural effusions. Around 15% of the patients of hepatic hydrothorax may be present as a case of spontaneous bacterial empyema. It should be suspected if patients develop fever, encephalopathy, or declining renal function. Large volumes of ascites are generally well tolerated by patients due to high compliance of the peritoneal cavity, but pleural fluid accumulation can cause significant symptoms as mentioned earlier.

Fluid Analysis

The diagnosis of hepatic hydrothorax can be made easily. Both ascitic fluid and pleural fluid tapping should be performed to discover that biochemical feature of both fluids (ascitic and pleural) are accordant to diagnosis and does not show any feature of exudative effusion. Further analysis of pleural fluid should be done to exclude out other diseases (heart, lung, or pleural) which cause effusion. In around 15% of the patients with cirrhosis and pleural effusion develop spontaneous bacterial empyema, which can also be detected with the help of thoracocentesis.

In one study, in patients with cirrhosis and pleural effusion, an alternate diagnosis was seen in 18 out of 60 patients (30%).[15] These diagnoses included spontaneous bacterial pleuritis in nine, tuberculosis in two, adenocarcinoma in two, parapneumonic effusion in two, and undiagnosed exudates in three.[15] These alternate diagnoses were kept in mind when there were no ascites or pleural effusion on the left side.[15]

The fluid is usually transudative. A study conducted by Bielsa et al.[20] concluded that pleural fluid analysis of 18 patients out of 102 (18%) met Light's criteria for exudates. The differential cell count may reveal predominantly polymorphonuclear leukocytes, small lymphocytes, or other mononuclear cells. Amylase levels should be determined and cytological examination performed on both fluid specimens to rule out pancreatic ascites or malignant disease.

The management of pleural effusions associated with cirrhosis and ascites should be directed toward the treatment of ascites because the hydrothorax is an extension of the peritoneal fluid. The patient should be put on a salt-restricted diet and diuretics should be administered. Liver transplant should be considered as a treatment of choice in those patients who are refractory to medical management and remain symptomatic.[21]

The next best treatment is the transjugular intrahepatic portosystemic shunt (TIPS) in which a stent is inserted to connect portal veins to hepatic veins which reduces pressure in the portal vein. A recent study demonstrated that this procedure was superior to serial thoracentesis in refractory cases.[22] If TIPS or liver transplant is not feasible due to any reason, probably the best alternative therapy is VATS closure of the diaphragmatic defects. Chemical pleurodesis can be performed along with it.[23,24] Intercostal chest drain (ICD) insertion in hepatic hydrothorax should not be done as it is associated with protein and electrolyte depletion, infection, bleeding, and increased mortality. However, if patients develop spontaneous bacterial empyema (SBEM), ICD insertion might be needed.[23]

Talc pleurodesis for cases refractory to treatment is a risky option due to its high periprocedural morbidity and complications of up to 45% of the cases. Patients may develop acute renal injury, pneumonias, pneumothorax, empyema, and rarely encephalopathy. Thoracoscopic pleural abrasion is a better option to talc pleurodesis.

If no other management strategy is practically feasible, a peritoneojugular shunt can be done with very limited success.

Peritoneal Dialysis

In recent years, continuous ambulatory peritoneal dialysis (CAPD) has been used by an increasing number of patients with chronic renal failure. CAPD can be one of the rare but important causes of transudative pleural effusions. Different studies suggested up to 2% of patients develop pleural effusion due to the movement of the dialysate from the peritoneal cavity into the pleural cavity through a similar mechanism as seen in hepatic hydrothorax in patients with CAPD.

Pleural effusion can develop as early as on first day of peritoneal dialysis or as late as 8 years of CAPD.[24] The pleural effusion occurs on the right side approximately 90% of the time, but it can be bilateral or left-sided.

Diagnosis

When a patient on CAPD develops a pleural effusion, thoracentesis, and pleural fluid analysis can diagnose the etiology easily due to its peculiarity of clear fluid with biochemical analysis (low protein and high glucose) of pleural fluid.[25] Sometimes it is also called "sweet" hydrothorax because of this high glucose concentration.[25,26] According to Chow a glucose gradient (pleural fluid glucose level minus simultaneous serum glucose level) of >50 mg/dL (2.7 mmol/L) has a 100% sensitivity and specificity to detect sweet hydrothorax,[25] but some patients had a lower glucose gradient, probably due to reabsorption of glucose by the pleural mesothelium.[27] Diagnosis can be established easily on the basis of clinical history and pleural fluid analysis, but in uncertain cases, diaphragmatic communication needs to be demonstrated with the help of further imaging modalities such as peritoneal scintigraphy and contrast-enhanced computed tomography (CECT) peritoneography.

Treatment

Temporary withholding of CAPD, for 1-4 months, and transfer of the patients on hemodialysis (HD) are considered as first-line treatment. Around half of the cases respond well to this conservative approach. If chest drain is in-situ chemical pleurodesis can be performed with talc, tetracycline, autologous blood, and other agents. Chemical pleurodesis was only successful in around 48% of the cases.[5] After pleurodesis window period of 10 days is advised before resuming the peritoneal dialysis.

Chemical pleurodesis can also be performed under video-assisted thoracoscopic guidance as talc insufflation and it was successful in around 90% (50–100%) of cases.[5] Peritoneal dialysis can be resumed after 3-4 weeks. Another benefit of VATS in these cases is that bigger diaphragmatic defects can be closed by suturing at the same time, and pleurodesis by pleurectomy or pleural abrasion could also be performed.

Some patients on peritoneal dialysis might develop exudative pleural effusions. In a retrospective study done by Kwan et al.,[28] they reviewed 82 chronic peritoneal dialysis patients that had pleural effusions and found that 22 of them had unexplained exudative effusions. When the dialysis therapy in these patients was intensified, the exudative effusion tended to resolve. So, the study concluded that these exudative effusions were uremic pleural effusions.[28]

Nephrotic Syndrome

The collection of fluid in the pleural cavity is commonly seen in a patient of nephrotic syndrome. In a study of 52 patients of nephrotic syndrome, 21% had pleural effusions, unlike hepatohydrothorax; this condition is associated with bilateral pleural effusions and fluid located in the infrapulmonary region.[29] The main mechanism responsible for the pleural fluid collection in patients of nephrotic syndrome is decreased plasma oncotic pressure due to low serum albumin levels. However, hydrostatic pressure is also increased due to salt retention which further contributes to excess pleural fluid formation.[6]

Diagnosis

A diagnostic pleural tapping should always be performed for the evaluation of pleural fluid. Usually, Pleural fluid secondary to nephrotic syndrome is transudative. Nephrotic syndrome leads to a hypercoagulable state which increases the chances of renal vein thrombosis and also pulmonary thromboembolism. The cause of the hypercoagulable state in patients with nephrotic syndrome is not well understood. In nephrotic syndrome, damage to the glomerular membrane results in increased filtration of small proteins such as antithrombin III, plasminogen, protein C, and protein S, and this in turn leads to increased coagulability. Further evaluation with D-dimer, coagulation profile, and CT angiograms should be done in all patients of nephrotic syndrome with pleural effusion for early diagnosis and timely intervention to prevent these complications.[30,31]

Treatment

The aim of treatment in pleural effusion associated with the nephrotic syndrome is to decrease the protein loss in the urine and to maintain plasma protein level which contributes to oncotic pressure. This is best achieved by administration of diuretics in conjunction with a low-sodium diet, angiotensin-converting enzyme inhibitors, and using nonsteroidal anti-inflammatory agents cautiously. The diet in patients with nephrotic syndrome is aimed to provide sufficient caloric and protein (1 g/kg/day) intake. Supplemental dietary proteins are of no proven value. A low-salt diet helps limit fluid retention and edema.[32] The principles of treatment in adults with acute nephrotic syndrome are not different from those for children. Diuretics, such as furosemide, spironolactone, and even metolazone, may be needed. Diuretic use may lead to volume depletion, which should be assessed by monitoring symptoms, weight, pulse, and blood pressure. In selected patients of secondary nephrotic syndrome ACE inhibitors and/or angiotensin 2 receptor blockers should be used. Serial thoracentesis are not advised as it can further deplete the protein content in the body which may cause deterioration. In refractory cases, pleurodesis with a sclerosing agent can be considered, though rarely needed.

TRANSUDATIVE MALIGNANT EFFUSION

Malignant pleural effusion (MPE) refers to pleural effusion with the presence of malignant cells in the pleural fluid or pleura, commonly seen in advanced neoplasm and associated with poor prognosis. Malignant pleural effusion mostly seen in lung and breast cancer account for 50–65% of all malignant effusions. Other malignancies such as lymphomas, gastrointestinal, and genitourinary tumors contribute for 25% and in around 7–15% of patients primary are unknown.[33] It has been thought that almost all MPE are exudative; however, some studies have reported transudative MPE in 1–10% of cases.[34] One Korean study retrospectively studied 229 consecutive patients with malignant pleural effusion, proven either cytologically or with biopsy. Transudative MPE was observed in seven (3.1%) of the 229 patients and was caused either by the malignancy itself (six patients) or by coexisting cardiac diseases (one patient). In almost all neoplasm pleural metastasis has been reported.[5]

Mechanism of excess pleural fluid formation in malignancy can be direct or indirect. Direct causes include invasion of pleura by tumor or increased capillary permeability due to local inflammatory changes, obstruction of pleural lymphatic vessels, thoracic duct obstruction, or bronchial obstruction while indirect causes are hypoproteinemia, pulmonary embolism, radiation therapy, etc. "Paramalignant effusions" are defined as effusions related to malignancy but negative on cytology. Factors causing paramalignant effusion include postbronchial obstructive pneumonia, postbronchial obstruction atelectasis, thoracic duct obstruction, treatment-related (drug-induced), etc.[35]

Transudative malignant effusion can be noted in early stages of MPE where pleural fluid protein level is low due to mediastinal lymph node involvement, endobronchial obstruction resulting in trapped lung, superior vena cava (SVC) obstruction and coexisting hypoalbuminemia, cardiac, renal, and hepatic failure.[36-38]

Management

To make the diagnosis of MPE, pleural fluid cytology is mandatory if clinical and radiological features are suggestive of malignancy and the yield of which is 62–90%. If pleural fluid cytology is negative pleural biopsy is indicated.[39] Presence of MPE associated with poor prognosis so management generally focused as palliative therapy to provide symptomatic relieve and improvement in quality of life. Asymptomatic MPE do not require thoracocentesis usually, while symptomatic large volume MPE should be drained for symptomatic relief. Along with drainage of pleural fluid, patients should also receive treatment for underlying malignancy. Recurrence of MPE is very common therefore most patients will require more definitive interventions, such as pleurodesis and intrapleural catheter (IPC).

Other Less Common Causes of Pleural Effusion

Percutaneous Transhepatic Coronary Vein Occlusion

In patients of chronic liver diseases with portal hypertension, esophageal varices bleeds are common. Gel foam or other materials are injected in coronary vein via transhepatic route for varices bleed management. Suggested theory is that the injected gel material will lodge in the esophageal veins and stop the variceal bleeding. In this procedure, the transhepatic route is taken through the diaphragm.[40] In a German study, percutaneous, transhepatic catheterization of the portal vein in order to occlude the gastric coronary vein was carried out in six patients with bleeding esophageal varices. Bleeding stopped in three patients, but in the other three ceased only temporarily. Complications were one pleural effusion and one haemothorax.[41] According to R Light's hypothesis the pleural effusion might be accumulating because of an iatrogenic diaphragmatic defect that allows ascitic fluid into the pleural space. The pleural fluid is transudative. The same mechanism might be responsible for the pleural effusion following percutaneous transhepatic cholangiography.

Obstruction of the Brachiocephalic Vein

The brachiocephalic vein may get thrombosed after interventions such as central venous catheter[42] and hemodialysis catheter.[43] Sometimes intrathoracic goiter can cause compression of this vein. Leading to transudative pleural effusion.[44]

Superior Vena Cava Obstruction

Superior vena cava obstruction can cause pleural effusion in 60% of the cases.[45] The nature of fluid depends on the etiology of SVC obstruction. SVC obstruction related to malignancies causes pleural effusions which are almost always exudates and around 18% of them are chylous.[45] Some reports show presence of transudative effusion, in a few cases the postoperative period of the SVC syndrome resulted in a persistent right-sided, transudative pleural effusion. It appears that the increased systemic venous pressure from left innominate thrombosis leading to SVC obstruction in association with chest tube drainage connected to suction (increased intrapleural negative pressure) produced hydrostatic imbalances that resulted in increased pleural fluid formation and collection.[46]

Pulmonary Veno-occlusive Disease

It is a clinical condition that occurs due to fibrosis of tunica intima of pulmonary veins and venule which further leads to their obstruction. It is a rare cause of pulmonary hypertension and recurrent pulmonary embolism. Pulmonary veno-occlusive disease (PVOD) can rarely cause pleural effusion. It is usually transudative, more commonly bilateral but can be unilateral. Obstruction of the pulmonary veins leads to increased interstitial fluid which is probably responsible for pleural effusion. A definite diagnosis of PVOD can be made only by lung biopsy. It has a poor prognosis and the only effective treatment is a lung transplant.[47]

Hypoalbuminemia

A prospective study done at the University of Oklahoma 7 of 104 patients in group 1, 2 of 45 patients in group 2, and 3 of 21 patients in group 3 had pleural effusions. Within each group, there were no significant differences in serum albumin concentration or plasma oncotic pressure between patients with and without pleural effusions. The study concluded that hypoalbuminemia is an uncommon cause of pleural effusion. The recognition of pleural effusions in patients with low serum albumin levels should prompt careful clinical evaluations to identify other potential causes for the effusions.[48]

Myxedema

Myxedema is an extreme but rare manifestation of hypothyroidism. It leads to increased expression of vascular endothelial growth factor (VEGF) which causes increased capillary permeability which leads to extravasation of fluid into the pleural spaces causing pleural effusion. Pleural effusions secondary to myxedema can be unilateral or bilateral and can be exudative or transudative in nature. Hypothyroidism and pleural effusion can coexist in many cases but in most of these cases some other coexisting disease may be the cause of effusion. Thyroid replacement in optimum dose is the treatment of pleural effusions secondary to myxedema.[49]

Glomerulonephritis

Pleural effusions in acute glomerulonephritis appear to be due to an increase in microvascular hydrostatic pressure and result in transudates. Edema and cardiomegaly are clinical accompaniments reflecting hypervolemia and salt and water excess.[50]

Urinothorax

Urinothorax is defined as presence of urine in pleural cavity. It is a rare cause of pleural effusions first recognized in canines in 1968 by Corriere et al. True prevalence is unknown as only case reports are available in the literature; however, this condition is underreported due to poor recognition by clinicians. The common cause for urinothorax is obstructive uropathy due to renal stone, urethral valve, ureteral stricture, and obstruction from renal cyst or tumor, surgery, and trauma. Accumulation of urine in pleural cavity can occur by a direct or indirect mechanism. Direct mechanisms include migration of urine into the pleural space through diaphragmatic pores, gradient difference between intra-abdominal and intrathoracic pressure helpful in the fluid movement. Besides, urine can also transfer directly into the pleural space after rupture of urinoma, a collection of urine in the retroperitoneal space which is formed sometimes after a urological procedure or intervention. An indirect mechanism includes the passage of urine through the retroperitoneal-pleural lymphatic connection.[51-53]

On chest X-ray, typical presentation is unilateral effusion on the side of trauma or genitourinary obstruction; however, bilateral or contralateral effusion is also reported. Diagnosis requires pleural fluid analysis (similar to urine) and is typically showed paucicellular, transudative effusion, which have protein levels <1 g/dL, and low LDH with a low pH. Pleural fluid may smell like urine. Confirmation of diagnosis is by simultaneous measurement of pleural fluid and serum creatinine levels. Pleural fluid to serum creatinine ratio >1.0 is supportive while >1.7 is diagnostic. Imaging studies such as CECT scan/ultrasonography (USG) of the abdomen, and technetium-m99 scan also performed to evaluate obstructive uropathy or urinoma. Initially, pleural fluid should be drain to provide symptomatic relief and prevention of infection. Definite treatment is to repair tract injury or obstruction to prevent recurrence. Notably, pleurodesis has not been found to be of beneficial.[54]

Glycinothorax

A case report by Baker and colleagues says postoperative accumulation of pleural effusion showing high levels of glycine. The fluid used for intra and postoperative bladder irrigation had leaked from the perforated bladder and collected in the pleural cavity leading to glycinothorax.[55]

Cerebrospinal Fluid Leak in Pleura

It is not uncommon for cerebrospinal fluid (CSF) to get accumulated in pleura causing pleural effusion. This can happen due to various reasons but more commonly due to ventriculopleural shunt, migration of ventriculoperitoneal (VP) shunt into the pleural cavity.[56,57] In other causes of subarachnoid pleural fistula include penetrating or nonpenetrating trauma, thoracic spine surgery. The fluid is clear, and colorless with very low protein content.

Even if CSF hydrothorax is rarely described, it should be suspected when respiratory failure, mechanical ventilation or oxygen requirement, and persistent pleural effusion are detected in VP-shunted patients in whom no adequate neurological examination can be carried on. Beta-2 transferrin assay and radionuclide shuntography are useful techniques to diagnose CSF pleural effusion and verify the shunt patency and course.[58]

Drug-induced

A drug as a causative factor of pleural effusion is usually a diagnosis of exclusion. When all possible causes are ruled out, the possibility of drug-induced pleural effusion can be considered. Thorough drug consumption history is important in such cases. This association can be supported if the resolved pleural effusion recurs after readministration of the same drug, this phenomenon is rare. Few case reports are available. In one report pleural effusion was associated with sodium valproate administration. The pleural fluid was neutrophilic and transudative.[59] In other report which was also sodium valproate-associated pleural effusion,[60] the fluid was transudative but eosinophilic. This patient also had blood eosinophilia. This eosinophilia and pleural effusion both got resolved after stopping sodium valproate. One case report presenting a patient with an accidental overdose of paracetamol (33 g) had transudative pleural effusion.[61] Many other drugs are known to cause pleural disease; they are discussed in Chapter 26 of this book.

Trapped Lung

The trapped lung or "nonexpandable lung" is a condition in which lung is unable to expand in their respective pleural cavities even after removal of pleural fluid due to thick, fibrosed visceral pleura which is usually seen when pleural inflammation heals with fibrosis. However, chronic atelectasis or an endobronchial lesion obstructing the bronchial lumen leading to lobar collapse also causes this condition. It is typically presenting as chronic stable pleural effusion. Due to negative intrapleural pressure the entry of fluid into pleural space is increased and reabsorption of pleural fluid through pleural lymphatics also reduced, leading to the formation of a chronic pleural effusion, so a steady state of fluid formation and removal is established, leads to pleural effusion of constant volume. The whole mechanism for persistence of the pleural effusion is mainly mechanical and can be considered a "pleural effusion ex vacuo."[62,63] Pleural fluid analysis showed a transudate nature of fluid or a protein-discordant exudate with mononuclear cell predominance with low LDH. The characteristic diagnostic clue is that after thoracentesis, the pleural fluid reaccumulates and the volume of pleural effusion remains remarkably constant over time. It can also be diagnosed via pleural manometry during thoracentesis. Management of the trapped lung depends upon the patient's symptoms, if the patient is asymptomatic no further treatment is indicated. In symptomatic patients, studies are in favor of decortication of thickened visceral pleura which allows reexpansion of trapped lung and resolution of symptoms; however, before performing decortication other causes of dyspnea should be ruled out first **(Box 1)**.

Transudative effusions have less protein content and are paucicellular. Though there are etiological factors that are almost distinct in their ability to cause a transudative effusion, there are some diseases that can lead to confusion by causing effusion of both the types, transudative, and exudative. Finding the etiology is important for the management, which should target not only the underlying cause but also the fluid itself.

BOX 1 Causes of transudative pleural effusion.

Etiologies that always cause transudative pleural effusion:

- Causes
    - Congestive cardiac failure
    - Hepatic hydrothorax
    - Nephrotic syndrome
    - Peritoneal dialysis
    - Cerebrospinal fluid leak into pleural space
    - Atelectasis
    - Hypoalbuminemia
    - Iatrogenic
    - Urinothorax
    - Pulmonary veno-occlusive disease
    - Obstruction of the brachiocephalic vein

Etiologies which may cause transudative pleural effusion (usually cause transudative effusion):

- Myxedema
- Amyloidosis
- Malignancy
- Sarcoidosis
- Superior vena cava obstruction

Miscellaneous:

- Drug-induced

KEY POINTS

- Unlike exudative pleural effusion, which is characterized by an inflammatory response and increased permeability of the pleura, transudative effusion is typically caused by imbalances in hydrostatic or oncotic pressures. This imbalance leads to the accumulation of a clear, protein-poor fluid in the pleural cavity.
- CCF is the most common cause of transudative pleural effusion. Around 80% of transudative effusions are due to CCF.
- In hepatic hydrothorax, the ascitic fluid in the abdomen enters the pleural cavity via defects in the diaphragm, because of the gradient between intraperitoneal and intrapleural pressure.
- Transudative pleural effusion secondary to peritoneal dialysis is also called "sweet" hydrothorax because of this high glucose concentration.
- In cases of transudative pleural effusion secondary to nephrotic syndrome, always rule out renal vein thrombosis and/or pulmonary thromboembolism.
- For about 1–10% of malignant effusions can be transudative, which may be due to mediastinal lymph node involvement or trapped lung.
- Urinothorax usually has transudative effusions with protein content < 1 g/dL.
- SVC obstruction, pulmonary veno-occlusive disease, myxedema, and cerebrospinal fluid leak in the pleura are some of the rare causes of transudative pleural effusion.

REFERENCES

1. Ferreiro L, Porcel JM, Valdés L. Diagnosis and management of pleural transudates. Arch Bronconeumol. 2017;53(11):629-36.
2. Hooper C, Lee YG, Maskell N; BTS Pleural Guideline Group. Investigation of a unilateral pleural effusion in adults: British Thoracic Society pleural disease guideline 2010. Thorax. 2010;65(Suppl 2):ii4-17.
3. Kataoka H. Pericardial and pleural effusions in decompensated chronic heart failure. Am Heart J. 2000;139(5):918-23.
4. Kinasewitz GT, Jones KR. Effusions from cardiac diseases. Textbook of Pleural Diseases, 2nd edition. London: Hodder Arnold; 2008. pp. 315-21.
5. Hall WJ, Mayewski RJ. Diagnostic thoracentesis and pleural biopsy in pleural effusions. Ann Intern Med. 1985;103(5):799-802.
6. Kinasewitz GT. Transudative effusions. Eur Respir J. 1997;10(3): 714-8.
7. Light RW, Macgregor MI, Luchsinger PC, Ball WC Jr. Pleural effusions: the diagnostic separation of transudates and exudates. Ann Intern Med. 1972;77(4):507-13.
8. Romero S, Candela A, Martín C, Hernández L, Trigo C, Gil J. Evaluation of different criteria for the separation of pleural transudates from exudates. Chest. 1993;104(2):399-404.
9. Broaddus VC. Diuresis and transudative effusions--changing the rules of the game. Am J Med. 2001;110(9):732-5.
10. Han ZJ, Wu XD, Cheng JJ, Zhao SD, Gao MZ, Huang HY, et al. Diagnostic accuracy of natriuretic peptides for heart failure in patients with pleural effusion: a systematic review and updated meta-analysis. PLoS One. 2015;10(8):e0134376.
11. Zhou Q, Ye ZJ, Su Y, Zhang JC, Shi HZ. Diagnostic value of N-terminal pro-brain natriuretic peptide for pleural effusion due to heart failure: a meta-analysis. Heart. 2010;96(15): 1207-11.
12. Romero-Candeira S, Hernández L, Romero-Brufao S, Orts D, Fernández C, Martín C. Is it meaningful to use biochemical parameters to discriminate between transudative and exudative pleural effusions? Chest. 2002;122(5):1524-9.
13. Chakko SC, Caldwell SH, Sforza PP. Treatment of congestive heart failure. its effect on pleural fluid chemistry. Chest. 1989;95(4):798-802.
14. Sudduth CD, Sahn SA. Pleurodesis for nonmalignant pleural effusions. recommendations. Chest. 1992;102(6):1855-60.
15. Xiol X, Castellote J, Cortes-Beut R, Delgado M, Guardiola J, Sesé E. Usefulness and complications of thoracentesis in cirrhotic patients. Am J Med. 2001;111(1):67-9.
16. Eisenberg B, Velchik MG, Alavi A. Pleuroperitoneal communication in a patient with right pleural effusion and ascites diagnosed by technetium-99m sulfur colloid imaging. Clin Nucl Med . 1988;13(2):99-101.
17. Lieberman FL, Hidemura R, Peters RL, Reynolds TB. Pathogenesis and treatment of hydrothorax complicating cirrhosis with ascites. Annals of Internal Medicine. 1966;64(2):341-51.
18. Rubinstein D, McInnes IE, Dudley FJ. Hepatic hydrothorax in the absence of clinical ascites: diagnosis and management. Gastroenterology. 1985;88(1 Pt 1):188-91.
19. Lazaridis KN, Frank JW, Krowka MJ, Kamath PS. Hepatic hydrothorax: pathogenesis, diagnosis, and management. Am J Med. 1999;107(3):262-7.
20. Bielsa S, Porcel JM, Castellote J, Mas E, Esquerda A, Light RW. Solving the Light's criteria misclassification rate of cardiac and hepatic transudates. Respirology. 2012;17(4):721-6.
21. Xiol X, Tremosa G, Castellote J, Gornals J, Lama C, Lopez C, et al. Liver transplantation in patients with hepatic hydrothorax. Transpl Int. 2005;18(6):672-5.
22. Rössle M, Ochs A, Gülberg V, Siegerstetter V, Holl J, Deibert P, et al. A comparison of paracentesis and transjugular intrahepatic portosystemic shunting in patients with ascites. N Engl J Med. 2000;342(23):1701-7.
23. Huang PM, Kuo SW, Lee JM. Thoracoscopic diaphragmatic repair for refractory hepatic hydrothorax: application of pleural flap and mesh onlay reinforcement. Thorac Cardiovasc Surg. 2006;54(1):47-50.

24. Nomoto Y, Suga T, Nakajima K, Sakai H, Osawa G, Ota K, et al. Acute hydrothorax in continuous ambulatory peritoneal dialysis—a collaborative study of 161 centers. Am J Nephrol. 1989;9(5):363-7.
25. Szeto CC, Chow KM. Pathogenesis and management of hydrothorax complicating peritoneal dialysis. Curr Opin Pulm Med. 2004;10(4):315-9.
26. Michel C, Devy A, Lavaud F, Lavaud S, Lebargy F. A "sweet" hydrothorax. Presse Med. 2001;30(28):1401-3.
27. Tang S, Chui WH, Tang AW, Li FK, Chau WS, Ho YW, et al. Video-assisted thoracoscopic talc pleurodesis is effective for maintenance of peritoneal dialysis in acute hydrothorax complicating peritoneal dialysis. Nephrol Dial Transplant. 2003;18(4):804-8.
28. Kwan BC, Chow KM, Pang WF, Leung CB, Li PK, Szeto CC. Unexplained exudative pleural effusion in chronic peritoneal dialysis patients. Perit Dial Int. 2010;30(5):534-40.
29. Cavina C, Vichi G. Radiological aspects of pleural effusions in medical nephropathy in children. Ann Radiol Diagn (Bolonga). 1958;31(3):163-202.
30. Llach F, Arieff AI, Massry SG. Renal vein thrombosis and nephrotic syndrome. A prospective study of 36 adult patients. Ann Intern Med. 1975;83(1):8-14.
31. Palmer BF. Nephrotic edema--pathogenesis and treatment. Am J Med Sci. 1993;306(1):53-67.
32. Appel GB. Improved outcomes in nephrotic syndrome. Cleve Clinic J Med. 2006;73(2):161-7.
33. Roberts ME, Neville E, Berrisford RG, Antunes G, Ali NJ, et al. Management of a malignant pleural effusion: British Thoracic Society pleural disease guideline 2010. Thorax. 2010;65(Suppl 2):ii32-40.
34. Alvarez M, Salud A, Vives M. Should a cytologic study be ordered in transudative pleural effusions? Chest. 1999;116(6):1836-7.
35. American Thoracic Society. Management of malignant pleural effusions. Am J Respir Crit Care Med. 2000;162(5):1987-2001.
36. Ryu JS, Ryu ST, Kim YS, Cho JH, Lee HL. What is the clinical significance of transudative malignant pleural effusion? Korean J Intern Med. 2003;18(4):230-3.
37. Fernandez C, Martín C, Aranda I, Romero S. Malignant transient pleural transudate: a sign of early lymphatic tumoral obstruction. Respiration. 2000;67(3):333-6.
38. Ashchi M, Golish J, Eng P, O'Donovan P. Transudative malignant pleural effusions: prevalence and mechanisms. South Med J. 1998;91(1):23-6.
39. Johnson L, Fakih HA, Daouk S, Saleem S, Ataya A. Transudative pleural effusion of malignant etiology: Rare but real. Respir Med Case Rep. 2017;20:188-91.
40. Widrich WC, Johnson WC, Robbins AH, Nabseth DC. Esophagogastric variceal hemorrhage: Its treatment by percutaneous transephatic coronary vein occlusion. Arch Surg. 1978;113(11): 1331-8.
41. Günther R, Kurtenbach P, Georgi M, Schmidt HD, Farack U. Perkutane transhepatische Thrombosierung der Vena coronaria ventriculi bei Ösophagusvarizenblutung. Rofo. 1977;126(1): 6-10.
42. Porcel JM. Unilateral pleural effusion secondary to brachiocephalic venous thrombosis: a rare complication of central vein catheterization. Respiration. 2002;69(6):569.
43. Muthuswamy P, Alausa M, Reilly B. Clinical problem-solving. The effusion that would not go away. N Engl J Med. 2001;345(10):756-9.
44. Gallelli A, Pelaia G, Calderazzo M, Roccia F, Vero G, Gallelli G, et al. Transudative right pleural effusion due to compression of the brachiocephalic vein caused by an intrathoracic goitre. Monaldi Archr Chest Dis. Monaldi Arch Chest Dis. 2000;55(3): 210-1.
45. Rice TW. Pleural effusions in superior vena cava syndrome: prevalence, characteristics, and proposed pathophysiology. Curr Opin Pulm Med. 2007;13(4):324-7.
46. Good Jr JT, Moore JB, Fowler AA, Sahn SA. Superior vena cava syndrome as a cause of pleural effusion. Am Rev Respir Dis. 1982;125(2):246-7.
47. Light RW, Lee GW. Effusions from vascular causes. Textbook of Pleural Diseases. London: Arnold; 2003. pp. 289-96.
48. Eid AA, Keddissi JI, Kinasewitz GT. Hypoalbuminemia as a cause of pleural effusions. Chest. 1999;115(4):1066-9.
49. Boulet LP, Milot JO, Boutet MI, St Georges F, Laviolette MI. Airway inflammation in nonasthmatic subjects with chronic cough. Am J Respir Crit Care Med. 1994;149(2):482-9.
50. Sahn SA, Miller KS. Obscure pleural effusion. Look to the kidney. Chest. 1986;90(5):631.
51. Austin A, Jogani SN, Brasher PB, Argula RG, Huggins JT, Chopra A. The urinothorax: a comprehensive review with case series. Am J Med Sci. 2017;354(1):44-53.
52. Toubes ME, Lama A, Ferreiro L, Golpe A, Álvarez-Dobaño JM, González-Barcala FJ, et al. Urinothorax: a systematic review. J Thorac Dis. 2017;9(5):1209-18.
53. Chawla AK, Chaudhary G, Chawla MK, Chawla R, Chawla PS. Case of urinothorax – A rare presentation. Lung India. 2020;37(1):53-6.
54. Ferreira PG, Furriel F, Ferreira AJ. Urinothorax as an unusual type of pleural effusion – Case report and review. Revista Portuguesa de Pneumologia (English Edition). 2013;19(2):80-3.
55. Barker L. Glycinothorax revisited. Anaesthesia. 2000;55(7):706-7.
56. Beach C, Manthey DE. Tension hydrothorax due to ventriculo-pleural shunting. J Emerg Mede. 1998;16(1):33-6.
57. Muramatsu H, Koike K. Pleural effusions appearing in the rehabilitation ward after ventriculoperitoneal shunts: a report of two adult cases and a review of the literature. Brain Inj. 2004;18(8):835-44.
58. Porcaro F, Procaccini E, Paglietti MG, Schiavino A, Petreschi F, Cutrera R. Pleural effusion from intrathoracic migration of a ventriculo-peritoneal shunt catheter: pediatric case report and review of the literature. Ital J Pediatr. 2018;44:42.
59. Tryfon S, Saroglou M, Kazanas K, Mermigkis C, Psathakis K, Galanis N. Sodium valproate as a cause of recurrent transudative pleural effusion: a case report. J Med Case Rep. 2009;3(1):51.
60. Kaufman J, O'Shaughnessy IM. Eosinophilic pleural effusion associated with valproic acid administration. South Med J. 1995;88(8):881-2.
61. Akbaş İ, Kocak AO, Utlu SG, Doğruyol S, Cakir Z. Paracetamol overdose may cause transudative pleural effusion in adults. J Emerg Med Case Rep. 2021;12(2):41-4.
62. Doelken P, Sahn SA. Trapped lung. Semin Respir Crit Care Med. 2001;22(6):631-6.
63. Pereyra MF, Ferreiro L, Valdés L. Unexpandable lung. Arch Bronconeumol. 2013;49(2):63-9.

CHAPTER

7

Tubercular Pleural Effusion

Saroj Meena, Anuj K Bhatnagar

INTRODUCTION

Tuberculosis (TB) is a significant global health concern and remains one of the leading causes of death from an infectious disease worldwide. The coronavirus disease 19 (COVID-19) pandemic has had a substantial impact on global health, but TB remains a major public health issue. In 2021, an estimated 10.6 million people worldwide developed TB, and 1.6 million died from the disease.[1] While TB primarily affects the lungs, it can also manifest as extrapulmonary TB, which accounts for approximately 15–20% of total TB cases in immunocompetent individuals. However, in individuals with compromised immune systems, such as those who are seropositive for human immunodeficiency virus (HIV), the incidence of extrapulmonary TB can be as high as 50%.[2] Following lymphatic engagement, tuberculous pleural effusion (TPE) emerges as the second most prevalent manifestation of extrapulmonary TB. Within regions where TB is endemic, TPE stands out as the primary underlying reason for pleural effusion occurrences. It arises when *Mycobacterium tuberculosis* (MTB) invades the pleural space, resulting in the buildup of fluid amid the layers of the pleura (the thin membranes surrounding the lungs).

PATHOGENESIS

Tuberculous pleural effusions can occur in connection with primary pulmonary TB or reactivation of latent TB, with the latter being more common. In cases of primary TB, the formation of pleural effusion occurs when a subpleural parenchymal focus ruptures, permitting the MTB antigen to enter the pleural space.[3] This leads to inflammation, heightened capillary permeability, and the generation of pleural fluid. Initially, there is a predominance of polymorphonuclear leukocytes, followed by an influx of macrophages that peak 3–4 days after the initial insult. During this phase, an effusion lymphocytic predominance emerges.[4] T-helper type 1 (TH1) cells orchestrate this robust immune response, which entails a delayed hypersensitivity reaction to MTB. The TH1-driven immune response releases adenosine deaminase (ADA) and interferon-gamma (IFN). Granuloma formation, orchestrated by monocyte macrophages, helps isolate the organisms and prevent further dissemination.[5] Due to the robust immune response, the bacteria are rapidly cleared, resulting in paucibacillary TPEs. When liquid culture media are used, these effusions yield positive cultures in 24–58% of cases.[6]

NATURAL HISTORY

Tubercular pleural effusion, if left untreated, can spontaneously resolve, but it is likely to recur in the future. This was demonstrated by Roper and Waring in the United States, who conducted a large study following up 141 military personnel with pleural effusion and a positive purified protein derivative (PPD) test from 1940 to 1944. For the majority of patients, the effusions resolved, and all remaining symptoms disappeared within a span of 2–4 months. Yet, out of the 141 individuals, 92 (65%) subsequently experienced some manifestation of active TB. None of the patients exhibited evident TB in the lungs or elsewhere within 8 months from the commencement of the initial pleurisy. The occurrence of subsequent TB stood at 60% among those whose initial pleural fluid cultures for TB were negative and at 65% among those with initially positive pleural fluid cultures. Furthermore, no correlation was found between the size of the initial effusions and the presence or absence of small radiologically repetitive pleural lymphosis concerning the subsequent development of active TB.[7] Therefore, it is crucial to promptly diagnose tuberculous pleuritis and initiate treatment. The use of antituberculous chemotherapy has reduced the incidence of subsequent TB. Additionally, treatment should be administered to patients with a high suspicion of TB, even when the diagnosis cannot be definitively established.

CLINICAL PRESENTATION

Patients with TPE typically present with an acute or subacute illness. The most common symptoms include unilateral pleuritic chest pain (approximately 75% of cases), cough (around 70% of cases), fever (approximately 85% of cases), night sweats (approximately 50% of cases), dyspnea (about 50% of cases), and weight loss (ranging from 25 to 85% of cases).[5] The dyspnea is caused by the presence of a large pleural effusion that compromises lung mechanics. In individuals who are HIV positive, the illness may be more disseminated and have a longer duration.

Tuberculous pleural effusion is typically unilateral but can occur on either side **(Fig. 1)**. In a study comprising 333 patients, pleural fluid was observed exclusively on the left side in 127 instances (38.1%), solely on the right side in 161 cases (48.4%), and both sides were impacted in 45 cases (13.5%).[2]

DIAGNOSIS

The definitive diagnosis of TPE involves the detection of MTB in the pleural fluid, pleural biopsy specimen, sputum, or the presence of granulomas in the pleura. A tentative diagnosis can also be reasonably established by assessing pleural fluid analysis and identifying heightened levels of ADA or IFN within the pleural fluid, combined with consideration of the clinical context **(Flowchart 1)**.

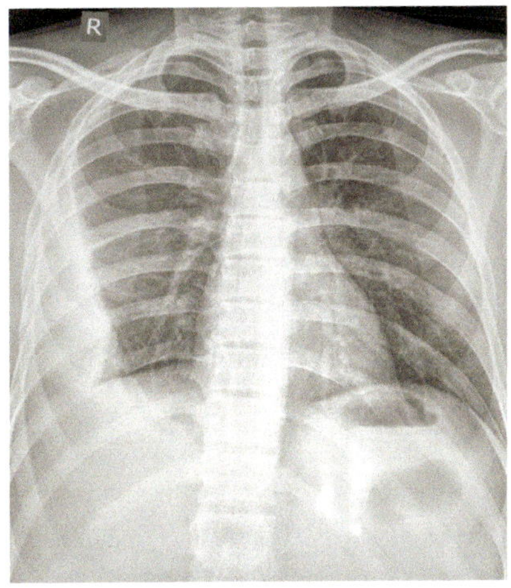

FIG. 1: Chest X-ray (CXR) anterior–posterior view of male patient with right pleural effusion.

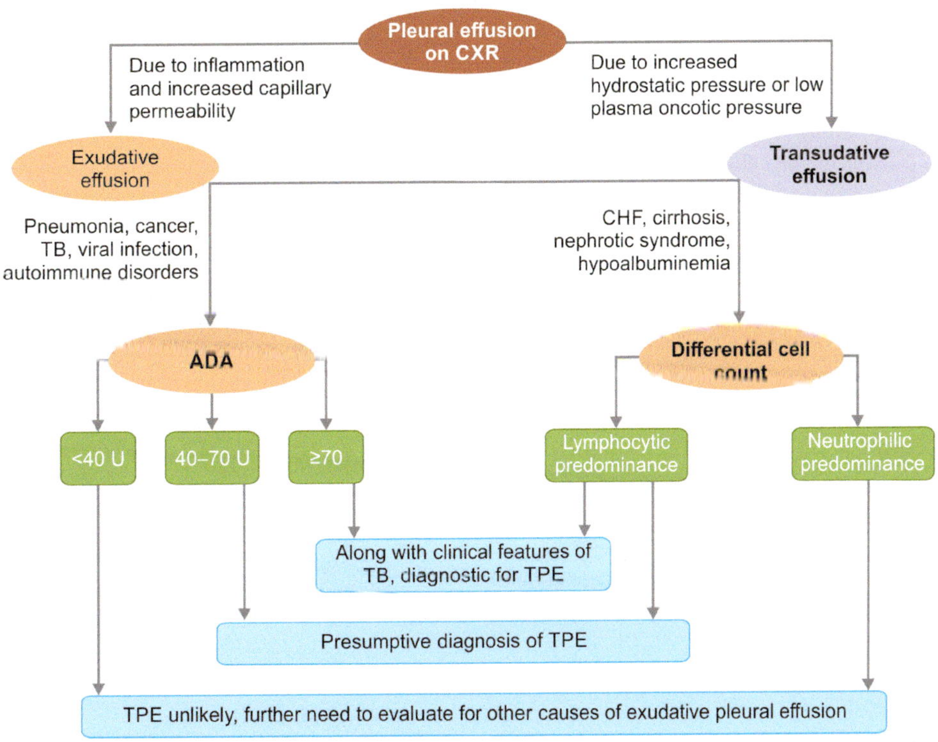

FLOWCHART 1: Approach to a patient with pleural effusion.

(ADA: adenosine deaminase; CHF: congestive heart failure; CXR: chest X-ray; TB: tuberculosis; TPE: tubercular pleural effusion)

Pleural Fluid Analysis

Tuberculous pleural effusion typically appears as a straw-colored fluid and is characterized as an exudate with a predominance of lymphocytes. Glucose levels in TPEs are usually low, although higher levels (ranging from 60 to 100 mg/dL) are not uncommon, especially in postprimary TB. The effusions also exhibit elevated levels of lactate dehydrogenase (LDH) and protein, consistent with an exudate based on the Light criteria. LDH levels frequently surpass 500 IU, and protein levels nearly always exceed 5 g/dL.[8] Additionally, the fluid's pH typically registers below 7.4.[3]

Diagnostic Markers

Adenosine Deaminase

Adenosine deaminase is an enzyme primarily found in T-lymphocytes that plays a role in converting adenosine and deoxyadenosine into inosine and deoxyinosine, respectively. ADA exists in two distinct molecular forms: ADA1 and ADA2. ADA1 is present in all cells, with its highest activity observed in lymphocytes and monocytes. In contrast, ADA2 is exclusively located in monocytes.

A meta-analysis comprising 16 studies and involving more than 4,000 patients revealed that ADA levels exhibit a sensitivity and specificity of approximately 90% for the diagnosis of TPE, irrespective of the diverse cutoff values employed in the studies (ranging between 23 and 45 U/L).[9] In another comprehensive meta-analysis conducted by Aggarwal et al., it was demonstrated that pleural fluid ADA exhibits a favorable sensitivity of 0.92 and specificity of 0.9 for the diagnosis of TPE.[10] Nevertheless, during the initial stages of pleural disease caused by TB, ADA levels might be diminished, leading to the need for repeated testing. It is worth noting that elderly patients and individuals who smoke could exhibit reduced ADA levels.[11]

Among patients with TPE, the pleural fluid ADA level is usually above 40 U/L, which is the widely recognized cutoff point for diagnosing TPE. Determining the optimal cutoff value for pleural fluid, ADA has been a topic of debate in the past. The extensive meta-analysis mentioned earlier demonstrated that pleural fluid ADA levels exceeding 70 U/L strongly indicate TPE. Conversely, levels below 40 U/L should lead to the consideration of a diagnosis other than TB. According to this meta-analysis, using a cutoff of 40 U/L yields a sensitivity of 0.93 and a specificity of 0.90, with a negative predictive value (NPV) of 0.93.[10] It is important to note that several other conditions can also result in elevated pleural fluid ADA levels, such as brucellosis, Q fever, lymphomas, rheumatoid arthritis, parapneumonic effusions, and empyema.[2]

Adenosine deaminase 2 is specifically found in monocytes, and in tuberculous pleural fluid, ADA2 is the predominant form. In other pleural fluids, ADA1 is more prevalent. While employing a ratio of ADA1 to total ADA activity lower than 0.42 can marginally enhance the sensitivity and specificity of ADA in the diagnosis of tuberculous pleuritis, the separation of isoenzymes is generally unnecessary in most instances.[12]

Assessing the pleural fluid ADA levels is a valuable tool in diagnosing tuberculous pleurisy. For individuals with lymphocytic pleural effusion, a pleural fluid ADA level exceeding 40 U/L strongly indicates the presence of tuberculous pleurisy. In cases where a lymphocytic pleural effusion is not caused by TB, the pleural fluid ADA level is typically below 40 U/L. Pleural fluid samples for ADA assay can be transported at normal room temperatures, provided that suitable preservatives are introduced into the fluid.[13]

Distinguishing between TPE and MPE can be challenging due to similar cytological and biochemical features, including ADA. A study conducted by Rabbi et al. evaluated the diagnostic accuracy of the ADA/CRP ratio in pleural fluid for differentiation. Out of the 59 participants, 31 had TPE, and 28 had MPE, those with TPE showed significantly higher pleural fluid ADA to serum CRP ratio and pleural fluid ADA levels. Serum CRP levels did not differ significantly between TPE and MPE patients. The ADA/CRP ratio enhances diagnostic accuracy beyond ADA alone in distinguishing between TPE and MPE.[14]

Interferon-gamma

Interferon-gamma, a cytokine with a vital role in T-cell-mediated granulomatous inflammation, has been investigated as a potential diagnostic marker for TPE. The elevated levels of IFN in TPE were first reported in 1988.[15]

A meta-analysis combining data from 22 studies, encompassing 782 individuals with TPE and 1,319 individuals with nontuberculous effusions, revealed that the IFN assay exhibited an overall sensitivity of 89% and an overall specificity of 97%. The highest combined sensitivity and specificity value achieved was 95%.[16] When evaluating sensitivity, specificity, positive likelihood ratio, negative likelihood ratio, and diagnostic odds ratio, the overall accuracy of IFN outperforms ADA as a diagnostic test for TPE.

However, despite its higher accuracy, the IFN assay is not commonly preferred over ADA for the diagnosis of TPE. This is mainly due to the simplicity and lower cost of the ADA test. ADA remains the preferred diagnostic test for TPE in clinical practice.[2]

Interferon-γ Release Assays

Interferon-gamma release assays (IGRAs) are laboratory tests conducted in controlled environments that quantify the discharge of gamma-interferon from sensitized T-cells found in peripheral blood or pleural fluid. These assays, such as QuantiFERON-TB Gold and T-SPOT.TB, are widely available tests. In a recent meta-analysis of seven studies involving 213 individuals with TPEs, the sensitivity and specificity of IGRA measurements in pleural fluid were evaluated. The findings showed that the sensitivity of IGRA in pleural fluid was 0.75 and the specificity was 0.82.[17] These results indicate that IGRAs have limitations in accurately diagnosing pleural TB when compared to other diagnostic tests.

Considering the significant difference in performance compared to ADA, IGRA is not recommended as a primary test for the diagnosis of pleural TB.

Polymerase Chain Reaction

Polymerase chain reaction (PCR) tests and other nucleic acid amplification test (NAAT) assays are molecular diagnostic techniques that amplify specific nucleic acid sequences of MTB for detection. These tests utilize nucleic acid samples, such as sputum or other clinical specimens, and amplify MTB-specific sequences for identification.

One such NAAT test is the Xpert MTB/RIF (Gene Xpert) assay, which has been developed to detect MTB and rifampin (RIF) resistance. This technique utilizes a hemi-nested real-time PCR assay to amplify a particular segment of the *rpoB* gene. Subsequently, this amplified segment is examined for mutations related to rifampin resistance through the application of molecular beacons.[18] One significant advantage of the Xpert MTB/RIF assay is its rapid turnaround time, with results available in as early as 2 hours. The sensitivity of the Xpert MTB/RIF assay is high, with a reported sensitivity of 99.8% for cases that are smear- and culture-positive and 90.2% for smear-negative but culture-positive patients. The approximate specificity of a solitary direct Xpert MTB/RIF assay performed on sputum is 99.2%.[19] Overall, PCR tests and NAAT assays, including the Xpert MTB/RIF assay, provide a sensitive and specific means of detecting MTB and RIF resistance, offering faster results compared to traditional culture-based methods.

Sputum Smears and Cultures

Sputum smear analysis is a frequently overlooked test in the process of diagnosing TPE. The rupture of local lung foci into the pleural space can result in the emergence of TPE, making sputum examination crucial for diagnosis **(Fig. 1)**. Conde et al. conducted a study in which they assessed the diagnostic effectiveness of acid-fast bacilli (AFB) smear and sputum culture in a prospective manner among 84 patients diagnosed with tuberculous pleuritis. They found that sputum studies were positive in 44 out of the 84 patients (52%). Among the positive cases, sputum smears were positive in 10 patients, while cultures were positive in all 44 patients (99%). Additionally, sputum induction was performed in 64 patients who exhibited a normal radiograph except for the presence of pleural effusion. Among these patients, sputum induction yielded positive results in 35 patients (55%).[20] These findings emphasize the importance of sputum examination, including AFB smear and culture, in the diagnosis of tuberculous pleuritis. Therefore, sputum examination should be considered in all patients presenting with pleural effusion, and if sputum production is not reported by the patient, sputum induction should be performed to improve the chances of detecting MTB in the respiratory tract.

Pleural Biopsy

Pleural biopsy is an important procedure for diagnosing tuberculous pleurisy. There are two methods commonly used to obtain pleural biopsy tissue: Blind biopsy of the pleura and medical thoracoscopy. Blind biopsy of the pleura, done by using Cope or Abram needle, is now considered outdated and involves obtaining pleural tissue samples without direct visualization. Medical thoracoscopy is a minimally invasive procedure that allows direct visualization and biopsy of the pleural space using a thoracoscope. A prospective study conducted by Wang et al. investigated exudative pleural effusions of unknown etiologies and found that among 833 patients with pleural effusion, 333 were confirmed to have tuberculous pleurisy. During thoracoscopy, the researchers observed various findings indicative of tuberculous pleurisy, including pleural nodules in 69.4% of patients, pleural adhesion in 66.7%, hyperemia in 60.7%, plaque-like lesions in 6.0%, and ulceration in 1.5% of patients. Pleural biopsy conducted during thoracoscopy verified the existence of MTB in pleural tissue or the revelation of cascating granulomas in 99.1% of cases (330 patients). This highlights the high diagnostic yield of pleural biopsy in detecting tuberculous pleurisy. Regarding complications, the study documented the absence of significant adverse events. The most prevalent minor complication observed was temporary chest discomfort experienced by 43.2% of patients due to the presence of the indwelling chest tube.[21]

Overall, medical thoracoscopy with pleural biopsy is a valuable diagnostic tool for tuberculous pleurisy, allowing direct visualization of the pleural space and obtaining tissue samples for histopathological examination and culture.

Tuberculin Skin Testing

Tuberculin skin test (also known as the Mantoux test) can provide supportive evidence in the diagnosis of tuberculous pleurisy, particularly in areas with low TB prevalence or where vaccination against TB is not common. A positive tuberculin skin test result indicates exposure to MTB antigens and the presence of a delayed hypersensitivity reaction, suggesting a previous or current TB infection. However, it is important to note that a positive result alone is not sufficient to confirm the diagnosis of tuberculous pleurisy, as other conditions, such as latent TB infection or prior Bacillus Calmette-Guérin (BCG) vaccination, can also lead to positive results. Conversely, a negative tuberculin skin test outcome does not definitively exclude the possibility of tuberculous pleurisy, given that around one-third of individuals[22] with this condition might still exhibit negative test results. There are several reasons why this can occur. Firstly, the tuberculin skin test relies on the immune response, and it may take several weeks to develop a positive reaction after initial infection. Therefore, if the test is performed early in the course of the disease before an adequate immune response has developed, a false-negative result may occur. Additionally, factors such as immunosuppression, malnutrition, and concurrent illnesses can weaken the immune response and reduce the sensitivity of the tuberculin skin test. It is important to interpret the test results in the context of the patient's clinical presentation, risk factors, and other diagnostic findings. If TB is suspected despite a negative tuberculin skin test, further investigations should be pursued to establish the diagnosis.

MANAGEMENT OF TUBERCULAR PLEURAL EFFUSION

The goals of the management of TPE should be as follows:

- *Alleviate symptoms*: The treatment should focus on relieving the symptoms associated with TPE.
- *Prevent future recurrences*: Efforts should be made to prevent the disease from recurring in the future, regardless of the specific type of TB.
- *Avoid complications*: Treatment should also aim to prevent any further complications that may arise due to persistent effusion in the pleural space.

Antitubercular Chemotherapy

The chemotherapy regimen for treating TPE is the same as that for pulmonary TB. It consists of an intensive phase lasting 2 months, during which four drugs are administered (rifampicin, isoniazid, ethambutol, and pyrazinamide). This is followed by a continuation phase lasting 4 months, during which three drugs are given (rifampicin, isoniazid, and ethambutol). These medications are provided under directly observed treatment short-course (DOTS) as per the guidelines of the National Tuberculosis Elimination Program (NTEP) for drug-sensitive TPE. In cases of multidrug-resistant (MDR) or extensively drug-resistant (XDR) TB, or any drug-resistant cases, treatment should be administered according to the national guidelines and the patient's specific drug resistance pattern.

Symptoms typically resolve within 2 weeks of starting treatment, although some patients may experience persistent symptoms for up to 2 months or longer. Therapeutic thoracocentesis can aid in the early resolution of symptoms, often within 4–5 days.[22]

Approximately 50% of patients may develop pleural thickening after 6–12 months of initiating treatment.[24] The presence of pleural thickening does not correlate with the initial findings of pleural fluid. Nevertheless, individuals with low glucose, elevated LDH, and heightened cytokine levels do exhibit a slightly elevated likelihood of experiencing residual pleural thickening.[23] Over time, the residual thickening gradually improves after the completion of treatment. There is no significant correlation between completely removing the fluid at the beginning of treatment and the development of residual pleural thickening. A randomized trial conducted by Lai et al., involving 118 patients, showed no difference in residual pleural thickening between a group receiving pigtail drainage until drainage decreased to <50 mL/day or ceased entirely, and a group without drainage, at the end of the treatment period.[24]

Corticosteroids

The use of corticosteroids in the treatment of tubercular pleurisy is a topic of debate and remains controversial. A recent Cochrane review conducted by Ryan et al., which included six trials with 590 participants, found that corticosteroids may have several beneficial effects. They concluded that corticosteroids could potentially reduce the time needed for resolution of pleural effusion, lower the risk of residual pleural effusion on chest X-rays, and decrease the likelihood of developing pleural thickening and adhesions. However, the review did not find any impact on long-term functional respiratory impairment in patients who received corticosteroids.[25] It is important to note that despite these findings, the current guidelines from the World Health Organization (WHO) and the national guidelines do not recommend the routine use of corticosteroids in patients with tubercular pleurisy.

There are apprehensions regarding the use of corticosteroids in individuals who are HIV-positive due to the potential heightened risk of opportunistic infections. In one randomized study involving 197 patients with HIV-associated tubercular pleurisy, the use of prednisolone (a corticosteroid) was linked to an increased likelihood of developing Kaposi sarcoma, a type of cancer commonly seen in HIV patients.[26] Because there is no evidence of a survival benefit and an increased risk of Kaposi sarcoma, the use of corticosteroids in HIV-associated tubercular pleurisy is currently not advised.

Surgical Intervention

Routine surgical intervention is not necessary for the management of TPE. In most cases, treatment with antitubercular chemotherapy is sufficient. However, in situations where the effusion is massive and causing significant dyspnea, therapeutic thoracocentesis may be considered.[27,28]

Pleural thickening resolves with appropriate treatment and passage of time. Decortication is not recommended as a routine approach and should only be considered for symptomatic individuals with persistent symptoms related to pleural thickening after completing the treatment.

Tuberculous Bronchopleural Fistula

Tuberculous bronchopleural fistulas (BPF) are uncommon complications of TB, particularly in the era of modern chemotherapy. These fistulas occur when a sinus passage develops between the bronchial tree and the pleural space. The presence of a BPF is typically suggested by the observation of an air-fluid level in the pleural space on a chest radiograph, along with varying levels of sputum production **(Fig. 2)**.

Bronchopleural fistula can further complicate by the spread of infection between the tracheobronchial tree and the pleural space, and vice versa. Initially, BPF can be managed conservatively by use of antituberculous therapy and intercostal drainage.[29]

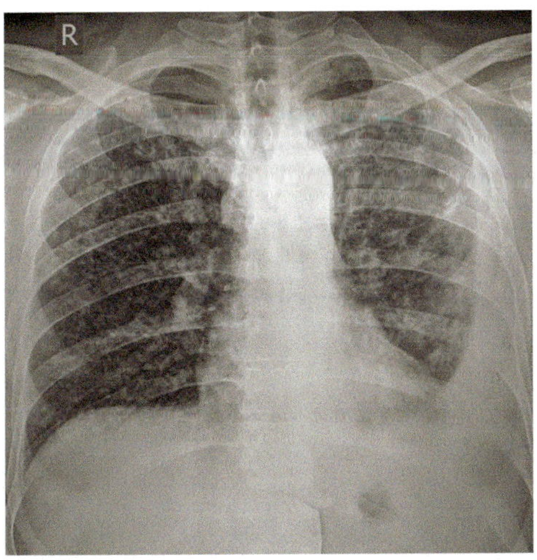

FIG. 2: Chest X-ray (CXR) anterior–posterior view of male patient with both pleural effusion and parenchymal infiltrates.

The treatment of BPF involves various surgical and medical procedures, with bronchoscopy playing a crucial role. Endoscopic interventions, such as the use of glues, coils, and sealants, can be considered depending on the localization and size of the fistula. The choice between surgical and endoscopic procedures depends on individual circumstances and the characteristics of the fistula. Definitive treatment for nonresolving BPF is decortication but should be considered only after administering chemotherapy for at least 3–4 months or until sputum conversion to negative.

KEY POINTS

- Tuberculosis remains a leading infectious disease globally, with millions of new cases and deaths each year. In 2021, 10.6 million people developed TB worldwide, resulting in 1.6 million deaths.
- TB primarily targets the lungs; approximately 15–20% of cases present as extrapulmonary TB.
- TPE ranks as the second most common form of extrapulmonary TB.
- Patients exhibit symptoms such as pleuritic chest pain, cough, fever, night sweats, dyspnea, and weight loss.
- TPE usually has unilateral presentation but can also manifest bilaterally in some cases.
- A conclusive diagnosis can be established by identifying MTB in pleural fluid, pleural biopsy, sputum, or pleural granulomas.
- Pleural fluid analysis reveals a lymphocyte-rich exudate with a straw-colored appearance, low glucose levels, elevated LDH, and increased protein content.
- ADA and IFN levels in pleural fluid are diagnostic markers.
- Tubercular skin testing can provide supportive evidence for the diagnosis, especially in regions with a low prevalence of TB, but it is not definitive on its own.
- The goals for the management of TPE should be to alleviate symptoms, prevent future recurrences, and avoid complications.
- The chemotherapy regimen for treating TPE is identical to that used for pulmonary TB after ruling out drug resistance.
- Routine use of corticosteroids is not advisable.
- For persistent pleural thickening, consider decortication, but after completing chemotherapy, as the thickening tends to gradually improve over time.
- Tuberculous BPF is an uncommon complication that necessitates a combination of surgical and medical interventions, where bronchoscopy plays a pivotal role in the management.
- Endoscopic interventions, such as the use of glues, coils, and sealants, can be considered depending on the localization and size of the fistula.

REFERENCES

1. Bagcchi S. WHO's Global Tuberculosis Report 2022. Lancet Microbe. 2023;4(1):e20.
2. Zhai K, Lu Y, Shi HZ. Tuberculous pleural effusion. J Thorac Dis. 2016;8(7):E486-94.
3. Lo Cascio CM, Kaul V, Dhooria S, Agrawal A, Chaddha U. Diagnosis of tuberculous pleural effusions: a review. Respir Med. 2021;188:106607.
4. Vorster MJ, Allwood BW, Diacon AH, Koegelenberg CFN. Tuberculous pleural effusions: advances and controversies. J Thorac Dis. 2015;7(6):981-91.
5. Shaw JA, Diacon AH, Koegelenberg CFN. Tuberculous pleural effusion. Respirology. 2019;24(10):962-71.
6. von Groote-Bidlingmaier F, Koegelenberg CF, Bolliger CT, Chung PK, Rautenbach C, Wasserman E, et al. The yield of different pleural fluid volumes for Mycobacterium tuberculosis culture. Thorax. 2013;68(3):290-1.
7. Roper WH, Waring JJ. Primary serofibrinous pleural effusion in military personnel. Am Rev Tuberc Pulm Dis. 1955;71(5):616-34.
8. Berger HW, Mejia E. Tuberculous pleurisy. Chest. 1973;63(1): 88-92.
9. Palma RM, Bielsa S, Esquerda A, Martínez-Alonso M, Porcel JM. Diagnostic accuracy of pleural fluid adenosine deaminase for diagnosing tuberculosis. Meta-analysis of Spanish studies. Arch Bronconeumol (Engl Ed). 2019;55(1):23-30.
10. Aggarwal AN, Agarwal R, Sehgal IS, Dhooria S. Adenosine deaminase for diagnosis of tuberculous pleural effusion: a systematic review and meta-analysis. PLoS One. 2019;14(3): e0213728.
11. Lee SJ, Lee SH, Lee TW, Lee HR, Cho YJ, Jeong YY, et al. Factors influencing pleural adenosine deaminase level in patients with tuberculous pleurisy. Am J Med Sci. 2014;348(5):362-5.
12. Pérez-Rodriguez E, Jiménez Castro D. The use of adenosine deaminase and adenosine deaminase isoenzymes in the diagnosis of tuberculous pleuritis. Curr Opin Pulm Med. 2000;6(4): 259-66.
13. Miller KD, Barnette R, Light RW. Stability of adenosine deaminase during transportation. Chest. 2004;126(6):1933-7.
14. Rabbi MF, Ahmed MN, Patowary MSA, Syed RH, SMA Razzaque, MA Hossain et al. Pleural fluid adenosine deaminase to serum C-reactive protein ratio for diagnosing tuberculous pleural effusion. BMC Pulm Med. 2023;23(1):349.
15. Ribera E, Ocaña I, Martinez-Vazquez JM, Rossell M, Español T, Ruibal A. High level of interferon gamma in tuberculous pleural effusion. Chest. 1988;93(2):308-11.
16. Jiang J, Shi HZ, Liang QL, Qin SM, Qin XJ. Diagnostic value of interferon-gamma in tuberculous pleurisy: a metaanalysis. Chest. 2007;131(4):1133-41.
17. Zhou Q, Chen YQ, Qin SM, Tao XN, Xin JB, Shi HZ. Diagnostic accuracy of T-cell interferon-γ release assays in tuberculous pleurisy: a meta-analysis. Respirol Carlton Vic. 2011;16(3): 473-80.
18. El-Hajj HH, Marras SAE, Tyagi S, Kramer FR, Alland D. Detection of rifampin resistance in Mycobacterium tuberculosis in a single tube with molecular beacons. J Clin Microbiol. 2001;39(11): 4131-7.
19. Boehme CC, Nabeta P, Hillemann D, Nicol MP, Shenai S, Krapp F, et al. Rapid molecular detection of tuberculosis and rifampin resistance. N Engl J Med. 2010;363(11):1005-15.
20. Conde MB, Loivos AC, Rezende VM, Soares SL, Mello FC, Reingold AL, et al. Yield of sputum induction in the diagnosis of pleural tuberculosis. Am J Respir Crit Care Med. 2003;167(5):723-5.
21. Wang Z, Xu LL, Wu YB, Wang XJ, Yang Y, Zhang J, et al. Diagnostic value and safety of medical thoracoscopy in tuberculous pleural effusion. Respir Med. 2015 Sep 1;109(9):1188-92.
22. Valdés L, Álvarez D, San José E, Penela P, Valle JM, García-Pazos JM, et al. Tuberculous pleurisy: a study of 254 patients. Arch Intern Med. 1998;158(18):2017-21.
23. Wyser C, Walzl G, Smedema JP, Swart F, Van Schalkwyk EM, Van de Wal BW. Corticosteroids in the treatment of tuberculous pleurisy: a double-blind, placebo-controlled, randomized study. Chest. 1996;110(2):333-8.
24. Gil V, Soler JJ, Cordero PJ. Pleural thickening in patients with pleural tuberculosis. Chest. 1994;105(4):1296.
25. Barbas CSV, Cukier A, de Varvalho CRR, et al. The relationship between pleural fluid findings and the development of pleural thickening in patients with pleural tuberculosis. Chest. 1 991;100:1264-1267.
26. Lai YF. Pigtail drainage in the treatment of tuberculous pleural effusions: a randomised study. Thorax. 2003;58(2):149-51.
27. Ryan H, Yoo J, Darsini P. Corticosteroids for tuberculous pleurisy. Cochrane Database Syst Rev. 2017;3(3):CD001876.
28. Elliott AM, Luzze H, Quigley MA, Nakiyingi JS, Kyaligonza S, Namujju PB, et al. A randomized, double-blind, placebo-controlled trial of the use of prednisolone as an adjunct to treatment in HIV-1-associated pleural tuberculosis. J Infect Dis. 2004;190(5):869-78.
29. Johnson TM, McCann W, Davey WN. Tuberculous bronchopleural fistula. Am Rev Respir Dis. 1973;107(1):30-41.

CHAPTER

8 Parapneumonic Effusions and Empyema

Roopanshi Jain, Rajkumar

INTRODUCTION

Infections of the pleural space constitute significant morbidity and mortality in major parts of the world.[1] Their incidence is increasing worldwide, despite a better understanding of the etiology, pathophysiology, and recent advances.[2,3]

Pleural complications of lung parenchymal infections occur mostly in the form of parapneumonic effusion (PPE) and empyema, which are among the leading causes of exudative effusion.

DEFINITIONS

Parapneumonic Effusion

Any pleural effusion associated with bacterial pneumonia, lung abscess, or bronchiectasis is called *PPE*.[4] They are further classified as uncomplicated, if treatable by antibiotic alone, and complicated if pleural drainage is required.[5,6]

Empyema

It refers to the macroscopic detection of purulent pleural fluid, i.e., pus in the pleural space or a positive pleural fluid Gram stain or culture.[7]

Empyema can be seen even in the absence of an underlying lung parenchymal infection (e.g., trauma, esophageal rupture, connective tissue diseases, such as rheumatoid arthritis, hematogenous spread of bloodstream infection, liver abscess, spine infection, and mediastinitis).

Pleural Infection

Pleural infection is defined as bacterial entry and their replication in the pleural space.[8] The term "pleural infection" includes both empyema and complicated parapneumonic effusion (CPPE).

PATHOPHYSIOLOGY

Initially from infected lung parenchyma, inflammatory cells are released in the pleura, leading to an inflammatory reaction inside the pleural space. This leads to the development of an exudative sterile pleural effusion (*uncomplicated PPE*).

In some cases, if an infection is not resolved, bacterial invasion can occur leading to the formation of *CPPE or empyema.*

With parapneumonic effusion:[9-11]

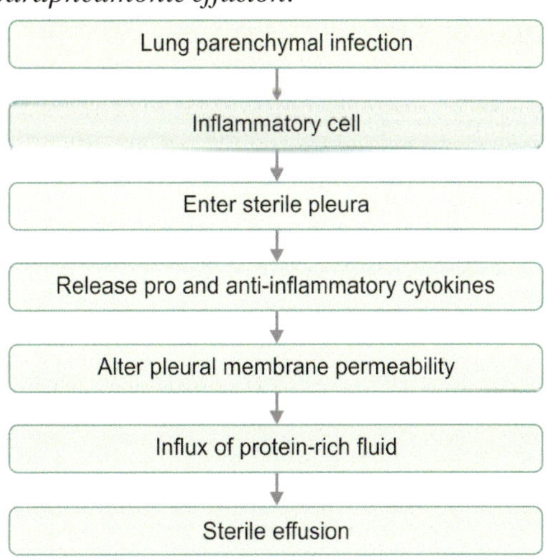

If bacterial invasion occurs:[12]

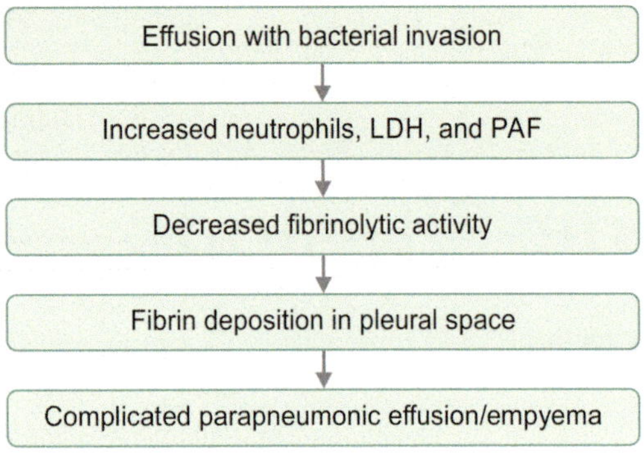

(LDH: lactate dehydrogenase; PAF: platelet-activating factor)

Pathophysiological Features

There are three stages for the development of PPE; however, each may not be distinct. They are as follows:[13]

1. *Exudative stage*: Fluid accumulation starts in the pleura. This fluid is sterile. The origin of the fluid is not exactly known. It is believed to originate either from interstitial spaces of the lung or capillaries of the visceral pleura. Pleural fluid is exudative with normal pH, normal glucose levels, low total leukocyte count (TLC), and low lactate dehydrogenase (LDH) levels. Treatment of lung parenchymal infection with antibiotics can prevent further progression.

   Effusion at this stage is also called *simple* or *uncomplicated PPE.*
2. *Fibropurulent stage*: In immunocompromised patients or if there is a delay in antibiotic course, bacteria from lung parenchyma may invade into the sterile pleural fluid. Neutrophil counts of the pleural fluid are raised. As the stage progresses, pleural fluid pH and glucose gradually decrease, and LDH increases. Bacteria and cellular debris may be found. Fibrin deposition starts on both visceral and parietal pleura-forming loculations, which may help to prevent the extension of the disease. Thoracocentesis or chest tube drainage may be needed.

   If frank pus is found, it is called *empyema;* otherwise this stage is called *CPPE.*
3. *Organizing stage*: With the disease progression, fibroblasts from the pleura grow into the exudate, leading to the formation of an inelastic membrane over the pleura called *pleural peel* or *fibrous peel.* This peel over the visceral pleura encases the lung parenchyma and prevents lung reexpansion. The pleural fluid becomes organized and difficult to drain.

   If the patient is left untreated, the fluid may drain spontaneously through the chest wall (*empyema necessitans*) or into the lung (*bronchopleural fistula*).

Table 1 summarizes the stages of the development of PPE or empyema.[1]

TABLE 1: Stages of a parapneumonic effusion/empyema.

Stage	Features
Exudative	Increased pleural membranes permeability with influx of inflammatory cells and protein-rich exudate *Treatment*: Antibiotics without pleural drainage
Early fibrino-purulent	• Increased procoagulant activity in the pleural space leading to fibrin deposition and septation • Pleural fluid becomes more viscous with increasing lactate dehydrogenase (LDH) and decreasing glucose and pH *Treatment*: Some patients may respond to antibiotics alone but drainage may be needed
Late fibrino-purulent	• Extensive fibrin deposition on pleural membrane: Loculations and pleural rind • Viable bacteria present. Markedly increase pleural fluid LDH and low glucose and pH Pleural fluid macroscopically appears purulent. *Treatment*: Pleural fluid drainage and possibly decortication
Organizing	Fibroblast proliferation leading to formation of fibrous pleural peel *Treatment*: Decortication (a trapped lung may occur if the empyema space is not obliterated)

RISK FACTORS

Pneumonia with PPE is more common in patients with immunosuppression, diabetes, cancer, alcoholism, poor dental hygiene, and high severity of pneumonia index.[14]

CLINICAL FEATURES

Patients usually present with the features of underlying lung parenchyma involvement, such as fever, cough, sputum, chest pain, and dyspnea. In elderly patients; however, these symptoms may be absent. They may present with generalized weakness and anemia and thus may be diagnosed at a later stage.

DIAGNOSIS

Investigations are done for the evaluation of the underlying lung parenchyma, pleura, and mediastinal lymph nodes. It also can help in the diagnosis of any other etiology like esophageal rupture and also to guide for pleural drain procedures.

Special investigations for diagnosis of underlying cause in cases of empyema without pneumonia are done on a case-by-case basis, for example, blood culture, ultrasound abdomen, etc.

Routine investigations include:

- *Chest X-ray*: This is the first investigation done in any patient with respiratory complaints. Finding depends on the site and extent of the disease. Commonly seen is obliteration of the costophrenic angle. Associated air bronchogram or mediastinal lymphadenopathy may be seen.[15]
- *Ultrasound chest*: This helps to evaluate for the quantity of pleural fluid, pleural septations, probable fluid consistency, and underlying lung consolidation. Semiquantitative to quantitative analysis of pleural fluid can be done with the measurement of pleural fluid thickness on ultrasound.
- *Contrast-enhanced computed tomography (CECT) of the chest*: It is needed in most of the cases. It gives a view of the underlying lung parenchymal involvement, mediastinal lymphadenopathy, visualizing septations, and a semiquantitative analysis of the free pleural fluid.
- *Pleural fluid analysis*: Thoracocentesis or an intercostal chest drain (ICD) insertion is done to get pleural fluid for analysis.
  Pleural fluid may appear to be clear in simple PPE. Turbid or frank pus can be seen in CPPE and empyema. A foul odor of the pleural fluid may indicate an anaerobic infection.[16,17] The presence of food particles indicates esophageal pleural fistula.[18] Microbiological yield of the pleural fluid can be increased by inoculating into the blood culture bottle media and by image-guided parietal pleural biopsy.[3]
  The following tests are routinely done **(Table 2)**.[1]
- *Sputum analysis or bronchoalveolar lavage*: It is a causative agent for pneumonia.
- *Pleural biopsy*: It is performed in certain undiagnosed cases.

ETIOLOGY

The knowledge of likely microbiological agents can help in selecting appropriate antibiotic therapy. Most of the community-acquired pleural infection is caused by gram-positive aerobic organisms. Anaerobic bacteria can be seen as a coinfection with aerobic organisms. Hospital-acquired pleural infections are caused mostly by resistant gram-positive organisms [e.g., methicillin-resistant *Staphylococcus aureus* (MRSA)] and gram-negative organisms with significant anaerobic involvement. Polymicrobial infection is rare. Fungal pleural infection is very rare (<1%),[19] and is usually seen in immunocompromised patients.[3] **Box 1** lists the common organisms responsible for pneumonia and effusion.[2]

TABLE 2: Common pleural fluid tests.

Test	Clinical significance
Cell count and differential	• Leukocyte counts vary depending on the stage of empyema formation (frank empyema may have low leukocyte counts because cells have undergone lysis) • The effusions are neutrophil predominant although (mononuclear cells may be high in partially treated PPE)
Protein	• Lights criteria to be applied • Values > 7.0 g/dL suggest Waldenström macroglobulinemia, multiple myeloma, or a cholesterol effusion
LDH	Defines an exudate in Light's criteria rule; (usually > 1,000 IU/L in empyema)
Microbiologic staining and culture	Cultures positive in ~60% of the patients who have signs of pleural infection
pH and glucose	• Pleural fluid pH and glucose decrease because of intrapleural bacterial metabolism and inflammatory cell activity that utilize glucose and release lactic acid • A PF pH < 7.20 and glucose < 60 mg/dL suggest that a PPE is complicated and requires drainage
Amylase (ordered in selected settings)	Empyema secondary to: • Esophageal rupture (elevated salivary isoenzyme of amylase) • Pancreaticopleural fistula (elevated pancreatic isoenzyme of amylase)

(PF: pleural fluid; PPE: parapneumonic effusion; LDH: lactate dehydrogenase)

BOX 1 Common microbiology of pleural infection.

- *Gram-positive bacteria:*
  - *Streptococcus pneumoniae*
  - *Staphylococcus aureus*
  - *Streptococcus pyogenes*
  - *Bacillus anthracis*
- *Gram-negative:*
  - *Escherichia coli*
  - *Klebsiella pneumoniae*
  - *Pseudomonas*
  - *Haemophilus influenzae*
  - *Proteus* species
  - *Legionella* species
- *Anaerobic bacteria:*
  - *Bacteroides*
  - *Peptostreptococcus*
  - *Fusobacterium*
  - *Prevotella*
  - *Clostridium*
- *Other organisms:*
  - Fungi
  - *Nocardia*
  - Parasite
  - Viral

TABLE 3: Renal, age, purulence, infection source, and dietary factors (RAPID) score.

Parameter	Measure	Score
Renal	Urea (mmol/L) < 5.0	0
	5.0–8.0	1
	> 8.0	2
Age	<50 years	0
	50–70 years	1
	>70 years	2
Purulence of pleural fluid	Purulent	0
	Nonpurulent	1
Infection source	Community-acquired	0
	Hospital-acquired	1
Dietary factor	Albumin (g/L) >27.0	0
	<27.0	1
Risk category	Score 0–2	Low risk
	Score 3–4	Medium risk
	Score 5–7	High risk

POOR PROGNOSTIC FACTORS

- Healthcare-acquired pleural infection
- The presence of septations on ultrasound
- High scores of CT scoring system of PPE
- Based on CT radiological features including pleural contrast enhancement, pleural microbubbles, increased attenuation of extrapleural fat, and pleural fluid volume > 400 mL, and diagnosis of CPPE can be made with a CT score ≥ 4.[20]
- Higher renal, age, purulence, infection source, and dietary factors (RAPID) scores **(Table 3)** indicate an increased risk of mortality and may indicate an increased length of hospital stay.[21]
- Higher Charlson Comorbidity Index Score (CCIS) is associated with an increased risk of mortality.

Pleural fluid characteristics indicating bad prognosis:[2]

- Pus present in pleural space
- Gram stain of pleural fluid positive
- Pleura fluid glucose below 40 mg/dL
- Pleura fluid culture-positive
- Pleura fluid pH < 7.0
- Pleura fluid lactate dehydrogenase (LDH) > 3× upper limit of normal for serum

MANAGEMENT

The management of PPE and empyema involves:[2]

- Selection of an appropriate antibiotic
- Management of the pleural fluid

Antibiotic

Most of the PPE can be resolved with the administration of sensitive antibiotics. However, initial antibiotic treatment starts before pleural fluid culture results are available. The initial antibiotic is usually based on the patient's clinical status and site of pneumonia acquisition. Due to geographic differences in microbiological pattern, the prevalence of the local flora has to be taken into account. Antibiotic penetration in the pleura should be considered as all antibiotics do not penetrate the pleura.

- Common antibiotics that can penetrate pleura include metronidazole, penicillin, clindamycin, vancomycin, ceftriaxone, and gentamicin.[22] A fair penetration of antibiotics such as quinolones, clarithromycin, azithromycin, linezolid, and ertapenem has also been found.[23-26]
- Initially, intravenous antibiotics are preferred, which can later be switched to oral.
- For patients with nonsevere community-acquired pneumonia, the recommended agents are a β-lactam (cefotaxime, ceftriaxone, ampicillin-sulbactam, or ertapenem) or a fluoroquinolone alone (levofloxacin and moxifloxacin).[27]
- In patients with severe community-acquired pneumonia, the recommended agents are a β-lactam plus either an advanced macrolide or a respiratory fluoroquinolone.[27]
- If a *Pseudomonas* infection is suspected, an anti-pseudomonal antibiotic such as piperacillin-tazobactam, imipenem, meropenem, and cefepime should be included.[27]
- Anaerobic coverage is recommended for all patients with PPE with either clindamycin or metronidazole.[28]
- *Hospital-acquired pleural infection*: Gram-negative bacteria and MRSA cover should be made (e.g., meropenem and vancomycin).[29]
- A positive culture test from pleural fluid or blood culture prompts targeted antibiotic treatment.

In general, a treatment of 2 and 6 weeks of antibiotic therapy is needed. Shorter courses may result in clinical relapse.[3]

Table 4 summarizes the usual empirical antibiotics.

Intrapleural Antibiotics

Instillation of intrapleural antibiotics is not recommended for patients with PPE due to a lack of randomized controlled trials (RCTs).

Options for Management of Pleural Fluid

Drainage of infected fluid from the pleural space is needed to achieve source control. Various methods by which the

TABLE 4: Empirical antibiotics as per the clinical settings.

Etiology	Antibiotic
Community-acquired pleural infection	• Second- or third-generation cephalosporin plus anaerobic cover (e.g., cefuroxime + metronidazole) • β-lactam (ampicillin–sulbactam) alone or with respiratory fluoroquinolones
Hospital-acquired pleural infection	Cover gram-negative organisms and potentially MRSA (e.g., meropenem + vancomycin)
Pseudomonas	• Piperacillin–tazobactam • Imipenem/meropenem • Cefepime
Anaerobes	• Metronidazole • Clindamycin

infected pleural fluid may be removed, ranges from simple percutaneous aspiration (thoracocentesis) to drainage via ICD tube placement to a more invasive thoracoscopic and surgical measures.[3]

Pleural fluid management:
- Observation
- Thoracentesis
- Tube thoracostomy (ICD)
- VATS with adhesiolysis and decortication
- Thoracotomy with adhesiolysis and decortication
- Intrapleural instillation of fibrinolytics

Observation

Observation is avoided because pleural fluid has to be examined to determine if its immediate drainage is required (e.g., empyema).[30] If drainage is delayed, loculations may develop.[16,31] If at all needed, observation can be done if the effusion is <10 mm in thickness on the decubitus chest radiograph, ultrasonography, or chest CT scan.[2]

Thoracocentesis

Thoracocentesis is done for pleural fluid examination especially culture and sensitivity. It can be diagnostic or therapeutic. In few cases, thoracocentesis along with broad-spectrum or sensitive antibiotics is enough to cure PPE. Daily therapeutic thoracentesis in patients with complicated PPE starting 48 hours after empyema induction may be beneficial in some.[32,33] Repeated thoracocentesis however can lead to septae formation in the pleural space.

Intercostal Drain Insertion

Intercostal chest drain (or tube thoracostomy) is widely used to drain CPPE and empyema. The tube is connected to a three-bottle connection system with water seal drainage. There is an arrangement for negative suction application, in case needed. Intercostal chest drain is positioned ideally in the largest locule or the most dependent region of the effusion. Presence of a pleural rind over visceral pleura may require application of a negative suction to the chest tube to aid expansion of the underlying lung.

Not only the presence of purulent pleural fluid but various other parameters may hint toward ICD placement. These include pleural fluid biochemistry (pH, LDH, and glucose) and radiological features [thoracic ultrasound (TUS) and CT].[3] Ultrasonography (USG) of the chest along with CECT chest may improve the detection of CPPE and guidance for ICD placement.

Pleural Fluid pH

Pleural fluid pH appears to have a good sensitivity and specificity for identifying patients who may develop CPPE or empyema and thus require ICD:[3]
- pH > 7.38—very low risk of CPPE
- pH ≤ 7.15—high risk of CPPE
- pH between 7.16 and 7.38—with increasing pH there is a decreasing risk of CPPE/pleural infection (especially with pH > 7.22)

Pleural fluid LDH or glucose measurements appear to be less accurate than pH. Since pleural fluid pH and glucose are highly correlated, where immediate or accurate pH measurement is not possible, glucose measurement may help. An initial glucose of 4.0 mmol/L (in the nondiabetic patient) may indicate a moderate to high likelihood of CPPE.

Before going for ICD insertion alternative diagnoses that can mimic PPE with a low pH and/or loculations should be ruled out, e.g., rheumatoid effusion, mesothelioma, etc. After drainage, pleural fluid should be examined as early as possible to avoid false pH. Pleural fluid should be free from anesthetic agents or heparin for proper pH measurement.

Recommendations

- For patients with PPE or suspected pleural infection, where diagnostic aspiration does not yield frank pus, immediate pH analysis should be performed. Intercostal chest drain placement is recommended if:
  - *pH ≤ 7.2*: ICD insertion (if the volume is enough)
  - pH > 7.2 and < 7.4 but pleural fluid LDH > 3 upper limit of normal (ULN), especially if other clinical

parameters support CPPE or pleural fluid glucose ≤ 4.0 mmol/L (specifically if symptomatic patient, i.e., fever, high pleural fluid volume, septation, or empyema such as features in CECT chest and ultrasound chest.
- If pH measurement is not available, pleural fluid glucose <3.3 may warrant ICD

Successful drainage of CPPE is evidenced by clinical and radiologic improvement within 24 hours of the placement. Improper placement of ICD may lead to failure of fluid drainage.[34] Failure can also be due to the presence of loculations that prevent complete pleural drainage, or the presence of pleural rind that prevents expansion of the underlying lung. If the drainage is inadequate, a CECT chest should be obtained and if multiple loculi of pleural fluid are present, the patient should be considered for video-assisted thoracoscopic surgery (VATS) decortication.

Chest Tube Bore Size

Different studies have shown that chest tube bore size has no effect on the length of the hospital stay, need for thoracic surgery or mortality rate. Rather a bore size > 14 F may increase posttreatment pain. Thus, it is a conditional recommendation by the British Thoracic Society (BTS) 2023 statement that initial drainage of pleural infection should be undertaken using a small-bore chest tube.

Duration[2]

There is no definite duration for ICD placement. In general, ICD is not removed until the volume of the pleural drainage is <50 mL for 24 hours.[35] Amount of pleural fluid sediment in the water seal drainage [representing white blood cells (WBCs) and debris] should be measured daily and ICD should not be removed until the collection is <5 mL. If the ICD becomes nonfunctional, i.e., no column movement is witnessed in the ICD, it should be removed. If the patient responds clinically and radiologically to ICD placement, but purulent drainage continues, thoracoscopy or thoracotomy should be considered.[35]

Surgery

A significant proportion of patients may fail to improve with optimal medical treatment and ICD. In these patients, surgical intervention may be required. Specific criteria for surgical referral are not defined.

Decortication is the most frequent surgery done in CPPE and empyema. In decortication, all the pus from the pleural space is evacuated and most of the fibrous tissue over the visceral and parietal pleura is removed.[36] Decortication helps in controlling pleural sepsis and allowing the underlying lung to expand. A CECT of the chest is always done before surgery to provide a guide about the anatomic extent and size of the empyema cavity and also the thickness of the pleural surface.[37]

Surgical approaches that can be used to access the infected pleural space include:
- Endoscopic technique—VATS
- Open techniques—thoracotomy

Video-assisted thoracoscopic surgery is preferred over thoracotomy because if the lung fails to expand, the VATS can be converted to a thoracotomy.

Video-assisted thoracoscopic surgery is very effective at treating incompletely drained PPEs. With this minimally invasive surgery, locules in the pleural space are disrupted and pleural space is drained. Pleural biopsy can be taken and ICD can be optimally placed.[37,38] If the lung is trapped, decortication can be attempted. In the acute stages, decortication should only be done to control the pleural infection and should not be considered just to remove the thickened pleura. This is so because such pleural thickening usually resolves itself over several months.[39,40] If it persists after 6 months and the patient's pulmonary function gets markedly reduced, decortication can be considered.

Less immediate postoperative pain and complications with a shorter hospital stay, are seen following VATS in comparison with thoracotomy. Postoperative mortality or the need for a repeat intervention are similar in either approach.

Intrapleural Therapies

These include the use of fibrinolytic with or without intrapleural enzyme therapy, saline irrigation, and intrapleural antibiotics.

Intrapleural Fibrinolytics

Pleural fluid loculations are difficult to drain. Intrapleural fibrinolytics destroy the fibrin membranes of the locules and thus facilitate drainage of the pleural fluid.[41] Earlier used intrapleural streptodornase for fibrinolysis was discouraged because its intrapleural injection was associated with systemic side effects such as fever, malaise, and leukocytosis.[42] In the landmark study on the use of intrapleural fibrinolytics for drainage of infected pleural fluid [Multicenter Intrapleural Sepsis Trial (MIST1)], the administration of streptokinase failed to improve mortality, need for surgery or length of hospitalization stay.[43]

It has been hypothesized that plasminogen levels in the pleural fluid are probably low, making streptokinase less effective. Direct plasminogen activators, such as tissue plasminogen activator (tPA), may overcome this problem.

The MIST2 study evaluated the efficacy of tPA and deoxyribonuclease (DNase), alone and in combination for the treatment of CPPE. The administration of the combination of tPA and DNase resulted in a significant reduction of the pleural opacity, less surgical referrals and a shorter hospital stay than did the administration of either alone.[44] Thus, a combination of tPA and DNase is recommended if one elects to use fibrinolytic therapy. Hemothorax is a rare complication.

A recommended regimen of tPA plus DNase is 10 mg tPA twice daily (10 mg BD) with 5 mg DNase twice daily (5 mg BD) for 3 days. However, consider reduced doses of tPA in patients with a potentially higher risk of bleeding.

Saline irrigation (250 mL saline TDS): It may reduce the need for thoracic surgery but does not reduce the length of the hospital day or have mortality benefits.

Open Procedures

In nonresolving empyema, chronic drainage of the pleural space may be needed. This is achieved with open drainage procedures.

Either of the two procedures can be performed:[45]

1. Resecting a few segments of one to three ribs overlying the lower part of the empyema cavity and making an open flap. After the rib resection, a skin and muscle flap is positioned in such a way that it lines with the tract between the pleural space and the surface of the chest[45] This open flap (Eloesser flap) creates a skin-lined fistula that provides drainage without tube. It can be easily managed by the patient at home. Cosmetic reasons are to be considered.
2. Inserting one or more short-length, large-bore tubes into the empyema is called *open drainage*. Daily irrigation of a mild antiseptic solution can be done. This tube can be connected to a colostomy bag placed if the drainage is needed. The advantage of this method is that the patient is freed from attachment to the ICD bottle. Before doing this procedure, the ICD is disconnected from the water seal drainage and is exposed to atmospheric pressure for a short period of time to evaluate for the development of lung collapse. If the two pleural spaces around the site of empyema have not fused, there may be development of a pneumothorax. If the lung does not collapse, this procedure can be attempted.

Table 5 shows the Light's classification of PPE and is based on the pleural fluid characteristics and the modalities discussed above.

TABLE 5: Light's classification of PPE.

Class	State	Description
Class 1	Nonsignificant pleural effusion	• <10 mm thick fluid collection on decubitus X-ray • *Rx*: No treatment is needed
Class 2	Typical PPE	• >10 mm thick fluid collection • Glucose > 40 mg/dL • pH >7.2 • LDH < 3 times ULN for serum • Gram stain and culture-negative • *Rx*: Antibiotic alone
Class 3	Borderline complicated pleural effusion	• pH < 7.20 but > 7.0 • LDH >3 times ULN for serum • Glucose > 40 mg/dL • Gram stain and culture-negative • *Rx*: Antibiotics + thoracocentesis
Class 4	Simple complicated pleural effusion	• pH < 7.0 • Glucose < 40 mg/dL • Gram stain and culture-positive • No pus • No loculations • *Rx*: Antibiotics + ICD
Class 5	Complex complicated pleural effusion	• pH < 7.0 • Glucose < 40 mg/dL • Gram stain and culture-positive • No pus • Multiple loculations • *Rx*: Antibiotics + ICD ± fibrinolysis (rarely thoracoscopy and decortication)
Class 6	Simple empyema	• Frank pus • Free-flowing • Rx: Antibiotics + ICD + decortication
Class 7	Complex empyema	• Frank pus • Multiple locules • Rx: Antibiotics + ICD ± fibrinolysis (mostly require thoracoscopy and decortication)

(ICD: intercostal chest drain; LDH: lactate dehydrogenase; PPE: parapneumonic effusion; Rx: medical prescription, ULN: upper limit of normal)

CONCLUSION

Being one of the most common causes of exudative pleural effusion, PPE, and empyema are to be diagnosed properly and treated on time. While management differs from clinician to clinician, BTS guidelines guide for a treatment protocol. **Flowchart 1** summarizes the management of PPE and empyema.

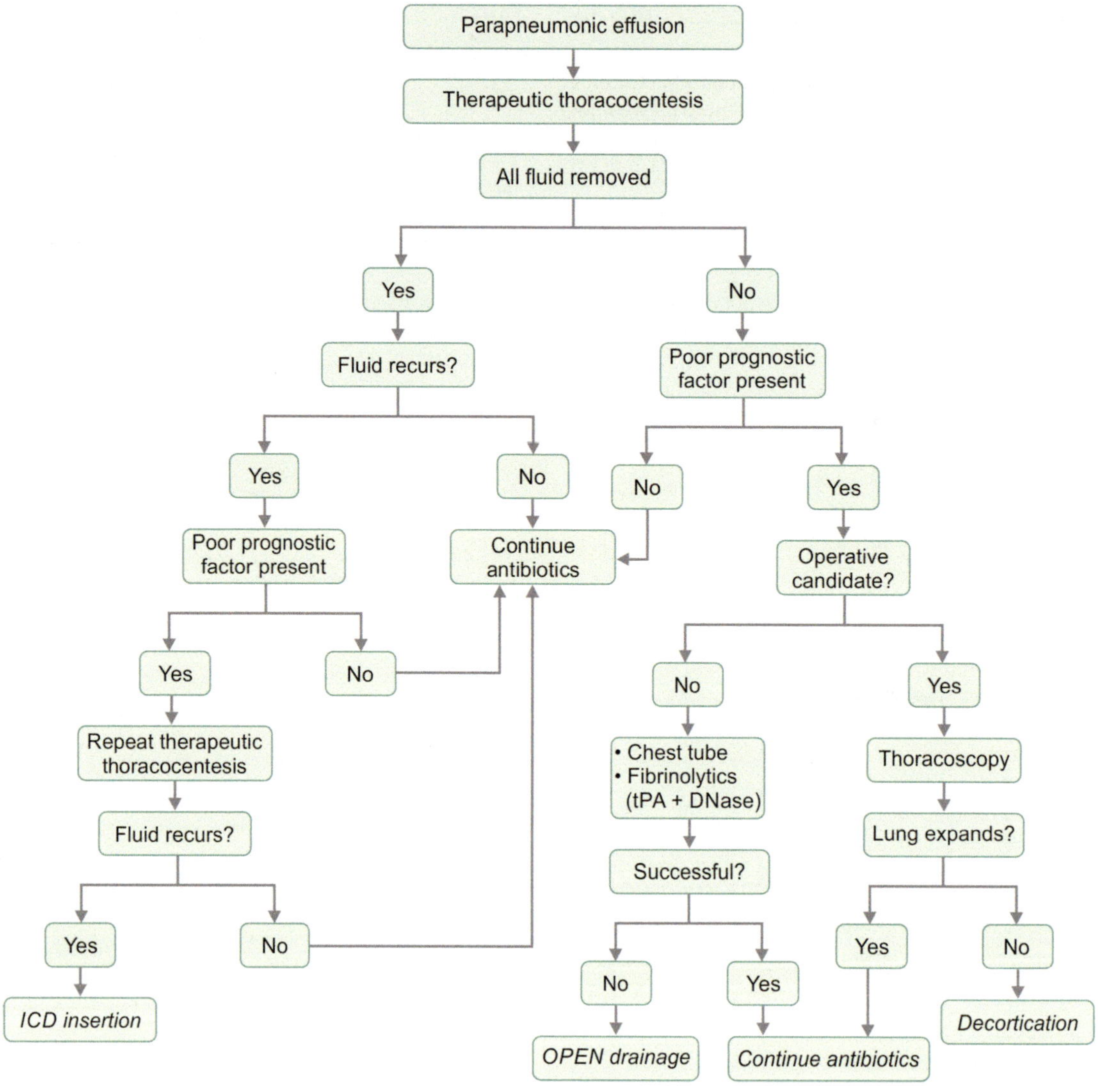

FLOWCHART 1: Management of PPE and empyema.

KEY POINTS

- It is to summarize that pleural effusion in many cases is just a PPE that resolves with pneumonia treatment.
- Parapneumonic pleural effusion with time may progress into CPPE or empyema.
- Thoracocentesis for biochemistry, cytological, and microbiological analysis of the pleural fluid should be done.
- Appropriate antibiotic treatment with thoracocentesis and/or intercostal drainage tube helps in the treatment of CPPE or empyema.
- Fibrinolytics (tPA + DNase) or surgical intervention is needed in certain cases.
- In nonexpanding lungs, thoracoplasty or open drainage can be attempted.

REFERENCES

1. Grippi MA, Antin-Ozerkis DE, Cruz CSD, Kotloff RM, Kotton C, Pack AI. Fishman's Pulmonary Diseases and Disorders, 6 edition. New York: McGraw Hill; 2023.
2. Light RW. Pleural Diseases, 6th edition. Philadelphia: Lippincott Williams and Wilkins; 2013.
3. Asciak R, Bedawi EO, Bhatnagar R, Clive AO, Hassan M, Lloyd H, et al. British Thoracic Society Clinical Statement on pleural procedures. Thorax. 2023;78(Suppl 3):s43-68.
4. Light RW, MacGregor MI, Ball WC Jr, Luchsinger PC. Diagnostic Significance of Pleural Fluid pH and Pco2. Chest. 1973;64(5): 591-6.
5. Colice GL, Curtis A, Deslauriers J, Heffner J, Light R, Littenberg B, et al. Medical and Surgical Treatment of Parapneumonic Effusions: An Evidence-Based Guideline. Chest. 2000;118(4):1158-71.
6. Davies HE, Davies RJ, Davies CW; BTS Pleural Disease Guideline Group. Management of pleural infection in adults: British Thoracic Society pleural disease guideline 2010. Thorax. 2010;65(Suppl 2):ii41-53.
7. Chen KY, Liaw YS, Wang HC, Luh KT, Yang PC. Sonographic septation: a useful prognostic indicator of acute thoracic empyema. J Ultrasound Med. 2000;19(12):837-43.
8. Chen JS, Chan WK, Tsai KT, Hsu HH, Lin CY, Yuan A, et al. Simple aspiration and drainage and intrapleural minocycline pleurodesis versus simple aspiration and drainage for the initial treatment of primary spontaneous pneumothorax: an open-label, parallel-group, prospective, randomised, controlled trial. Lancet. 2013;381(9874):1277-82.
9. Sahn SA. Diagnosis and management of parapneumonic effusions and empyema. Clin Infect Dis. 2007;45(11):1480-6.
10. TaryleDA, Potts DE, Sahn SA. The incidence and clinical correlates of parapneumonic effusions in pneumococcal pneumonia. Chest. 1978;74(2):170-3.
11. Light RW, Girard WM, Jenkinson SG, George RB. Parapneumonic effusions. Am J Med. 1980;69(4):507-12.
12. Menendez R, Torres A, Zalacain R, Aspa J, Martín Villasclaras JJ, Borderías L, et al. Risk factors of treatment failure in community acquired pneumonia: implications for disease outcome. Thorax. 2004;59(11):960-5.
13. Andrews NC, Parker EF, Shaw RR, Wilson NJ, Webb WR. Management of nontuberculous empyema: a statement of the subcommittee on surgery. Am Rev Respir Dis. 1962;85:935-6.
14. Hooper CE, Edey AJ, Wallis A, Clive AO, Morley A, White P, et al. Pleural irrigation trial (PIT): a randomised controlled trial of pleural irrigation with normal saline versus standard care in patients with pleural infection. Eur Respir J. 2015;46(2):456-63.
15. Kearney SE, Davies CW, Tattersall DJ, Gleeson FV. The characteristics and significance of thoracic lymphadenopathy in parapneumonic effusion and empyema. Br J Radio. 2000;73(870): 583-7.
16. Bartlett JG, Finegold SM. Anaerobic infections of the lung and pleural space. Am Rev Respir Dis. 1974;110(1):56-77.
17. Sullivan KM, O'Toole RD, Fisher RH, Sullivan KN. Anaerobic empyema thoracis. Arch Intern Med. 1973;131:521-7.
18. Landay MJ, Christensen EE, Bynum LJ, Goodman C. Anaerobic pleural and pulmonary infections.] AJR Am J Roentgenol. 1980;134(2):233-40.
19. Cho S, Ryu KM, Jheon S, Sung SW, Kim BH, Huh DM. Additional mechanical pleurodesis after thoracoscopic wedge resection and covering procedure for primary spontaneous pneumothorax. Surg Endosc. 2009;23(5):986-90.
20. Chew R, Gerhardy B, Simpson G. Conservative versus invasive treatment of primary spontaneous pneumothorax: A retrospective cohort study. Acute Med Surg. 2014;1(4):195-9.
21. Rahman NM, Kahan BC, Miller RF, Gleeson FV, Nunn AJ, Maskell NA. A clinical score (RAPID) to identify those at risk for poor outcome at presentation in patients with pleural infection. Chest. 2014;145(4):848-55.
22. Teixeira LR, Sasse SA, Villarino MA, Nguyen T, Mulligan ME, Light RW. Antibiotic levels in empyemic pleural fluid. Chest. 2000;117(6):1734-9.
23. Liapakis IE, Kottakis I, Tzatzarakis MN, Tsatsakis AM, Pitiakoudis MS, Ypsilantis P, et al. Penetration of newer quinolones in the empyema fluid. Eur Respir. 2004;24(3):466-70.
24. Liapakis IE, Light RW, Pitiakoudis MS, Karayiannakis AJ, Giamarellos-Bourboulis EJ, Ismailos G, et al. Penetration of clarithromycin in experimental pleural empyema model fluid. Respiration. 2005;72(3):296-300.
25. Saroglou M, Ismailos G, Tryfon S, Liapakis I, Papalois A, Bouros D. Penetration of azithromycin in experimental pleural empyema fluid. Eur J Pharmacol. 2010;626(2-3):271-5.
26. Saroglou M, Tryfon S, Ismailos G, Liapakis I, Tzatzarakis M, Tsatsakis A, et al. Pharmacokinetics of linezolid and ertapenem in experimental parapneumonic pleural effusion. J Inflamm (Lond). 2010;7:22.
27. Mandell LA, Barltett JG, Dowell SF, File TM Jr, Musher DM, Whitney C. Update of practice guidelines for the management of community-acquired pneumonia in immunocompetent adults. Clin Infect Dis. 2003;37(11):1405-33.
28. Rahman NM, Chapman SJ, Davies RJ. The approach to the patient with a parapneumonic effusion. Clin Chest Med. 2006;27(2):253-66.
29. Wrightson JM, Davies RJ. The approach to the patient with a parapneumonic effusion. Semin Respir Crit Care Med. 2010;31(6):706-15.
30. Light RW, Girard WM, Jenkinson SG, George RB. Parapneumonic effusions. Am J Med. 1980;69(4):507-11.
31. Cham CW, Haq SM, Rahamim J. Empyema thoracis: a problem with late referral. Thorax. 1993;48(9):925-7.
32. Sasse S, Nguyen T, Teixeira LR, Light R. The utility of daily therapeutic thoracentesis for the treatment of early empyema. Chest. 1999;116(6):1703-8.
33. Storm HKR, Krasnik M, Bang K, Frimodt-Møller N. Treatment of pleural empyema secondary to pneumonia: thoracocentesis regimen versus tube drainage. Thorax. 1992;47(10):821-4.
34. Kerr A, Vasudevan VP, Powell S, Ligenza C. Percutaneous catheter drainage for acute empyema. Improved cure rate using CAT scan, fluoroscopy, and pigtail drainage catheters. N Y State J Med. 1991;911:4-7.
35. Sherman MM, Subramanian V, Berger RL. Management of thoracic empyema. Am Surg. 1977;133(4):474-9.
36. Thurer RJ. Decortication in thoracic empyema. Indications and surgical technique. Chest Surg Clin N Am. 1996;6(3):461-90.

37. Silen ML, Naunheim KS. Thoracoscopic approach to the management of empyema thoracis. Indications and results. Chest Surg Clin N Am. 1996;6(3):491-9.
38. Bilgin M, Akcali Y, Oguzkaya F. Benefits of early aggressive management of empyema thoracis. ANZ J Surg. 2006;76(3): 120-2.
39. Neff CC, Van Sonnenberg E, Lawson DW, Patton PS. CT follow-up of empyemas: pleural peels resolve after percutaneous catheter drainage. Radiology. 1990;176(1):195-7.
40. Jimenez Castro D, Diaz G, Perez-Rodriguez E, Light RW. Prognostic features of residual pleural thickening in parapneumonic pleural effusions. Europ Respir J. 2003;21(6):952-5.
41. Rahman NM. Intrapleural agents for pleural infection: fibrinolytics and beyond. Curr Opin Pulm Med. 2012;18(4): 326-32.
42. Light RW, Nguyen T, Mulligan ME, Sasse SA. The in vitro efficacy of varidase versus streptokinase or urokinase for liquefying thick purulent exudative material from loculated empyema. Lung. 2000;178(1):13-8.
43. Maskell NA, Davies CW, Nunn AJ, Hedley EL, Gleeson FV, Miller R, et al. U.K. controlled trial of intrapleural streptokinase for pleural infection. N Engl Med. 2005;352(9):865-74.
44. Rahman NM, Maskell NA, West A, Teoh R, Arnold A, Mackinlay C, et al. Intrapleural use of tissue plasminogen activator and DNase in pleural infection. N Engl Med. 2011;365(6):518-26.
45. Deslauriers, Jacques LF, Gregoire J. Role of Eloesser flap and thoracoplasty in the third millennium. Chest Surg Clin N Am. 2002;12(3):605-23.

CHAPTER 9

Pleural Effusion Secondary to Fungal, Nocardia, and Parasitic Infections

Sonam Singla, Manan Bedi

INTRODUCTION

Empyema thoracis is an infection of the pleural space. Empyema is common and a leading cause of morbidity and mortality worldwide. Empyema usually occurs due to an underlying infection of the lung parenchyma, but can also be caused by a blood-borne infection, chest surgery, trauma, abdominal infection, or neoplasm. The most common infectious cause of empyema is bacterial (anaerobic and aerobic); however, *Mycobacterium tuberculosis*, fungi, *Nocardia* species, are increasingly isolated due to increased awareness and improved diagnostic facilities.

FUNGAL INFECTION OF PLEURA

Fungal infection of pleura is a rare and emerging entity associated with high morbidity and mortality.[1] The various predisposing factors such as use of broad-spectrum antibiotics, immunocompromised states in individuals with leukemia, lymphoma, human immunodeficiency virus (HIV), posthematopoietic stem cell transplantation (HSCT), prolonged use of steroid therapy, and rarely postoperative cases of lobectomy/pneumonectomy, bronchopleural fistula formation, and lung procedures have increased the likelihood of development of fungal infections of the pleura.[2] Hence, a high clinical suspicion, early diagnosis, and management of fungal infections will prevent morbidity and mortality.[3]

Fungal pulmonary infections are more commonly a parenchymal problem; however, fungal empyema thoracis is usually acquired in the hospital. In a study, 84% patients acquired fungal pleural infections mostly in intensive care units (ICUs), and the overall mortality accounted for 73%.[4] Candidiasis accounts for most of the cases of fungal empyema thoracis; other fungi as causative organisms are rare and only a few cases have been reported. Pleural cryptococcosis and *Aspergillus* empyema thoracis have also been reported as a result of a ruptured aspergilloma cavity or as a complication of a preexisting chronic empyema but it is extremely rare to isolate fungi in pleural fluid.[5]

Unlike bacterial infections of the pleura, which may spread to the pleural effusions from parenchymal lung infections like pneumonia; fungal infections require breach of the pleura to enter the pleural space.[6] Fungal empyema thoracis occur as a parapneumonic process and can also occur as a complication of medical procedures.[5]

Clinical factors leading to increase incidence of fungal lung infections: The increasing trend in the incidence of opportunistic fungal pathogens is due to various factors. Following are some of the factors:

- Increase in number of susceptible hosts. This is due to increased indications for hematological transplantation procedures, including the use of CD341 selected autografts.
- Evolving solid organ and stem cell transplantation practices has contributed to the increased prevalence of fungal infections.
- Antimicrobial prophylactic regimens for immunosuppressed patients including the use of fluconazole antifungal prophylaxis, antivirals, and the wide use of fluoroquinolones for gram-negative bacterial prophylaxis, has rendered the host at greater risk for colonization with more resistant fungal species, enhancing the incidence of invasive fungal infection.

- Increase awareness and suspicion of fungal infections among clinicians, in addition to improved laboratory diagnostic methods.[3]
- The criteria for diagnosis fungal empyema thoracis is as following:
  - Isolation of a fungal species from the pleural fluid
  - Significant signs of infection, such as fever (body temperature > 38.3°C) and leukocytosis (white blood cell > 10,000/mL)
  - Isolation of the same fungal species from pleural effusion on more than one occasion, or from pleural effusion and other specimens such as blood, sputum, and surgical wounds that showed evidence of tissue invasion.[7]

Candida

Invasive candidiasis has emerged as an important nosocomial infection, especially in critical patients. According to a data from the Centre of Disease Control (CDC) between 1980 and 1990, *Candida* species emerged as the sixth most common nosocomial pathogen (7.2% of total).[8] In an analysis from Taiwan from 1990 to 1997, 67 of the patients with fungal pleural infection were identified. It was observed that *Candida* species was isolated in 60 of 73 isolates.[4]

In another study, *Candida* was responsible for 44% of pleural space infections in a series of consecutive lung transplant recipients whose pleural fluid was sampled in the 90 days after transplantation.[9]

The common risk factors include abdominal disease or gastrointestinal perforation, insertion of drainage tube, and immunocompromised status.[1] It usually presents as superadded infection with bacterial infection. Such cases of effusions can lead to empyema. The clinical presentation of empyema is septicemia, followed by breathlessness and effusion.

Diagnostic workup is done by thoracocentesis which may reveal exudative effusion with budding yeasts cells with pseudohyphae on microscopy. Treatment is mainly focused on the surgical closure of the perforation along with appropriate antifungal and antibiotic coverage and catheter drainage in cases of empyema. Conventional treatment is done with 400 mg/day of fluconazole or 0.7 mg/kg of amphotericin B.[6,10]

Aspergillus

Aspergillus species are ubiquitous saprophytic fungi that are present in the air, water, soil, and decaying vegetables. *Aspergillus* species encompass a wide-spectrum of human diseases with pulmonary aspergillosis the most important and of clinical significance.[11] *Aspergillus* empyema is relatively uncommon entity amongst the spectrum of invasive *Aspergillus* infection. The most common causative pathogen seen in pleural aspergillosis is *Aspergillus fumigatus* although *Aspergillus flavus*, *Aspergillus niger*, and *Aspergillus terreus* has also been isolated.[6]

Pleural aspergillosis is a rarely reported disease; however, it is associated with a high risk of mortality, mostly due to late or missed diagnosis and lack of safe and effective treatment.[12] The most common preceding conditions associated with pleural aspergillosis are preexisting tuberculosis, development of bronchopulmonary fistulas, pleural drainage, and lung resection.[13] The presence of a direct communication between the airway and the pleural space allows seeding of the pleura by inhaled *Aspergillus* conidia or direct endobronchial spread of infection in patients with preexisting disease. The presence of a necrotic exudate and an aerobic environment provide conditions in which the organism may thrive. The comorbidities includes diabetes, long-term oral steroid use, cirrhosis, solid organ transplant, in human immunodeficiency virus (HIV), and alcohol abuse.[13]

Clinical presentation includes anorexia, weight loss, productive cough of chronic duration and low-grade fever. Pleural thickening and air fluid levels are observed on imaging. Suspicious cases can be diagnosed with fungal culture which is time consuming.[6]

The histological diagnosis of invasive aspergillosis requires the presence of invasion of the lung tissue by fungus of the *Aspergillus* species.[14]

Serological markers including galactomannan assay may be detectable in pleural fluid. *Aspergillus* specific immunoglobulin G (IgG) can also be done.[11]

Optimal treatment to prevent invasion and destruction of lung is excision of the pleura with resection of the involved lobe or lung at the earliest with preoperative and postoperative coverage with antifungals such as itraconazole and voriconazole to reduce the chances of *Aspergillus* infection of the pleura.[6] Patients who are not fit for surgery can be given intrapleural antifungal therapy (amphotericin B/nystatin) via intercostal drain. In view of the good pleural space penetration, micafungin and voriconazole can also be used.[10] The surgical resection and thoracoplasty as treatments for pleural aspergillosis are prone to many complications and should be avoided.[14]

Histoplasmosis

Histoplasma capsulatum is a dimorphic fungi mostly found in soil around poultry, farms, caves, or the construction sites. Infection is acquired from inhalation of such contaminated dust. Pleural involvement in histoplasmosis is very uncommon and is seen in immunocompromised cases or disseminated histoplasmosis.

It commonly presents as subpleural nodules or infiltrate with acute or chronic presentation. Pleural effusion can be seen with pleural nodules presenting subacutely with low-grade fever, malaise, and pleuritic chest pain.[6,10]

Clinical suspicion followed by radiological evidence of nodules or infiltrate with effusion can be confirmed with pleural fluid analysis showing exudative etiology with lymphocyte predominance, fungal culture of the pleural fluid, and sputum or biopsy material demonstrating the organism. Noncaseating granulomas can be seen on pleural biopsy with raised antibody titers of *Histoplasma* using complement fixation (CF) serological test. Pleural effusion usually resolves spontaneously with time. Rarely, the treatment with amphotericin B is required with dissemination or drainage/decortication is required in cases of empyema if occurs.[6]

Coccidioides

Coccidioidomycosis refers to the spectrum of disease caused by the dimorphic fungi *Coccidioides immitis*. The infection is acquired by inhalation of arthroconidia causing primary pulmonary coccidioidomycosis. With recent increase in domestic and international travel, a detailed travel history must be taken to consider *Coccidioides* infection as a differential diagnosis.[15]

Pulmonary coccidioidomycosis commonly presents as community-acquired pneumonia. Pleural effusions can be associated with pulmonary foci in 10% of the patients.[16]

It produces either primary pleural disease presenting as mild to moderate exudative effusion with chest pain and fever, or causes cavity formation which ruptures into the pleural space resulting in hydropneumothorax or bronchopleural fistula (BPF) having an acute presentation. The diagnosis is made by pleural fluid analysis with exudative picture with eosinophilia, fungal culture, pleural biopsy, and additional cocci skin test titers. Treatment of primary pleural effusion is conservative with only disseminated cases requiring systemic antifungal therapy. However with hydropneumothorax or BPF, treatment is done with intercostal chest drain (ICD) placement with systemic antifungals followed by which the surgery for cavity removal and BPF closure may be required.[17,18]

Cryptococcosis

Cryptococcosis is an opportunistic fungal disease caused by *Cryptococcus neoformans*, an encapsulated dimorphic fungus.[19] The common source of exposure involves contact with soil contaminated with bird droppings. The infection spread by inhalation, and despite the fact that the virus most commonly enters the body through the lungs, meningoencephalitis is the most common clinical manifestation of the infection.[20] Pulmonary cryptococcosis (PC) is diagnosed with increasing incidence in recent years in both immunocompromised and immunocompetent patients.[19,21] Pulmonary cryptococcosis presents with a wide range of radiological patterns such as nodules, consolidation, pneumonia, and miliary lesions, and rarely pleuritis.[22] Till date, only 50 cases of cryptococcal pleuritis in relation to the lung and disseminated disease has been reported.[19,21]

The diagnosis of cryptococcal pleural infection requires isolation of *Cryptococcus* species in the effusion or pleura and is typically established by examination of pleural biopsy or fluid culture.[20] However, the yield from a pleural fluid culture for *Cryptococcus* is approximately 50% due to the small amount of organisms present in the pleural fluid.[22]

India ink staining is the traditional method for identifying *Cryptococcus* by delineating the refractile mucinous capsule surrounding the organism, giving the organism a characteristic "starry night" appearance.[23] Another method for diagnosis is the detection of cryptococcal antigen in the pleural fluid. The antigenemia could be due to dissemination of the fungus via subpleural pulmonary lesions.[22] Detecting *Cryptococcus neoformans* by histopathological examination is the gold standard for confirming the diagnosis. There are 100% detection rates of *Cryptococcus neoformans* with Gomori methenamine silver stain and periodic acid–Schiff stain.[20]

Because of the diagnostic difficulty of cryptococcal pleural infection, there have been similar case reports of these patients who were initially treated for the pleural tuberculosis because of the raised adenosine deaminase (ADA) levels in exudative lymphocytic pleural effusions. Adenosine deaminase is useful in the diagnosis of pleural tuberculosis due to its high sensitivity, where a negative result helps to exclude tuberculosis, and a high level lymphocytic effusion strongly favors tuberculosis.[21]

Patients with pleural cryptococcosis not always require treatment. Many patients with pleural infection recover spontaneously without the treatment, while those with symptoms and positive cryptococcal antigen in blood in immunosuppressed cases require treatment with fluconazole in a dose of 400 mg/day for 6 months, while those with cryptococcal antigen positive in cerebrospinal fluid (CSF) therapy treatment with amphotericin B and flucytosine is recommended. Rarely, tube thoracostomy may be required in severe cases.[6]

Blastomyces

Blastomyces dermatitidis is the etiologic agent of blastomycosis. The infection is usually acquired after the inhalation of conidia or inoculation.[24]

Empyema caused by blastomycosis are usually associated with acute airspace pneumonia.[25] Of a series of the 26 patients with pulmonary blastomycosis, 23 (88%) showed radiographic evidence of blastomycotic pleural disease; of these, only four patients had pleural effusions and the patients responded well to amphotericin B therapy.[26]

The pleural effusions are usually small and cause blunting of the costophrenic angle on X-ray. The cytological examination of pleural fluid may aid in the diagnosis of pleural effusion if the characteristic broad-based budding yeasts are seen. Fungal cultures of the pleural fluid are more reliable but take time. Treatment consists of itraconazole in patients with localized disease while in patients with disseminated infection; liposomal amphotericin B is the treatment of choice.[6,25]

Others

Pneumocystis jirovecii is rarely seen to cause pleural effusion in human immunodeficiency virus (HIV) cases which is usually an extension of the pneumonia. *Pneumocystis* pneumonia-associated bilateral pleural effusions have been reported after hematopoietic stem cell transplantation (HSCT); however, identification of *Pneumocystis* pneumonia (PCP) from pleural fluid is rare.[5]

Rare cases of pleural effusion with *Sporothrix schenckii*, *Paracoccidioides brasiliensis*, and *Talaromyces* (previously known as *Penicillium marneffei*) *marneffei* has been reported.[5]

PARASITIC INFESTATION OF PLEURA

Pleural parasitic infestation (PPI) is an extremely rare pleural disease caused by a variety of parasites, such as the lung fluke *Paragonimus westermani*, *Toxocara* species, *Clonorchis sinensis*, *Spirometra* species, and *Taenia solium*. Pleural parasitic infestation may only have pleural involvement, or other nonspecific pulmonary manifestations.

Lung diseases caused by parasites is either due to transient passage in the lung or as a result of an immunologic reaction.[27] There are different pleural manifestations in patients with PPI, such as pleural thickening, pleural effusion, empyema, and chylothorax. The clinical manifestations are nonspecific and many patients are initially treated for tuberculosis or misdiagnosed as lung cancer.[28] With increasing globalization, it is important to consider parasitic infections in the differential diagnosis of the lung diseases.

Echinococcosis (Hydatid Disease)

Causative organism is the tapeworm *Echinococcus granulosus*. The transmission is via definitive host like dogs/wolves, which ingest meat containing larvae and their feces contain eggs of parasite which after ingestion in humans are lodged in tissues and cause the disease. It commonly presents as pulmonary or hepatic hydatid cyst which ruptures into the pleural space causing effusion and very rarely pulmonary hydatid cyst enlarge to cause pleural involvement. Symptoms of acute rupture are sudden severe chest pain, breathlessness, coughing of pus or cyst material such as cyst membranes and shock if the cyst gets ruptured. Radiological features such as single and multiple well-defined round cysts or cyst with air fluid level in cases of secondary infection support the diagnosis.[29]

On examination, peripheral and pleural fluid eosinophilia is seen; demonstration of scolices with hooklets in pleural fluid establishes diagnosis with serology being less sensitive in pulmonary hydatid than hepatic disease. Casoni skin test and Weinberg complement fixation test (CFT) is seen positive in many cases. Patients are usually asymptomatic and are incidentally found to have hydatid cysts. Treatment of hydatid disease is elective surgical resection of the cyst however in cases of rupture urgent thoracotomy with drainage of cyst and antiprotozoal therapy with albendazole 400 mg twice a day for 28 days is given. Decortication may be required in cases of the delayed surgical intervention.

Amoebiasis

Low socioeconomic or poor sanitary conditions favor amoebiasis. *Entamoeba histolytica* is the common infecting species. It has a fecal-oral route of transmission via the ingested cysts. These cysts proliferate to form trophozoites, which inhabit the large intestine and are the potent forms to cause invasion to the portal circulation and cause hepatic abscess.[30]

Pleural effusion is commonly seen due to irritation of diaphragm with sympathetic stimulation by the abscess; however, can also be seen with rupture of the hepatic abscess into the pleural space via diaphragm. Rupture of abscess produces anchovy paste which is a mixture of cytolyzed liver parenchyma with blood. Clinical presentation is usually right upper abdominal pain and tenderness with right-sided pleuritic chest pain with sepsis and shock occurring in severe cases. Peripheral eosinophilia with deranged liver function tests is usually seen. Serology testing is helpful in diagnosis along with radiological evidence via ultrasound (USG), chest X-ray, and computerized tomography (CT) abdomen. Treatment in reactive effusion is with metronidazole 500–750 mg TDS for 10 days.[31] In cases with a large effusion or rupture of abscess, a pigtail catheter drainage with medical therapy is advised.

Paragonimiasis

The causative agents are lung flukes of the *Paragonimus* genus. Most cases are caused by *Paragonimus westermani* and other species include *Paragonimus miyazakii, Paragonimus mexicanus,* and *Paragonimus skrjabini.* Humans are infected by eating crayfish or water crab containing larvae which migrates from small intestine to the lung. Migration of the warm causes pleural effusion, pneumothorax, and chronic pleural thickening. As the worm resides, it causes cystic lesion with ischemic infarction and intraluminal occlusion by the worm. Patient's presents with pleuritic chest pain, fever, or chronic cough with rusty expectoration and hemoptysis if the cyst erodes the bronchi.[32]

Diagnosis is done by demonstration of the eggs in stool, sputum, bronchoalveolar lavage (BAL) or biopsy material. Serological diagnosis is done by identifying specific antibody. Peripheral eosinophilia with raised immunoglobulin E (IgE) levels are seen. Pleural fluid analysis showing exudative picture, eosinophilia, raised interleukin-5 (IL-5) levels, raised levels of IgE and IgG levels specific to parasite. Cholesterol crystals with pseudochylothorax are also seen in pleura fluid. Treatment is done by praziquantel in the dose of 25 mg/kg thrice for 3 days. Treatment involves surgical intervention in patients with pneumothorax, empyema, or pleural thickening.

Others

Parasitic infections may disseminate and involve the pleura in HIV infected patients. Microsporidia, *Trypanosoma cruzi* (Chagas disease), *Leishmania donovani*, and *Leishmania chagasi* (visceral leishmaniasis) have been isolated in the pleural fluid in such patients.[5]

Tropical pulmonary eosinophilia is caused by reaction to microfilaria along with *Strongyloides*, *Toxocara*, and ascariasis. They may have allergic or inflammatory pleural effusion being associated with the primary illness.[33,34]

NOCARDIA

Nocardia species, belong to *Actinomycetes* group, are ubiquitous in the environment, especially in soil, organic matter, and water. It is a normal oral flora, in gingiva and periodontal pockets along with other species such as *Actinomyces* and *Streptomyces.*[35]

Nocardia are gram-positive filamentous bacteria causing opportunistic infection in the patients with long-term corticosteroid exposure, malignancy, human immunodeficiency virus (HIV) infection, and history of transplantation. However, infection in immunocompetent patients has also been reported.[36]

Nocardia infection can be classified as acute, subacute, and chronic infection. The infection is commonly acquired through inhalation and manifest as pulmonary, central nervous system, and cutaneous infections.[37] Hematogenous spread from cutaneous or pulmonary site can lead to disseminated nocardiosis. Pulmonary nocardiasis constitutes up to 70% of the total incidences of nocardiosis and this is due to the fact that the route of infection is by inhalation. *Nocardia asteroides* complex is the most common cause of pleuropulmonary nocardiosis while *Nippostrongylus brasiliensis* is an uncommon pulmonary pathogen.[38] Pleural involvement was observed in 36% cases of the pulmonary nocardiosis.[39] Pleural involvement occurs through direct spread from the chest wall or the lung parenchyma and pleural fluid may be the only source of diagnosis.

Pulmonary nocardiosis usually presents with subacute onset, but may manifest as an acute or chronic pneumonitis. It produces an indolent progressive pneumonia and shows a granulomatous lesion mimicking tuberculosis in immunocompetent subjects. In immunocompromised hosts, the lesions develop rapidly causing an acute pyogenic necrotizing pneumonia. The symptoms are nonspecific including weight loss, malaise, night sweats, and fever (low grade to spiking with chills). Pulmonary symptoms are cough, copious purulent/bloody sputum, pleuritic chest pain, and dyspnea. The pleural fluid is exudative, ranging from serous fluid to frank pus.

Radiologic finding on CT chest reveals multiple pulmonary infiltrates, solitary pulmonary nodule, lung abscess, and pleural involvement resulting in pleural thickening, pleural effusions and empyema.[35]

The diagnosis of *Nocardia* is difficult as the growth on culture media is slow and also there is a lack of serologic test for nocardiosis. Gram stain is useful for early diagnosis of nocardiosis. Gram-positive branching filaments with characteristic "beaded" staining is suggestive of *Nocardia.* It appears acid fast when stained with Modified Ziehl-Neelsen method using 1% sulfuric acid.

The isolation of *Nocardia* on routine culture media takes 3–5 days but usually negative bacterial culture are discarded within 72 hours leading to missed cases.[40]

Hence, a longer incubation is required before discarding the culture plates as negative for the isolation and identification of *Nocardia*.[38]

The drug of choice includes trimethoprim-sulfamethoxazole and more recently, along with trimethoprim-sulfamethoxazole (TMP-SMX), surgical drainage is done when required. The drugs such as minocycline, amikacin, imipenem, and linezolid are effective for the treatment of nocardiosis. The other effective drugs are ciprofloxacin, amoxyclav, the extended-spectrum cephalosporins, and azithromycin. The duration of the treatment is generally for 6–12 months.[38]

ACTINOMYCOSIS

Actinomyces israelii is a gram-positive anaerobic bacterium that inhabits the oropharynx, gastrointestinal tract, and urogenital tract. The sources of infection are dental caries, gum infection, or infected tonsils. The most common type of actinomycosis is cervicofacial followed by pulmonary or abdominopelvic followed by the cutaneous type.[41]

The clinical presentation of pulmonary actinomycosis has changed as in the past; it is mainly presented with pain in the chest along with multiple cutaneous sinus and fistulas. However, with judicial use of antibiotics, better oral hygiene and early disease diagnosis, it presents now either with features of chronic suppurative lung disease or radiological features mimicking lung malignancy. At times the pulmonary disease may get disseminated to cause multiple abscesses in skin, muscles, or peripheral tissues. Pleural space gets thickened with the extension of pulmonary infection beyond the chest wall to form sinus or abscess. Pleural effusion is mild and serous and may further get infected to cause empyema. Radiological workup with CT scan is beneficial with consolidation in patches, cavitation, multiple nodules, pleural thickening, or pleural effusions and hilar and/or mediastinal lymphadenopathy with more specific finding of rib erosion or osteomyelitis.[42]

Diagnosis is confirmed by microbiology or histopathology in suspected cases with pleural fluid. The microbiological examination by Gram stain and isolation of the bacteria from an infected specimen or histopathological evidence of sulfur granules. Pleural fluid analysis can be exudative with eosinophilia.

Treatment is done with injectable penicillin 10 million units/day for 4–6 weeks duration followed by oral therapy for next 12–18 months. Other alternatives such as macrolides, tetracycline, and clindamycin can be used in cases with hypersensitivity to the penicillin. In rare cases of empyema intercostal drainage may be required or decortication may be needed in severe cases. Prognosis of pulmonary actinomycosis is not good hence an early diagnosis and treatment is required.

KEY POINTS

- It is to summarize that in undiagnosed cases of the pleural effusion with suppressed immunity and with additional history of exposure, there should always be a high level of suspicion for secondary causes of empyema.
- Hence pleural fluid should be sent for cytological analysis, staining, and culture for diagnosing pleural effusion.
- The clinical picture should dictate additional testing by serology markers, molecular assays, or pleural biopsy.
- All high-risk and immunocompromised cases with undiagnosed etiology of pleural should undergo screening for fungal infections.
- Epidemiological trend and increased susceptibility for fungal infections is emerging in the current times.
- Although it is rarely seen but mortality rate associated with fungal empyema (FE) is around 70%; hence, early diagnosis and management is the key.

REFERENCES

1. Subramanian K, Ch Toi P, Siddaraju N. Fungal Empyema Thoracis due to Candida species: A diagnosis on fine needle aspiration cytologya. Eurasian J Pulmonol. 2022;24:144-6.
2. Ruff H. Fungal Infections, Pleural. In: Allen TC, Suster S (Eds). Pathology of the Pleura and Mediastinum. Encyclopedia of Pathology. Cham: Springer; 2018. pp. 117-9.
3. Limper AH. The changing spectrum of fungal infections in pulmonary and critical care practice: clinical approach to diagnosis. Proc Am Thorac Soc. 2010;7(3):163-8.
4. Ko SC, Chen KY, Hsueh PR, Luh KT, Yang PC. Fungal empyema thoracis: an emerging clinical entity. Chest. 2000;117(6):1672-8.
5. Bennett JE, Dolin R, Blaser MJ. Mandell, Douglas, and Bennett's Principles and Practice of Infectious Diseases, 9th edition. Amsterdam: Elsevier; 2019.
6. Degryse A, Light RW. Pleural Effusions-Infectious Disease and Antimicrobial agents. [online] Available from http://www.antimicrobe.org/e29.asp# [Last accessed October, 2023].
7. Baradkar VP, Mathur M, Kulkarni SD, Kumar S. Thoracic empyema due to Candida albicans. Indian J Pathol Microbiol. 2008;51(2):286-8.
8. Pal N, De A, Mondal M, Maiti PK. Candida albicans as a Rare Causative Agent of Pyopneumothorax. Int J Curr Microbiol App Sci. 2015;4(7):716-9.
9. Wahidi MM, Willner DA, Snyder LD, Curl J, Hardison JL, Chia JY, et al. Diagnosis and outcome of early pleural space infection following lung transplantation. Chest. 2009;135(2):484-91.
10. Senger SS, Thompson GR, Samanta P, Ahrens J, Clancy CJ, Nguyen MH. Candida empyema thoracis at two academic

medical centers: New Insights into treatment and outcomes. Open Forum Infect Dis. 2021;8(4):ofaa656.

11. Chang KM, Kim AC, Jurado JE, Donaghy HJ. Aspergillus pleural empyema in a chronic smoker: A case report and review of literature. J Mycol Med. 2022;32(4):101299.
12. Bhatnagar T, Bhatnagar AK. Pleural Aspergillosis in an otherwise healthy individual. Lung India. 2014;31(2):155-7.
13. Abreu I, Guedes M, Duro R, Lopes S, Maciel J, Santos L. Pleural Aspergillosis in a patient with recurrent spontaneous pneumothorax: The challenge of an optimal therapeutic approach. Med Mycol Case Rep. 2020;28:4-7.
14. Denning DW, Riniotis K, Dobrashian R, Sambatakou H. Chronic cavitary and fibrosing pulmonary and pleural aspergillosis: case series, proposed nomenclature change, and review. Clinic Inf Dis. 2003;37(Suppl-3):265-80.
15. Afshar K, Boydking A, Sharma OP. Exudative pleurisy of coccidioidomycosis: a case report and review of the literature. J Med Case Rep. 2008;2:291.
16. Thompson GR 3rd, Sharma S, Bays DJ, Pruitt R, Engelthaler DM, Bowers J, et al. Coccidioidomycosis: adenosine deaminase levels, serologic parameters, culture results, and polymerase chain reaction testing in pleural fluid. Chest. 2013;143(3):776-81.
17. Lin J, Hamill RJ. Coccidioidomycosis Pulmonary Infection. Curr Infect Dis Rep. 2001;3(3):274-8.
18. Merchant M, Romero AO, Libke RD, Joseph J. Pleural effusion in hospitalized patients with Coccidioidomycosis. Respir Med. 2008;102(4):537-40.
19. Zhang Y, Zhang SX, Trivedi J, Toll AD, Brahmer J, Hales R, et al. Pleural fluid secondary to pulmonary cryptococcal infection: a case report and review of the literature. BMC Infect Dis. 2019;19(1):710.
20. Georgakopoulou VE, Damaskos C, Sklapani P, Trakas N, Gkoufa A. Pleural involvement in cryptococcal infection. World J Clin Cases. 2022;10(16):5510-4.
21. Wee ACR, Seet JE, Venkatalacham J, Tan SK. Cryptococcal pleural infection in a recurrent pleural effusion: a case report. Respirol Case Rep. 2018;6(3):e00294.
22. Toranzo M, Arrojo M, Gonzalez A, Fielle M. Pleural effusion as a manifestation of pulmonary cryptococcosis. Univ Louisville J Respir Infect. 2020;4(2):Article 2.
23. Chen M, Wang X, Yu X, Dai C, Chen D, Yu C, et al. Pleural effusion as the initial clinical presentation in disseminated cryptococcosis and fungaemia: an unusual manifestation and a literature review. BMC Infect Dis. 2015;15:385.
24. Tadi LJ, Uma B, Ariyanachi K, Reddy NC. Disseminated Blastomycosis: A Case Report. J Case Rep Stud. 2001;9(2):204.
25. Eldaabossi S, Saad M, Aljawad H, Almuhainy B. A rare presentation of blastomycosis as a multi-focal infection involving the spine, pleura, lungs, and psoas muscles in a Saudi male patient: a case report. BMC Infect Dis. 2022;22(1):228.
26. Kinasewitz GT, Penn RL, George RB. The spectrum and significance of pleural disease in blastomycosis. Chest. 1984;86(4):580-4.
27. Al-Tawfiq JA, Kim H, Memish ZA. Parasitic lung diseases. Eur Respir Rev. 2022;31(166):220093.
28. Wang J, Luo W, Shen P, He J, Zeng Y. Retrospective study of pleural parasitic infestations: a practical diagnostic approach. BMC Infect Dis. 2019;19(1):576.
29. Aribas OK, Kanat F, Gormus N, Turk E. Pleural complications of hydatid disease. J Thorac Cardiovasc Surg. 2002;123(3):492-7.
30. Lyche KD, Jensen WA, Kirsch CM, Yenokida GG, Maltz GS, Knauer CM. Pleuropulmonary manifestations of hepatic amebiasis. West J Med. 1990;153(3):275-8.
31. Shamsuzzaman SM, Hashiguchi Y. Thoracic amebiasis. Clin Chest Med. 2002;23(2):479-92.
32. Strobel M, Veasna D, Saykham M, Wei Z, Tran DS, Valy K, et al. Pleuro-pulmonary paragonimiasis. Med Mal Infect. 2005;35(10):476-81.
33. Roberts PP. Parasitic infections of the pleural space. Semin Respir Infect. 1988;3(4):362-82.
34. Lal C, Huggins JT, Sahn SA. Parasitic diseases of the pleura. Am J Med Sci. 2013;345(5):385-9.
35. Sethy HK, Meher B, Pradhan S, Patro M. Pleuroplumonary Nocardiosis in an Immunocompetent Host. SAS J Med. 2016;2(4):79-83.
36. Zia K, Nafees T, Faizan M, Salam O, Asad SI, Khan YA, et al. Ten year review of pulmonary nocardiosis: A series of 55 cases. Cureus. 2019;11(5):e4759.
37. Sukahri S, Zainudin LD, Hadi MF, Firdaus MA, Hafidz MI. Recurrent empyema thoracic secondary to pulmonary nocardiosis in immunocompetent patients. Case Rep Pulmonol. 2020;2020:8840920.
38. Das AK, Nandy S, Dudeja M, Tiwari R, Alam S. The incidence of nocardiosis at pulmonary and extra-pulmonary sites. J Clin Diagn Res. 2013;7(7):1427-9.
39. Hui CH, Au VWK, Rowland K, Slavotinek JP, Gordon DL. Pulmonary nocardiosis re-visited: experience of 35 patients at diagnosis. Respir Med. 2003;97(6):709-17.
40. Gowrinath K, Rao PS, Mohapatra AK, Prakash PY. Pleural nocardiosis. Indian J Chest Dis Allied Sci. 2009;51:169-71.
41. Ghisalberti M, Madioni C, Ghinassi G, Maccari U, Corzani R, Meniconi F, et al. A Strange Case of Traumatic Pleural Effusion: Pleural Empyema due to Actinomyces meyeri, a Case Report. Life (Basel). 2023;13(7):1450.
42. Mabeza GF, Macfarlane J. Pulmonary actinomycosis. Eur Respir J. 2003;21(3):545-51.

CHAPTER

10 Pleural Diseases in HIV

Vikas Deswal, Sandeep K Mittal

INTRODUCTION

Pleural effusions are commonly observed in patients with acquired immunodeficiency syndrome (AIDS). Among hospitalized patients with AIDS, the prevalence of pleural effusion varied from 7 to 27%.[1,2] A wide range of prevalence can be explained by stage of the human immunodeficiency virus (HIV) infection and the techniques used to detect pleural effusion. Almost two-thirds of the pleural effusions in patients with HIV infection are caused by infections; however, approximately a third are due to noninfectious causes also.[3]

Majority of the data regarding prevalence come from hospitalized patients with advanced HIV infection in the prepotent antiretroviral therapy (ART) era which may not reflect the true prevalence in the current era of potent ART. With advancement in diagnostics, we can establish the etiology of most of the pleural effusion in patients with AIDS; however, a small percentage remains undiagnosed, as is the case in the non-AIDS population.[3]

INFECTIOUS CAUSES

We usually consider opportunistic infections of the pleura in patients with a CD4 count below 150 cells/mL, as these patients have an increased risk of opportunistic infection, possibly approaching that of prepotent ART patients. Many of the same infectious agents that cause lung parenchymal disease in AIDS should be considered as potential etiologies of pleural effusion.

Bacteria

Bacterial pneumonia is the cause of pleural effusion in almost one-third of hospitalized AIDS patients.[1,2] In patients with community-acquired pneumonia, HIV-infected patients had a higher rate of parapneumonic effusions than non-HIV-infected patients.[4] *Streptococcus pneumoniae* is the leading cause of parapneumonic effusions accounting for >50% of all cases. *Staphylococcus aureus* is the next most common etiologic organism, and less frequent causes include *Haemophilus influenzae, Mycoplasma pneumoniae, Legionella,* and *Nocardia.*[3]

With advent of potent ART, the incidence of bacterial pneumonia[5] and the complication of parapneumonic effusion have decreased in HIV-infected patients.[6]

Majority of the parapneumonic effusions are small and confined to the ipsilateral side of the pneumonia. The fluid is exudative and generally nucleated cell counts are low[3] **(Table 1)**. Empyema is common and, compared to immunocompetent patients, *S. aureus* was significantly more often isolated from pleural fluid culture in patients with AIDS.[4,7]

Pneumocystis jirovecii

Pneumocystis jirovecii (*P. jirovecii*) is an uncommon cause of pleural effusion in HIV-infected patients. The incidence of pleural effusion in HIV infection varies from 3 to 15% among hospitalized patients.[1,3] It is postulated that pleural effusion due to *P. jirovecii* is more common in patients receiving aerosolized pentamidine prophylaxis.[8] Pleural fluid is exudative and has poor cellular response **(Box 1)**.

TABLE 1: Stages of parapneumonic effusion and empyema: Diagnosis and management.

Stage	Stage 1 Uncomplicated/simple	Stage 2 Complicated/fibropurulent	Stage 3 Complicated/organized
Timing	Early (days)	Late (days to weeks)	Late (week to months)
Pleural fluid characteristics	• Exudative characteristics • Low to moderately elevated WBC • LDH level < 1,000 IU/L • Normal pH and glucose levels • No bacterial organisms	• Exudative characteristics • High WBC • LDH > 1,000 IU/L • pH < 7.20 • Glucose < 40 mg/dL *OR* • Bacterial organisms present	• Fluid may be difficult to obtain • Bacterial organisms may or may not be present
Imaging characteristics	• Generally small to moderate in size • Free flowing	Generally large and free flowing, loculated, and/or with associated pleural thickening with contrast enhancement	• May be large, loculated, and/or with pleural thickening (may be extensive and demonstrate a pleural rind) • Pleural calcification may be evident
Treatment	• Typically resolves with antibiotic therapy alone • Drain if symptomatic	• Antibiotics plus drainage • Fibrinolytics/DNase may be required	• Antibiotics plus drainage • Fibrinolytics/mucolytics *or VATS* may be required

(LDH: lactate dehydrogenase; VATS: video-assisted thoracoscopic surgery; WBC: white blood cell)

BOX 1 Characteristics of pleural fluid in *Pneumocystis jirovecii*.

- Small to moderate in size
- Can be either unilateral or bilateral
- Serous to bloody in appearance
- *Exudative in nature*:
  - Normal pH
  - Elevated lactate dehydrogenase (LDH): Pleural fluid to serum LDH ratio > 1
  - Pleural fluid to serum protein ratio < 0.5
  - Glucose and amylase—similar to serum values
- *Cellular response*:
  - Total leukocyte count (TLC)—low
  - Differential leukocyte count (DLC)—predominantly lymphocytic

A definitive diagnosis requires demonstration of the trophozoite or cyst forms of *Pneumocystis* in the pleural fluid. Grocott silver staining will show the cysts. A *P. jirovecii* polymerase chain reaction (PCR) on pleural fluid may be performed. The diagnosis of pleural effusion due to *Pneumocystis* can be made presumptively if the organisms are identified in bronchoalveolar lavage (BAL) fluid and the effusion resolves following treatment for *Pneumocystis jirovecii* pneumonia (PJP).

Neither the treatment nor the prognosis of PJP is altered by the development of a pleural effusion; however, the development of pneumothorax in these patients is often a sinister sign and usually indicates the need for prolonged chest tube drainage. Treatment of *P. jirovecii* pleural effusion is similar to PJP pulmonary parenchymal disease. The pleural fluid resolves as the interstitial infiltrate clears. ART should be started within 2 weeks after initiation of PJP treatment and once the patient has stabilized on it; however, in those already on ART, it should be continued.

Nocardia

Nocardia asteroides has been identified in about 3% of pleural effusions in patients with AIDS.[3,9] It is usually associated with advanced disease and almost all have AIDS-defining illness before or concurrently with nocardiosis.

The diagnosis of nocardiosis should be suspected when there is involvement of skin, lung cavities, pulmonary infiltrates, nodules, pleural effusion, and brain parenchyma (abscess or ring-enhancing lesion) in a host with a cell mediated immune defect like advanced HIV, organ transplant recipients and exposed to high dose systemic steroids. Pleural fluid analysis is exudative with low pH and glucose and is like an empyema. Prior to obtaining specimens for testing, laboratory personnel should be notified that *Nocardia* is suspected so they can take special measures to optimize results. Pleural fluid, sputum samples, and BAL if performed should be sent to a laboratory for Gram stain, modified Zeil Neilson stain. *Nocardia* species usually appear as delicate, branching, and filamentous, sometimes beaded gram-positive bacilli on Gram stain.[10] Among the various branching gram-positive bacilli, only *Nocardia* species will stain positive by modified acid-fast staining.[11] When no pathogen has been identified using traditional microbiologic testing and clinical suspicion remains for *Nocardia,* PCR or whole-genome sequencing on pleural fluid at reference laboratories may identify the organism.

With evidence of direct spread from the lung to the pleura, chest wall, or another contiguous organ, it will be managed like severe pulmonary disease. We suggest that patients with severe infection that does not involve the central nervous system (CNS) be treated initially with TMP-SMX trimethoprim/sulfamethoxazole [15 mg/kg intravenous (IV) of the TMP component per day in three or four divided doses] plus amikacin (7.5 mg/kg IV every 12 hours).

Duration of treatment: Initial injectable induction therapy—3–6 weeks, followed by 6–12 months of oral therapy.

Cryptococcus

Cryptococcus neoformans and *Cryptococcus laurentii* have been identified as causative agents of pleural effusion in HIV.[12,13] An isolated pleural effusion may be the initial presentation of disseminated disease. It is more severe and presents acutely than in a non-HIV host. Cryptococcal effusions are exudative with low total leukocyte count (TLC). Culture may yield the diagnosis in 41% cases. Serum and pleural fluid cryptococcal antigen should be performed in all AIDS patients with pleural effusion. Antigen tests may help in early diagnosis and prevent dissemination of disease. Pleural fluid culture should be incubated for 2 weeks before labeling it as negative; in select cases, pleural biopsy would yield definitive diagnosis.[14] Optimal treatment strategies are not well defined and are extrapolated from cryptococcal pulmonary or disseminated disease. Initial therapy with liposomal amphotericin (5 mg/kg for 7 days or single dose 10 mg/kg) should be followed by fluconazole 400 mg daily for 6–12 months. The decision to stop treatment should be made once the patient has immune reconstituted (CD4 > 100) on stable ART regimen, and serum cryptococcal antigen has turned negative.

Histoplasma

Pleural effusion due to *Histoplasma capsulatum* is rarely seen in both AIDS and non-AIDS patient.[15] It is usually seen as part of disseminated disease, contiguous spread, hypersensitivity pleuritis, and pericarditis. The effusion is serous with a low TLC. A cytocentrifuged pleural fluid specimen stained with Wright–Giemsa stain will demonstrate intracellular yeast typical of *H. capsulatum.* Isolated pleural disease due to *Histoplasma* may resolve spontaneously; however, disseminated disease would need treatment. Initial treatment is with liposomal amphotericin B (3–5 mg/kg) for 10 days followed by itraconazole for 1 year. Voriconazole and posaconazole can be used as an alternative to itraconazole.

Toxoplasma gondii

Toxoplasma gondii is a rare cause of pleural effusion. Pleural effusion may be unilateral or bilateral. A cytocentrifuged Wright–Giemsa-stained specimen of pleural fluid will demonstrate *T. gondii* tachyzoites within neutrophils. Tachyzoites can also be found in BAL fluid when there is concomitant pulmonary parenchymal disease.

MALIGNANT CAUSES

Kaposi's Sarcoma

Pleuropulmonary involvement is seen in 20% of AIDS patients with Kaposi's sarcoma.[1] There is a poor correlation between the extent of skin lesions and systemic involvement; thoracic Kaposi's sarcoma invariably would have concomitant skin lesions. Pleuritic chest pain is absent because the parietal pleura is spared and only visceral pleura is involved.

Pleural effusions are predominantly bilateral and are massive in size with or without alveolar infiltrates. 25–60% of patients with pleuropulmonary Kaposi's sarcoma would have associated hilar and mediastinal adenopathy.

Pleural fluid is exudative, low cell counts which is lymphocytic predominant with normal glucose concentration. Pleural fluid cytology is generally noncontributory. Chylous effusions have been increasingly recognized in Kaposi's sarcoma, but the hemorrhagic nature of the effusion may mask the typical appearance of a chylothorax. Pleural fluid triglyceride concentration will confirm the diagnosis if it is >110 mg/dL.[16] Since lesions are not present on parietal pleura, pleural biopsy is not helpful in establishing diagnosis. Lung biopsy is gold standard and often establishes the diagnosis. Bronchoscopic visualization of typical cherry-red endobronchial lesions may lead us to diagnosis in an appropriate clinical setting. Pleuropulmonary Kaposi's sarcoma has poor outcomes and combination chemotherapy, and ART may lead to partial clinical response.

Lymphoma

In AIDS, the prevalence of B-cell lymphoma is 5–10%. Mediastinal and hilar adenopathy is typically absent in AIDS-related lymphomas. Isolated pleural effusion can be the only manifestation of AIDS-related lymphoma. AIDS-related lymphoma-associated pleural effusion tends to be large, unilateral, and serosanguineous.[16] Pleural fluid is exudative, lymphocytic cellular response with normal glucose concentration. Pleural biopsy and pleural fluid cytology establish the diagnosis. Pleural fluid flowcytometric examination may yield the diagnosis in cases where pleural fluid cytology is noncontributory. Pleural effusion usually responds to chemotherapy and ART.

KEY POINTS

- Pleural effusion can be due to both infectious and noninfectious causes in patients with HIV.
- Consider opportunistic infections of the pleura in patients with a CD4 count below 150 cells/mL.
- The incidence of pleural diseases in HIV has decreased in the potent ART era.
- Tuberculosis (TB) and bacterial infection are common causes of pleural diseases in HIV.
- Common malignant causes include lymphoma and Kaposi's sarcoma.
- Pleural fluid analysis and pleural biopsy yield diagnosis in majority of cases.

REFERENCES

1. Afessa B. Pleural effusions and pneumothoraces in AIDS. Curr Opin Pulm Med. 2001;7(4):202-9.
2. Afessa B. Pleural effusion and pneumothorax in hospitalized patients With HIV Infection: The pulmonary complications, ICU support, and prognostic factors of hospitalized patients with HIV (PIP) study. Chest. 2000;117(4):1031-7.
3. Joseph J, Strange C, Sahn SA. Pleural effusions in hospitalized patients with AIDS. Ann Intern Med. 1993;118(11):856-9.
4. Suay VG, Cordero PJ, Martinez E, Soler JJ, Perpina M, Greses JV, et al. Parapneumonic effusions secondary to community-acquired bacterial pneumonia in human immunodeficiency virus-infected patients. Eur Respir J. 1995;8(11):1934-9.
5. Grau I, Pallares R, Tubau F, Schulze MH, Llopis F, Podzamczer D, et al. Epidemiologic changes in bacteremic pneumococcal disease in patients with human immunodeficiency virus in the era of highly active antiretroviral therapy. Arch Intern Med. 2005;165(13):1533-40.
6. Schlossbauer T, Schmidt GP, Bogner JR, Sing A, Reiser MF, Becker-Gaab C. Pulmonary radiological characteristics in patients with HIV infection at the time of highly active antiretroviral therapy (HAART). Eur J Med Res. 2007;12(8):341-6.
7. Coker RJ. Empyema thoracis in AIDS. J R Soc Med. 1994;87(2):65-7.
8. Horowitz MI, Schiff M, Samuels J, Russo R, Schnader J. Pneumocystis carinii Pleural effusion: Pathogenesis and pleural fluid analysis. Am Rev Respir Dis. 1993;148(1):232-4.
9. Uttamchandani RB, Daikos GL, Reyes RR, Fischl MA, Dickinson GM, Yamaguchi E, et al. Nocardiosis in 30 patients with advanced human immunodeficiency virus infection: clinical features and outcome. Clin Infect Dis. 1994;18(3):348-53.
10. Brown-Elliott BA, Brown JM, Conville PS, Wallace RJ. Clinical and laboratory features of the Nocardia spp. based on current molecular taxonomy. Clin Microbiol Rev. 2006;19(2):259-82.
11. Mohanty S, Mohanty M. Modified Acid-Fast Stain in the Diagnosis of Nocardia Infection: A Revisit. Am J Med Sci. 2021;361(1):e7-8.
12. Cartwright E, Rouphael N, Jain S, Ilksoy N. Pleural effusion in a patient with AIDS. Clin Infect Dis. 2008;46(12):1887-8.
13. Shankar EM, Kumarasamy N, Bella D, Renuka S, Kownhar H, Suniti S, et al. Pneumonia and Pleural effusion due to Cryptococcus laurentii in a clinically proven case of AIDS. Can Respir J. 2006;13:275-8.
14. Katz AS, Niesenbaum L, Mass B. Pleural effusion as the initial manifestation of disseminated cryptococcosis in acquired immune deficiency syndrome: Diagnosis by pleural biopsy. Chest. 1989;96(2):440-1.
15. Marshall BC, Cox JK jr, Carroll KC, Morrison RE. Case Report: Histoplasmosis as a cause of pleural effusion in the acquired immunodeficiency syndrome. Am J Med Sci. 1990;300(2):98-101.
16. Bhattacharya AK. Pleural effusion in aids. Lung India. 2005;22(3):101-4.

CHAPTER

11

Malignant Pleural Effusion

Manoj K Goel, Ajay Kumar, Gargi Maitra

INTRODUCTION

Malignant pleural effusion (MPE) is characterized by the presence of malignant cells in the pleural fluid and is suspected in a patient with a recurrent hemorrhagic pleural effusion. MPE, when present, is a sign of an advanced stage of either a thoracic or an extrathoracic malignancy. MPE usually occurs in patients with a history of advanced malignant disease, affecting 15% of oncologic patients,[1] but could also be the first presenting feature of malignancy. It is associated with a lower life expectancy, with the median survival ranging from 4 to 7 months, depending on the type of malignancy, tumor characteristics, the extent of disease, comorbidities, and the composition of the MPE.[2] It is a very disabling condition with a huge impact on quality of life (QOL).[3]

CLINICAL PRESENTATION

The clinical presentation of MPE is variable. Dyspnea on effort is the most common presenting symptom of MPE. Some cases present with acute respiratory distress needing urgent thoracocentesis. Other symptoms include cough, chest pain, weight loss, anorexia, and malaise.[3,4] The severity of the symptoms does not necessarily correlate with the volume of the pleural effusion. Factors such as underlying collapse of the lung parenchyma, consolidation and lymphangitis carcinomatosis due to underlying malignancy, and other pulmonary or cardiac comorbidities may affect symptomatology. Patients with mesothelioma may present with dull chest pain which is nonpleuritic.[5] Up to 25% of patients are asymptomatic.[3,4]

DIAGNOSTIC APPROACH

The diagnosis of MPE needs multiple modalities, including various imaging, pleural fluid examination, and pleural biopsy along with clinical correlation.

Imaging

Various imaging modalities are used for recognizing the presence of pleural effusion and guiding the invasive procedures for establishing the diagnosis while minimizing the risks of complications.

Chest X-ray

A posteroanterior chest X-ray (CXR) is the first imaging modality. Eighty percent of patients with MPE who present with dyspnea will demonstrate a moderate-to-large pleural effusion on CXR, 10% will have a massive pleural effusion, and 10% will present with an MPE of <500 mL.[6] A massive pleural effusion and underlying collapse of the ipsilateral lung is suggestive of MPE.

Thoracic Ultrasound

Thoracic ultrasound (US) findings suggestive of an MPE are pleural thickening (>1 cm), diaphragmatic nodules, pleural irregularity, and nodularity.[7] US is also the standard of care to identify the appropriate site for thoracocentesis and to guide intrapleural interventions such as chest-tube drainage.[8-10]

Contrast-enhanced Computed Tomography

Contrast-enhanced computed tomography (CT) of chest is useful in diagnosing the presence of a pleural effusion and associated mediastinal and parenchymal lesions. The CT scan may help differentiate between benign and malignant pleural disease as the CT finding suggestive of malignancy includes presence of pleural lesions > 1 cm, medial pleural and interlobar fissure thickening and nodularity, liver metastases, and a lung mass or nodule > 1 cm.[11,12]

Positron Emission Tomography

Positron emission tomography (PET) scans are performed as part of the staging evaluations for malignancy. The PET-CT findings are similar to those in the contrast-enhanced CT of chest, but in addition, the pleural lesions appear fluorodeoxyglucose (FDG) avid. PET-CT in the workup of an MPE also helps to determine anatomic sites of the pleura to biopsy. The PET imaging may be negative in the early stage tumors. It may be difficult to differentiate accurately between the malignancy and conditions such as inflammatory pleuritis only on the basis of PET-CT findings.[13]

Thoracic Magnetic Resonance Imaging

The clinical value of magnetic resonance imaging is yet to be determined as a diagnostic tool, and its use is limited to highly selected cases and research studies.

Diagnostic Thoracocentesis

Ultrasound-guided thoracentesis can be used for diagnosis of MPE. The majority of MPEs are lymphocyte-rich exudates, with approximately 5–10% being transudates.[14,15] Although the pleural fluid biochemistry is neither characteristic nor specific for MPE, pleural fluid cytology is the initial test with an overall diagnostic yield close to 60%.[16] The cytology has a high sensitivity for adenocarcinomas (79%) but very low for mesothelioma (6%).[17] It seems that a volume of 20–40 cc of pleural fluid is sufficient for cytological evaluation.[16] Pleural fluid aspiration can be safely performed in patients who have mild-to-moderate coagulopathy, renal disease, and thrombocytopenia.[18,19]

Pleural Biopsy

When the yield of pleural fluid cytology for diagnosis is nondiagnostic or low in a suspected case of MPE, the further approach is pleural biopsy, which is done either image guided or blindly. The gold standard procedure in diagnosing MPE is pleural biopsy.[20]

Percutaneous Blind Pleural Biopsy

Abraham's and Cope's needles have been traditionally used for the percutaneous blind pleural biopsies without imaging guidance. The blind pleural biopsies reportedly have a lower sensitivity as compared to cytology, as malignant parietal pleura infiltrates have a patchy pattern (46%),[14] but can improve the diagnostic sensitivity of pleural fluid cytology by 7–27%.[6] The complication rates of blind pleural biopsy are as high as 14.4%, with a 9.4% incidence of pneumothorax.[21] Blind pleural biopsy is performed in areas where the expertise or equipment for image-guided biopsies, pleuroscopy, or video-assisted thoracoscopic surgery (VATS) is not available.

Image-guided Pleural Biopsy

Ultrasound and CT-guided biopsies improve the sensitivity and specificity of diagnosing malignancy compared with blind closed biopsy up to 87–94%.[22,23] US-guided biopsies have a sensitivity ranging from 70 to 94%, whereas CT-guided biopsy has a reported sensitivity of 76–88% and a specificity of up to 100% for the diagnosis of malignant pleural thickening.[6]

When pleural thickening is >1 cm, the diagnostic sensitivity of CT-guided pleural biopsy is similar to that of thoracoscopic biopsy (96 vs. 95%).[24] If pleural thickening is millimetric or the imaging access is difficult, then pleural biopsy should be performed by thoracoscopy.

Pleuroscopy

Medical thoracoscopy, also termed pleuroscopy, allows for direct visualization and biopsy of suspicious pleural abnormalities such as thickening, nodularity, and masses. Pleuroscopy has the advantage of both establishing a definitive diagnosis and therapeutic drainage of the pleural fluid as well as pleurodesis if needed. It is usually performed by the pulmonary physicians in an endoscopic suite with local anesthesia and moderate sedation and is associated with a low complication rate. Pleuroscopy is less invasive than VATS but has a sensitivity of 92.6% for the diagnosis of malignant disease.[25] It is usually a safe procedure. The major complications of pleuroscopy have been reported in 1.8% of cases,[26] which include empyema, hemorrhage, bronchopleural fistula, pneumothorax, air leak, and port site tumor growth, especially in mesothelioma patients.

MANAGEMENT

The management of MPE is primarily a palliative care with the objective of relief of symptoms, preventing MPE reoccurrence, and improving the QOL with minimal interventions and hospitalizations. The treatment modality should be individualized based on the patient's functional status, type of tumor, access to medical services, and expected survival. Some tools have been developed to assess the risk of mortality, such as the LENT score.[27] The therapeutic modality should also consider the individual patient's preferences, comorbid conditions, frequency of recurrence, the presence of loculations, or a trapped lung.[28] Asymptomatic patients with a limited survival may be managed with supportive care, whereas more invasive procedures are reserved for symptomatic patients. Pleurodesis and indwelling pleural catheter (IPC) are more definitive pleural procedures compared to repeat thoracentesis, which result in fewer subsequent pleural procedures, complications, and emergency procedures.[29] In patients with lymphoma, small-cell carcinoma, and breast cancer, chemotherapy alone may control the pleural effusion.[30]

Therapeutic Thoracocentesis

The initial step in the management of a symptomatic patient with MPE is US-guided therapeutic thoracentesis.[4,5] The advantages of thoracentesis are that it is simple and can be performed in an outpatient setting. The main drawback is the development of reexpansion pulmonary edema when large amounts of pleural fluid are drained rapidly, producing excessively negative intrapleural pressures. Thoracentesis may be the best option in frail patients with a limited life expectancy of few weeks and in those who are not candidates for pleurodesis or an IPC.[4] Repeated thoracentesis may be performed to relieve symptoms, but ensuring that not >1.5 L of fluid is removed in a single procedure.[4,31] There are no absolute contraindications for thoracentesis. There is no increased risk of bleeding due to mild to moderate coagulopathy and thrombocytopenia, renal disease, thrombocytopenia, and use of clopidogrel.[18,19]

Thoracic Drainage and Pleurodesis

Pleurodesis induces an inflammatory response in the pleura that forces the fusion of both parietal and visceral pleura, obliterating the pleural space and preventing the accumulation of pleural fluid. Pleurodesis as compared to repeated thoracocentesis improves dyspnea, increases survival,[32] and reduces the hospital stay as well as frequent future interventions.[33-38] It is ideal in patients who show complete lung expansion after thoracocentesis but can be performed in patients with incomplete lung expansion with partial apposition of the parietal and visceral pleural membranes.[3] In patients with MPE and <25% nonexpandable lung, talc slurry pleurodesis may improve QOL and breathlessness. Pleurodesis is likely to be unsuccessful in patients who have trapped lung, which is reported in 30% of cases,[39,40] and in those with multiloculated pleural effusion.

Pleurodesis is performed through the intrapleural instillation of a sclerosing agent after complete evacuation of the pleural fluid by intercostal chest tube drainage or during thoracoscopy. Talc is the most widely used sclerosing agent for chemical pleurodesis.[41] It can be administered during the thoracoscopy using an atomizer termed talc poudrage or via a chest tube as a slurry. Other sclerosing agents such as tetracycline, doxycycline, bleomycin, silver nitrate, iodopovidone, and *Corynebacterium parvum* have also been used through an intercostal chest tube. A meta-analysis[1] of 62 randomized trials suggests that talc insufflation is the most effective method of pleurodesis. In a systemic review[42] involving 1,168 patients with recurrent symptomatic MPE, the authors reported that a complete response was achieved in 64% of patients undergoing chemical pleurodesis and that talc was the most effective sclerosing agent, with a success rate of 93%. The British Thoracic Society reports that the efficacy of the talc poudrage and talc slurry procedures is similar.[4] In a study, the overall rate of success of pleurodesis was 81.4%, which included 84.9% for nonmesotheliomas and 73% for mesotheliomas.[43] It is recommended to instill large-particle talc (>15 μm) to prevent the risk of developing acute respiratory distress syndrome.[44,45] The most common complications of pleurodesis are fever and chest pain, which can be easily managed.

Large-bore chest tubes are preferred in performing pleurodesis as TIME-1 (1st Therapeutic Interventions in Malignant Effusion) trial revealed that large-bore tubes (24F) are superior to small-bore tubes (12F).[33] The 12F versus 24F chest tubes were reportedly associated with higher rates of pleurodesis failure (30 vs. 24%).[46,47]

Effective pain management is important after pleural procedures. Nonsteroidal anti-inflammatory drugs for pain relief need not be avoided in patients undergoing pleurodesis for MPE,[20,46] owing to fears that their anti-inflammatory effect may reduce pleurodesis success. In addition, rotation of the patient does not improve the rate of successful pleurodesis.[48]

Indwelling Pleural Catheter

Indwelling pleural catheters are inserted percutaneously to maintain lung expansion by intermittently draining pleural fluid. IPC placement is performed in patients with a trapped lung and in those who are not stable enough to undergo pleurodesis. In patients with a radiologically significant (>25%) nonexpandable lung, prefer an IPC rather than talc pleurodesis. IPC reduces hospital stay and avoids repeated pleural procedures.[49] IPCs are as effective as pleurodesis as a first-line treatment of MPE.[33,38] A systematic review of 19 studies reported symptomatic relief with IPC in 95% of cases[50] with MPE. IPC can cause pleurodesis in 46–70% of patients, leading to full lung expansion. This is caused by local inflammation induced by the IPC.[50,51] In five studies involving 133 patients with MPE and a trapped lung, symptoms improved by >94% in patients with an IPC.[52-56] The AMPLE-2 trial, which involved 87 patients treated with an IPC, revealed a higher success rate of pleurodesis compared with repeated thoracocentesis in MPE.[57] Pleurodesis may occur within 54–90 days, depending on the frequency of drainage.[6] The complications of IPC include drain blockade or malposition (<5%),[58] catheter rupture,[59] cellulitis, pleural infections (0–12%), and seeding of the catheter tract (5%).[60-62] These complications generally do not cause significant morbidity.[38]

Surgical Pleurodesis

Many surgeons perform pleural abrasion followed by talc insufflation for pleurodesis. Surgical pleurodesis is currently not routinely done because this is no more effective than talc.[63]

Antitumor Therapy

The intrapleural instillation of a monoclonal antibody, bevacizumab, in patients with nonsmall cell lung cancer and MPE, achieved a greater reduction in the size of pleural effusion and a higher survival rate in two randomized phase II studies.[64,65] In malignant mesotheliomas, gene therapy and immunotherapy were found to be useful.[66] The current literature is limited, and no conclusions can be drawn on the value of antitumor treatment in MPE management.[20]

Intrapleural Fibrinolysis

Intrapleural instillation of urokinase in patients with multiloculated MPE does not reduce dyspnea or improve success of pleurodesis compared with placebo.[67] Intrapleural fibrinolytics can be considered in highly selected symptomatic patients with MPE and septated effusion to try to improve breathlessness.

Thoracic Surgery

Surgery can be considered for palliation of symptoms in a minority of patients with significantly septated MPE and associated symptoms and otherwise good prognosis and performance status.

TRAPPED LUNG

The word trapped lung is used to describe a situation when the lung is unable to fully expand, leaving the parietal and visceral pleura either partly or completely unopposed. Trapped lung can occur either as a result of pleural thickening causing encasement of the lung or due to the proximal endobronchial obstruction causing distal lung collapse or because of prolonged atelectasis. IPCs appear to be an effective option in the management of MPE with trapped lung. Decortication surgery may improve pleurodesis success in selected patients with MPE and nonexpandable lung, but the risks and benefits of IPC and surgical treatment should be discussed with patients and treatment individualized according to circumstances (e.g., fitness to undergo thoracic surgery).

MULTILOCULATED MALIGNANT PLEURAL EFFUSION

Loculated MPE is defined as MPE with multiple loci, i.e., there is more than one fluid collection, or the effusion is divided into multiple separate pockets of fluid.[68] Loculations can prevent complete drainage of the pleural space and limit lung reexpansion. Therefore, loculated MPE is potentially a contraindication of pleurodesis while there is insufficient symptomatic relief with IPCs. Intrapleural fibrinolytic agents increase the volume of fluid drainage. However, they have no effect on clinical outcomes, such as dyspnea or pleurodesis success. Alternatives, however, are limited for patients with loculated MPE for whom surgery is not suitable.[20]

CONCLUSION

Malignant pleural effusion usually presents with recurrent hemorrhagic pleural effusion. Diagnosis can be established by pleural fluid examination, but image guided or thoracoscopic pleural biopsy is highly sensitive and specific. Optimal management of patients with MPE is still unclear and should be individualized with a multidisciplinary approach. The goal of management is to use the less-invasive approaches, minimal repeated interventions, and hospitalization. Both talc pleurodesis and IPC are effective in reducing repeated pleural fluid accumulation and in the relief from dyspnea. Pleurodesis is preferred when lung shows full expansion, and IPC is considered in patients with a trapped lung. Palliation of symptoms and ambulatory care remain the cornerstone in the management of MPE **(Flowchart 1)**.

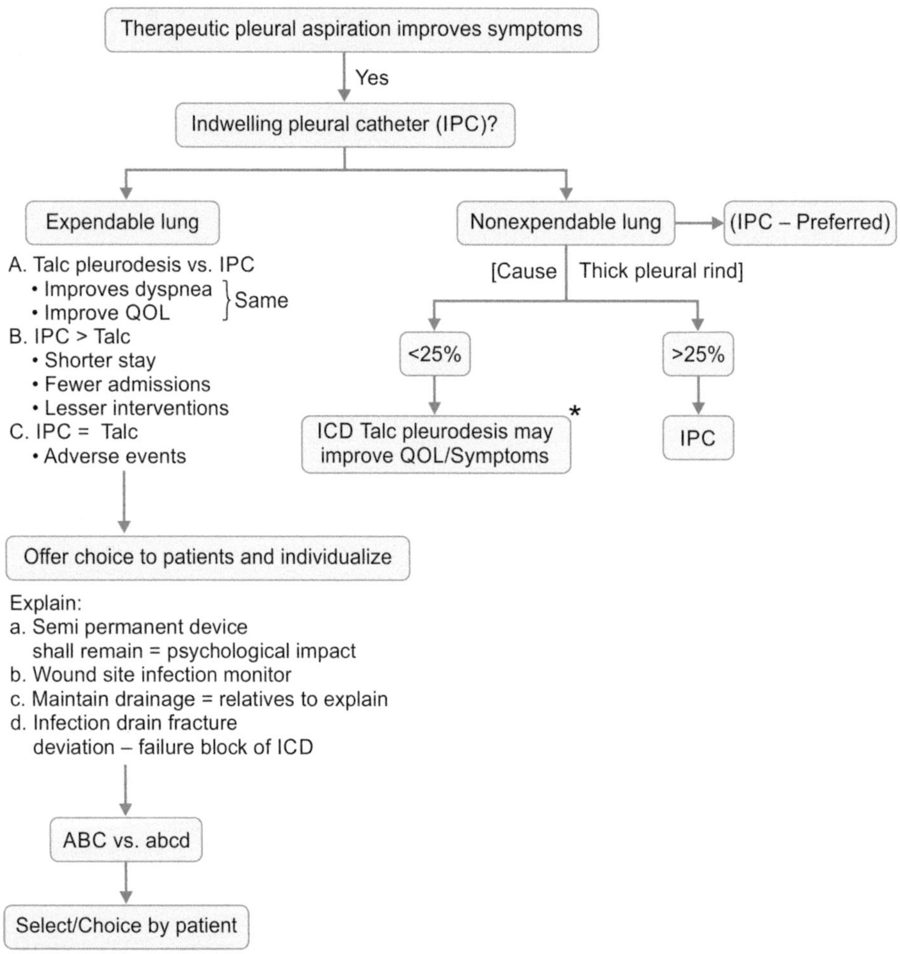

* Decortication: If fit and long survival.

Notes:

A. If proximal growth obstructing bronchus
- Intraluminal/Extraluminal

Treat: As pleural procedures will not alone benefit ("No lung = No breath")

B. Lymphangitis, Imminent

Early death = Symptomatic aspirations

FLOWCHART 1: Malignant effusion: Treatment approach.
(IPC: indwelling pleural catheter)
Courtesy: Dr Anand Jaiswal.

KEY POINTS

- MPE usually occurs in patients with a history of advanced malignant disease.
- It usually presents with recurrent hemorrhagic pleural effusion and dyspnea as the most common symptom.
- The management of MPE is primarily palliative care.
- Pleurodesis and IPC are more definitive pleural procedures compared to repeat thoracentesis.

REFERENCES

1. Clive AO, Jones HE, Bhatnagar R, Preston NJ, Maskell N. Interventions for the management of malignant pleural effusions: a network meta-analysis. Cochrane Database Syst Rev. 2016;5:CD010529.
2. Burrows CM, Mathews WC, Colt HG. Predicting survival in patients with recurrent symptomatic malignant pleural effusions: an assessment of the prognostic values of physiologic, morphologic, and quality of life measures of extent of disease. Chest. 2000;117:73-8.
3. Terra RM, Dela Vega AJ. Treatment of malignant pleural effusion. J Vis Surg. 2018;4:110.
4. Roberts ME, Neville E, Berrisford RG, Antunes G, Ali NJ. Management of a malignant pleural effusion: British Thoracic Society pleural disease guideline 2010. Thorax. 2010;65:ii32-40.
5. American Thoracic Society. Management of malignant pleural effusions. Am J Respir Crit Care Med. 2000;162:1987-2001.
6. Desai NR, Lee HJ. Diagnosis and management of malignant pleural effusions: state of the art in 2017. J Thoracic Dis. 2017;9(Suppl. 10):S1111-22.
7. Porcel JM, Light RW. Pleural effusions. Dis Mon. 2013;59:29-57.
8. Mercaldi CJ, Lanes SF. Ultrasound guidance decreases complications and improves the cost of care among patients undergoing thoracentesis and paracentesis. Chest. 2013;143:532-8.
9. Diacon AH, Brutsche MH, Soler M. Accuracy of pleural puncture sites: a prospective comparison of clinical examination with ultrasound. Chest. 2003;123:436-41.
10. Grogan DR, Irwin RS, Channick R, Raptopoulos V, Curley FJ, Bartter T, et al. Complications associated with thoracentesis: a prospective, randomized study comparing three different methods. Arch Intern Med. 1990;150:873-7.
11. Porcel JM, Pardina M, Bielsa S, González A, Light RW. Derivation and validation of a CT scan scoring system for discriminating malignant from benign pleural effusions. Chest. 2015;147:513-9.
12. Wang ZJ, Reddy GP, Gotway MB, Higgins CB, Jablons DM, Ramaswamy M, et al. Malignant pleural mesothelioma: evaluation with CT, MR imaging, and PET. Radiographics. 2004;24:105-19.
13. Porcel JM, Hernández P, Martínez-Alonso M, Bielsa S, Salud A. Accuracy of fluorodeoxyglucose-PET imaging for differentiating benign from malignant pleural effusions: a meta-analysis. Chest. 2015;147:502-12.
14. Sahn SA. State of the art. The pleura. Am Rev Respir Dis. 1988;138:184-234.
15. Ferreiro L, Gude F, Toubes ME, Lama A, Suárez-Antelo J, San-José E, et al. Predictive models of malignant transudative pleural effusions. J Thorac Dis. 2017;9:106-16.
16. Hooper C, Lee YCG, Maskell N, BTS Pleural Guideline Group. Investigation of a unilateral pleural effusion in adults: British Thoracic Society pleural disease guideline 2010. Thorax. 2010;65(Suppl. 2):ii4-17.
17. Arnold DT, Fonseka DD, Perry S, Morley A, Harvey JE, Medford A, et al. Investigating unilateral pleural effusions: the role of cytology. Eur Respir J. 2018;52(5):1801254.
18. Puchalski JT, Argento AC, Murphy TE, Araujo KLB, Pisani MA. The safety of thoracentesis in patients with uncorrected bleeding risk. Ann Am Thorac Soc. 2013;10:336-41.
19. Zalt MB, Bechara RI, Parks C, Berkowitz DM. Effect of routine clopidogrel use on bleeding complications after ultrasound-guided thoracentesis. J Bronchol Interv Pulmonol. 2012;19:284-7.
20. Bibby AC, Dorn P, Psallidas I, Porcel JM, Janssen J, Froudarakis M, et al. ERS/EACTS statement on the management of malignant pleural effusions. Eur Resp J. 2018;52:1800349.
21. Pereyra MF, San-Jose E, Ferreiro L, Golpe A, Antúnez J, González-Barcala FJ, et al. Role of blind closed pleural biopsy in the management of pleural exudates. Can Respir J. 2013;20:362-6.
22. Maskell NA, Gleeson FV, Davies RJO. Standard pleural biopsy versus CT guided cutting-needle biopsy for diagnosis of malignant disease in pleural effusions: a randomised controlled trial. Lancet. 2003;361:1326-30.
23. Hallifax RJ, Corcoran JP, Ahmed A, Nagendran M, Rostom H, Hassan N, et al. Physician-based ultrasound-guided biopsy for diagnosing pleural disease. Chest. 2014;146:1001-6.
24. Metintas M, Ak G, Dundar E, Yildirim H, Ozkan R, Kurt E, et al. Medical thoracoscopy vs CT scan-guided Abrams pleural needle biopsy for diagnosis of patients with pleural effusions: a randomized, controlled trial. Chest. 2010;137:1362-8.
25. Rahman NM, Ali NJ, Brown G, Chapman SJ, Davies RJO, Downer NJ, et al. Local anaesthetic thoracoscopy: British Thoracic Society pleural disease guideline 2010. Thorax. 2010;65 (Suppl. 2):ii54-60.
26. Medford AR, Agrawal S, Bennett JA, Free CM, Entwisle JJ. Thoracic ultrasound prior to medical thoracoscopy improves pleural access and predicts fibrous septation. Respirology. 2010;15:804-8.
27. Clive AO, Kahan BC, Hooper CE, Bhatnagar R, Morley AJ, Zahan-Evans N, et al. Predicting survival in malignant pleural effusion: development and validation of the LENT prognostic score. Thorax. 2014;69:1098-104.
28. Lui MMS, Fitzgerald DB, Lee YCG. Phenotyping malignant pleural effusions. Curr Opin Pulm Med. 2016;22:350-5.
29. Ost DE, Niu J, Zhao H, Grosu HB, Giordano SH. Quality gaps and comparative effectiveness of management strategies for recurrent malignant pleural effusions. Chest. 2018;153:438-52.
30. Asciak R, Rahman NM. Malignant pleural effusion: from diagnostics to therapeutics. Clin Chest Med. 2018;39:181-93.

31. Feller-Kopman DJ, Reddy CB, DeCamp MM. Management of malignant pleural effusions. An official ATS/STS/STR clinical practice guideline. Am J Resp Crit Care Med. 2018;198:839-49.
32. Hassan M, Mercer RM, Maskell NA, Asciak R, McCracken DJ, Bedawi EO, et al. Survival in patients with malignant pleural effusion undergoing talc pleurodesis. Lung Cancer. 2019;137: 14-8.
33. Davies HE, Mishra EK, Kahan BC, Wrightson JM, Stanton AE, Guhan A, et al. Effect of an indwelling pleural catheter vs chest tube and talc pleurodesis for relieving dyspnea in patients with malignant pleural effusion: the TIME2 randomized controlled trial. JAMA. 2012;307:2383-9.
34. Boshuizen RC, Vd Noort V, Burgers JA, Herder GJM, Hashemi SMS, Hiltermann TJN, et al. A randomized controlled trial comparing indwelling pleural catheters with talc pleurodesis (NVALT-14). Lung Cancer. 2017;108:9-14.
35. Hunt BM, Farivar AS, Vallières E, Louie BE, Aye RW, Flores EE, et al. Thoracoscopic talc versus tunneled pleural catheters for palliation of malignant pleural effusions. Ann Thorac Surg. 2012;94:1053-7.
36. Putnam Jr JB, Walsh GL, Swisher SG, Roth JA, Suell DM, Vaporciyan AA, et al. Outpatient management of malignant pleural effusion by a chronic indwelling pleural catheter. Ann Thorac Surg. 2000;69:369-75.
37. Srour N, Amjadi K, Forster AJ, Aaron SD. Management of malignant pleural effusions with indwelling pleural catheters or talc pleurodesis. Can Respir J. 2013;20:106-10.
38. Fysh ETH, Waterer GW, Kendall PA, Bremner PR, Dina S, Geelhoed E, et al. Indwelling pleural catheters reduce inpatient days over pleurodesis for malignant pleural effusion. Chest. 2012;142:394-400.
39. Dresler CM, Olak J, Herndon 2nd JE, Richards WG, Scalzetti E, Fleishman SB, et al. Phase III intergroup study of talc poudrage vs talc slurry sclerosis for malignant pleural effusion. Chest. 2005;127:909-15.
40. Bibby AC, Halford P, De Fonseka D, Morley AJ, Smith, S, Maskell NA. The prevalence and clinical relevance of nonexpandable lung in malignant pleural mesothelioma. A prospective, single-center cohort study of 229 patients. Ann Am Thorac Soc. 2019;16:1273-9.
41. Lee YCG, Baumann MH, Maskell NA, Waterer GW, Eaton TE, Davies RJO, et al. Pleurodesis practice for malignant pleural effusions in five English-speaking countries: survey of pulmonologists. Chest. 2003;124:2229-38.
42. Walker-Renard PB, Vaughan LM, Sahn SA. Chemical pleurodesis for malignant pleural effusions. Ann Intern Med. 1994;120:56-64.
43. Mercer RM, Macready J, Jeffries H, Speck N, Kanellakis NI, Maskell NA, et al. Clinically important associations of pleurodesis success in malignant pleural effusion: analysis of the TIME1 data set. Respirology. 2020;25:750-55.
44. Maskell NA, Lee YCG, Gleeson FV, Hedley EL, Pengelly G, Davies RJO. Randomized trials describing lung inflammation after pleurodesis with talc of varying particle size. Am J Respir Crit Care Med. 2004;170:377-82.
45. Janssen JP, Collier G, Astoul P, Tassi GF, Noppen M, Rodriguez-Panadero F, et al. Safety of pleurodesis with talc poudrage in malignant pleural effusion: a prospective cohort study. Lancet. 2007;369:1535-9.
46. Rahman NM, Pepperell J, Rehal S, Saba T, Tang A, Ali N, et al. Effect of opioids vs NSAIDs and larger vs smaller chest tube size on pain control and pleurodesis efficacy among patients with malignant pleural effusion: the TIME1 randomized clinical trial. JAMA. 2015;314:2641-53.
47. Hayek SM, Lawrence MM. Size matters in chest tubes—efficacy of analgesia and pleurodesis in patients with malignant pleural effusion. JAMA Oncol. 2016;2:1643-4.
48. Mager HJ, Maesen B, Verzijlbergen F, Schramel F. Distribution of talc suspension during treatment of malignant pleural effusion with talc pleurodesis. Lung Cancer. 2002;36:77-81.
49. Iyer NP, Reddy CB, Wahidi MM, Lewis SZ, Diekemper RL, Feller-Kopman D, et al. Indwelling pleural catheter versus pleurodesis for malignant pleural effusions. A systematic review and meta-analysis. Ann Am Thor Soc. 2019;16:124-31.
50. Tremblay A, Mason C, Michaud G. Use of tunnelled catheters for malignant pleural effusions in patients fit for pleurodesis. Eur Respir J. 2007;30:759-62.
51. Van Meter MEM, McKee KY, Kohlwes RJ. Efficacy and safety of tunneled pleural catheters in adults with malignant pleural effusions: a systematic review. J Gen Intern Med. 2011;26:70-6.
52. Warren WH, Kalimi R, Khodadadian LM, Kim AW. Management of malignant pleural effusions using the PleurX catheter. Ann Thorac Surg. 2008;85:1049-55.
53. Pien GW, Gant MJ, Washam CL, Sterman DH. Use of an implantable pleural catheter for trapped lung syndrome in patients with malignant pleural effusion. Chest. 2001;119:1641-6.
54. Qureshi RA, Collinson SL, Powell RJ, Froeschle PO, Berrisford RG. Management of malignant pleural effusion associated with trapped lung syndrome. Asian Cardiovasc Thorac Ann. 2008;16(2):120-3.
55. Van den Toorn LM, Schaap E, Surmont VFM, Pouw EM, Van der Rijt KCD, Van Klaveren RJ. Management of recurrent malignant pleural effusions with a chronic indwelling pleural catheter. Lung Cancer. 2005;50:123-7.
56. Burgers JA, Olijve A, Baas P. Chronic indwelling pleural catheter for malignant pleural effusion in 25 patients. Ned Tijdschr Geneeskd. 2006;150:1618-23.
57. Muruganandan S, Azzopardi M, Fitzgerald DB, Shrestha R, Kwan BCH, Lam DCL, et al. Aggressive versus symptom-guided drainage of malignant pleural effusion via indwelling pleural catheters (AMPLE-2): an open-label randomised trial. Lancet Respir Med. 2018;6:671-80.
58. Wrightson JM, Fysh E, Maskell NA, Lee YCG. Risk reduction in pleural procedures: sonography, simulation and supervision. Curr Opin Pulm Med. 2010;16:340-50.
59. Fysh ETH, Wrightson JM, Lee YCG, Rahman NM. Fractured indwelling pleural catheters. Chest. 2012;141:1090-4.
60. Fysh ETH, Tremblay A, Feller-Kopman D, Mishra EK, Slade M, Garske L, et al. Clinical outcomes of indwelling pleural catheter-related pleural infections: an international multicenter study. Chest. 2013;144:1597-602.
61. Lui MMS, Thomas R, Gary Lee YC. Complications of indwelling pleural catheter use and their management. BMJ Open Respir Res. 2016;3:e000123.
62. Porcel JM, Torres M, Pardina M, Civit C, Salud A, Bielsa S. Predictors of indwelling pleural catheter removal and infection: a single-center experience with 336 procedures. J Bronchol Interv Pulm. 2020;27:86-94.
63. Rintoul RC, Ritchie AJ, Edwards JG, Waller DA, Coonar AS, Bennett M, et al. Efficacy and cost of video-assisted thoracoscopic partial pleurectomy versus talc pleurodesis in patients with malignant pleural mesothelioma (MesoVATS): an open-label, randomised, controlled trial. Lancet. 2014;384:1118-27.

64. Qi N, Li F, Li X, Kang H, Zhao H, Du N. Combination use of paclitaxel and avastin enhances treatment effect for the NSCLC patients with malignant pleural effusion. Medicine (Baltimore). 2016;95(47):e5392.

65. Du N, Li X, Li F, Zhao H, Fan Z, Ma J, et al. Intrapleural combination therapy with bevacizumab and cisplatin for non-small cell lung cancer-mediated malignant pleural effusion. Oncol Rep. 2013;29:2332-40.

66. Sterman DH, Alley E, Stevenson JP, Friedberg J, Metzger S, Recio A, Moon EK, et al. Pilot and feasibility trial evaluating immuno-gene therapy of malignant mesothelioma using intrapleural delivery of adenovirus-IFNα combined with chemotherapy. Clin Cancer Res. 2016;22:3791-800.

67. Mishra EK, Clive AO, Wills GH, Davies HE, Stanton AE, Al-Aloul M, et al. Randomized controlled trial of urokinase versus placebo for nondraining malignant pleural effusion. Am J Respir Crit Care Med. 2018;197:502-8.

68. Olfert JAP, Penz ED, Manns BJ, Mishra EK, Davies HE, Miller RF, et al. Cost-effectiveness of indwelling pleural catheter compared with talc in malignant pleural effusion. Respirology. 2017;22(4):764-70.

CHAPTER

12 Mesothelioma and Other Primary Pleural Tumors

Siddharth Chatterjee, Ashok Vaid

INTRODUCTION

The most common tumor of the pleura is metastatic neoplasm, mainly originating from breast, colon, and lungs. It is extremely rare for primary tumors to arise from the pleura per se and are further divided into benign and malignant forms, the cells of origin being numerous.

Leading in the list of primary malignant tumors of pleura is malignant mesothelioma, a sinister neoplasm with a bleak outcome appearing from the mesothelial surface of the pleural cavity.

ASBESTOSIS

Asbestos exposure has been undoubtedly recognized as a major etiological association with malignant mesothelioma. Almost three-fourths of the cases (70%) are linked with documented exposure. Around 8–13% of asbestos workers stand at an increased risk of suffering from mesothelioma.[1] A latent period of nearly 30–40 years from first exposure to asbestos till the occurrence of mesothelioma has been documented. It is still uncertain, if a dose-response association between asbestos exposure and advancing toward mesothelioma exists.[2]

Asbestos is a name given to a commercial form comprising a group of hydrated magnesium silicate fibrous minerals, which are further classified into:

A. Serpentines chrysotile fibers: Around 95% of the asbestos. Formerly utilized for the purpose of industrial needs, these spiral-shaped, flexible fibers, break easily, and are solvable in tissues.
B. Amphiboles (crocidolite, amosite, anthophyllite, actinolite, and tremolite): Unbending, extended, needle-like, with a long persistence when compared with above fibers.[3,4]

The carcinogenic potential of asbestos is assumed to be influenced by the dose, biodurability, surface reactivity, and its various other physical properties. Fibers having a high length-to-width ratio, for example, crocidolite, penetrate easily up to the pleural surface, are thought to have higher carcinogenicity. The remaining types of fibers, amosite has an in-between risk, while Chrysotile has the lowest.[3,4] All the fiber types, however, have an oncogenic potential. Apart from asbestos miners/workers, other occupations such as plumbers/pipefitters, mechanical engineers, ship/boat repairing/building happen to be more vulnerable. The risk of malignant mesothelioma can be predictable from the following mathematic equation:

$$R = K \times F \times TP$$

Where,

R is the risk of mesothelioma.

K is a coefficient dependent on the fiber size and type (highest for crocidolite and lowest for chrysotile).

F is the number of fibers per milliliter.

T is the time after the first exposure.

P is the exponent that is thought to be between 3 and 4.

The most current estimates for K for chrysotile and crocidolite are 0.013 and 1.0, respectively.[5,6]

The exact pathogenesis pathway by which these fibers result in malignant changes is yet to be known. The major causes of genotoxicity are:

- Production of reactive oxygen species
- Mechanical processes, namely meddling with mitotic spindle formutation, also the exclusion of chromosomes 17 and 18. It can also result in destruction of the cellular DNA, and if these cells carrying the destructed DNA avoid the apoptosis or

cell cycle arrest, will lead to a malignant alteration, nevertheless, till now no reliable aberrations in suppressor or oncogenes genes have been observed in mesothelioma.[5]

- Quite a few growth factors, exuded by mesothelioma cells, are involved in different stages of the tumor genesis, namely:
  - Platelet-derived growth factors A and B (PDGF-A and B)
  - Insulin-like growth factors 1 and 2 (IGF-1 and IGF-2)
  - Basic fibroblast growth factor (bFGF)
  - Vascular endothelial growth factor (VEGF)
  - Hepatocyte growth factor, and
  - Transforming growth factor β1, β2, and β3 (TGF-β1, -β2, and -β3) together acts as a stimuli for cell proliferation and also the beginning of tumor angiogenesis.[7,8] These mechanisms have been simplified in flowcharts that are written below **(Flowchart 1)**.

VIRAL ONCOGENES

This is a polyoma virus, i.e., Simian virus 40 (SV-40) with an oncogenic ability. It inhibits tumor suppressor genes, with the peptide called as the SV-40 large T antigen (Tag). The examples are retinoblastoma gene (Rb) and wild-type p53 (wt p53). In brain tumors, lymphomas and osteosarcomas, Simian virus-40 DNA sequences have been recognized.[9] It is a solitary cause resulting in malignant conversion of primary mesothelial cells in vitro.[10] In unprotected exposure of cell lines to SV-40 as well as asbestos fibers, the degree of oncogenic change surges ominously. Both crocidolite asbestos and SV-40 are cocarcinogens, which is also validated in the animal studies.[11] Nevertheless, Tag intervention with Rb and wt p53 could well perform an additional part in the oncogenesis of mesothelioma. This postulates when accepted, unique approaches of vaccination/immunization to thwart mesothelioma and also for timely initial diagnosis can be possible.[12]

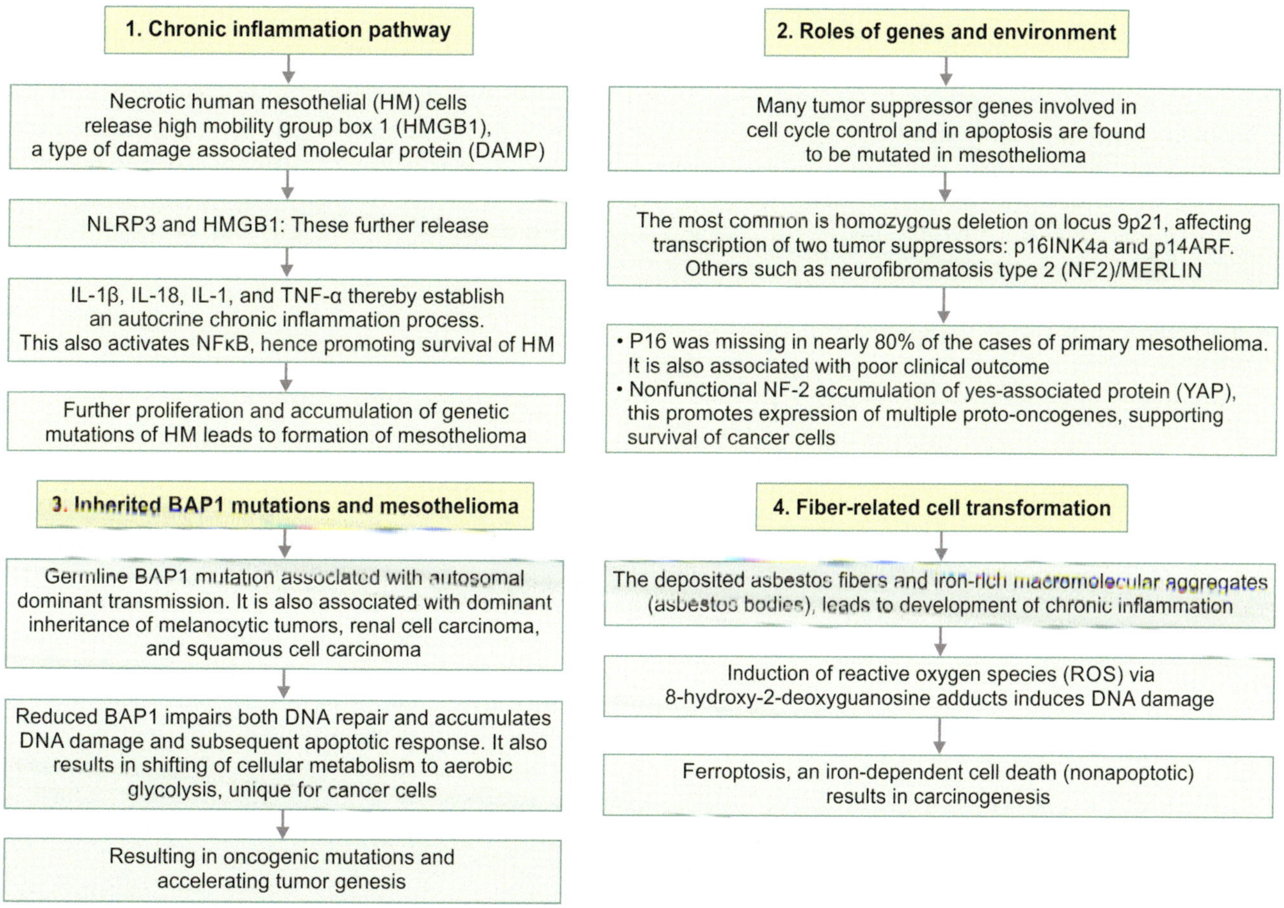

FLOWCHART 1: Mechanisms of development of mesothelioma.
(IL: interleukin; TNF: tumor necrosis factor)

ADDITIONAL CAUSES

Progression to malignant mesothelioma is also seen in sporadic instances in etiologic causes, such as treatment with ionizing irradiation at supradiaphragmatic fields, intrapleural Thorotrast, and also with inhalation of other fibrogenic silicates, for example, erionite.[13,14]

HISTOPATHOLOGY

The revised 2021 WHO classification of pleural tumors suggests: Three main histologic subtypes:[15]

1. *Epithelioid:* This subtype is most common. The histologic variants consist of tubulopapillary, trabecular, micropapillary, and solid. Some of the less common variants include adenomatoid, rhabdoid, deciduoid, small cell, and signet ring patterns. A myxoid matrix could be misguided for mucin, but this milieu is essentially hyaluronate and displays staining with Alcian blue, which is hyaluronidase-sensitive.

   Pleomorphic features—precisely anaplastic/bizarre nuclei and multinucleated giant cells—can be perceived in the epithelioid type and ought to be described as a pointer of aggressive behavior.

   Lymphohistiocytoid features—described mainly by dense lymphoid infiltrates, primarily of $CD8^+$ T cells, obscuring the malignant histiocytoid appearing tumor cells should be reported.[15]
2. *Sarcomatoid*: The most commonly found configuration is of fibroblastic-like spindle cells that mimic a fibrosarcoma. organized in storiform, fascicular, or haphazard. A few of this type of mesothelioma show "heterologous elements", for instance, rhabdomyosarcoma, chondrosarcoma, and osteosarcoma.[15]
3. *Biphasic*: Biphasic mesotheliomas denote about 30% of cases. These mesotheliomas have both epithelioid and sarcomatoid components. Collectively, the components should be at least 10% of the tumor for the label of biphasic mesothelioma in the specimens. Nevertheless, a tumor can be labelled as biphasic irrespective of the proportion of each constituent in a small biopsy sample. Whether a smaller biopsy sample or a larger resection, the proportion of the sarcomatoid part should be looked at, because of the probable affect on the treatment possibilities and prognosis.[15]

Formerly known as "well-differentiated papillary mesothelioma" has been deleted from the mesothelioma grouping and is now a separate entity. This precise entity is now known as "well-differentiated papillary mesothelial tumor" and is limited to an exceptionally sporadic and unique mesothelial tumor that consists of papillary stromal formations enclosed by cytologically bland mesothelial cells missing invasion.[15]

Common immunohistochemical (IHC) markers, if found positive, can provide a supportive diagnosis of malignant mesothelioma. These IHC markers are, viz., calretinin, CK5/6, the Wilms tumor 1 (WT1) antigen, and D2-40. These markers help in limiting the gap in the diagnosis between malignant epithelioid mesothelioma and primary pulmonary adenocarcinoma.[16] In order to support a diagnosis of adenocarcinoma, markers such as MOC31, CEA, Ber-EP4, thyroid transcription factor 1 (TTF-1), and napsin A are commonly employed.[16]

SYMPTOMS AND SIGNS

Around 65% of patients are among the age limit of 40–70 years, and a majority of them carry a potential past contact to asbestos for at least 20 years. Patients primarily experience the gradual onset of chest pain or dyspnea. The symptoms are present for several months before a physician is consulted.[17,18] Some patients have intermittent periods of low-grade fever. The chest pain is most often nonpleuritic in nature and because of diaphragmatic involvement, it is mainly referred to the upper abdomen or shoulder. As the disease evolves, there is a weight loss, a dry hacking cough and an increasing dyspnea.[17]

Physical examination might reveal clubbing. In chest examination, the associated hemithorax has an occasional reduction in size besides sometimes, a retraction of the intercostal spaces is seen. Physical signs of a pleural effusion can also be perceived.

RADIOLOGY

Chest Radiograph (Fig. 1)

It shows a pleural effusion in approximately 90% of patients.[19] This effusion is commonly moderate to gross, inhabiting 50% or more of the hemithorax and concealing the pleural tumor. In about a third of the patients, pleural plaques are apparent in the opposite hemithorax.[20] With further evolution of the disease, the tumor encloses the ipsilateral lung and thus results in a mediastinal shift to the same side of the effusion and consequently causes a loculated pleural effusion. In the later stages, it reveals enlargement of the cardiac shadow owing to intrusion of the pericardium, and destruction of soft-tissue masses, ribs, and there is also a mediastinal widening. The disease is unilateral in almost all cases.[21]

CT Scan

The pleura is thick, unequal, and frequently has a nodular internal margin that aids in making a distinction from other kinds of pleural thickening. These findings are utmost marked on the base. It also generally discloses increased thickening of the major fissure owing to a blend of tumor, fibrosis, and related bud. Due to tumor infiltration of the fissure, it may also appear nodular.[20] Features suggesting malignant mesothelioma rather than metastatic pleural disease are namely rind-like mediastinal pleural involvement, and pleural thickness >1 cm.[22] It should be highlighted, though, the opposite side of mediastinal shift is seen in approximately 15–25% of cases, it is typically owed to a larger effusion.[19]

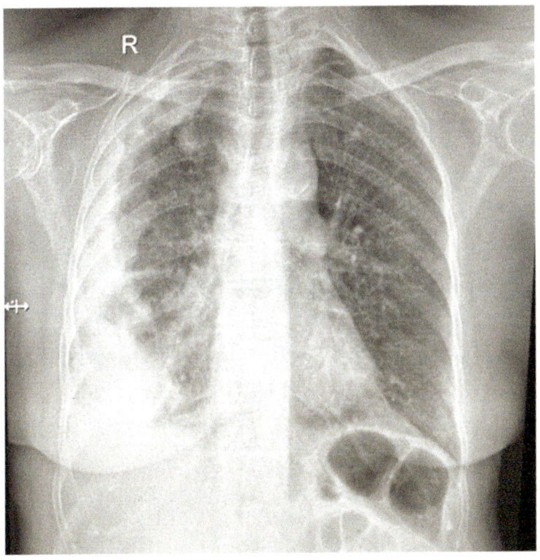

FIG. 1: Chest X-ray (PA view) in a 68-year-old female patient with mesothelioma (before treatment).

CT scan also signifies the disease further than the pleura and thus helping in the staging. It often discloses intrapulmonary nodules that are not very much seen on the standard chest radiograph. It may also show chest wall and diaphragmatic incursion, or extension of the tumor to the liver or retroperitoneal space.[20]

Some of the limitation of CT scans are that it is unable to recognize chest wall and mediastinal incursion in few cases, which have undergone surgical interventions **(Figs. 2A to C)**.[23] Often, it is very tough to differentiate pleural disease from accompanying pericardial disease.

Widespread pleural disease regularly encloses and conceals the nodal anatomy in the middle mediastinal and hilar nodal groups.[24]

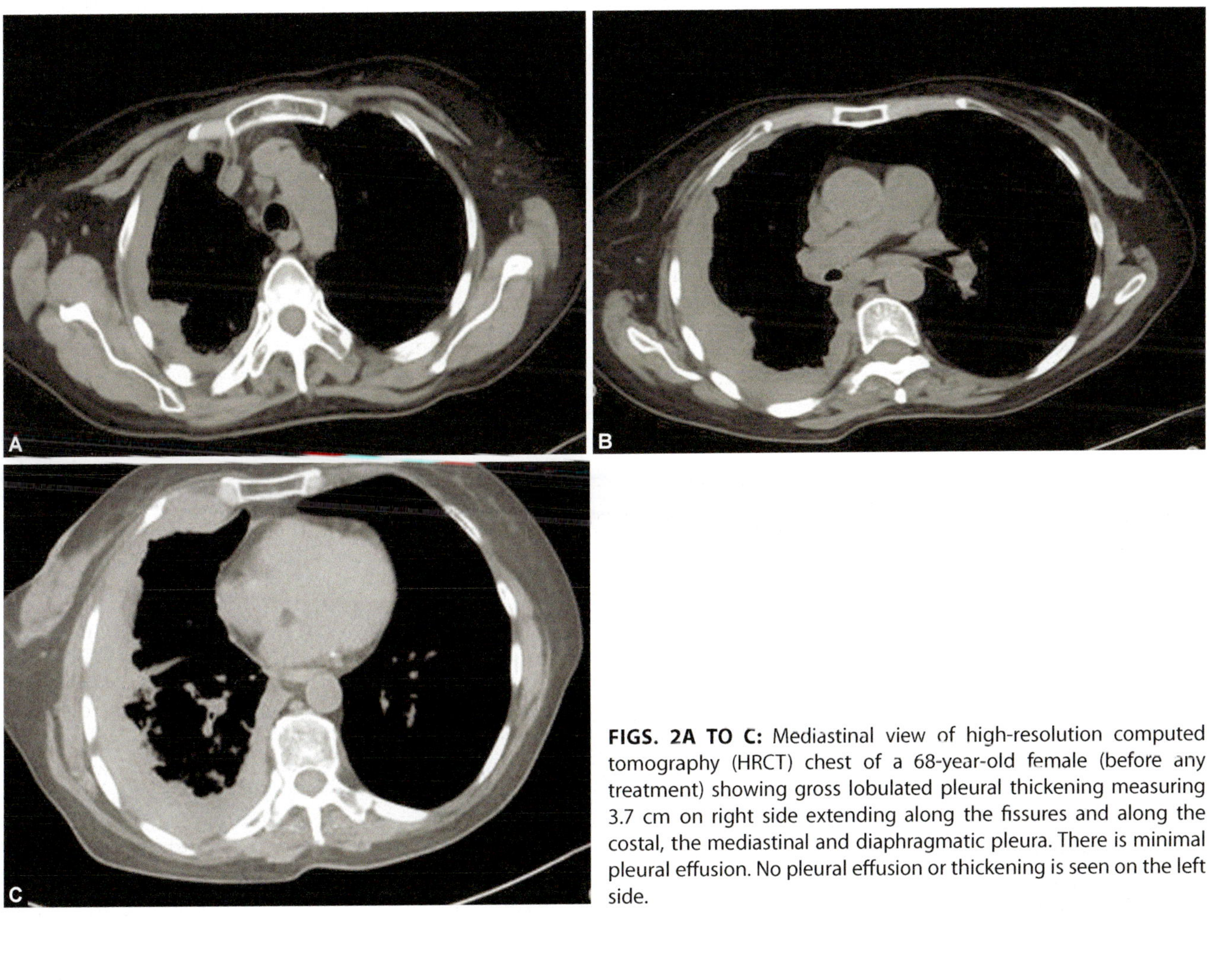

FIGS. 2A TO C: Mediastinal view of high-resolution computed tomography (HRCT) chest of a 68-year-old female (before any treatment) showing gross lobulated pleural thickening measuring 3.7 cm on right side extending along the fissures and along the costal, the mediastinal and diaphragmatic pleura. There is minimal pleural effusion. No pleural effusion or thickening is seen on the left side.

Magnetic Resonance Imaging and Fluorodeoxyglucose Positron Emission Tomography

MRI is better than CT in determining the degree of a malignant mesothelioma chiefly when the tumor invades local structures, for example, the ribs and the diaphragm.[25] Positron emission tomography (PET) CT is helpful in distinguishing malignant pleural disease from that of the benign forms **(Figs. 3A to C)**.[26]

PLEURAL FLUID

This fluid is exudative in nature. In about 30% of patients, the glucose level is <50 mg/dL and the pH level is <7.20.[27] Low pH or glucose level is likely to have not so good prognosis.[27] Cytology reveals a mixture of normal mesothelial cells, differentiated and undifferentiated malignant mesothelial cells, and varying numbers of lymphocytes and polymorphonuclear leukocytes.[28]

The presence of increased levels of soluble mesothelin related protein (SMRP) is helpful in supporting the diagnosis for mesothelioma.[29,30] Sometimes, the fluid of the patients is viscous due to existence of increased quantity of hyaluronate. However, the amount of SMRP in subjects having sarcomatoid mesothelioma is low.[30]

The cut-off for hyaluronate is kept at 75 mg/L. Hence, the specificity was 100% and the sensitivity was 56%.[31] Lactate dehydrogenase (LDH) levels are often more than malignant pleural effusions with levels being >600 IU/L.[27]

The cytokine profile is slightly exclusive, such that the tumor basically yields increased levels of:

- *Interleukin 6 (IL-6)*: Anticipated to cause generalized symptoms, viz., cachexia, fever, and thrombocytosis.[32,33]
- Transforming growth factor-β (TGF-β)

Quite decreased levels of:

- Tumor necrosis factor alpha (TNF-α)
- Interleukin (IL)-1β

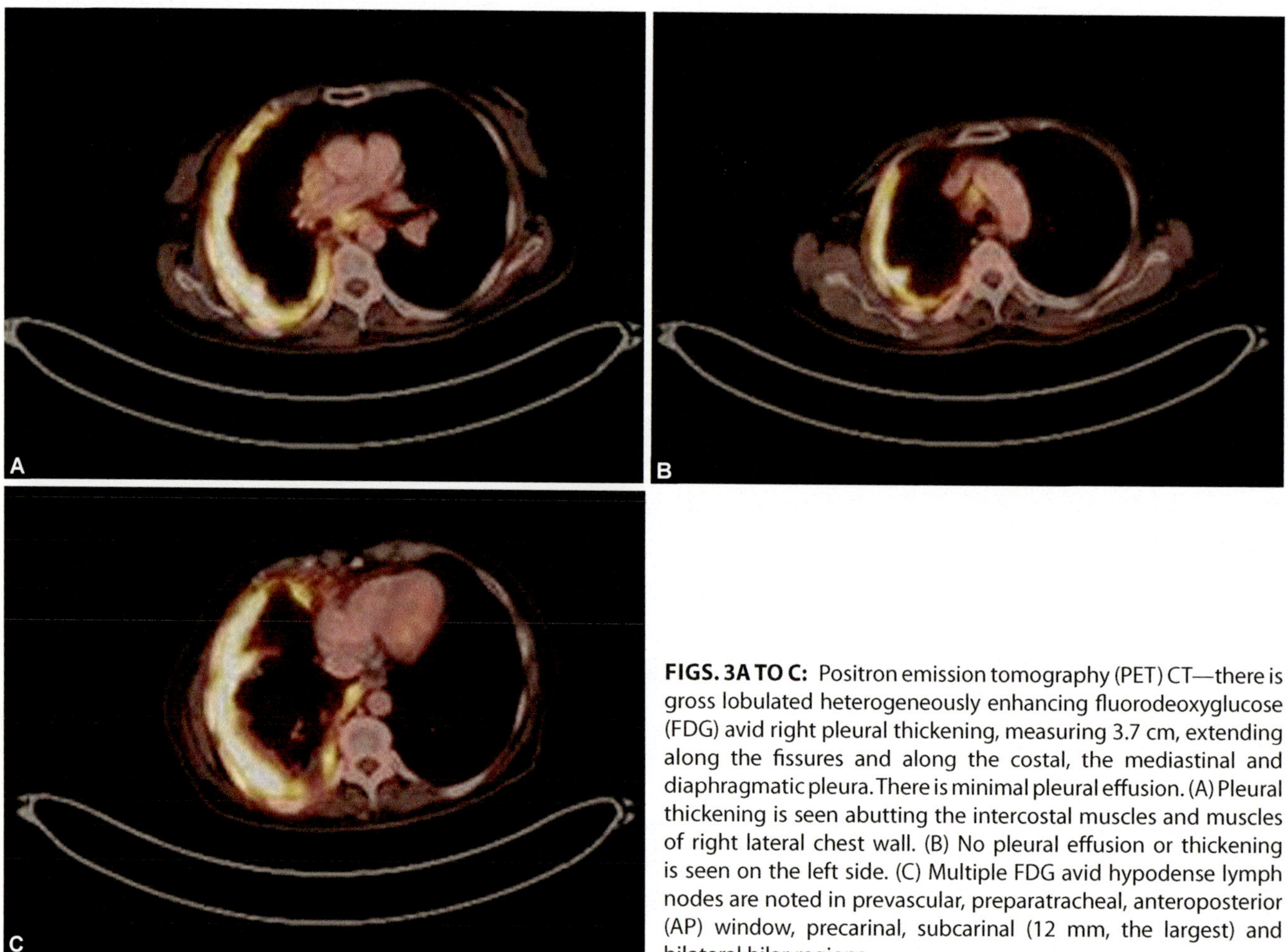

FIGS. 3A TO C: Positron emission tomography (PET) CT—there is gross lobulated heterogeneously enhancing fluorodeoxyglucose (FDG) avid right pleural thickening, measuring 3.7 cm, extending along the fissures and along the costal, the mediastinal and diaphragmatic pleura. There is minimal pleural effusion. (A) Pleural thickening is seen abutting the intercostal muscles and muscles of right lateral chest wall. (B) No pleural effusion or thickening is seen on the left side. (C) Multiple FDG avid hypodense lymph nodes are noted in prevascular, preparatracheal, anteroposterior (AP) window, precarinal, subcarinal (12 mm, the largest) and bilateral hilar regions.

Mesothelin and Other Serum Markers

- Mesothelin, mainly SMRP, is a 40-kDa glycoprotein, that is seen in reduced levels on the cell surface of normal mesothelial cells, such as lining the pleura, peritoneum, pericardium, and tunica vaginalis. It is produced in higher amounts in mesothelioma, pancreatic cancer, and ovarian cancer cells.[34,35] Currently, SMRP levels mainly have accessory role in the diagnosis of the mesothelioma.
- Osteopontin, a glycoprotein, involved in mediating cell-matrix interactions, is increasingly expressed in numerous kinds of malignancies, including malignant mesothelioma.[36]
- Fibulin-3 is an extracellular glycoprotein, which is encoded by the epidermal growth factor-containing fibulin-like extracellular matrix protein 1 (EFEMP1) gene. Increased concentration of fibulin-3 has high sensitivity and specificity of 97% and 96%, respectively. This distinguishes those patients with pleural mesothelioma from those with having an exposure history to asbestos but devoid of mesothelioma and from those with other benign or malignant causes of pleural effusion. Those patients with mesothelioma who underwent surgical resection had decreased levels of fibulin-3. For its role as a biomarker for early diagnosis and monitoring of patients who went through the treatment, additional studies are required.[37]

STAGING OF MALIGNANT MESOTHELIOMA (TABLE 1)

TNM staging as per the American Joint Committee on Cancer (AJCC), 8th edition.[38]

TABLE 1: TNM staging.

T1	Tumor limited to the ipsilateral parietal pleura with or without involvement of: Visceral pleura, mediastinal pleura, and diaphragmatic pleura
T2	Tumor involving each of the ipsilateral pleural surfaces with at least one of the following features: (1) Involvement of diaphragmatic muscle (2) Extension of tumor from visceral pleura into the underlying pulmonary parenchyma
T3	Describes locally advanced but *potentially resectable* tumor. Tumor involving all the ipsilateral pleural surfaces with at least one of the following features: (1) Involvement of the endothoracic fascia (2) Extension into the mediastinal fat (3) Solitary, completely resectable focus of tumor extending into the soft tissues of the chest wall (4) Nontransmural involvement of the pericardium
T4	Describes locally advanced *technically unresectable* tumor. Tumor involving all the ipsilateral pleural surfaces with at least one of the following features: (1) Diffuse extension or multifocal masses of tumor in the chest wall, with or without associated rib destruction (2) Direct transdiaphragmatic extension of tumor to the peritoneum (3) Direct extension of tumor to the contralateral pleura (4) Direct extension of tumor to mediastinal organs (5) Direct extension of tumor into the spine (6) Tumor extending through to the internal surface of the pericardium with or without a pericardial effusion, or tumor involving the myocardium
N0	No regional lymph nodes metastases
N1	Metastases in the ipsilateral bronchopulmonary, hilar, or mediastinal (including the internal mammary, peridiaphragmatic, pericardial fat pad, or intercostal) lymph nodes
N2	Metastases in the contralateral mediastinal, ipsilateral, or contralateral supraclavicular lymph nodes
M0	No distant metastasis
M1	Distant metastasis present

Staging

Stage Ia	T1N0M0
Stage Ib	T2N0M0, T3N0M0
Stage II	T1-2N1M0
Stage IIIA	T3N1M0
Stage IIIB	T1-3N2M0, T4N0-2M0
Stage IV	Any T, any N, any M1

Treatment

Surgery

The surgical management of mesothelioma is associated with considerable morbidity, but it has made noteworthy advances in palliating the chief symptoms and possibly showing some progression in survival for selected patients. The augmented employment of video-assisted thoracic surgery (VATS), along with novel biomarkers, has helped early diagnosis, at which point they could be potential candidates for more proactive efforts at "definitive" surgical management (along with other therapies).

Nevertheless, the definitive surgical management is possible in a small proportion of subjects. Besides, <25% of those undergoing proactive surgical management will be alive at 5 years, and also lesser will be disease free at that point of time.[39]

Extrapleural pneumonectomy (EPP) is a radical surgical method, which involves complete removal of the ipsilateral lung besides the parietal and visceral pleura, pericardium, with parts of the phrenic nerve, and significant part of the hemidiaphragm. This results in maximum amount of cytoreduction, also since the lung has been removed, causes increased radiation dosages to be delivered at the ipsilateral hemithorax. It is the one and only debulking process done, when a thick tumor rind obliterates the pleural space.[40] Limitation of EPP with adjuvant chemotherapy ± local radiotherapy is that, it is restricted to patients such as those with early-stage disease, noninvolvement of the mediastinal lymph nodes and epithelioid histology. Patients with other histologic types (biphasic or sarcomatoid) and/or mediastinal or hilar node involvement have a gloomy prognosis.[41] Although EPP alone has no impact on survival without adjuvant therapy, but EPP alone is an exceptional way of palliating the symptoms, such as profound dyspnea and orthopnea related with severe ventilation/perfusion mismatch due to lung encasement by mesothelioma.[42,43]

Complete parietal and visceral pleurectomy, known as extended pleurectomy/decortication or radical pleurectomy (EPD/RP), is intended to accomplish utmost cytoreduction while keeping the ipsilateral lung untouched. It comprises complete resection of whole parietal and visceral pleura plus the diaphragmatic pleura and encompasses the hilum to involve and resect the pleural surfaces of the interlobar fissures. This also includes dissection and removal of mediastinal, hilar, intercostal, and internal mammary lymph nodes. This has mainly become standard of care for surgical management of resectable malignant mesothelioma, though it has not shown to prolong the survival.[44]

Chemotherapy

The first-line chemotherapy in good performance status and unresectable mesothelioma is combination treatment with pemetrexed and cisplatin.

Pemetrexed is an antifolate targeting multiple enzymes such as thymidylate synthase, the rate-limiting step in the synthesis of thymidylate, which is essential for DNA synthesis. Thymidylate synthase is also the enzyme inhibited by the cytotoxic agents 5-fluorouracil and raltitrexed. If cisplatin toxicity is a specific concern, pemetrexed plus carboplatin may be another regimen mainly in aged or those patients with compromised renal function. Addition of vitamin B12 and folic acid to chemotherapy caused in decrease in the severity and occurrence of hematologic and nonhematologic toxicities. In EMPHACIS study, 456 patients planned to receive cisplatin (75 mg/m^2) treatment and randomized to receive either pemetrexed (500 mg/m^2) or a placebo once every 3 weeks. Time to progression (5.7 against 3.9 months), the objective response rate (41% vs. 17%), and the median survival (12.1 vs. 9.3 months) were all enhanced for the combination **(Figs. 4A to C)**.[45,46]

The Mesothelioma Avastin Cisplatin Pemetrexed Study (MAPS) trial in 2016 was the first trial to exhibit the efficacy of antiangiogenesis in the management of mesothelioma. Bevacizumab when combined with standard chemotherapy resulted in significantly longer survival than those with only the first line chemotherapy (overall survival 18.8 months vs. 16.1 months). The limitation in adding bevacizumab is a rise in adverse events (71% vs. 62%), mainly vascular adverse events.[47]

The combination of gemcitabine and cisplatin or carboplatin is also an effective first-line option in the management of mesothelioma due to its suitable toxicity profile, better response rate, and palliative effects.[48]

Currently, there is no standard of care for second-line chemotherapy, after the management with cisplatin and pemetrexed. The most commonly used second-line regimens comprise of gemcitabine or other drugs with single-agents such as vinorelbine.[49]

Radiation Therapy

Mesothelioma also involves the regions of intercostal drainage tube insertion sites, biopsies, thoracoscopy trocars, and incisions, resulting in subcutaneous nodules. The radiation may play a role by thwarting these relapses and refining the native control after pleurectomy or EPP, by prophylactic radiotherapy **(Fig. 5)**. In a randomized trial, Boutin et al. revealed a 21-Gy given in three daily fractions, 10–15 days after thoracoscopy, reduced local relapse from 40 to 0%. These findings have also been established by other investigators too.[50-52]

There has also been interest in employing tumor treating fields (TTF), a technology that uses discontinuous electric fields to cause an antimitotic effect. The STELLAR trial was a phase 2, multicenter, single-arm trial which combined TTF with standard chemotherapy of pemetrexed and cisplatin or carboplatin as primary treatment for unresectable pleural mesothelioma. In the study population, there was a high percentage with nonepithelioid histology, and largely survival of 18.2 months was achieved. This survival outcome was higher than the controls of standard chemotherapy alone. The limitation is that the device is to be worn in the form of external vest along with a battery pack for roughly around 18 hours/day, somewhat affecting the quality of life.[53]

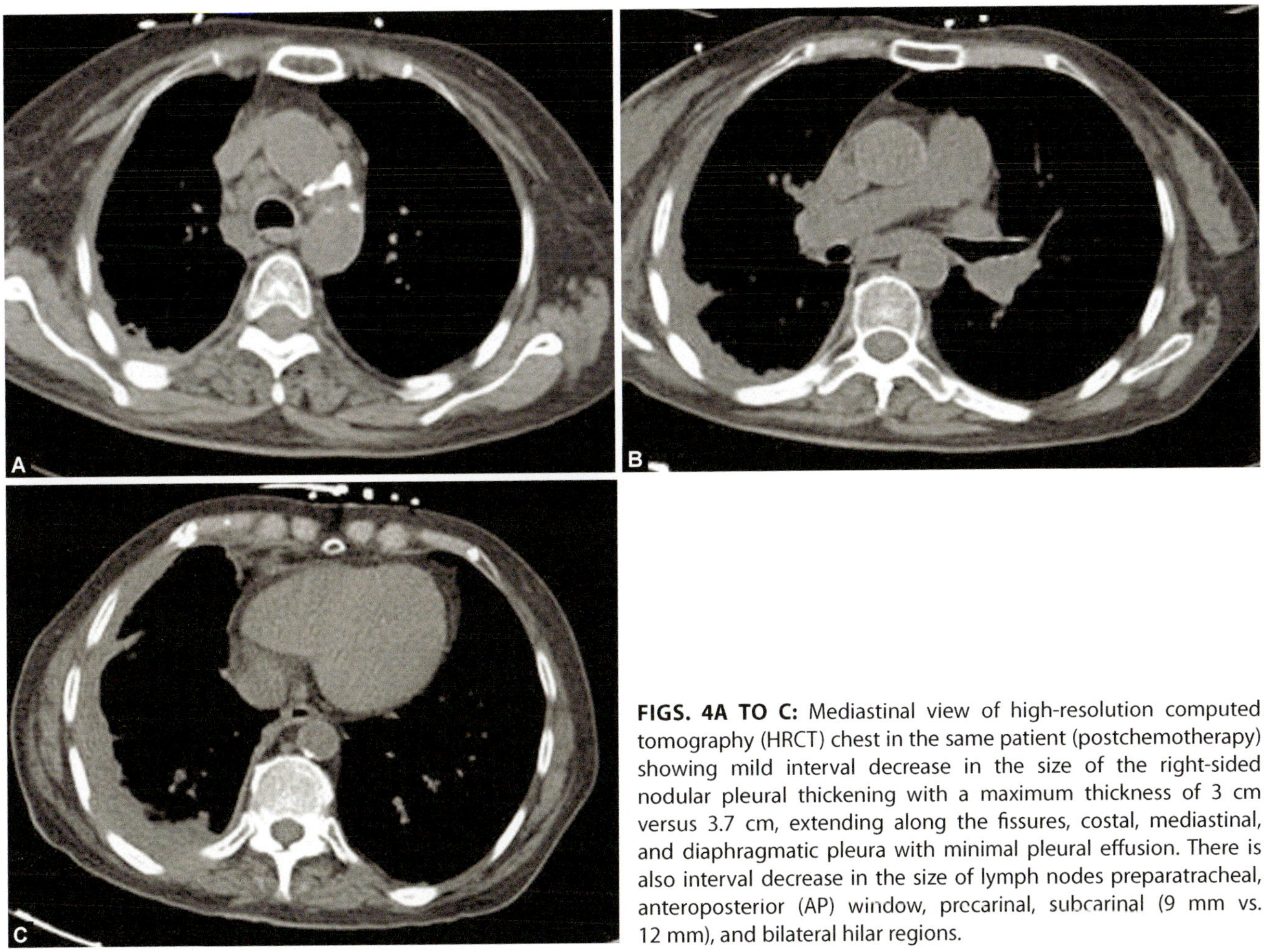

FIGS. 4A TO C: Mediastinal view of high-resolution computed tomography (HRCT) chest in the same patient (postchemotherapy) showing mild interval decrease in the size of the right-sided nodular pleural thickening with a maximum thickness of 3 cm versus 3.7 cm, extending along the fissures, costal, mediastinal, and diaphragmatic pleura with minimal pleural effusion. There is also interval decrease in the size of lymph nodes preparatracheal, anteroposterior (AP) window, precarinal, subcarinal (9 mm vs. 12 mm), and bilateral hilar regions.

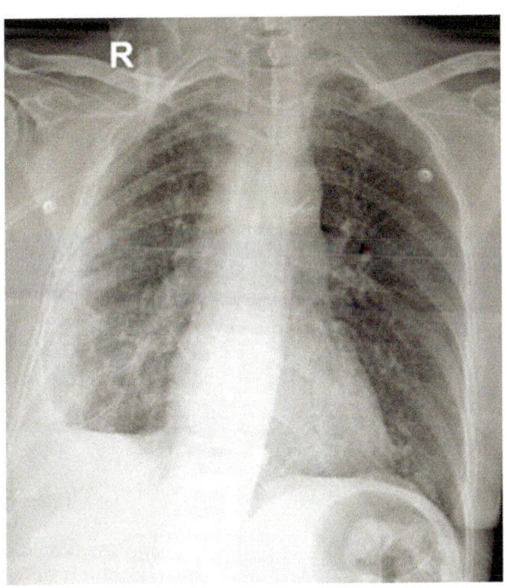

FIG. 5: Chest X-ray [posteroanterior (PA) view] of the same patient after chemotherapy.

OTHER EVOLVING APPROACHES

Immunotherapy

Many immunotherapies have been commenced in subjects with mesothelioma, containing IL-2 and interferon (IFN)-γ, both of which had limited usefulness along with substantial side effects. The major limitation of these cytokines is that they can besides have anti-inflammatory end-results. For instance, IL-2 supports the activity of T regulatory cells. Additionally, IFN-γ can result in downregulation of MHC molecules and upregulation of checkpoint ligands on tumor cells.[54]

Boutin et al., in Marseilles, France, initiated the intrapleural supervision of immunostimulants to manage mesothelioma and revealed noteworthy local tumor response with intrapleural IL-2 and IFN-γ. Most striking was the result of intrapleural IFN-γ in early-stage mesothelioma. A total of 89 patients were managed over 46 months with a response rate of 20%. In all, eight patients had histologically established thorough responses, and nine patients had responses which were somewhat >50% reduction in tumor volume. Overall, stage I disease had a response rate of 45%. The effectiveness of IFN-γ against mesothelioma was due to: (i) direct inhibitory effects on mesothelioma cell growth and (ii) decreased intrapleural production of IL-6, which results in tumor directed macrophages and cytotoxic T lymphocytes.[55,56]

In the past decade, application of immune checkpoint inhibitors (CPI) has transformed the treatment model of mesothelioma. The milestone phase 3 trial CheckMate 743 revealed, considerably increased survival with first-line combination PD-L1/CTLA4 CPI (Nivolumab + Ipilimumab) versus standard chemotherapy (Platinum + Pemetrexed) in subjects with untreated unresectable mesothelioma, predominantly in those with sarcomatoid and biphasic histologic subtypes and >1% PD-L1 expression. At a median follow-up of 30 months, the median overall survival (OS) was 18 months versus 14 months respectively. 2-year OS rates were 41 versus 27%, respectively. Subsequently reported 3-year OS results were 23% versus 15%, respectively. This regimen was permitted by the Food and Drug Administration (FDA) in 2020—first immunotherapy regimen permitted for the management of mesothelioma of any given stage.[57]

Single-agent management with nivolumab in earlier enrolled subjects managed, better survival and resulted in FDA endorsement as second-line therapy. 164 managed with avelumab, a PD-L1 inhibitor, in previously managed patients and first-line treatment with durvalumab, a PD-1 inhibitor, in combination with standard chemotherapy revealed robust responses in early-stage trials, prompting ongoing study.[58,59]

Targeted Therapy

Clinical trials have been carried out with novel targeted agents, for example, antiangiogenic agents, viz., thalidomide and bevacizumab, and copper-chelating agent tetrathiomolybdate, reduces copper, an important cofactor in angiogenesis. The copper-chelating compound did show any obvious benefit till date in human trials. Presently, there are many clinical trials of combinations of targeted agents to see if it could have synergistic effects upon growth of mesothelioma in advanced stage.[60-62]

Further pathways of cellular metabolism, targeted in mesothelioma, the most convincing of which is intracellular consumption of arginine. Szlosarek et al. published the first trial of arginine deficit in cancer, explicitly managing the subjects with arginosuccinate synthetase 1 (AS1)-deficit tumors with pegylated arginine deiminase (ADI-PEG20).[63] When comparing with standard supportive care, they revealed an improved progression-free survival, and the subgroup with approximately 75% reduction in AS1 had both progression-free survival and overall survival.[63] Beddowes et al. carried out an increment in dose study with pegylated arginine deiminase in combination with standard chemotherapy in subjects with mesothelioma or a nonsmall-cell lung cancer, no dose-limiting toxicity was illustrated; however, it succeeded with partial responses in seven out of nine patients.[64] Currently multicenter, randomized, controlled trial reviewing the combination of ADI-PEG20 with standard chemotherapy in mesothelioma is ongoing.[65]

Gene Therapy

Mesothelioma remains confined at the outset and pleural access to the tumor is easy and safe. Several methods have been used in cell culture and in animal models. Gene therapy vectors have involved liposomal/DNA complexes and vaccinia, modified herpes and adenoviruses. Transgenes included suicide genes, cytokines, tumor suppressor genes (e.g., *p53*), and proapoptotic genes.[66,67]

Other gene therapy methodologies are being studied by various groups trying to reach increased-amounts of expression of other cytokines such as IL-2 and IL-12, GM-CSF, and TNF. Phase 1 trials of intrapleural delivery of oncolytic viruses, for example, measles, herpes simplex viruses, and vaccinia viruses, all of them have shown substantial antitumor action against mesothelioma in vitro and in preclinical models.[66]

SOLITARY FIBROUS TUMOR OF THE PLEURA

Solitary fibrous tumor is a mesenchymal tumor of fibroblastic origin, and alike tumors have been defined in other extrathoracic sites. There is no significant exposure is seen with asbestos or environmental agent. While the peak age range is comparable to that of mesothelioma (40–70 years), it can affect patients of all ages, which also includes children as young as 5 years old.[15]

Signs and Symptoms

Patients are commonly asymptomatic and the diagnosis is established incidentally by routine chest radiography, but can exist with dyspnea, nonpleuritic chest pain, cough, or pleural effusion. A substantial percentage (up to 40%) of subjects present with symptomatic hypoglycemia, known as Doege–Potter syndrome. It is assumed to be due to elaboration of insulin-like growth factors. This amplified manufacture of insulin-like substance causes an augmented glucose consumption by peripheral tissues and diminished production of glucose by the liver. It can present commonly with clubbing of fingers and toes, diffuse arthralgias, but the occurrence of pulmonary hypertrophic osteoarthropathy is debatable.[68-70]

Radiography

They typically present radiographically as large, rounded, well-circumscribed, pleura-based mass, but occasionally could appear as intraparenchymal. These masses sometimes can be very large (>30 cm in diameter) resulting in clinically significant compression of the lung. 17% of the subjects come with an ipsilateral pleural effusion.[68-71]

Pathology

Histologically, these have been described as a "patternless pattern". Alternating areas of hypocellularity and hypercellularity with short fascicles of interlacing spindle cells are seen, hence forming a storiform pattern. These fascicles are scattered between areas of erratically collagenized tissue. Histologic criteria predicting a malignant course includes increased cellularity, cytologic atypia, infiltrative growth, a mitotic rate with >2 mitoses/ mm^2 and necrosis. Immunohistochemical stains clinch the diagnosis. These are CD34 and STAT6 positive but CK negative.[15]

Treatment

Surgical resection of solitary fibrous tumors of the pleura is beneficial with very low risk of relapse. There is classically a distinctive separation between the tumor and underlying compressed lung, so widespread pulmonary resection is typically avoidable.

In most subjects, complete resection results in favorable prognosis in malignant solitary fibrous tumors of the pleura. In one study, complete resection was done in >90% of subjects, with disease-free survival rates at 5 and 10 years was at 72% and 61%, respectively.[72]

KEY POINTS

- Leading in the list of primary malignant tumors of pleura is malignant mesothelioma, a sinister neoplasm with a bleak outcome appearing from the mesothelial surface of the pleural cavity.
- Asbestos exposure has been undoubtedly recognized as major etiological association with malignant mesothelioma.
- Progression to malignant mesothelioma is also seen in sporadic instances in etiologic causes, such as treatment with ionizing irradiation at supradiaphragmatic fields, intrapleural Thorotrast, and also with inhalation of other fibrogenic silicates, for example, erionite.
- Common immunohistochemical (IHC) markers, if found positive, can provide a supportive diagnosis of malignant mesothelioma. These IHC markers are, viz., calretinin, CK5/6, the Wilms tumor 1 (WT1) antigen, and D2-40. These markers help in limiting the gap in the diagnosis between malignant epithelioid mesothelioma and primary pulmonary adenocarcinoma. In order to support a diagnosis of adenocarcinoma, markers such as MOC31, CEA, Ber-EP4, thyroid transcription factor 1 (TTF-1), and napsin A are commonly employed.
- CT scan signifies the disease further than the pleura and thus helps in the staging. It often discloses intrapulmonary nodules that are not very much seen on the standard chest radiograph. It may also show chest wall and diaphragmatic incursion, or extension of the tumor to the liver or retroperitoneal space.
- MRI is better than CT in determining the degree of a malignant mesothelioma chiefly when the tumor invades local structures, for example, the ribs and the diaphragm.
- Pleural fluid is exudative in nature. In about 30% of patients, the glucose level is <50 mg/dL and the pH level is <7.20. Low pH or glucose level is likely to have not so good prognosis. Cytology reveals a mixture of normal mesothelial cells, differentiated and undifferentiated malignant mesothelial cells, and varying numbers of lymphocytes and polymorphonuclear leukocytes.
- The surgical management of mesothelioma is associated with considerable morbidity, but it has made noteworthy advances in palliating the chief symptoms and possibly showing some progression in survival for selected patients.
- The first-line chemotherapy in good performance status and unresectable mesothelioma is combination treatment with pemetrexed and cisplatin.
- Many evolving therapies are also developing, these are: Immunotherapy, target therapy, and gene therapy.
- Solitary fibrous tumor is a mesenchymal tumor of fibroblastic origin, and alike tumors have been defined in other extrathoracic sites. There is no significant exposure is seen with asbestos or environmental agent.

REFERENCES

1. Selikoff IJ, Hammond EC, Seidman H. Latency of asbestos disease among insulation workers in the United States and Canada. Cancer. 1980;46(12):2736-40.
2. Hansen FR, Schroll M, Westphall K. Influence of environmental changes on elderly patients. Ugeskr Laeger. 1988;150(4):221-4.
3. Hodgson JT, McElvenny DM, Darnton AJ, Price MJ, Peto J. The expected burden of mesothelioma mortality in Great Britain from 2002 to 2050. Br J Cancer. 2005;92(3):587-93.
4. Antman KH. Natural history and epidemiology of malignant mesothelioma. Chest. 1993;103(4 Suppl):373S-376S.
5. Lee A, De Klerk B, Henderson DW. Malignant Mesothelioma. In: Hendrick DJ, Beckett W, Burge PS, Churg A (Eds). Occupational Disorders of the Lung: Recognition, Management and Prevention. Saunders; 2002. pp.359-79.
6. Berman DW, Crump KS. Technical support document for a protocol to assess asbestos-related risk. EPA. 2003;9345:4-6.
7. Jean D, Daubriac J, Le Pimpec-Barthes F, et al. Molecular changes in mesothelioma with an impact on prognosis and treatment. Arch Pathol Lab Med. 2012;136(3):277-93.
8. Rascoe PA, Jupiter D, Cao X, Littlejohn JE, Smythe WR. Molecular pathogenesis of malignant mesothelioma. Expert Rev Mol Med. 2012;14:e12.
9. Butel JS. Patterns of polyomavirus SV40 infections and associated cancers in humans: a model. Curr Opin Virol. 2012;2(4):508-14.
10. Carbone M, Burck C, Rdzanek M, Rudzinski J, Cutrone R, Bocchetta M. Different susceptibility of human mesothelial cells to polyomavirus infection and malignant transformation. Cancer Res. 2003;63(19):6125-9.
11. Kroczynska B, Cutrone R, Bocchetta M, Yang H, Elmishad AG, Vacek P, et al. Crocidolite asbestos and SV40 are cocarcinogens in human mesothelial cells and in causing mesothelioma in hamsters. Proc Natl Acad Sci U S A. 2006;103(38):14128-33.
12. Gazdar AF, Carbone M. Molecular pathogenesis of malignant mesothelioma and its relationship to simian virus 40. Clin Lung Cancer. 2003;5(3):177-81.
13. Tward JD, Wendland MM, Shrieve DC, Szabo A, Gaffney DK. The risk of secondary malignancies over 30 years after the treatment of non-Hodgkin lymphoma. Cancer. 2006;107(1):108-15.
14. Travis LB, Fosså SD, Schonfeld SJ, McMaster ML, Lynch CF, Storm H, et al. Second cancers among 40,576 testicular cancer patients: Focus on long-term survivors. J Natl Cancer Inst. 2005;97(18):1354-65.
15. Borczuk AC, Cooper WA, Dacic S. Tumors of the pleura and pericardium. In: WHO Classification of Tumours Editorial Board (Ed). Thoracic Tumours: WHO Classification of Tumours, 5th edition. Geneva, Switzerland: World Health Organization; 2021. p. 500.
16. Husain AN, Colby TV, Ordóñez NG, Allen TC, Attanoos RL, Beasley MB, et al. Guidelines for pathologic diagnosis of malignant mesothelioma 2017 update of the consensus statement from the international mesothelioma interest group. Arch Pathol Lab Med. 2018;142(1):89-108.
17. Suzuki Y. Pathology of human malignant mesothelioma. Semin Oncol. 1981;8:268-82.
18. Pisani RJ, Colby TY, Williams DE. Malignant mesothelioma of the pleura. Mayo Clin Proc. 1988;63:1234-44.
19. Yilmaz UM, Utkaner G, Yalniz E, Kumcuoglu Z. Computed tomographic findings of environmental asbestos-related malignant pleural mesothelioma. Respirology. 1998;3:33-8.
20. Kreel L. Computed tomography in mesothelioma. Semin Oncol. 1981;8:302-12.
21. Aisner J, Wiernik PH. Malignant mesothelioma: current status and future prospects. Chest. 1978;74:438-44.
22. Metintas M, Ucgun I, Elbek O, Erginel S, Metintas S, Kolsuz M, et al. Computed tomography features in malignant pleural mesothelioma and other commonly seen pleural diseases. Eur J Radiol. 2002;41:1-9.
23. Ng CS, Munden RF, Libshitz HI. Malignant pleural mesothelioma: the spectrum of manifestations on CT in 70 cases. Clin Radiol. 1999;54:15-21.
24. Kawashima A, Libshitz HI. Malignant pleural mesothelioma: CT manifestations in 50 cases. Am J Roentgenol. 1990;155:965-9.
25. Wang ZJ, Reddy GP, Gotway MB, Higgins CB, Jablons DM, Ramaswamy M, et al. Malignant pleural mesothelioma: evaluation with CT, MR imaging, and PET. Radiographies. 2004;24:105-19.
26. Nowak AK, Armato SG 3rd, Ceresoli GL, Yildirim H, Francis RJ. Imaging in pleural mesothelioma: a review of imaging research presented at the 9th International Meeting of the International Mesothelioma Interest Group. Lung Cancer. 2010;70:1-6.
27. Gottehrer A, Taryle DA, Reed CE, Sahn SA. Pleural fluid analysis in malignant mesothelioma. Chest. 1991;100:1003-6.
28. Klempman S. The exfoliative cytology of diffuse pleural mesothelioma. Cancer. 1962;15:691-704.
29. Scherpereel A, Grigoriu B, Conti M, Gey T, Grégoire M, Copin MC, et al. Soluble mesothelin-related protein in the diagnosis of malignant pleural mesothelioma. Am J Respir Crit Care Med. 2006;173:1155-60.
30. Davies HE, Sadler RS, Bielsa S, Maskell NA, Rahman NM, Davies RJ, et al. The clinical impact and reliability of pleural fluid mesothelin in undiagnosed pleural effusions. Am J Respir Crit Care Med. 2009;180:437-44.
31. Nurminen M, Dejmek A, Mårtensson G, Thylen A, Hjerpe A. Clinical utility of liquid-chromatographic analysis of effusions for hyaluronate content. Clin Chem. 1994;40:777-80.
32. Hegmans JP, Hemmes A, Hammad H, Boon L, Hoogsteden HC, Lambrecht BN. Mesothelioma environment comprises cytokines and T-regulatory cells that suppress immune responses. Eur Respir J. 2006;27(6):1086-95.
33. Vlaeminck-Guillem V, Bienvenu J, Isaac S, Grangier B, Golfier F, Passot G, et al. Intraperitoneal cytokine level in patients with peritoneal surface malignancies. A study of the RENAPE (French Network for Rare Peritoneal Malignancies). Ann Surg Oncol. 2013;20(8):2655-62.
34. Chang K, Pai LH, Pass H, Pogrebniak HW, Tsao MS, Pastan I, et al. Monoclonal antibody K1 reacts with epithelial mesothelioma but not with lung adenocarcinoma. Am J Surg Pathol. 1992;16(3):259-68.
35. Ordóñez NG. Value of mesothelin immunostaining in the diagnosis of mesothelioma. Mod Pathol. 2003;16(3):192-7.

36. Pass HI, Lott D, Lonardo F, Harbut M, Liu Z, Tang N, et al. Asbestos exposure, pleural mesothelioma, and serum osteopontin levels. N Engl J Med. 2005;353(15):1564-73.
37. Pass HI, Levin SM, Harbut MR, Melamed J, Chiriboga L, Donington J, et al. Fibulin-3 as a blood and effusion biomarker for pleural mesothelioma. N Engl J Med. 2012;367(15):1417-27.
38. Amin MB, Greene FL, Edge SB, Compton CC, Gershenwald JE, Brookland RK, et al., (Eds). American Joint Committee on Cancer (AJCC) Cancer Staging Manual, 8th edition. Chicago: Springer; 2017.
39. Sugarbaker DJ, Strauss GM, Lynch TJ, Richards W, Mentzer SJ, Lee TH, et al. Node status has prognostic significance in the multimodality therapy of diffuse, malignant mesothelioma. J Clin Oncol. 1993;11(6):1172-8.
40. Sugarbaker DJ, Flores RM, Jaklitsch MT, Richards WG, Strauss GM, Corson JM, et al. Resection margins, extrapleural nodal status, and cell type determine postoperative long-term survival in trimodality therapy of malignant pleural mesothelioma: Results in 183 patients. J Thorac Cardiovasc Surg. 1999;117(1):54-63; discussion 63-5.
41. Grondin SC, Sugarbaker DJ. Pleuropneumonectomy in the treatment of malignant pleural mesothelioma. Chest. 1999;116(6 Suppl):450S-454S.
42. Rusch VW, Piantadosi S, Holmes EC. The role of extrapleural pneumonectomy in malignant pleural mesothelioma. A Lung Cancer Study Group trial. J Thorac Cardiovasc Surg. 1991;102(1):1-9.
43. Rusch VW, Venkatraman E. The importance of surgical staging in the treatment of malignant pleural mesothelioma. J Thorac Cardiovasc Surg. 1996;111(4):815-25; discussion 825-6.
44. van Ruth S, Baas P, Zoetmulder FAN. Surgical treatment of malignant pleural mesothelioma: a review. Chest. 2003;123(2): 551-61.
45. Vogelzang NJ, Rusthoven JJ, Symanowski J, Denham C, Kaukel E, Ruffie P, et al. Phase III study of pemetrexed in combination with cisplatin versus cisplatin alone in patients with malignant pleural mesothelioma. J Clin Oncol. 2003;21(14):2636-44.
46. van Meerbeeck JP, Gaafar R, Manegold C, Van Klaveren RJ, Van Marck EA, Vincent M, et al. Randomized phase III study of cisplatin with or without raltitrexed in patients with malignant pleural mesothelioma: an intergroup study of the European Organisation for Research and Treatment of Cancer Lung Cancer Group and the National Cancer Institute of Canada. J Clin Oncol. 2005;23(28):6881-9.
47. Zalcman G, Mazieres J, Margery J, Greillier L, Audigier-Valette C, Moro-Sibilot D, et al. Bevacizumab for newly diagnosed pleural mesothelioma in the Mesothelioma Avastin Cisplatin Pemetrexed Study (MAPS): a randomised, controlled, open-label, phase 3 trial. Lancet. 2016;387(10026):1405-14.
48. Castagneto B, Zai S, Dongiovanni D, Muzio A, Bretti S, Numico G, et al. Cisplatin and gemcitabine in malignant pleural mesothelioma: a phase II study. Am J Clin Oncol. 2005;28(3): 223-6.
49. Paik PK, Krug LM. Histone deacetylase inhibitors in malignant pleural mesothelioma: preclinical rationale and clinical trials. J Thorac Oncol. 2010;5(2):275-9.
50. Aisner J. Current approach to malignant mesothelioma of the pleura. Chest. 1995;107(6 Suppl):332S-344S.
51. Maggi G, Casadio C, Cianci R, Rena O, Ruffini E. Trimodality management of malignant pleural mesothelioma. Eur J Cardiothorac Surg. 2001;19(3):346-50.
52. Boutin C, Rey F, Viallat JR. Prevention of malignant seeding after invasive diagnostic procedures in patients with pleural mesothelioma. A randomized trial of local radiotherapy. Chest. 1995;108(3):754-8.
53. Ceresoli GL, Aerts JG, Dziadziuszko R, Ramlau R, Cedres S, van Meerbeeck JP, et al. Tumour treating fields in combination with pemetrexed and cisplatin or carboplatin as first-line treatment for unresectable malignant pleural mesothelioma (STELLAR): a multicentre, single-arm phase 2 trial. Lancet Oncol. 2019;20(12):1702-9.
54. Astoul P, Picat-Joossen D, Viallat JR, Boutin C. Intrapleural administration of interleukin-2 for the treatment of patients with malignant pleural mesothelioma: a phase II study. Cancer. 1998;83(10):2099-104.
55. Boutin C, Viallat JR, Van Zandwijk N, Douillard JT, Paillard JC, Guerin JC, et al. Activity of intrapleural recombinant gamma-interferon in malignant mesothelioma. Cancer. 1991;67(8):2033-7.
56. Boutin C, Nussbaum E, Monnet I, Bignon J, Vanderschueren R, Guerin JC, et al. Intrapleural treatment with recombinant gamma-interferon in early-stage malignant pleural mesothelioma. Cancer. 1994;74(9):2460-7.
57. Baas P, Scherpereel A, Nowak AK, Fujimoto N, Peters S, Tsao AS, et al. First-line nivolumab plus ipilimumab in unresectable malignant pleural mesothelioma (CheckMate 743): a multicentre, randomised, open-label, phase 3 trial. Lancet. 2021;397(10272):375-86.
58. Hassan R, Thomas A, Nemunaitis JJ, Patel MR, Bennouna J, Chen FL, et al. Efficacy and safety of avelumab treatment in patients with advanced unresectable mesothelioma: Phase 1b results from the JAVELIN solid tumor trial. JAMA Oncol. 2019;5(3):351-7.
59. Nowak AK, Lesterhuis WJ, Kok PS, Brown C, Hughes BG, Karikios DJ, et al. Durvalumab with first-line chemotherapy in previously untreated malignant pleural mesothelioma (DREAM): a multicentre, single-arm, phase 2 trial with a safety run-in. Lancet Oncol. 2020;21(9):1213-23.
60. Dubey S, Jänne PA, Krug L, Pang H, Wang X, Heinze R, et al. A phase II study of sorafenib in malignant mesothelioma: results of Cancer and Leukemia Group B 30307. J Thorac Oncol. 2010;5(10):1655-61.
61. Pass HI, Brewer GJ, Dick R, Carbone M, Merajver S. A phase II trial of tetrathiomolybdate after surgery for malignant mesothelioma: final results. Ann Thorac Surg. 2008;86(2):383-9; discussion 390.
62. Baas P, Boogerd W, Dalesio O, Haringhuizen A, Custers F, van Zandwijk N. Thalidomide in patients with malignant pleural mesothelioma. Lung Cancer. 2005;48(2):291-6.
63. Szlosarek PW, Steele JP, Nolan L, Gilligan D, Taylor P, Spicer J, et al. Arginine deprivation with pegylated arginine deiminase in patients with argininosuccinate synthetase 1-deficient malignant pleural mesothelioma: a randomized clinical trial. JAMA Oncol. 2017;3(1):58-66.
64. Beddowes E, Spicer J, Chan PY, Khadeir R, Corbacho JG, Repana D, et al. Phase 1 dose-escalation study of pegylated arginine deiminase, cisplatin, and pemetrexed in patients with argininosuccinate synthetase 1-deficient thoracic cancers. J Clin Oncol. 2017;35(16):1778-85.
65. Szlosarek PW, Baas P, Ceresoli GL, Fennell DA, Gilligan D, Johnston A, et al. ATOMIC-Meso: A randomized phase 2/3 trial of ADI-PEG20 or placebo with pemetrexed and cisplatin in patients with argininosuccinate synthetase 1-deficient non-epithelioid mesothelioma. J Clin Oncol. 2017;35(15 Suppl):TPS8582.

66. Vachani A, Moon E, Wakeam E, Albelda SM. Gene therapy for mesothelioma and lung cancer. Am J Respir Cell Mol Biol. 2010;42(4):385-93.
67. Robinson BW, Mukherjee SA, Davidson A, Morey S, Musk AW, Ramshaw I, et al. Cytokine gene therapy or infusion as treatment for solid human cancer. J Immunother. 1998;21(3):211-7.
68. Wignall OJ, Moskovic EC, Thway K, Thomas JM. Solitary fibrous tumors of the soft tissues: review of the imaging and clinical features with histopathologic correlation. AJR Am J Roentgenol. 2010;195(1):W55-W62.
69. Cardillo G, Lococo F, Carleo F, Martelli M. Solitary fibrous tumors of the pleura. Curr Opin Pulm Med. 2012;18(4):339-46.
70. Lahon B, Mercier O, Fadel E, Ghigna MR, Petkova B, Mussot S, et al. Solitary fibrous tumor of the pleura: outcomes of 157 complete resections in a single center. Ann Thorac Surg. 2012;94(2):394-400.
71. Lee KS, Im JG, Choe KO, Kim CJ, Lee BH. CT findings in benign fibrous mesothelioma of the pleura: pathologic correlation in nine patients. AJR Am J Roentgenol. 1992;158(5):983-6.
72. Lococo F, Cesario A, Cardillo G, Filosso P, Galetta D, Carbone L,et al. Malignant solitary fibrous tumors of the pleura: retrospective review of a multicenter series. J Thorac Oncol. 2012;7(11):1698-706.

CHAPTER

13 Pneumothorax and Bronchopleural Fistula

Pralhad P Prabhudesai, Bhaumik J Kamdar, Nafeesath PCP

PNEUMOTHORAX

INTRODUCTION

The abnormal presence of air in the pleural cavity, separating the visceral from the parietal pleura is known as *pneumothorax*. The term "pneumothorax" was first coined by Itard in 1803, and the full clinical picture was first described by Laennec in 1819. Kjaergaard, in 1932, provided the first modern description of primary spontaneous pneumothorax (PSP) in young people.

CLASSIFICATION (FLOWCHART 1)

Pneumothorax has been divided into spontaneous and traumatic. Spontaneous pneumothorax is further subclassified as PSP and secondary spontaneous pneumothorax (SSP). The distinction between the two is based on the underlying etiopathology. PSP refers to spontaneous pneumothorax occurring in a clinically normal lung. SSP refers to pneumothorax as a consequence of underlying lung disease, most commonly chronic obstructive pulmonary disease (COPD), asthma, tuberculosis (TB), and interstitial lung disease (ILD). However, it has been proposed that PSP frequently happens in the context of undetected lung disease due to the rupture of subpleural blebs.[1-3]

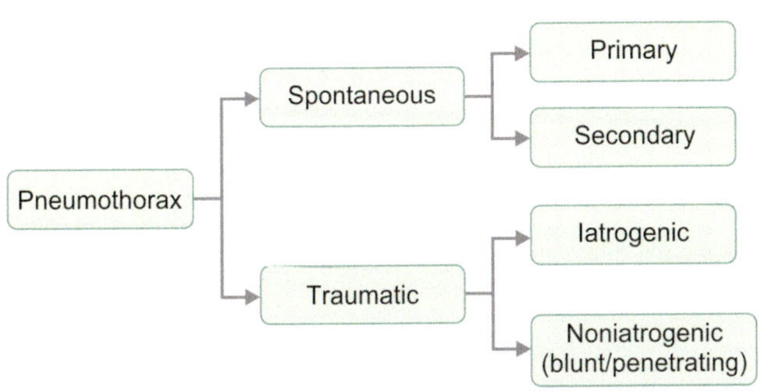

FLOWCHART 1: Classification of pneumothorax.

Traumatic pneumothorax, as the name suggests, occurs secondary to any form of blunt or penetrating trauma. Often, it occurs secondary to medical procedures, such as central line insertion, thoracocentesis, and mechanical ventilation.

Tension pneumothorax is a medical emergency that occurs when the intrapleural pressure becomes greater than the atmospheric pressure throughout all the phases of respiration, leading to cardiopulmonary compromise.

PATHOPHYSIOLOGY

Even though the pressure within the pleural space is negative with respect to alveolar pressure during the entire respiratory cycle, air does not normally exist within the pleural cavity as the partial pressure of alveolar air is 760 mm Hg (at the sea level during the end inspiration) and the partial pressure of all the gases in the venous blood is 706 mm Hg, thereby driving the net movement of alveolar air into the capillaries and not the pleural space. Under physiological conditions, healthy individuals do not generate a net negative inspiratory force of –54 mm Hg.[4]

The negative intrapleural pressure is not uniform throughout the pleural space and is influenced by gravitational force, a person's height and weight, etc. It is more negative at the apex of the lung and gradually tapers down at the base, causing more distension of the alveoli at the apex. There exists a vertical pressure gradient from the apex to the base of the lung of 0.25 cm of water.

The air enters the pleural cavity by one of the three events:

1. Communication between the pleura and the alveoli
2. Communication between the atmosphere and the pleura
3. Presence of a gas-producing organism within the pleura[4]

When an aberrant communication develops, air will move until there is equalization of pressure between the two structures or the communication is sealed. As the air enters the pleural cavity, it causes collapse of the lung. If unabated enough air may enter the pleural space to cause mediastinal shift and hemodynamic compromise leading to tension pneumothorax.

The exact mechanism responsible for PSP is not completely understood. Primary spontaneous pneumothorax is thought to be caused by a subpleural bleb or bulla, also known as emphysema-like changes (ELC), rupturing into the pleural space.[5] Air can be dissected along the bronchovascular sheath, leading to pneumomediastinum or subcutaneous emphysema.

The physiological impact of pneumothorax depends upon the quantity of air that has entered the pleural cavity, causing the collapse of the lung. It can cause a decrease in vital capacity (VC) and a decrease in partial pressure of oxygen in arterial blood (PaO_2). The reduction in arterial PaO_2 appears to be caused by a low ventilation–perfusion (V/Q) ratio, an anatomical shunt, and alveolar hypoventilation.[6] Maintenance of perfusion to the collapsed lung leads to a pulmonary shunt, which causes significant hypoxemia. If the perfusion to the collapsed lung is reduced by hypoxic vasoconstriction, hypoxemia may be minimal. The total lung capacity, functional residual capacity, and diffuse capacity may also be affected. Generally, if the pneumothorax involves around 25% of the hemithorax there is no significant shunt.[7] In a healthy individual with preserved functional residual capacity (FRC) and VC, a decrease in PaO_2 is well tolerated.

The main factors determining gaseous reabsorption are the pressure gradient across the pleural space and the venous blood, the diffusion properties of different gases, the contact area, and the permeability of different gases through the pleural surface. The total gas pressure in the pneumothorax is similar to the atmospheric pressure (760 mm Hg), and that of systemic venous blood is around 706 mm Hg, creating a pressure gradient of only 54 mm Hg so that the reabsorption of the gas into the venous blood is limited. Thus, the inhalation of 100% oxygen, which has no nitrogen content, substantially reduces the total gas pressure to 146 mm Hg vis-à-vis the 706 mm Hg of the capillary blood.

PRIMARY SPONTANEOUS PNEUMOTHORAX

Primary spontaneous pneumothorax refers to pneumothorax occurring in an apparently normal lung without any known obvious lung disorder.

Epidemiology

The annual incidence of PSP ranges from 7.4 to 18 cases per 100,000 population in males and 1.2–6 cases per 100,000 population in females. It is an increasing problem, with annual hospital admission rates rising from 9.1 to 14.1 per 100,000 population in the last 50 years. The male-to-female ratio is almost 3:1. The peak incidence occurs in the fifth decade of life.[8,4] The characteristic patient with PSP is a tall, thin male in his third to fifth decade of life. Tobacco smoking increases the risk ninefold.[9] The number of cigarettes smoked has a direct relationship with the incidence of pneumothorax. The relative risk of PSP increases by 20-fold in men who smoke half a pack of cigarettes per day and 100-fold in men who smoke one pack per day as compared to nonsmokers.

Etiology of Primary Spontaneous Pneumothorax

As mentioned earlier, PSP is a sort of misnomer because, in the majority of cases, there is an underlying unknown lung pathology or some rare genetic syndrome. Rupture of the subpleural bleb or bullae leads to the communication of the alveolar space with the pleural space. The subpleural blebs and bullae are referred to as emphysema-like changes. No causal relationship has been established between PSP and these blebs; however, they are often present in PSPs, and in 80% of the cases, abnormalities are found on a CT scan of the chest. Another important term that needs to be clarified is "pleural porosity."[4] It is believed that the mesothelial cells of the visceral pleura are replaced by inflammatory cells, which increase the permeability of the pleura.[10] The exact mechanism by which the rupture occurs is unknown; airway inflammation secondary to cigarette smoking can be one of the causes.

Primary spontaneous pneumothorax also has a strong genetic component; their mode of inheritance is unclear. Genetic risk factors that have been associated with PSP include the haplotype A_2B_{40}, the alpha-1 antitrypsin phenotypes M1M2, and the *FBN1* gene mutations causing connective tissue abnormalities.[11,12] Familial spontaneous pneumothorax (FSP) accounts for almost 12% of all the cases. They are associated with mutations in the *FLCN* gene.[13,14] The recurrence rate is high in FSP compared to sporadic cases.

The rate of recurrence in PSP is approximately 25% and it usually occurs within 1–2 years after the first episode.[15] As in most other lung pathologies, the rate of recurrence increases with each successive pneumothorax which accounts for 60% after a second pneumothorax and 83% after a third pneumothorax. The mortality rate of PSP is very low (0.06–0.09%).[16]

SECONDARY SPONTANEOUS PNEUMOTHORAX

Pneumothorax in a patient with a known underlying lung disorder is known as *secondary spontaneous pneumothorax*. It is more severe than PSP because the patient already has an underlying lung disease compromising the pulmonary reserve. The incidence of SSP is similar to PSP; however, mortality rates and recurrence rates are much higher than PSP.

Etiology of Secondary Spontaneous Pneumothorax

Although chronic obstructive pulmonary disease (COPD) is the most common cause of SSP followed by cystic fibrosis (CF) and severe asthma, a wide spectrum of pulmonary disease has been associated with SSP **(Box 1)**.

BOX 1 Causes of secondary spontaneous pneumothorax.

- Obstructive lung disease:
  - COPD
  - Asthma
- Interstitial lung disease:
  - IPF
  - NSIP
  - Langerhans cell histiocytosis
  - Lymphangioleiomyomatosis
  - Sarcoidosis
- Infections:
  - *Pneumocystis jirovecii* pneumonia
  - Tuberculosis
  - Acute bacterial pneumonia (*Staphylococcus*)
- Malignancy:
  - Primary lung cancer
  - Metastasis
  - Complication of chemotherapy
- Connective tissue disorder:
  - Rheumatoid arthritis
  - Ankylosing spondylitis
  - Marfan's syndrome
  - Ehlers–Danlos syndrome
- Others:
  - Catamenial pneumothorax
  - Pulmonary infarction
  - Pulmonary alveolar proteinosis

Chronic Obstructive Pulmonary Disease

It is the most common cause of SSP according to the Western data. It tends to occur in moderate to severe COPD. Rupture of the bullae at the apical zone is the most common cause. Almost, 25–30% of patients have FEV_1 below 1 L and a mean forced expiratory volume (FEV_1)/forced vital capacity (FVC) ratio of 57%.[17] Persistent bronchopleural fistula (BPF), a complication of pneumothorax is also commonly found in COPD patients. Another study found that SSP increased the mortality of age-matched COPD patients by 3.5-fold.[18]

Cystic Fibrosis

Pneumothorax is common in CF patients and is a poor prognostic factor. The pathophysiology of pneumothorax in CF can be understood from the nature of the disease itself. It leads to significant air trapping, chronic airway obstruction, and uncleared inspissated secretions with eventual inflammation of the pleural surface leading to its rupture. On expected lines, with increasing age and decreasing FEV_1, the risk of pneumothorax increases in CF patients. Along with these, the presence of *Pseudomonas aeruginosa, Burkholderia cepacia, or Aspergillus* in the airways can be considered an independent risk factor for the development of pneumothorax in a CF patient. The use of dornase alfa and noninvasive positive pressure ventilation (NIV) are also risk factors. A potential point of debate is whether airway clearance measures be deployed in a case of pneumothorax in CF. If the pneumothorax is small, it can be continued except for positive pressure ventilation, but if it is large, then airway clearance modalities should be withheld. Recurrence rates are much higher in CF patients. Therefore, pleurodesis should also be considered for large recurrent pneumothoraces.

Malignancy

Malignancies account for 16–18% of cases of SSP. Primary lung malignancy is a common cause of SSP than metastases. The underlying pathology is tumor necrosis with endobronchial obstruction and air trapping. There can be the development of necrotizing cysts which predisposes the patient to develop pneumothorax.

Necrotizing Infections

Pneumocystis jirovecii, TB, bacteria, and less often fungi or other microorganisms, including severe acute respiratory syndrome coronavirus-2 (SARS-CoV-2) can complicate an ongoing pneumonia. The underlying mechanism being necrotizing destruction of the underlying lung tissue.

- *Pneumocystis carinii pneumonia (PCP)*: The underlying pathology being the presence of subpleural cysts and subpleural necrosis associated with this infection. Extensive invasion of the interstitial tissue is common with PCP. These lesions are more common at the apex compared to the base. Due to the necrotizing nature of this infection, it is difficult to treat. Surgical intervention may be indicated in such patients.
- *TB*: In the Indian context, TB remains one of the common causes of secondary pneumothorax. Western data states COPD to be the most common cause of SSP, however, as far as Indian data is concerned, in our experience, TB remains one of the most common causes of SSP. Tuberculosis lesions are notoriously common at the apex of the lung due to poor ventilation at the apex.

IATROGENIC PNEUMOTHORAX

The rate of iatrogenic pneumothorax has risen significantly due to an increase in the use of invasive diagnostic and therapeutic techniques. The leading cause of iatrogenic pneumothorax is transthoracic needle aspiration followed by central venous catheterization, mainly in the subclavian vein followed by the internal jugular vein. Routine use of ultrasound (USG)-guided catheterization reduces the risk of developing complications. Other procedures such as transbronchial needle aspiration, intercostal nerve blocks, and tracheostomy also increase the risk of iatrogenic pneumothorax.

Mechanical ventilation is also a potential risk factor for developing pneumothorax. Increased positive end-expiratory pressure, right mainstem intubation, inflammatory conditions like aspiration pneumonia, and acute respiratory distress syndrome (ARDS) increase the risk of pneumothorax. When a patient on mechanical ventilation displays significant decompensation while being ventilated, a high index of suspicion is warranted. An increase in peak and plateau pressures, patient-ventilator dyssynchrony, and an increase in respiratory rate should all be seen as red flag signs.

CLINICAL FEATURES OF PNEUMOTHORAX

Chest pain and dyspnea are the main symptoms of pneumothorax, and they are experienced by 85–95% of the patients. The pain is pleuritic in nature and is restricted to the affected side.

In PSP, the patient tolerates the symptoms well, and they typically subside within 24–48 hours. This is one of the reasons why there is a delay in patients with PSP approaching the healthcare facility. Patients with SSP typically experience more severe symptoms than those with PSP. Secondary spontaneous pneumothorax often presents with tachycardia, tachypnea, and significant respiratory distress, which may be out of proportion to the size of the pneumothorax. Pneumothorax rarely presents with symptoms, such as cough, hemoptysis, orthopnea, and Horner syndrome.[7,19] A small percentage of patients are asymptomatic and only complain of generalized malaise and fatigue. In catamenial pneumothorax, women in the reproductive age-group may develop recurrent pneumothorax within 48 hours of menstruation, which is more common on the right side. Tension pneumothorax is a medical emergency wherein patients present with respiratory distress, marked hypoxemia, and hypotension, often requiring mechanical ventilation and cardiopulmonary resuscitation.

Small pneumothoraces are usually undetectable on physical examination. Examination of the chest shows the affected side moves less with respiration. Tactile fremitus is reduced or absent, percussion notes are hyperresonant, and breath sounds are reduced or absent on the affected side. In tension pneumothorax, there is severe tachycardia often > 140 BPM, hypotension, and cyanosis; breath sounds are absent and there is a shift of the trachea and mediastinum to the opposite side.

Arterial blood gas often shows changes such as mild hypoxemia and hypocarbia resulting from hypoventilation. Severe hypoxemia is noted if pneumothorax involves > 25% of the lung. Patients with SSP already have diminished pulmonary reserves and can have life-threatening hypoxemia and hypercapnia due to a pulmonary shunt.

IMAGING IN PNEUMOTHORAX

Chest Radiograph

It is the most commonly used diagnostic modality for pneumothorax. An erect, posteroanterior chest radiograph in full inspiration is ideal. The outer margin of the visceral pleura is separated from the parietal pleura by a lucent space devoid of lung markings. The visible visceral pleural edge is seen as a thin, sharp, and white line. A shift of the mediastinum to the opposite side can be observed in cases of tension pneumothorax. Lung collapse, subcutaneous emphysema, and pneumomediastinum may be present. On a supine chest radiograph (in an intensive care unit or as a part of a trauma radiograph), a deep sulcus sign can be seen. Chest X-ray is also useful in quantification of pneumothorax **(Fig. 1)**.

Chest Computed Tomography

It is the gold standard of investigation and can detect even a small pneumothorax. A CT scan is especially useful to appreciate underlying lung pathologies. A routine CT scan is suggested in cases of chest wall trauma **(Fig. 2)**.

Lung Ultrasound

Sonographic signs of pneumothorax include the absence of lung sliding, the lung point sign, the barcode, or the stratosphere sign. Extended-focused assessment with sonography in trauma (eFAST) is the use of bedside ultrasonography in an emergency setting to rule out major pneumothorax **(Figs. 3A and B)**.

MANAGEMENT OF PNEUMOTHORAX

Management of pneumothorax depends on the size of the pneumothorax, the clinical status of the patient, the underlying lung disease, and the rate of recurrence. Treatment of pneumothorax has two goals: (1) Evacuation of air and (2) prevention of recurrence.

Conservative Management

In selected patients with a small pneumothorax (<20% of hemithorax) with minimal or no symptoms and good access to medical care in case of deterioration, observation alone may be appropriate. The administration of supplemental oxygen has been shown to increase the resorption of a pneumothorax. If the pneumothorax remains stable or decreases in size in the follow-up chest

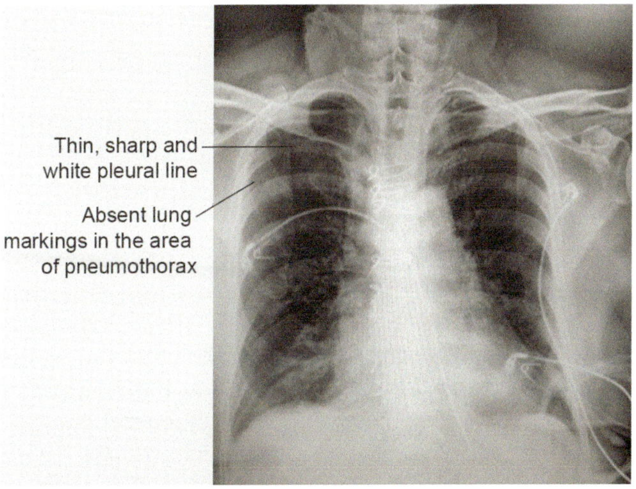

FIG. 1: Chest X-ray posteroanterior (PA) view of a 57-year-old male patient showing left-sided pneumothorax.

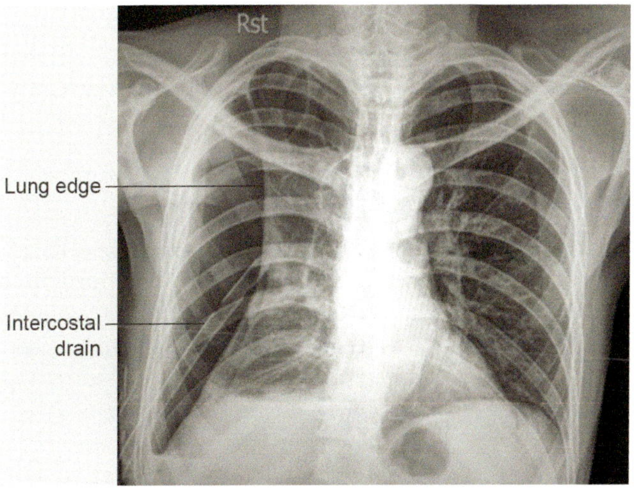

FIG. 2: Chest X-ray frontal view showing right-sided hydro-pneumothorax with intercostal drain tube in situ. A bulla is noted in the right apical region.

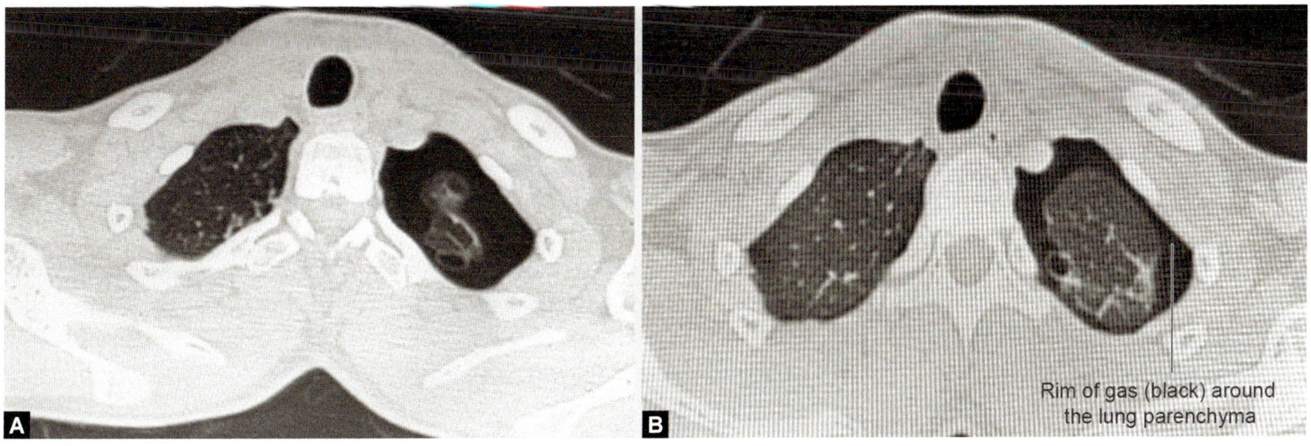

FIGS. 3A AND B: High-resolution computed tomography (HRCT) chest, axial view lung window showing left-sided pneumothorax.

X-ray and the patient does not report any significant symptoms, intervention may be deferred. Patients should be discouraged from airline travel or underwater diving until at least 1 week after radiographic resolution of spontaneous pneumothorax and 2 weeks after a traumatic pneumothorax. Cessation of smoking should be strongly encouraged.

Percutaneous needle aspiration or thoracic drain?
British Thoracic Society (BTS) and American College of Clinical Pharmacy (ACCP) guidelines differ in their view of the utility of needle aspiration, with BTS guidelines suggesting aspiration as an initial intervention in patients with a large or symptomatic primary pneumothorax and ACCP guidelines suggesting catheter drainage. When performed, aspiration should proceed until 2.5 L of air is aspirated or increased resistance is encountered. In general, small-bore (≤14F) chest tubes are preferred to large-bore (>14F) chest tubes for the management of pneumothorax. If the lung does not completely reexpand after 24–48 hours, suction may be considered to aid in visceral-parietal pleural apposition.

Thoracotomy or Video-assisted Thoracoscopic Surgery

Thoracotomy is increasingly being replaced by video-assisted thoracoscopic surgery VATS. VATS is preferred for recurrent PSP or SSP, particularly in pediatric patients. It has been shown to have better recovery and outcomes.

Indications for surgery in pneumothorax:
- Persistent air leak for longer than 7 days
- Recurrent, ipsilateral pneumothorax
- Bilateral pneumothorax
- First-time presentation in a patient with a high-risk occupation (e.g., diver and pilot)
- Patients with acquired immunodeficiency syndrome (AIDS) (often because of extensive underlying necrosis)
- Unacceptable risk of recurrent pneumothorax for patients with plans for extended stays at the remote sites[20]
- Lymphangiomyomatosis, a condition causing a high risk of recurrent pneumothorax

Pleurodesis

In patients with recurrent pneumothoraces who are surgically unfit, pleurodesis can be considered. Talc (5–10 g in 250 mL sterile isotonic solution) is commonly used for chemical pleurodesis.

Chemical Pleurodesis

It refers to the obliteration of the pleural space by the induction of pleural inflammation and fibrosis using a sclerosant (most commonly talc). The preferred method is via a small-bore chest tube rather than via thoracoscopy because the former is as effective, less invasive, and better tolerated.
- *Talc (hydrated magnesium silicate)*: It contains varying amounts of calcium, aluminum, iron, and lead. Talc is also cheap and readily available. The highest recommended dose is about 10 g. Talc causes an intense inflammatory response leading to the production of cytokines and adhesion molecules, such as interleukin-8 (IL-8), vascular endothelial growth factor (VEGF), and transforming growth factor-beta (TGF-β). Talc can be instilled through a chest tube as talc slurry or during thoracoscopy as talc poudrage.
- The tetracycline derivative doxycycline is an alternative sclerosant with reported success rates of about 80%.[21]
- Other sclerosing agents such as bleomycin, silver nitrate, and povidone–iodine, fluorouracil, autologous blood, mitomycin C, and interferon beta have also been used, however very rarely.

Mechanical/Surgical Pleurodesis

It is the mechanical abrasion of the parietal pleura during medical thoracoscopy, VATS, or open thoracotomy.

ALGORITHM FOR MANAGEMENT OF PRIMARY SPONTANEOUS PNEUMOTHORAX

Refer to **Flowchart 2** for details.

SECONDARY PNEUMOTHORAX

In general, SSP requires more aggressive management than PSP because of a higher rate of recurrence. Tube thoracostomy is indicated in most of the cases of pneumothorax in COPD patients. If the patient is not fit for surgery, chemical pleurodesis can be done and in those who are good candidates for surgery, aggressive therapy such as VATS and thoracotomy with mechanical pleurodesis should be considered. This approach provides a more effective way of reducing recurrence.

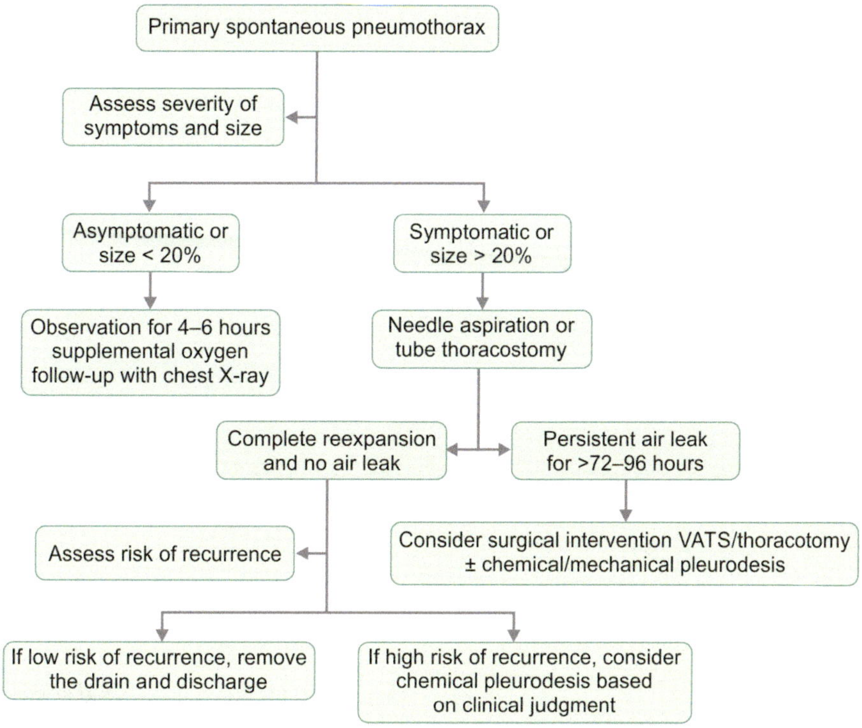

FLOWCHART 2: Management of primary spontaneous pneumothorax.

TENSION PNEUMOTHORAX

It is a medical emergency where a delay in diagnosis may cause hemodynamic compromise. In such cases, needle decompression in the second intercostal space in the midaxillary line should immediately be performed.

IATROGENIC AND TRAUMATIC PNEUMOTHORAX

Aspiration is the technique of choice. Traumatic pneumothorax is well-treated with a chest tube. Tubes are attached to one way valves.

CATAMENIAL PNEUMOTHORAX

OCP are excellent in the management of catamenial pneumothorax. Rarely it requires surgery.

COMPLICATIONS OF PNEUMOTHORAX

Refer to **Box 2** for details.

BOX 2 Complications of pneumothorax.

- Hypoxemic respiratory failure
- Respiratory or cardiac arrest
- Hemopneumothorax
- Bronchopulmonary fistula
- Reexpansion pulmonary edema
- Empyema
- Pneumomediastinum
- Pneumopericardium
- Pneumoperitoneum
- Pyopneumothorax

PNEUMOMEDIASTINUM

INTRODUCTION

Pneumomediastinum or mediastinal emphysema was first described by Laennec in 1819. It is defined as the presence of air in the mediastinum. Spontaneous pneumomediastinum, also known as *Hamman syndrome* occurs without any provoking cause and was first reported in 1939 by Hamman. It is a rare, self-limiting condition most commonly affecting young males. The risk of pneumomediastinum is increased by the use of recreational drugs, such as cocaine, marijuana, and methamphetamine. Secondary pneumomediastinum occurs as a complication of primary lung injury, blunt or penetrating chest trauma, endoscopic procedure of the airway or esophagus, neonatal lung disease, mechanical ventilation, chest surgery, or other invasive procedures **(Box 3)**.

PATHOPHYSIOLOGY

Sequence of events in the development of pneumomediastinum is as follows: The dissection of free air may not be confined solely to the mediastinum. It communicates with the submandibular space, the retropharyngeal space, and vascular sheaths within the neck. Other two routes of communication with the retroperitoneum have been noted: via a tissue plane extending through the sternocostal attachment to the diaphragm, as well as periaortic and periesophageal fascial planes. As a result, air present within the mediastinum may be dissected through these tissue planes, causing pneumopericardium, pneumothorax, subcutaneous emphysema, pneumoperitoneum, or pneumoretroperitoneum. Tension pneumomediastinum has been reported in which elevated mediastinal pressure leads to diminished cardiac output because of direct cardiac compression or reduced venous return. In the presence of extensive mediastinal gas or emphysematous gas, there can be significant airway compression.

BOX 3 Complications occurring in surgical procedures.

Complications of surgical procedures:

- Failure to cure the problem
- Acute respiratory distress
- Infection of the pleural space
- Cutaneous or systemic infection
- Persistent air leak
- Pain at the site of chest tube insertion
- Prolonged tube drainage and hospital stay

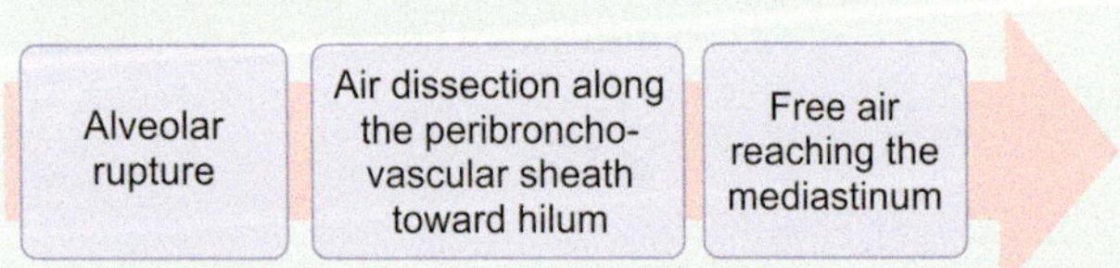

ETIOLOGY OF PNEUMOMEDIASTINUM

Refer to **Table 1** for details.

CLINICAL FEATURES

Spontaneous pneumomediastinum almost always presents with chest pain (50–90% of cases). Typically, it is substernal in location, often pleuritic which may radiate to shoulders and back and be worsened by inspiratory maneuvers.[22,23]

Additional symptoms that may occur include dyspnea, dysphagia, odynophagia, and dysphonia. Fever may occur following cytokine release that is associated with air leak. However, mediastinitis or infectious/inflammatory disorders should be included in the differential diagnosis when fever is present.

Subcutaneous crepitations: It is the unusual crackling sensation (crepitus) felt on palpation as the gas is pushed through the tissue.

Hamman sign: Crunching or clicking sound heard over the pericardium, synchronous with the heartbeat.

Rhinolalia: High-pitched nasal tone, which occurs because of the dissection of air into the soft palate and subcutaneous tissues of the neck.

DIAGNOSIS

The characteristic feature of pneumomediastinum in a chest X-ray is a thin radiolucent streak along the

TABLE 1: Etiology of pneumomediastinum.

Air from outside the body	• Penetrating or blunt injury • *Iatrogenic*: Tracheostomy, mediastinoscopy, sternotomy, and laparoscopy with pneumoperitoneum
Spontaneous alveolar rupture	Forceful coughing, vigorous crying, forceful vomiting or retching, Valsalva maneuver, scuba diving, and mechanical ventilation
Respiratory disease	• *Upper respiratory tract*: Trauma to hypopharynx or larynx, head and neck infections, and dental procedures • *Lower respiratory tract*: Asthma, bronchiolitis, trauma, bronchoscopy procedures, surgery, foreign body, and bronchopulmonary dysplasia
Gastrointestinal system	• Rupture of esophagus • Perforated viscus
Infection	Acute mediastinitis and descending necrotizing mediastinitis

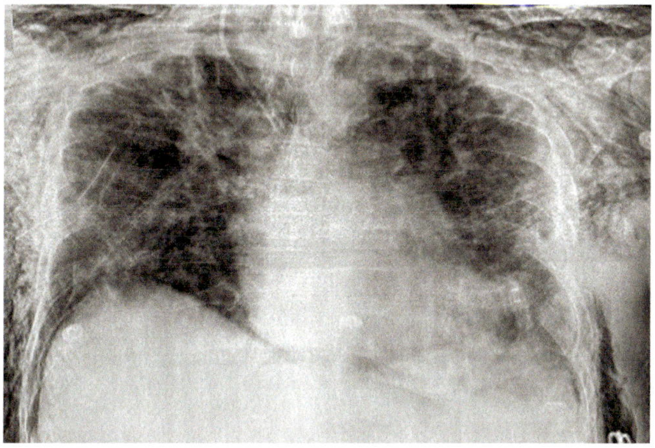

FIG. 4: Chest X-ray frontal view suggestive of pneumomediastinum and extensive subcutaneous emphysema.

mediastinal plane representing free air most commonly tracking along the margins of the heart, within the retrosternal space, or surrounding the trachea. Air outlining normal anatomic structures as it tracks from the mediastinum produces characteristic radiographic features, such as the thymic sail sign, ring around the artery sign, tubular artery sign, double bronchial wall sign, continuous diaphragm sign, and the extrapleural sign **(Fig. 4)**.

A CT scan of the chest confirms the diagnosis in suspicious cases with an inconclusive chest X-ray and can provide information on causative factors or alternative diagnoses. Additional diagnostic procedures such as bronchoscopy and esophagogastroduodenoscopy may be required if aerodigestive injuries are suspected as the cause of the pneumomediastinum. Contrast studies have been recommended when esophageal perforation is suspected in patients with pneumomediastinum.

MANAGEMENT

Treatment of spontaneous pneumomediastinum is supportive and is primarily directed at pain relief and reassurance. It is important to implement appropriate care for contributory factors, such as foreign bodies, asthma, and parenchymal pulmonary disorders. To rule out other causes of mediastinal emphysema and to look for potential pneumothorax, the patient should be monitored clinically and radiographically. Supplemental oxygen to hasten reabsorption (similar to that proposed for pneumothorax) has been reported but is probably not necessary. Only a short period of monitoring in the emergency room is necessary for patients who arrive with modest symptoms and a definite triggering cause (such as coughing). Some patients require admission for a short period of pain control and observation, with an excellent prognosis. Recurrence is rare.

Needle aspiration or skin incision to relieve subcutaneous emphysema is almost never necessary and is discouraged. Prophylactic tube thoracostomy is unnecessary. The use of mediastinoscopy in alleviating life-threatening pneumomediastinum has been reported in a small number of cases.

COMPLICATIONS AND PROGNOSIS

Spontaneous pneumomediastinum is usually a self-limited condition that rarely produces significant or life-threatening symptoms. The pneumomediastinum is almost invariably benign, with morbidity or mortality principally attributable to the associated or precipitating condition. Recurrence is rare.

Although rare, tension pneumomediastinum may occur, leading to compression of the great veins, compromising venous return, which may result in hypotension and hypoxemia secondary to ventilation-perfusion mismatch.

BRONCHOPLEURAL FISTULA

DEFINITION

BPF refers to a sinus fistula between the major, lobar, or segmental bronchus and the pleural space. Alveolopleural fistula is a communication between the lung parenchyma (distal to the level of the subsegmental bronchus) and the pleural space.

It can be a potentially fatal complication following pneumonectomy or other pulmonary surgical resections. Morbidity ranges between 25 and 71%, and diagnosis and management are often challenging for physicians.[24] Bronchopleural fistula is most commonly encountered after lung resection surgery (pneumonectomy, lobectomy, and segmentectomy), with a frequency ranging from 4.5 to 20% after pneumonectomy and 0.5–1% after lobectomy.[21]

ETIOLOGY

BPF is most commonly seen in the postoperative setting. Right-sided pneumonectomy and right lower lobectomy are more commonly associated with BPF. The proposed mechanism being that the residual stump of the tissue is predisposed to ischemic necrosis with bacterial colonization. Several risk factors are associated with BPF in the postoperative setting:[25-29]

- Right-sided surgery
- Pneumonectomy

- Diabetes mellitus
- Heavy smoking
- Residual tumor at the bronchial margin
- A large diameter bronchial stump (>25 mm)
- Extensive lymph node dissection
- Older age (>60 years)
- Male sex
- Prolonged postoperative mechanical ventilation

Other causes of BPF include chemotherapy, radiation therapy, chest trauma, bullous lung disease, tuberculosis, necrotizing pneumonia, empyema, barotrauma, etc.[21]

PATHOPHYSIOLOGY AND CLINICAL FEATURES

Broadly, BPF may be classified into three categories:

1. Acute
2. Subacute
3. Chronic

A BPF can happen at any point throughout the postoperative period, although it usually happens 8–12 days following surgery. The acute form is related to surgical dehiscence postoperatively and requires immediate surgical intervention. Acute BPF can be life-threatening as it can lead to tension pneumothorax and/or asphyxiation. Patients present with the sudden appearance of dyspnea, hypotension, subcutaneous emphysema, cough with expectoration of purulent fluid, tracheal or mediastinal shift, persistent air leak, and a reduction or disappearance of pleural effusion on the chest radiograph.

The subacute and chronic forms are primarily related to infection and are often seen in immunocompromised or debilitated patients with multiple comorbidities and are characterized by wasting, malaise, and fever.

DIAGNOSIS

The diagnosis of BPF is made using a combination of clinical, radiographic, and bronchoscopic findings that confirm an air leak from a major, lobar, or segmental bronchus to the pleural space.

Chest Radiography

Radiological features that suggest the presence or the development of a BPF include an increase in the intrapleural airspace, the appearance of a new air-fluid level, changes in an already present air-fluid level, development of tension pneumothorax, and a drop in the air-fluid level exceeding 2 cm.

While imaging features are often apparent on the chest radiograph, they are better appreciated on chest CT. The CT scan of the chest can demonstrate actual fistulous communication as well as evidence of pneumothorax, pneumomediastinum, and underlying lung pathology. Three-dimensional (3D) reconstruction using the spiral technique has also been used successfully to demonstrate BPF in its entirety.

Bronchoscopy

Bronchoscopy is critical for the diagnosis and localization of BPF. Bronchoscopy additionally allows proper evaluation of the surgical site, assessment of fistula size, and exclusion of other etiologies. Continuous bubbling at the surgical site when saline is instilled during bronchoscopy suggests the presence of BPF. Inflation of a balloon-tipped catheter into selected airways can aid in localization, as balloon occlusion decreases or eliminates an air leak. Localization of the BPF can also be done by the instillation of methylene blue into the pleural space through the chest tube with simultaneous bronchoscopic visualization of dye in the tracheobronchial tree.

Computed tomography bronchography (CTB) has been utilized in the diagnosis of a difficult BPF. Standard ventilation scintigraphy has been used to diagnose and localize moderate-sized peripheral BPF.

Differential Diagnosis

In patients who have had lung resection (especially pneumonectomy), acute findings of tension pneumothorax are almost pathognomonic of BPF. Although other conditions such as postoperative tension chylothorax or hemorrhage into the pleural space may also cause similar findings, the affected hemithorax gets filled with fluid rather than air.

Although a fall in the postpneumonectomy fluid level is considered a sign of a BPF, a few patients may have a condition described as the benign emptying of the postpneumonectomy space (BEPS). To make a diagnosis of this condition, all patients should undergo an exhaustive evaluation and fulfill the following criteria:

- Asymptomatic with no fever
- Leukocytosis
- Fluid expectoration
- Negative pleural fluid culture
- No evidence of BPF on bronchoscopy and/or ventilation scintigraphy

Ultimately, bronchoscopic findings of a bronchial defect will distinguish BPF from other competing etiologies.

MANAGEMENT AND PROGNOSIS

First-line therapy should address any immediate, life-threatening conditions, for example, endobronchial contamination, pulmonary flooding, and tension pneumothorax.

General Supportive Care

The following therapies should be performed when indicated:

- *Chest tube (minimize suction)*: The first intervention for BPF should be drainage of air (and fluid) from the pleural space by chest tube thoracostomy (if not already in place), which is usually placed in supra-diaphragmatic/midaxillary line under ultrasound guidance. Pleural fluid should be sent for cell count, pH, total protein, lactate dehydrogenase, glucose, cytology, triglycerides, Gram stain, and culture (in blood culture bottles) to assess for or rule out concomitant pleural infection.
- *Assess and treat for potential pleural space infection*:
    - Broad-spectrum intravenous antibiotics against gram-positive, gram-negative, and anaerobic microorganisms should be given to all patients until Gram stain, cultures, and sensitivities are available.
    - Intrapleural enzyme therapy may be appropriate for patients with infected multiloculated effusions where the chest tube is unable to completely drain the pleural cavity.
    - *Postural drainage*: If postural drainage is performed, there are some prerequisites that need to be fulfilled to prevent contralateral spillage of infection:
        - The patient should be able to expectorate
        - Complete drainage of chest cavity and chest tube drainage should be <30 mL/day
        - Technique is done with concomitant pleural irrigation[30]
- Patients should receive adequate nutrition, and therapy for comorbidities should also be optimized.
- For patients who are mechanically ventilated, lowering the level of positive pressure and selective intubation of the healthy lung is appropriate.

Postlung Resection

Surgical Repair (Curative)

Most patients who develop BPF following lung resection, particularly those who develop BPF in the early postoperative period (<14 days), should undergo surgical repair provided that the patient is fit for surgery, the bronchial stump is not diseased, and postoperative extubation is expected. Late dehiscence can be more technically challenging to repair because of diminished tissue quality, the development of a matured fistula tract, and significant pleural contamination and scarring. In patients who are on mechanical ventilation for significant hypoxia or hemodynamic instability, it is generally preferable to wait until they are extubated since positive pressure ventilation might interfere with stump healing.

Surgical repair involves revision of the stump with debridement of necrotic tissue and suture reclosure of the bronchial stump with vascularized flap tissue, such as omentum and muscle.[31]

For those who present later in the postoperative course (>14 days), surgery is generally indicated but may need to be delayed if the patient requires therapy to treat a complicating empyema or improve their physical strength and nutritional status.

In patients with small fistulas (<8 mm), each strategy may theoretically result in fistula closure; however, preferably bronchoscopic methods must be adopted based upon the rationale that this approach likely eliminates lengthy periods of hospitalization and reduces morbidity in this population.

In patients who are unable to tolerate bronchial stump revision or if an early repair fails, open-window thoracostomy (OWT), such as the Eloesser flap or Clagett procedure, should be considered as adequate drainage allows most BPFs to close over time. The duration of OWT usually depends on the response to antibiotic therapy, obliteration of the empyema cavity, and nutrition status.[32]

Patients not Surgically Fit

For postoperative patients with BPF who are at high risk for surgery (e.g., suppurative pleuropulmonary disease, hemodynamic instability, and severe hypoxemia), patients who need a bridge to surgery, or patients with advanced malignancy, bronchoscopic management is typically indicated.

Nonlung Resection Patients (Bronchoscopic Intervention)

In general, patients with BPF for reasons other than lung resection (e.g., those directly caused by malignancy and infection) are treated with bronchoscopic methods since in most cases, the bronchial stump is affected by disease and therefore stump revision is not feasible (e.g., advanced malignancy).

Bronchoscopic management is largely targeted at temporary fistula closure but can be used as a bridge to curative surgery in the event that the underlying cause is reversible.

Fistulas ≥8 mm—fistula closure with airway stents, coils, or Amplatzer devices are options in patients with larger BPF.

Fistulas <8 mm—while stents, coils, and Amplatzer devices can be used to seal smaller fistulas, other methods have also been reported as successful and are considered less invasive, making them suitable for closing small fistulas, among which occlusive materials are the most commonly employed. In general, occlusive material should be injected through a catheter passed inside the working channel of the bronchoscope since they all have the potential to occlude and damage the bronchoscope. A few case series have reported successful closure of small BPFs using endobronchial injection of sclerosants, such as ethanol, polidocanol, and tetracycline followed by autologous blood.[33-35] Argon plasma coagulation and neodymium-doped yttrium aluminum garnet (Nd:YAG) laser have been described for patients with small BPF with very limited experience.[36,37]

Prognosis

Bronchopleural fistulas are associated with significant morbidity and mortality that range from 21 to 71% in the setting of postpneumonectomy empyema.[38] Since most BPFs occur early in the postoperative period and are not infected, most patients undergo surgical repair with excellent success. Bronchoscopic approaches have variable success rates, and prognosis may be determined by the underlying illness or morbid state that prevents surgery.

KEY POINTS

- Pneumothorax can be defined as the presence of abnormal air in the pleural cavity.
- Management of pneumothorax depends upon the quantity of air that is present in the pleural cavity.
- A significant amount of pneumothorax (>20%) can cause hemodynamic instability.
- Tension pneumothorax is a medical emergency, it requires immediate decompression.
- In an emergency presentation, pneumothorax is largely a clinical diagnosis.
- Management ranges from close observation, supplemental observations, intercostal drainage (ICD) insertion, bullectomy, VATS with pleurodesis, or even open thoracotomy.
- Pneumomediastinum is the presence of abnormal air in the mediastinal cavity.
- Pneumomediastinum can be secondary to trauma or even spontaneously.
- Management depends upon the clinical status of the patient, because many patients may be asymptomatic, surgical intervention is reserved for patients who are hemodynamically unstable.
- BPF is an abnormal connection between the main stem bronchus, or segmental bronchus with pleural space.
- BPF management-first-line therapy should address any immediate, lifethreatening conditions, for example, endobronchial contamination, pulmonary flooding, and tension pneumothorax.

REFERENCES

1. Donahue DM, Wright CD, Viale G, Mathisen DJ. Resection of pulmonary blebs and pleurodesis for spontaneous pneumothorax. Chest. 1993;104(6):1767-9.
2. Lesur O, Delorme N, Fromaget JM, Bernadac P, Polu JM. Computed tomography in the etiologic assessment of idiopathic spontaneous pneumothorax. Chest. 1990;98(2):341-7.
3. MacDuff A, Arnold A, Harvey J. BTS Pleural Disease Guideline Group. Management of spontaneous pneumothorax: British Thoracic Society pleural disease guideline 2010. Thorax. 2010;65(Suppl 2):ii18-31.
4. Noppen M. Spontaneous pneumothorax: epidemiology, pathophysiology and cause. Eur Respir Rev. 2010;19(117):217-9.
5. Macklin MT, Macklin CC. Malignant interstitial emphysema of the lungs and mediastinum as an important occult complication in many respiratory diseases and other conditions: interpretation of the clinical literature in the light of laboratory experiment. Medicine. 1944;23(4):281-358.
6. Anthonisen NR. Regional lung function in spontaneous pneumothorax. Am Rev Respir Dis. 1977;115(5):873-6.
7. Walker S, Maskell N. Pneumothorax. ERS Monogr. 2016;2016(1):1-14.
8. Melton LJ, Hepper NGG, Offord KP. Incidence of spontaneous pneumothorax in Olmsted county, Minnesota: 1950 to 1974. Am Rev Respir Dis. 1979;120(6):1379-82.
9. Bense L, Eklund G, Odont D, Wiman LG. Smoking and the increased risk of contracting spontaneous pneumothorax. Chest. 1987;92(6):1009-12.
10. Haynes D, Baumann MH. Pleural controversy: aetiology of pneumothorax. Respirology. 2011;16(4):604-10.
11. Sharpe IK, Ahmad M, Braun W. Familial spontaneous pneumothorax and HLA antigens. Chest. 1980;78(2):264-8.
12. Cardy CM, Maskell NA, Handford PA, Arnold AG, Davies RJ, Morrison PJ, et al. Familial spontaneous pneumothorax and FBN1 mutations. Am J Respir Crit Care Med. 2004;169(11):1260-2.
13. Abolnik IZ, Lossos IS, Zlotogora J, Brauer R. On the inheritance of primary spontaneous pneumothorax. Am J Med Genet. 1991;40(2):155-8.
14. Ren H-Z, Zhu C-C, Yang C, Chen SL, Xie J, Hou YY, et al. Mutation analysis of the FLCN gene in Chinese patients with sporadic and familial isolated primary spontaneous pneumothorax. Clin Genet. 2008;74(2):178-83.

15. O'Rourke JP, Yee ES. Civilian spontaneous pneumothorax. Treatment options and long-term results. Chest. 1989;96(6):1302-6.
16. Gupta D, Hansell A, Nichols T, Dyong T, Ayres JG, Strachan D. Epidemiology of pneumothorax in England. Thorax. 2000;55(8):666-71.
17. Baumann MH. Do blebs cause primary spontaneous pneumothorax? Pro: blebs do cause primary spontaneous pneumothorax. J Bronchol. 2002;9(4):313-8.
18. Videm V, Pillgram-Larsen J, Ellingsen O, Andersen G, Ovrum E. Spontaneous pneumothorax in chronic obstructive pulmonary disease: complications, treatment and recurrences. Eur J Respir Dis. 1987;71(5):365-71.
19. Kansal S, Chawla R. Pleural Diseases. In: ICU Protocols. Singapore: Springer Singapore; 2020. pp.129-38.
20. Lippert HL, Lund O, Blegvad S, Larsen HV. Independent risk factors for cumulative recurrence rate after first spontaneous pneumothorax. Eur Respir J. 1991;4(3):324-31.
21. Lois M, Noppen M. Bronchopleural fistulas: an overview of the problem with special focus on endoscopic management. Chest. 2005;128(6):3955-65.
22. MacKnight JM, Mistry DJ. Chest Pain in the Athlete: Differential Diagnosis, Evaluation, and Treatment. In: Lawless CE (Ed). Sports Cardiology Essentials, 1st edition. New York: Springer; 2011. pp. 115-40.
23. Kim KS, Jeon HW, Moon Y, Kim YD, Ahn MI, Park JK, et al. Clinical experience of spontaneous pneumomediastinum: diagnosis and treatment. J Thorac Dis. 2015;(10):1817-24.
24. Nagahiro I, Aoe M, Sano Y, Date H, Andou A, Shimizu N. Bronchopleural fistula after lobectomy for lung cancer. Asian Cardiovasc Thorac Ann. 2007;15(1):45-8.
25. Wright CD, Wain JC, Mathisen DJ, Grillo HC. Postpneumonectomy bronchopleural fistula after sutured bronchial closure: incidence, risk factors, and management. J Thorac Cardiovasc Surg. 1996;112(5):1367-71.
26. Farkas EA, Detterbeck FC. Airway complications after pulmonary resection. Thorac Surg Clin. 2006;16(3):243-51s.
27. Li SJ, Zhou XD, Huang J, Liu J, Tian L, Che GW. A systematic review and meta-analysis-does chronic obstructive pulmonary disease predispose to bronchopleural fistula formation in patients undergoing lung cancer surgery? J Thorac Dis. 2016;8(7):1625-38.
28. Okuda M, Go T, Yokomise H. Risk factor of bronchopleural fistula after general thoracic surgery: review article. Gen Thorac Cardiovasc Surg. 2017;65(12):679-85.
29. Toufektzian L, Patris V, Sepsas E, Konstantinou M. Does postoperative mechanical ventilation predispose to bronchopleural fistula formation in patients undergoing pneumonectomy? Interact Cardiovasc Thorac Surg. 2015;21(3): 379-82.
30. Mao R, Ying PQ, Xie D, Dai C-Y, Zha J-Y, Chen T, et al. Conservative management of empyema-complicated post-lobectomy bronchopleural fistulas: experience of consecutive 13 cases in 9 years. J Thorac Dis. 2016;8(7):1577-86.
31. Liberman M, Cassivi SD. Bronchial stump dehiscence: update on prevention and management. Semin Thorac Cardiovasc Surg. 2007;19(4):366-73.
32. Litle VR. Management of Post-pneumonectomy Bronchopleural Fistula: A Roadmap for Rescue. Semin Thorac Cardiovasc Surg. 2018;30(1):114-5.
33. Takaoka K, Inoue S, Ohira S. Central bronchopleural fistulas closed by bronchoscopic injection of absolute ethanol. Chest. 2002;122(1):374-8.
34. Varoli F, Roviaro G, Grignani F, Vergani C, Maciocco M, Rebuffat C. Endoscopic treatment of bronchopleural fistulas. Ann Thorac Surg. 1998;65(3):807-9.
35. Martin WR, Siefkin AD, Allen R. Closure of a bronchopleural fistula with bronchoscopic instillation of tetracycline. Chest. 1991;99(4):1040-2.
36. Aynaci E, Kocatürk CI, Yildiz P, Bedirhan MA. Argon plasma coagulation as an alternative treatment for bronchopleural fistulas developed after sleeve pneumonectomy. Interact Cardiovasc Thorac Surg. 2012;14(6):912-4.
37. Kiriyama M, Fujii Y, Yamakawa Y, Fukai I, Yano M, Kaji M, et al. Endobronchial neodymium:yttrium-aluminum garnet laser for noninvasive closure of small proximal bronchopleural fistula after lung resection. Ann Thorac Surg. 2002;73(3):945-8; discussion 948-9.
38. Bribriesco A, Patterson GA. Management of Postpneumonectomy Bronchopleural Fistula: From Thoracoplasty to Transsternal Closure. Thorac Surg Clin. 2018;28(3):323-35.

CHAPTER

14 Hemothorax

Aditi Singh, Pinky Goyal, Bornali Datta

INTRODUCTION

The term hemothorax literally translates to "blood in the pleural cavity."

But not all bloody effusions are hemothorax. Usually, such effusions have a hematocrit of <5%.[1,2] For diagnosing a bloody effusion as hemothorax, the hematocrit of pleural fluid should be ≥50% of the peripheral blood hematocrit's value.[3] If for some reason, the pleural fluid could not be sent for hematocrit quantification, another way to estimate hematocrit is by dividing the pleural fluid red blood cell (RBC) count by 100,000.

ETIOLOGY

The etiology of hemothorax is broadly divided into three types: Traumatic, iatrogenic, and nontraumatic **(Box 1)**.

Traumatic

An injury to the thoracic wall, diaphragm, mediastinum, and lung, is the most common cause of hemothorax. These injuries could be penetrating or blunt injuries. Traumatic hemothorax is frequently accompanied by pneumothorax. Massive hemothorax can be seen in aortic rupture, myocardial rupture, injuries to hilar structures, and lung parenchyma. Hemothorax is more common in case of a displaced rib fracture.

BOX 1 Etiology of hemothorax.

- Traumatic
- Iatrogenic
- Nontraumatic

Diagnosis

Any patient with a history of trauma to the chest should be investigated for hemothorax. It is possible that it may not be apparent in the first chest radiograph and might take a few hours to days to become obvious, especially in case of a blunt injury.[4]

Chest ultrasound has great sensitivity and specificity (92 and 100%, respectively) with a negative predictive value (98%) and a faster performance time, but it is operator-dependent.[5] Ultrasonography (USG) chest characteristically shows homogeneously echogenic effusion and plankton signs.[6] Hematocrit sign is seen in older collections[7] **(Box 2)**.

Computed tomography (CT) thorax differentiates simple fluid from blood using attenuation value which lies typically between 35 and 70 Hounsfield unit (HU).[8] Hyperdensity on CT scan points toward a hematoma. It should be performed on a person with a thoracic injury because it additionally tells us about lung contusions and fractures.

Management

Hemothoraces that are small (<300 mL), and clinically insignificant can be subjected to needle aspiration or even expectant management as these collections will often be reabsorbed spontaneously.[9] A volume > 300–500 mL or

BOX 2 Signs of hemothorax on ultrasonography (USG) chest.

- Homogeneous echogenic effusion
- Plankton sign
- Hematocrit sign (in older effusion)

symptomatic hemothorax calls for a tube thoracostomy (preferably in the triangle of safety) immediately.[10] This not only helps evacuate blood but also opposes the two pleural membranes and aids in stopping bleeding, helps in quantifying blood loss, and prevents complications such as retained blood clot and fibrothorax.

As far as possible, insertion of the chest tube should be image-guided as the ipsilateral diaphragm might be elevated due to either atelectasis or phrenic nerve palsy. When this is not feasible, then a chest tube should be inserted in the fourth and fifth intercostal space in the midaxillary line in order to protect the diaphragm. Traditionally, large-bore chest tubes (24–36 Fr) are recommended for hemothorax to avoid blot clots in the tube, but some of the recent studies have come to the conclusion that smaller-bore chest tubes (14–22 Fr) have the same efficacy and chances of failure.[11]

Immediate drainage of 1.5 L of blood into the chest tube or continuous drainage of 200 mL/h for 4 hours or more or hemodynamic instability should prompt for immediate surgical intervention.[12] Thoracotomy has largely been replaced by video-assisted thoracoscopic surgery (VATS) with thoracotomy reserved for massive acute hemothorax, hemodynamically unstable patients, diaphragm injury, and >900 mL of retained blood.[13] Pleura is inspected for a bleeding vessel which can be controlled by electrocautery, ligation via a suture, stapling, or lung resection.

Patients draining ≥ 200 mL/h can be subjected to contrast-enhanced CT scan of the thorax which helps in identifying the bleeder, and transcatheter arterial embolization can then be performed to stop the bleeding.[14]

It comes with its share of possible complications such as spinal cord ischemia due to embolic material displacement and collateral vessel rupture leading to hemoptysis[15] **(Table 1)**.

TABLE 1: Management of hemothorax.

Quantified blood in pleural cavity/ICD drain	Management
<300 mL/clinically insignificant	Needle aspiration Expectant management
>300–500 mL/ symptomatic	Tube thoracoscopy
Immediate drainage of 1.5 L of blood/continuous drainage of 200 mL/h for 4 or more hours/ hemodynamically unstable	Surgical intervention (VATS/ open thoracotomy)
Continuous drainage of 200 mL/h	Can consider performing CECT chest followed by transcatheter arterial embolization

(CECT: contrast-enhanced computerized tomography; VATS: video-assisted thoracoscopic surgery)

Complications

Complications of hemothorax are given in **Box 3**:

- *Retention of blood clots*: Small residual clotted blood does not pose any risk but if it occupies ≥30% of the hemithorax[16] it needs to be evacuated. A decision to go ahead should be made after a CT scan.[17] The best time to remove clots is between 3 and 7 days as after that these start to organize, adhere to the pleura, and become difficult to remove.[18] Thoracoscopy can be used successfully to remove these retained clots though VATS is considered the mainstay of management. An alternative method is the placement of a second drainage tube, but it has been found that VATS significantly reduces the hospital stay and the duration of the chest tube in situ.[19] Fibrinolytic agents (streptokinase, urokinase) can be tried, but there is no randomized controlled trial available that compares these with conservative or surgical management. They are used if the patient is not in the condition to tolerate surgery.[20]
- *Empyema*: About 1–4% of patients develop empyema post-traumatic pneumothorax,[21] especially those with gross contamination of pleura, long-standing chest tubes, associated abdominal injuries, and who are admitted with shock.[22,23] The risk increases to as high as 26.8% with a residual blood clot as it acts as a good culture medium[24] and persistent bronchopleural fistula with direct injury to the lung. The need for additional interventions such as removal of retained blood is also a predictor of empyema. Administration of antibiotics to patients with hemothorax with chest tube in situ prevents pleural infection.[25] An empyema complicating hemothorax needs to be treated like any bacterial infection of the pleural cavity.
- *Pleural effusion*: In around 10% of patients, pleural effusion is observed once the chest tube is removed.[16,21] A thoracocentesis should be performed just to see if this effusion is infected. Most such effusions resolve spontaneously.
- *Fibrothorax*: It develops in <1% of patients with hemothorax.[16] It takes months to develop a diffuse pleural thickening. It is more often associated with

BOX 3 Complications of hemothorax.

- Retention of blood clots
- Empyema
- Pleural effusion
- Fibrothorax

hemopneumothorax or an infected hemothorax.[26] The definitive treatment is decortication. But in most cases, this thickening diminishes with time and decortication should be attempted after several months of injury if the pleural thickening still remains unresolved.

Iatrogenic

The most common cause of iatrogenic hemothorax is thoracic surgery.[27] Other causes include perforation of a central vein while inserting a percutaneous catheter, percutaneous lung biopsy, thoracocentesis, tube thoracostomy, transbronchial biopsy, sclerotherapy for esophageal varices, or postcardiopulmonary resuscitation.

In patients in the intensive care unit with chronic renal failure, hemothorax is more common. Management of iatrogenic hemothorax remains similar to traumatic hemothorax.

Nontraumatic Hemothorax

This is a relatively uncommon etiology for hemothorax. Spontaneous pneumothorax is the most common cause of nontraumatic hemothorax and constitutes 2–7% of cases in this category, the usual reasons being torn adhesions or vascular bulla rupture.[28] Rupture of intrathoracic vessels [aortic aneurysm, aneurysm of the pulmonary artery, coarctation of the aorta, subpleural *arteriovenous* (AV) malformations, patent ductus arteriosus], neurofibromatosis, thoracic endometriosis syndrome leading to catamenial hemothorax (seen in 14% of these women and is usually seen in the right hemithorax),[29,30] bronchopulmonary sequestration, intrathoracic extramedullary hematopoiesis, and pleural metastasis are some other causes. Abdominal pathologies such as splenic artery aneurysm, pancreatic pseudocyst rupturing through the diaphragm, and hepatocellular carcinoma can lead to hemothorax.

Anticoagulant therapy with warfarin/heparin [both unfractionated and *low molecular weight* (LMW)] and systemic thrombolytic therapy can get complicated due to hemothorax which usually can be seen by day 4–7 but also much later sometimes.[31] Similarly, intrapleural fibrinolytic therapy can have similar effects.[32]

The association between the risk of bleeding with thoracocentesis complicated with coagulopathy or anticoagulation administration was studied. Though a randomized controlled trial is not available yet, current studies suggest that there is no correlation.[15]

General management of nontraumatic hemothorax remains similar to traumatic hemothorax. In case of hemothorax complicating anticoagulant therapy, immediate discontinuation of anticoagulant therapy is required. In case of catamenial hemothorax, co-occurrence with menstruation is noted. An association with pelvic and abdominal endometriosis is seen. Suppressing ovulation by oral contraceptive pills and progesterone-only pills and suppression of gonadotropins or gonadotropin-releasing hormones are the modalities of treatment. If hormonal therapy fails, then chemical pleurodesis and ultimately total hysterectomy with bilateral salpingo-oophorectomy are the options available.[33]

KEY POINTS

- Hemothorax literally translates to blood in the pleural cavity.
- For diagnosis of hemothorax, hematocrit of pleural fluid should be ≥50% of the peripheral blood hematocrit's value.
- The etiology of hemothorax is divided into three types: (1) Traumatic, (2) iatrogenic, and (3) nontraumatic.
- Penetrating or blunt injuries to the thoracic wall, diaphragm, mediastinum, and lung are the most common causes of traumatic hemothorax and are commonly accompanied by pneumothorax.
- The most common cause of iatrogenic hemothorax is thoracic surgery.
- Nontraumatic hemothorax constitutes 2–7% of cases, the usual reasons being torn adhesions or vascular bulla rupture. Anticoagulant therapy with warfarin/heparin and intrapleural fibrinolytic therapy can have similar effects.
- USG chest (homogeneous echogenic effusion/plankton sign/hematocrit sign) and CT chest (hyperdensity with attenuation value between 35 and 70 HU) are good modalities to diagnose hemothorax.
- Hemothorax that is small (<300 mL) or clinically insignificant can be subjected to expectant management or needle aspiration can be attempted.
- A volume > 300–500 mL or symptomatic hemothorax calls for a tube thoracostomy.
- Immediate drainage of 1.5 L of blood into the chest tube or continuous drainage of 200 mL/h for 4 hours or more or hemodynamic instability should prompt immediate surgical intervention.
- Patients draining ≥ 200 mL/h can be subjected to a contrast-enhanced CT scan and transcatheter arterial embolization can then be performed.
- In case of catamenial hemothorax, modalities such as oral contraceptive pills and progesterone-only pills can be tried. If hormonal therapy fails, then chemical pleurodesis and surgery are the only options.
- Complications of hemothorax include retention of blood clots, pyothorax, pleural effusion, and fibrothorax.

REFERENCES

1. Porcel JM, Madronero AB, Pardina M, Vives M, Esquerda A, Light RW. Analysis of pleural effusions in acute pulmonary embolism: radiological and pleural fluid data from 230 patients. Respirology. 2007;12(2):234-9.
2. Kakaris S, Athanassiadi K, Vassilikos K, Skottis I. Spontaneous hemopneumothorax: a rare but life-threatening entity. Eur J Cardiothorac Surg. 2004;25(5):856-8.
3. Azfar Ali H, Lippmann M, Mundathaje U, Khaleeq G. Spontaneous hemothorax: a comprehensive review. Chest. 2008;134(5): 1056-65.
4. Drummond DS. Traumatic hemothorax: complications and management. Am Surg. 1967;33(5):403-8.
5. Brooks A, Davies B, Smethhurst M, Connolly J. Emergency ultrasound in the acute assessment of haemothorax. Emerg Med J. 2004;21(1):44-6.
6. Soni NJ, Franco R, Velez MI, Schnobrich D, Dancel R, Restrepo MI, et al. Ultrasound in the diagnosis and management of pleural effusions. J Hosp Med. 2015;10(12):811-6.
7. Connolly JA, Dean AJ, Hoffmann B, Jarman RD (Eds). Emergency Point-Of-Care Ultrasound. New York: Wiley; 2017.
8. Kaewlai R, Avery LL, Asrani AV, Novelline RA. Multidetector CT of blunt thoracic trauma. Radiographics. 2008;28(6):1555-70.
9. Gilbert RW, Fontebasso AM, Park L, Tran A, Lampron J. The management of occult hemothorax in adults with thoracic trauma: A systematic review and meta-analysis. J Trauma Acute Care Surg. 2020;89(6):1225-32.
10. Choi J, Villarreal J, Andersen W, Min JG, Touponse G, Wong C, et al. Scoping review of traumatic hemothorax: Evidence and knowledge gaps, from diagnosis to chest tube removal. Surgery. 2021;170(4):1260-7.
11. Kulvatunyou N, Bauman ZM, Zein Edine SB, de Moya M, Krause C, Mukherjee K, et al. The small (14 Fr) percutaneous catheter (P-CAT) versus large (28-32 Fr) open chest tube for traumatic hemothorax: A multicenter randomized clinical trial. J Trauma Acute Care Surg. 2021;91(5):809-13.
12. Karmy-Jones R, Jurkovich GJ, Nathens AB, Shatz DV, Brundage S, Wall MJ Jr, et al. Timing of urgent thoracotomy for hemorrhage after trauma: a multicenter study. Arch Surg. 2001;136(5):513-8.
13. DuBose J, Inaba K, Demetriades D, Scalea TM, O'Connor J, Menaker J, et al. Management of post-traumatic retained hemothorax: a prospective, observational, multicenter AAST study. J Trauma Acute Care Surg. 2012;72(1):11-24.
14. Hagiwara A, Yanagawa Y, Kaneko N, Takasu A, Hatanaka K, Sakamoto T, et al. Indications for transcatheter arterial embolization in persistent hemothorax caused by blunt trauma. J Trauma. 2008;65(3):589-94.
15. Chemelli AP, Thauerer M, Wiedermann F, Strasak A, Klocker J, Chemelli-Steingruber IE. Transcatheter arterial embolization for the management of iatrogenic and blunt traumatic intercostal artery injuries. J Vasc Surg. 2009;49(6):1505-13.
16. Wilson JM, Boren CH Jr, Peterson SR, Thomas AN: Traumatic hemothorax: is decortication necessary? J Thorac Cardiovasc Surg. 1979;77(4):489-95.
17. Velmahos GC, Demetriades D, Chan L, Tatevossian R, Cornwell EE 3rd, Yassa N, et al. Predicting the need for thoracoscopic evacuation of residual traumatic hemothorax: chest radiograph is insufficient. J Trauma. 1999;46(1):65-70.
18. Carrillo EH, Richardson JD: Thoracoscopy in the management of hemothorax and retained blood after trauma. Curr Opin Pulm Med. 1998;4(4):243-6.
19. Meyer DM, Jessen ME, Wait MA, Estrera AS: Early evacuation of traumatic retained hemothoraces using thoracoscopy: a prospective, randomized trial. Ann Thorac Surg. 1997;64(5): 1396-1400.
20. Mowery NT, Gunter OL, Collier BR, Diaz JJ Jr, Haut E, Hildreth A, et al. Practice management guidelines for management of hemothorax and occult pneumothorax. J Trauma. 2011;70(2): 510-8.
21. Beall AC Jr, Crawford HW, De Bakey ME: Considerations in the management of acute traumatic hemothorax. J Thorac Cardiovasc Surg. 1966;52(3):351-60.
22. Griffith GL, Todd EP, McMillin RD, Zeok JV, Dillon ML, Utley JR, et al. Acute traumatic hemothorax. Ann Thorac Surg. 1978;26(3):204-7.
23. Light RW. Pleural controversy: optimal chest tube size for drainage. Respirology. 2011;16(2):244-8.
24. DuBose J, Inaba K, Okoye O, Demetriades D, Scalea T, O'Connor J, et al. Development of posttraumatic empyema in patients with retained hemothorax: results of a prospective, observational AAST study. J Trauma Acute Care Surg. 2012;73(3):752-7.
25. Brunner RG, Vinsant GO, Alexander RH, Laneve L, Fallon WF Jr. The role of antibiotic therapy in the prevention of empyema in patients with an isolated chest injury (ISS 9-10): a prospective study. J Trauma. 1990;30(9):1148-53.
26. Maxwell RA, Campbell DJ, Fabian TC, Croce MA, Luchette FA, Kerwin AJ, et al. Use of presumptive antibiotics following tube thoracostomy for traumatic hemopneumothorax in the prevention of empyema and pneumonia: a multi-center trial. J Trauma. 2004;57(4):742-8.
27. Waller DA, Edwards JG, Martin-Ucar AE. Surgery of the pleural cavity. In: Light RW, Lee YCG (Eds). Textbook of Pleural Diseases. London: Hodder Arnold; 2003. pp. 513-25.
28. Lin FC, Li RY, Tung YW, Jeng KC, Tsai SC. Morbidity, mortality, associated injuries, and management of traumatic rib fractures. J Chin Med Assoc. 2016;79(6):329-34.
29. Bobbio A, Canny E, Mansuet Lupo A, Lococo F, Legras A, Magdeleinat P, et al. Thoracic Endometriosis Syndrome Other Than Pneumothorax: Clinical and Pathological Findings. Ann Thorac Surg. 2017;104(6):1865-71.
30. Rawala MS, Khaliq MF, Iqbal MA, Naqvi STS, Farhan K, Myers A, et al. A Rare Case of Cyclical Hemothorax: Thoracic Endometriosis Syndrome. Case Rep Pulmonol. 2018;2018:9830797.
31. Mrug M, Mishra PV, Lusane HC, Cunningham JM, Alpert MA. Hemothorax and retroperitoneal hematoma after anticoagulation with enoxaparin. South Med J. 2002;95(8):936-8.
32. Kalomenidis IT. Effusions due to drugs. In: Light RW, Lee YCG (Eds). Textbook of Pleural Diseases. London: Hodder Arnold; 2003. pp. 383-93.
33. Shepard MK, Mancini MC, Campbell GD Jr, George R. Right-sided hemothorax and recurrent abdominal pain in a 34-year-old woman. Chest. 1993;103(4):1239-40.

CHAPTER

15 Chylothorax

Vidhi Jobanputra, Abhijeet Khandelwal

INTRODUCTION

Chylothorax is a rare but potentially serious pleural disease characterized by the accumulation of chyle, a milky lymphatic fluid, within the pleural cavity. The word "chyle" is derived from a Greek word "chylos," which means "juice." It is a milky fluid made of lymph, emulsified fats, and free fatty acids. This condition arises from disruptions to the thoracic duct or its tributaries, leading to the leakage of chyle into the pleural space.[1]

The term should not be confused with pseudochylorax which is a high-cholesterol-containing effusion formed due to chronic inflammatory processes. It is similar in appearance grossly and hence, it is crucial to differentiate between the two as the management significantly varies.[2,3]

The incidence of chylothorax is relatively low, accounting for approximately 1% of all pleural effusions.[4] Despite its rarity, understanding the pathophysiology, diagnosis, and management of chylothorax is crucial due to its potential for significant morbidity and mortality. This chapter aims to provide a comprehensive overview of chylothorax, including its etiology, clinical presentation, diagnostic approach, and treatment strategies.

To understand the etiology of chylothorax it is essential to know about the anatomy of the thoracic duct and its relation to the surrounding structures.

The thoracic duct is a crucial component of the lymphatic system, responsible for draining lymphatic fluid from the lower half of the body and the left upper half of the body. Its anatomy and function play a significant role in the development of chylothorax.

ANATOMY OF THE THORACIC DUCT

The thoracic duct is the largest lymphatic vessel in the human body, measuring about 2–3 mm in diameter. It originates from the cisterna chyli, an enlarged sac-like structure located just below the diaphragm at the level of the second lumbar vertebra. The cisterna chyli serves as a storage reservoir for lymphatic fluid that originates from the intestinal lacteals, the right and left lumbar trunks, and the intestinal trunk[5] **(Fig. 1)**.

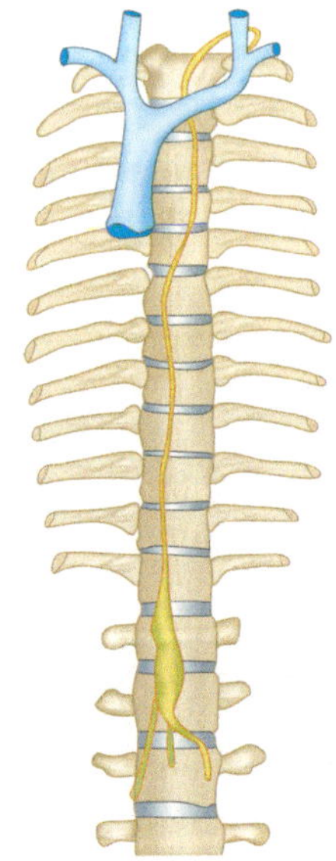

FIG. 1: Pathway of the thoracic duct. It originates from the cisterna chyle at level L1 and L2 and ascends upward on the right side and arches toward the left at the level of D5.

COURSE OF THE THORACIC DUCT

From its origin in the cisterna chyli, the thoracic duct ascends through the posterior mediastinum, passing through the aortic hiatus in the diaphragm. It then arches posterior to the esophagus and anterior to the vertebral bodies, reaching the level of the fifth thoracic vertebra. At this point, the thoracic duct often tapers and becomes more tortuous. It then crosses to the left side of the vertebral column and ascends into the superior mediastinum.[6]

DRAINAGE AREAS

The thoracic duct is responsible for draining lymphatic fluid from a vast region of the body. It receives lymph from the following areas **(Fig. 2)**:

- *Left upper limb*: The thoracic duct drains lymph from the left arm and hand, as well as the left side of the head and neck.
- *Left side of the thorax*: Lymphatic fluid from the left side of the chest wall and left lung is drained into the thoracic duct.
- *Abdominal organs*: The thoracic duct collects lymph from the abdominal organs, including the stomach, spleen, liver, pancreas, and intestines.
- *Left lower limb*: Lymph from the left leg and foot also enters the thoracic duct.[6,7]

ETIOLOGY

Chylothorax can be classified into two major categories based on its etiology—traumatic and nontraumatic chylothorax.

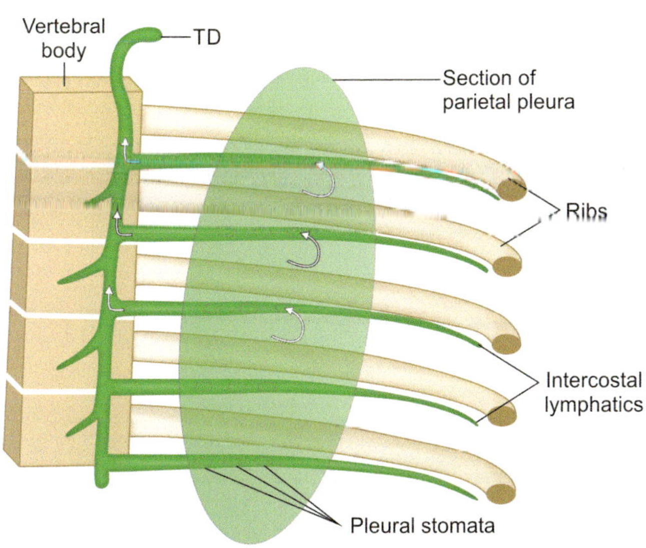

FIG. 2: Pleural stomata are present in the intercostal lymphatics on the lower border of the ribs.[8]
(TD: thoracic duct)

Traumatic Chylothorax

Traumatic chylothorax often results from thoracic trauma, such as iatrogenic injury during surgery or penetrating chest injuries. It occurs when the thoracic duct or its major branches are damaged, leading to the leakage of chyle into the pleural cavity. Common iatrogenic causes include complications during thoracic surgeries involving the esophagus, heart, or lungs, as well as central venous catheterization. Noniatrogenic traumatic causes such as trauma, straining, coughing, and vomiting have also been reported **(Box 1)**.

Nontraumatic Chylothorax

Nontraumatic chylothorax may occur due to various underlying conditions that directly or indirectly damage the thoracic duct and its drainage **(Table 1)**.

Some of the common causes include:

- *Malignancies*: Lymphoma, particularly Hodgkin's lymphoma and metastatic cancers can obstruct or infiltrate the thoracic duct, causing chylothorax.

BOX 1 Traumatic causes of chylothorax.

Surgical:
- Esophageal surgery
- Congenital heart surgery
- Mediastinal lymph node dissection
- Lobectomy
- Pneumonectomy
- Lung transplant
- Cardiovascular surgery
- Neck surgery
- Thyroidectomy
- Sympathectomy
- Diaphragmatic hernia repair
- Gastric banding
- Thymectomy
- Tube thoracostomy
- Nephrectomy
- Central venous catheterization
- Radiation

Nonsurgical:
- Thoracic radiation
- Childbirth
- Vomiting
- Sneezing
- Stretching
- Blunt trauma
- Thoracolumbosacral orthosis
- Knife wound
- Gunshot wound

TABLE 1: Nontraumatic causes of chylothorax.

Malignancy	Infectious	Lymphatic disorder	Miscellaneous	Chylous ascites
Lymphomatous	Tuberculosis	LAM	SVC thrombosis	Cirrhosis
Leukemia	Filariasis	Lymphangiectasis	Fibrosing mediastinitis	Nephrotic syndrome
Lung cancer		Lymphangiomatosis	Gorham–Stout syndrome	Idiopathic
Mediastinal		Lymphangioma	Yellow nail syndrome	
Kaposi sarcoma			Sarcoidosis	
Myeloma			Amyloidosis	

(LAM: lymphangioleiomyomatosis; SVC: superior vena cava)

- *Idiopathic*: In some cases, the cause of chylothorax remains unknown and it is termed "idiopathic chylothorax." Approximately, 6–14% of chylothoraxes are idiopathic in nature.
- *Congenital*: Rarely, chylothorax may be present at birth due to congenital abnormalities of the lymphatic system.
- *Infections*: Inflammatory conditions, such as tuberculosis and fungal infections, can cause inflammation, mediastinal lymphadenopathy, and obstruction of lymphatic vessels, leading to chyle leakage.
- *Miscellaneous*: Lymphatics disorder like LAM and other disorders. Though LAM associated with chylothorax occurs mostly in females, there are case reports of LAM in male with chylothorax.[9] Apart from LAM other lymphatics disorders are also cause of chylothorax. Rarely it may be associated with chyluria[10,11] and chyloperitoneum.[12] Other miscellaneous conditions such as, thoracic outlet aneurysms, filariasis, thyroid goiter.[13-15]

CLINICAL PRESENTATION

The clinical presentation of chylothorax can vary based on its underlying cause and the rate of chyle accumulation. The duration of symptoms may also vary according to the underlying cause. The onset may be gradual in nontraumatic etiologies. Common symptoms and signs include:

Symptoms

- *Dyspnea*: Gradual or sudden onset of breathlessness is a common presenting complaint in chylothorax patients. Majority of patients present with dyspnea due to the mechanical effect of pleural effusion. This may be associated with other symptoms of "chest uneasiness and heaviness."
- *Cough*: Patients may experience a persistent cough, often associated with the presence of an underlying lung disease. The cough is usually dry in patients with no other parenchymal abnormalities.
- *Chest pain*: It is uncommon in chylothorax as the fluid is chylous; it does not provoke an inflammatory response and is rarely infected.
- *Fever*: It is equally uncommon as the fluid is sterile and does not have any bacteriostatic dues to the presence of immunoglobulins in it.[16]
- *Symptoms of malnutrition*: Since the chyle fluid consists of a large number of proteins and fat, malnutrition is fairly common. It may be associated with vitamin deficiencies such as A, D, E, and K due to their fat-soluble nature. These deficiencies are more likely to occur when a large amount of chylous fluid is drained rather than its plain accumulation.
- *Repeated infections*: Chyle is rich in immunoglobulins and thus, immune suppression due to loss of immunoglobulins can make the individual more prone to repeated infections.
- *Chyloptysis*: An extremely rare symptom is chyloptysis, i.e., expectorating chylous fluid is reported. This can happen when an abnormal communication exists between the bronchial tree and the lymphatic channel or due to a bronchopleural fistula in the presence of a chylous effusion.[17]

Signs

- *Signs of underlying condition*: Depending on the underlying cause, patients may exhibit other signs related to malignancies or infections.
- *Decreased breath sounds*: On auscultation, decreased breath sounds may be noted over the affected hemithorax.
- Dull note on percussion and presence of all the signs of pleural effusion.
- *Arrythmias*: A relatively rare sign of presentation may be arrhythmias in patients on digoxin and amiodarone, as these drugs are carried through the chyle and their concentration may be decreased in the presence of a chylothorax leading to arrhythmias.[18]

DIAGNOSTIC APPROACH (FLOWCHART 1)

The diagnosis of chylothorax involves a systematic approach to evaluate the pleural effusion and identify its chylous nature.

Imaging Studies

- *Chest X-ray*: Initial evaluation usually includes a chest X-ray which may show a pleural effusion with characteristic features of a homogenous white opacity in the pleural space. This effusion is usually unilateral, more commonly involving the right side. Signs of the underlying cause may also be evident such as the presence of mediastinal masses or other parenchymal lesions[19] **(Fig. 3)**.
- *Chest computed tomography (CT) scan*: It provides more detailed information about the pleural effusion and any underlying lung or mediastinal pathology. The thoracic duct which is not visible on a plain radiograph may be identified on a CT and can also be traced along its course. The location of the chylothorax is influenced by the exact place of thoracic duct trauma or obstruction. For example, a right-sided chylothorax is seen in injury or obstruction just below the fifth thoracic vertebra. This is because the thoracic duct crosses over to the left side beyond this point. In the presence of disruption of multiple lymphatics, a bilateral chylothorax may also be seen.

  Other mediastinal masses, lymph nodes, and infections leading to parenchymal consolidations may also be clearly evident on a CT scan[20] **(Fig. 4)**.
- *Thoracic ultrasound*: As in the evaluation of all pleural effusions, thoracic ultrasound helps to quantify the amount of pleural fluid and identify the presence of septations and loculations. A chylothorax appears isodense on ultrasound without septations and loculations. However, it cannot be used alone to diagnose chylorax as its appearance is similar to all other effusions.

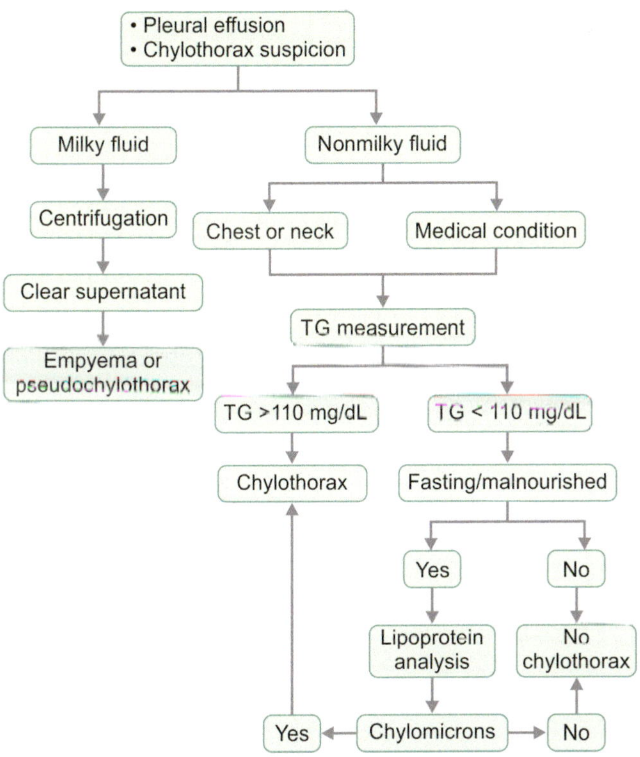

FLOWCHART 1: Diagnostic approach to chylothorax.
(TG: triglyceride)

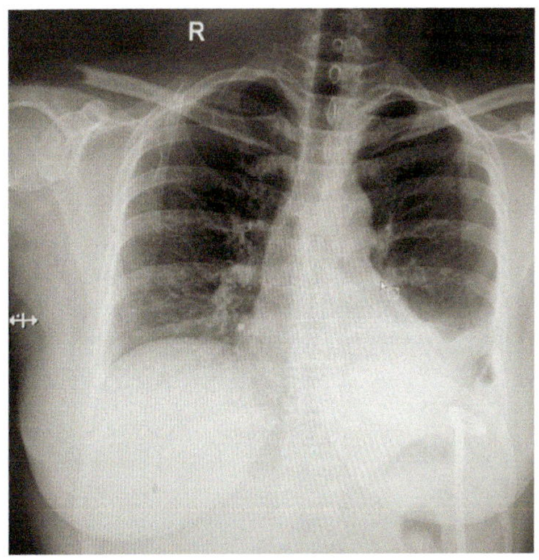

FIG. 3: Chest X-ray of a patient with chylothorax suggestive of left costophrenic (CP) angle blunting with intercostal drain in situ.

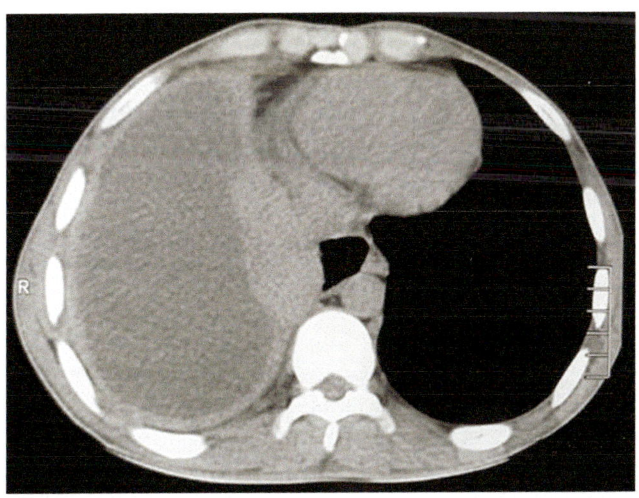

FIG. 4: Computed tomography image showing a pleural effusion on the right side.

Laboratory Tests

No particular laboratory test is diagnostic for chylorax. Electrolyte losses in chylothorax may result in hyponatremia, hypocalcemia, and metabolic acidosis. Rarely, hypoproteinemia and hypoalbuminemia may be seen. Immunoglobulin and serum triglyceride levels may be normal despite the loss.

Pleural Fluid Analysis

- *Thoracentesis*: Pleural fluid aspiration via thoracentesis is essential to confirm the presence of chyle in the pleural cavity.
- *Chyle examination*: A milky appearance of the pleural fluid highly suggests the presence of chyle, but additional tests are required for confirmation. The milky fluid of chylothorax can be differentiated from the white fluid of empyema by centrifugating the fluid. The white blood cells present in an empyema settle after centrifugation. Also, the milky fluid of chylothorax may clear after a fast **(Fig. 5)**.
- *Cell count and differential*: Examination of pleural fluid cells and their differential can provide insights into the underlying cause of chylothorax. A vast majority of chyloraxes are lymphocyte-rich in nature.
- *Proteins and electrolytes*: The protein and electrolyte levels in chyle are similar to that of plasma. Most of the chylothoraxes are exudative in nature.
- *pH*: Chylous fluid usually has a pH ranging from 7.40 to 7.80. It may be influenced by the underlying cause of chylothorax.

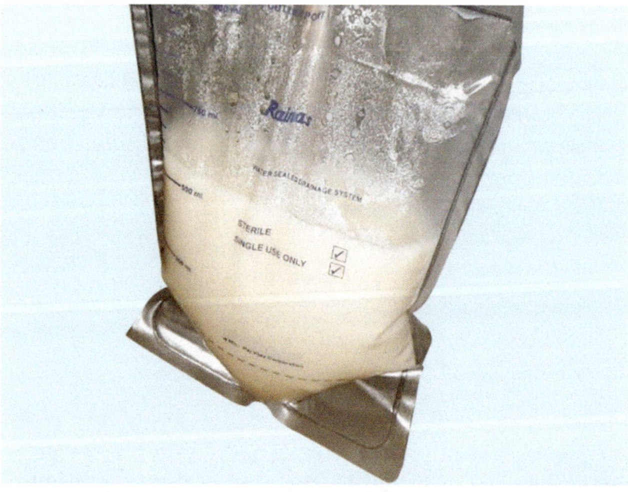

FIG. 5: Image showing the milky appearance of chylous fluid.

- *Glucose levels*: Plasma glucose levels reflect the chylous effusion glucose levels. Low glucose levels are classically seen in empyemas.
- *Lactate dehydrogenase (LDH) levels*: Chyle has low LDH levels usually. It may be increased depending on the underlying cause of chylothorax.
- *Triglyceride levels*: Measuring triglyceride levels in the pleural fluid is crucial. A triglyceride level > 110 mg/dL (1.24 mmol/L) is diagnostic of chylothorax. Though the cutoff value of 110 mg/dL is most frequently used, it should be interpreted in a clinical context to support the diagnosis of chylothorax because triglyceride levels may be influenced by the fat content in diet.
- *Cholesterol levels*: They are typically low in chylothorax compared to other pleural effusions. Levels < 200 mg/dL are suggestive of chylothorax. Higher cholesterol levels are seen in pseudochylothorax.
- *Chylomicrons*: Lipid electrophoresis detects chylomicrons in pleural fluid, giving the definitive diagnosis of chylothorax. Though not routinely performed as the first test, these tests are expensive and laborious.
- *Sudan III staining*: Fat globules can be seen in chylothorax with the help of Sudan III stains which stains chylomicrons orange.[21-24]

Other Investigations

- *Lymphangiography*: It is a specialized imaging technique that can identify the site of chyle leakage, aiding in planning potential interventions. Lymphangiography is rarely used in recent times due to the availability of safer and less invasive methods. It involves instillation of dye through the small vessels of the toes. The lymphatic vessel is isolated with the help of methylene blue dye. It is dissected further and 10 mL of lipoidal dye is injected through the vessel at a rate of 0.2–0.4 mL/s. The dye used is radiopaque and its path is visualized with the help of fluoroscopy or magnetic resonance imaging (MRI). If MRI is used, then it is called MRI lymphangiography. Serial images using fluoroscopy show the exact path and defect in the thoracic duct.[25-27]
- *Lymphoscintigraphy*: In this test, Tc99m labeled human diethylenetriaminepentaacetic acid (HAS-DTPA) is injected in the dorsum of the foot subcutaneously. Sequential images are then taken with the help of a gamma camera and the lymphatic pathways and subsequent leak is identified. This technique when combined with low-dose CT with single-photon emission CT (SPECT) provides a more accurate localization.[28]

BOX 2 Management of chylothorax.

Nonsurgical management:
- Thoracocentesis
- Chest tube drainage
- *Dietary modification*:
  - Fat-free diet
  - Medium-chain triglyceride diet
  - Total parenteral nutrition
- *Medical management*:
  - Somatostatins and analogs
  - Midodrine

Surgical management:
- Percutaneous embolization of thoracic duct
- VATS-assisted thoracic duct ligation
- *Pleurodesis*:
  - Chemical or mechanical
  - Chest tube or thoracoscopic
- Thoracotomy
- Pleuroperitoneal and pleurovenous shunts

(VATS: video-assisted thoracoscopic surgery)

MANAGEMENT (BOX 2)

The management of chylothorax is multifaceted and depends on the underlying cause, the patient's clinical status, and the rate of chyle leakage. The main therapeutic strategies include:

Conservative Management

Conservative management helps significantly when dealing with small defects in the thoracic duct. It is usually successful when the rate of chyle formation is <1,000 mL/day. It can be remembered like 4D's [Diet, Drainage, Desis (pleurodesis) and Drugs].

- *Dietary modifications*: Patients are often advised to adopt a high-protein, low-fat diet supplemented with medium-chain triglycerides (MCTs) that are absorbed directly into the portal system and bypass the lymphatic system, reducing chyle production. Long-chain fatty acids are mainly responsible for the formation of chyle in humans; hence, its elimination leads to a decreased formation of chyle and hence helps in resolution. However, this may not be practical in cases of a large defect as long-term avoidance of fats leads to malnutrition. A dietary intake of <5 kcal from fats in each meal is recommended. In cases where a long-term avoidance is required, the long-chain fatty acids can be administered intravenously instead. Complete parenteral nutrition can also be started in postoperative cases of chylothorax until proper surgical intervention is done.[29,30]
- *Pleural **D**rainage (Thoracentesis)*: Therapeutic thoracentesis can be performed to relieve respiratory distress and maintain lung expansion while conservative measures are employed. Intermittent drainage of fluid allows the patients to be dyspnea-free and also avoid malnutrition caused by continuous drainage. It is typically used as the first-line management in nontraumatic and nonsurgical chyloraxes.[29]
- *Pleuro**desis***: Chemical pleurodesis with agents such as talc may be considered to prevent recurrent chylothorax in nontraumatic cases. Pleurodesis is relied upon when repeated thoracocentesis is unsuccessful and the chylothorax is caused to due malignant causes especially when patient is not fit for surgical interventions. Pleurodesis along with thoracic duct ligation has an excellent success rate. Pleurodesis can be done with the help of talc slurry or other agents such as bleomycin, doxycycline, etc. through an intercostal drain or via direct instillation through video thoracoscopy. The details of pleurodesis and its technique have been discussed elsewhere.[17]
- ***D**rugs Somatostatin/octreotide*: Somatostatin is a hormone that is produced by the paracrine cells of gastrointestinal tract. It mainly inhibits the gastrointestinal endocrine secretions. Octreotide is a long-acting analogue of somatostatin. The role of these hormones in the management of chylothorax is controversial, and hence these are usually used as an adjunct to other conservative measures or when conservative measures are unsatisfactory. They inhibit the gastric and pancreatic secretions and hence reduce chyle formation and accumulation in the thoracic cavity. Optimal dosage is not yet known. Currently used dosages are as follows:

  Somatostatin: Intravenous (IV) infusion—6 mg/kg for 2 weeks

  Subcutaneous—50 μ every 8 hourly

  Octreotide: 50–200 μ every 8 hourly for 2–14 days

  Side effects: Nausea, diarrhea, flushing, deranged liver function tests, transient hypothyroidism, and injection site pain.[31]
- *Midodrine*: It is an alpha 1 adrenergic agonist that reduces lymph drainage by causing vasoconstriction of the lymphatic system. There have been very few case reports where this drug is used and its results are yet to be proven.[32]

Interventional Procedures

Interventional procedures are usually required in high-output chylothorax, where the rate of fluid production is >1,000 mL/day. Such high-out chylothorax is usually encountered more frequently postoperatively. This is why patients in the postoperative period who are likely to have a risk of chylothorax should be closely monitored. Esophagectomy has the highest risk of postoperative complication of developing a chylothorax.

Selection of the interventional procedure depends upon the underlying etiology of chylothorax as well as its rate of formation.

- *Thoracic duct embolization*: Lymphangiography-guided embolization of the thoracic duct can be performed to occlude the site of chyle leakage, allowing the duct to heal. Patients who usually do not respond to 3–5 days of conservative management require embolization. In this procedure, cisterna chyle cannulation is done percutaneously and it is advanced into the thoracic duct while simultaneously instilling a contrast dye. The leak is thus identified and is then embolized with the help of a coil or glue.

  The thoracic duct, cisterna chyle, or other lymphatic tributaries may be disrupted to decrease the lymphatic flow. Such a procedure is called thoracic duct disruption.[34-36]
- *Surgical ligation*: In cases where conservative measures and embolization fail, surgical ligation of the thoracic duct may be considered. Surgical ligation of the thoracic duct is the gold standard for high-output chylothorax. It may be done with the help of video thoracoscopy or open thoracotomy depending upon the surgeons' choice and feasibility. A variety of radiological tests and lymphangiography may be required for the accurate identification of the duct preoperatively. Injection of indocyanine green dye intraoperatively in bilateral inguinal region may help isolate the damaged site during thoracotomy. If the exact site of leak cannot be identified, sutures and clips may be placed on either side of the duct. Excessive dissection to identify the exact site of leak is not encouraged as this leads to multiple injuries and further damage to the thoracic duct.[33,37]
- *Pleuroperitoneal shunts*: When all the measures fail, a pleuroperitoneal shunt may be formed to drain the chyle fluid from the pleura. This prevents malnutrition, as well as the loss of immunoglobulins is reduced as it is postulated that the peritoneal omentum reabsorbs the chyle.[38]

  Pleurovenous shunts have also been attempted in which a shunt is created between the pleura and the subclavian or jugular vein.
- *Indwelling pleural catheter (IPC)*: The use of a tunneled IPC is generally not recommended in cases of chylothorax due to the potential complications such as malnutrition and decreased immunity and also the potential risk of having a hemodynamic instability. However, its use has been done in few cases of benign persistent chylothorax with success.[39]

Management of Underlying Cause

- *Treatment of malignancies*: Chemotherapy, radiation therapy, or surgical resection may be necessary to manage chylothorax secondary to lymphoma or metastatic cancers.
- *Treatment of infections*: Appropriate antimicrobial therapy is required to manage chylothorax associated with infections.

  Once the underlying cause is identified, appropriate measures can be taken to reduce the chyle formation while simultaneously treating the primary cause. Usually, a combination of measures is done simultaneously for best results.

COMPLICATIONS (TABLE 2)

- *Malnutrition*: It occurs due to loss of fats and essential proteins. Long-standing chylothorax usually leads to malnutrition deficiencies, which need to be actively

TABLE 2: Difference between chylothorax and pseudochylothorax.[41]

	Chylothorax	Pseudochylothorax
Cause	Neoplasm and trauma of thoracic duct	Long-standing pleural effusion—tubercular, rheumatoid arthritis, and poorly treated empyema
Frequency	Uncommon	Rare
Presentation	Acute or subacute	Chronic
Computed tomography (CT)	Normal pleural layers	Thick pleural layers
Appearance of pleural fluid	Milky, serous, and turbid	Milky and shiny
Triglycerides	>110 mg/dL	<110 mg/dL (usually <50 mg/dL)
Cholesterol	<200 mg/dL	>200 mg/dL
Cholesterol crystals	Absent	Often present
Chylomicrons	Present	Absent

managed. Protein loss also leads to hypoalbuminemia.
- *Infection*: Loss of immunoglobulins through the chylous fluid leads to increased susceptibility to infections.
- *Respiratory compromise*: This can occur in larger chylothoraxes due to mechanical factors as well as due to the underlying cause of the chylothorax.
- Longer postoperative recovery and ventilator dependence.[40]

PROGNOSIS

The prognosis of chylothorax depends on various factors, including the underlying cause, the patient's general health, and the response to treatment. Traumatic chylothorax, if promptly managed, usually has a favorable prognosis. However, nontraumatic chylothorax may have a more guarded outlook, especially when associated with malignancies or severe underlying diseases.

CONCLUSION

Chylothorax is a rare pleural disease that poses diagnostic and therapeutic challenges. A thorough understanding of its etiology, clinical presentation, and management is crucial for healthcare professionals to optimize patient outcomes. Early recognition and appropriate intervention can improve the prognosis and enhance the quality of life for individuals affected by chylothorax. Further research and advancements in diagnostic and therapeutic modalities are necessary to enhance our knowledge and refine the management of this rare condition.

KEY POINTS

- Chylothorax is a rare but potentially serious pleural disease characterized by the accumulation of chyle, a milky lymphatic fluid, within the pleural cavity caused due to disruption of the thoracic duct.
- Chylothorax can be classified into two major categories based on its etiology: traumatic and nontraumatic chylothorax.
- Traumatic chylothorax often results from thoracic trauma, such as iatrogenic injury during surgery or penetrating chest injuries.
- Nontraumatic chylothorax can be caused due to malignancies, infections and other miscellaneous conditions like SVC obstruction.
- The diagnosis of chylothorax involves a systematic approach to evaluate the pleural effusion and identify its chylous nature. Imaging studies such as chest X-ray and CT chest help us identify the presence of an effusion, however, the diagnosis of chylothorax can only be made by identifying a high triglyceride level and the presence of chylomicrons in the milky pleural fluid.
- Lymphangiography and lymphoscintigraphy have been proven beneficial in diagnosing and identifying the exact location of thoracic duct disruption.
- Once the site of leak has been identified, it can be managed either conservatively with, 4D's [Diet, Drainage, Desis (pleurodesis) and Drugs].
- Dietary modifications such as a low-fat diet and giving somatostatins.
- However, larger chylothorax may require surgical interventions such as pleurodesis, thoracic duct embolization and/or thoracic duct ligation.
- Many other surgical options are available, but the ultimate treatment is to address the underlying cause of chylothorax.

REFERENCES

1. Bhardwaj R, Vaziri H, Gautam A, Ballesteros E, Karimeddini D, Wu GY. Chylous Ascites: A Review of Pathogenesis, Diagnosis, and Treatment. J Clin Transl Hepatol. 2018;6(1):105-13.
2. Lama A, Ferreiro L, Toubes ME, Golpe A, Gude F, Álvarez-Dobaño JM, et al. Characteristics of patients with pseudochylothorax—a systematic review. J Thorac Dis. 2016;8(8):2093-101.
3. Agrawal V, Sahn SA. Lipid pleural effusions. Am J Med Sci. 2008;335:16-20.
4. Rudrappa M, Paul M. Chylothorax. In: StatPearls [Internet]. Treasure Island (FL): StatPearls Publishing; 2023.
5. Schuenke M, Schulte E, Schumacher U, Ross LM, Lamperti ED, Voll M, et al. Thieme Atlas of Anatomy: Neck and internal organs. Uttar Pradesh, India: Thieme Medical and Scientific Publishers Private Limited; 2007. p. 136.
6. Ndiaye A, Di-Marino V, Ba PS, Ndiaye A, Gaye M, Nazarian S. Anatomical variations in lymphatic drainage of the right lung: applications in lung cancer surgery. Surg Radiol Anat. 2016; 38(10):1143-51.
7. Jacob S (Ed). Thorax. Atlas of Human Anatomy. Michigan: Churchill Livingstone; 2002. pp. 51-70.
8. Cholet C, Delalandre C, Monnier-Cholley L, Le Pimpec-Barthes F, El Mouhadi S, Arrivé L. Nontraumatic Chylothorax: Nonenhanced MR Lymphography. Radiographics. 2020;40(6):1554-73.
9. Prakash AK, Chatterjee S, Datta B, Jaiswal A. Cystic lung disease lymphangioleiomyomatosis (LAM) in a male patient BMJ Case Reports CP 2023;16:e251513.
10. Jha S, Mamnoon F, Prabhudesai P, Khandelwal A, Maniar M, Prakash A. A Rare Cause of Chyluria and Recurrent Chylothorax: Lymphatic Dysplasia Syndrome. Chest. 2014;146(4):477A.

11. Turpin S, Lambert R. Lymphoscintigraphy of Chylous Anomalies: Chylothorax, Chyloperitoneum, Chyluria, and Lymphangiomatosis-15-Year Experience in a Pediatric Setting and Review of the Literature. J Nucl Med Technol. 2018;46(2):123-8.
12. Pui MH, Yueh TC. Lymphoscintigraphy in chyluria, chyloperitoneum and chylothorax. J Nucl Med. 1998 Jul;39(7): 1292-6. PMID: 9669413.
13. Doerr CH, Allen MS, Nichols FC 3rd, Ryu JH. Etiology of Chylothorax in 203 Patients. Mayo Clin Proc. 2005;80(7):867-70.
14. Beghetti M, La Scala G, Belli D, Bugmann P, Kalangos A, Le Coultre C. Etiology and management of pediatric chylothorax. J Pediatr. 2000;136(5):653-8.
15. McGrath EE, Blades Z, Anderson PB. Chylothorax: Aetiology, diagnosis, and therapeutic options. Respir Med. 2010;104(1):1-8.
16. Boffa DJ, Sands MJ, Rice TW, Murthy SC, Mason DP, Geisinger MA. A critical evaluation of a percutaneous diagnostic and treatment strategy for chylothorax after thoracic surgery. Eur J Cardiothorac Surg. 2008;33:435-9.
17. Nair SK, Petko M, Hayward MP. Aetiology and management of chylothorax in adults. Eur J Cardiothorac Surg. 2007;32(2):362-9.
18. Zarei M, Montazer M, Shakeri Bavil Oliyaei S, Jahanshahlou F, Hosseini MS. Postesophagectomy chylothorax: a review of the risk factors, diagnosis, and management (Lond). 2023;85(6): 2781-6.
19. Soto-Martinez M, Massie J. Chylothorax: Diagnosis and management in children. Paediatr Respir Rev. 2009;10(4):199-207.
20. Sachs PB, Zelch MG, Rice TW, Geisinger MA, Risius B, Lammert GK. Diagnosis and localization of laceration of the thoracic duct: usefulness of lymphangiography and CT. AJR Am J Roentgenol. 1991;157(4):703-5.
21. Maldonado F, Hawkins FJ, Daniels CE, Doerr CH, Decker PA, Ryu JH. Pleural fluid characteristics of chylothorax. Mayo Clin Proc. 2009;84(2):129-33.
22. Agrawal V, Doelken P, Sahn SA. Pleural fluid analysis in chylous pleural effusion. Chest. 2008;133(6):1436-41.
23. Staats BA, Ellefson RD, Budahn LL, Dines DE, Prakash UB, Offord K. The lipoprotein profile of chylous and nonchylous pleural effusions. Mayo Clin Proc. 1980;55(11):700-4.
24. Skouras V, Kalomenidis I. Chylothorax: diagnostic approach. Curr Opin Pulm Med. 2010;16(4):387-93.
25. McGraw JR, Itkin M, Kovach SJ 3rd. Lymphangiography-Guided Thoracic Duct Surgical Lymphovenous Bypass for Distal Thoracic Duct Occlusion. J Vasc Interv Radiol. 2023;34(8):1472-3.
26. Iio K, Soneda K, Shimotakahara A, Hataya H, Kono T. Effective method of evaluating infantile chylothorax. Pediatr Int. 2019; 61(2):203-5.
27. Choe J, Koo HJ, Ahn Y, Lee GD, Yang DH, Kang JW, et al. Evaluation of Chylothorax Using Dynamic Contrast-enhanced Magnetic Resonance Lymphangiography after Lung Cancer Surgery. Lymphat Res Biol. 2023;21(4):343-50.
28. Zhang L, Zhang X, Wen Z, Tong G, Hao K, Qiu Y, et al. Lymphoscintigraphy findings in patients with chylothorax: influence of biochemical parameters. EJNMMI Res. 2023; 13(1):72.
29. Papoulidis P, Vidanapathirana P, Dunning J. Chylothorax, new insights in treatment. J Thorac Dis. 2018;10(Suppl 33):S3976-7.
30. Sriram K, Meguid RA, Meguid MM. Nutritional support in adults with chyle leaks. Nutrition. 2016;32:281-6.
31. Lim KA, Kim SH, Huh J, Kang IS, Lee HJ, Jun TG, et al. Somatostatin for postoperative chylothorax after surgery for children with congenital heart disease. J Korean Med Sci. 2005;20(6): 947-51.
32. Liou DZ, Warren H, Maher DP, Soukiasian HJ, Melo N, Salim A, et al. Midodrine: a novel therapeutic for refractory chylothorax. Chest. 2013;144(3):1055-7.
33. Chovanec V, Drugda J, Lojík M, Vodárek P, Žák P, Hanke I, et al. Chylothorax treatment with thoracic duct embolization. Rozhl Chir. 2022 Winter;101(12):607-11. English.
34. Robinson CL. The Management of Chylothorax. Ann Thorac Surg. 1985;39(1):90-5.
35. Lampson RS. Traumatic Chylothorax: A Review of the Literature and Report of a Case Treated by Mediastinal Ligation of the Thoracic Duct. J Thorac Surg. 1948;17(6):778-91.
36. Ferguson MK, Little AC, Skinner DB. Current concepts in the management of postoperative chylothorax. Ann Thorac Surg. 1985;40:542-5.
37. Milsom JW, Kron IL, Rheuban KS, Rodgers BM. Chylothorax: an assessment of current surgical management. J Thorac Cardiovasc Surg. 1985;89:221-7.
38. Costa R, Magalhães T, Rocha G, Fernandes P, Salgueiro E. A Unique Shunt for Treatment of a Postoperative Chylothorax. Port J Card Thorac Vasc Surg. 2022;29(3):63-5.
39. DePew ZS, Iqbal S, Mullon JJ, Nichols FC, Maldonado F. The role for tunneled indwelling pleural catheters in patients with persistent benign chylothorax. Am J Med Sci. 2013;346(5): 349-52.
40. Wasmuth-Pietzuch A, Hansmann M, Bartmann P, Heep A. Congenital chylothorax: lymphopenia and high risk of neonatal infections. Acta Paediatr. 2004;93:220-4.
41. Hillerdal G. Chylothorax and pseudochylothorax. Eur Respir J. 1997;10(5):1157-62.

CHAPTER

16

Thoracocentesis

Shweta Bansal, Ashwani Prakash

INTRODUCTION

Thoracocentesis, also known as pleural tap or pleural puncture, is a medical procedure used to diagnose and treat various respiratory conditions, primarily pleural effusion. This life-saving procedure involves the insertion of a needle or catheter into the pleural space to drain excess fluid, providing relief to patients experiencing breathing difficulties and allowing healthcare providers to identify the underlying causes of pleural effusions. In this chapter, we will explore the indications of thoracocentesis, its contraindications, the procedure itself, potential risks, and its role in patient care.

DEFINITION

Thoracentesis is a procedure to remove fluid or air from the thoracic cavity for both diagnostic and/or therapeutic purposes. It is also known as thoracocentesis, pleural tap, needle thoracostomy, or needle decompression.[1]

Thoracocentesis can be small- or large-volume thoracocentesis. A small volume (20–50 mL) is generally used for diagnostic purposes for cytological and other investigations for the evaluation of pleural effusion.[2]

Large-volume thoracentesis involves the removal of more than 1 L of pleural fluid for relieving dyspnea and symptomatic relief.

INDICATIONS[1]

Diagnostic

- For undiagnosed exudative lymphocytic effusions
- For diagnosis of chylous and chylothorax
- Diagnostic needle thoracocentesis for primary pneumothorax

Therapeutic

- To relieve dyspnea in large or massive pleural effusion
- Therapeutic needle thoracocentesis for primary pneumothorax

CONTRAINDICATIONS[1,3]

- *Absolute contraindications*: None
- *Relative contraindications*:
    - Bleeding disorder or anticoagulation
    - Thrombocytopenia < 25,000/mm^3
    - Altered chest wall anatomy
    - Cellulitis or herpes zoster at the site of thoracentesis puncture
    - Pulmonary disease is severe enough to make complications life threatening.
    - Uncontrolled coughing or an uncooperative patient

Preprocedural routine blood investigations may be done as part of the evaluation of pleural effusions.

Coagulation profile is not recommended for all cases according to the *British Thoracic Society* (BTS) guidelines, unless the patient has history of any coagulopathy or is on anticoagulant drugs.

PREREQUISITES AND CHECKLIST[4]

- Patient's name and details should be verified.
- Explain the procedure to the patient.
- Informed consent should be taken. Written information should be provided to the patients.

- Look for any contraindications.
- Investigations—chest X-ray and coagulation profile
- Warfarin should be stopped for 5 days before an elective procedure, direct oral anticoagulant (DOAC) for 24–48 hours before the procedure, clopidogrel and prasugrel should be stopped 5 days pre-elective procedure and ticagrelor 7 days pre procedure. Aspirin therapy and prophylactic dose heparin can be continued.[5] (2B)
- Ensure there is recent chest radiology to see the amount and side of pleural fluid.
- Look for history of allergies to any drug
- Procedure should preferably be performed in a dedicated room as per the BTS guidelines. Bedside thoracentesis should be avoided.
- Equipment check should be done; monitors, oxygen supply, emergency crash cart, and presence of ultrasonography (USG) machine should be there.

MATERIALS REQUIRED

- Sterile gloves, eye protection, and face mask
- Sterile drapes or towels
- *Chlorhexidine or betadine*: 5, 10, and 20 mL
- Sterile drapes and gauze pieces
- 18 G and 21 G intravenous catheter
- Three-way valve
- Sample containers
- *Thoracentesis kits*:
  - Arrow-Clark™ Pleura-Seal® Thoracentesis Kit[7]—catheter-over-needle design, self-sealing valve that closes upon needle removal, reduces the risk of pneumothorax associated with open catheters and a reliance on thumb or finger occlusion.
  - Rocket® Thoracentesis Set 6Fg:[8] It has a 6Fg catheter mounted on an 18G needle—the catheter remains in situ whereas the needle helps in insertion and needs lesser force. There is a mounted aspiration syringe for collection of a pleural fluid sample and a soft stitch round plate to secure the catheter in position with the help of tape or sutures. To allow for aspiration, an extension of the tubing and three-way tap are provided with the kit **(Fig. 1)**.
  - Argyle™ Turkel™ Safety Thoracentesis System, 3.5in L Catheter, 8Fr

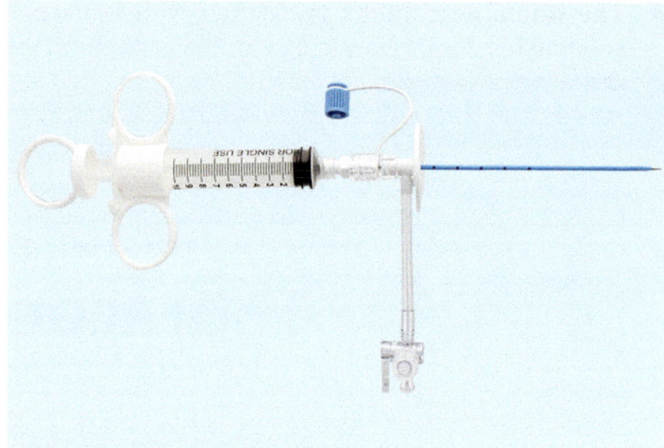

FIG. 1: Rocket® Thoracentesis Set 6Fg.[8]

PROCEDURE STEPS[6]

Patients should be monitored throughout the procedure.

- *Positioning of the patient*:
  - Patient sits on the side or foot of the bed.
  - His arms and head should rest on one or more pillows on a bedside table and feet rested on a footstool.
  - The patient should not stoop, so the bed may be elevated to the level of the table. If he/she leans forward too much, there may be no fluid posteriorly as the lowest part of hemithorax moves anteriorly.
  - If the patient cannot sit, the bed may be propped up maximally and thoracocentesis performed in semirecumbent position.
  - He/she may lie in lateral decubitus position with the pleural effusion side at the edge of the table.
- *Selection of the thoracocentesis site*:
  - Physical examination of the chest and radiology plays an important role which helps in determining and confirming both the side and site of the pleural tap.
  - The rib spaces may be full on the side of pleural effusion, tactile fremitus will be absent, note will be stony dull, and chest sounds absent.
  - The pleural tap should be done one space below where the note turns dull from resonant.
  - Thoracentesis should be performed above a rib to minimize the risk of damage to the neurovascular bundle.[4]
  - USG chest is more useful and superior to chest X-ray to confirm the diagnosis, quantification of fluid and its characteristics, and determination of site of thoracocentesis.
  - The BTS has recommended that thoracic ultrasound be used for all thoracenteses.[4]
- Once the site of thoracentesis is confirmed by USG, the site is marked with a skin marking pen or with the cap of syringe or pen, the skin is indented to leave a small mark.
- The patient is explained the procedure.
- He/she is placed in the appropriate position as explained.

- The whole hemithorax is cleaned with antiseptic solution betadine followed by alcohol, going from the center toward outside, at least 4 inches from the site marked. The area is then draped with a sterile drape.
- The skin, subcutaneous tissue, periosteum, bone, and parietal pleura are then anesthetized with 2% lidocaine solution. Some fluid may be aspirated into the lidocaine syringe to confirm the diagnosis and the right site. The needle is then withdrawn.
- The 18G plastic intravenous canula or thoracocentesis kit catheter with needle is then inserted into the pleural space while aspirating continuously and stopping when the fluid starts coming. The needle is then withdrawn. A finger is kept on the tip to prevent air from going into the pleural cavity (this step is not needed if thoracocentesis kits are used as they do not allow to enter into pleural cavity once the needle is withdrawn), and a three-way canula is attached.
- Small-bore needles are preferably used so as to minimize the complications.[4]
- If >60 mL fluid is aspirated, especially if diagnostic thoracocentesis is planned, a catheter should be used rather than a needle alone. The aspiration should be done either manually with the help of syringe or under the effect of gravity with the help of tubing and bottle. Use of wall suction or vacuum bottles is not recommended.[4]
- Use of the Veress needle is recommended.[4]
- In case only diagnostic fluid is to be obtained, 30–40 mL fluid may be aspirated. In case therapeutic aspiration needs to be done, 1–1.5 L may be aspirated. The patient should be monitored continuously, and the maximum amount aspirated should not exceed 1.5 L to prevent re-expansion pulmonary edema. The pleural aspiration should also be stopped if the patient feels sudden chest pain, shortness of breath, or no fluid could be aspirated.
- In cases of suspected pleural infections, immediate pleural fluid pH should be obtained (not to be mixed with heparin or local anesthetic) and sample should be sent in plain as well as blood culture bottles.[9]
- In case of suspected malignancy, at least 20–50 mL of fluid should be sent,[9] and cell blocks should be prepared.
- Serum NT-proBNP (N-terminal prohormone of brain natriuretic peptide) should be considered to support a diagnosis of heart failure in patients with unilateral pleural effusion suspected of having heart failure.

COMPLICATIONS[4,6]

- Pneumothorax may occur either due to air flowing into the pleural space when the needle is removed and syringe attached or due to injury to lung during aspiration.
- Chest radiograph should be done 1–2 hours after the pleural aspiration to detect this complication at an early stage.
- Infection of the pleural space
- Hemothorax due to laceration of intercostal artery
- Vasovagal response
- Cough
- Re-expansion pulmonary edema
- Failed pleurodesis/dry tap
- Symptomatic hypotension
- Organ puncture—laceration of spleen or liver
- Infection of the soft tissue due to seeding of the needle tract with bacteria or spread of tumor cells
- Adverse reactions to the local anesthetic
- Pain

CONCLUSION

Thoracocentesis plays a crucial role in diagnosing and treating pleural effusion, a condition that can significantly impair a patient's breathing and overall well-being. This procedure not only provides immediate relief but also helps healthcare providers identify the underlying causes of pleural effusion, guiding further treatment. While it carries some risks, the benefits of thoracocentesis in improving patient outcomes and quality of life are undeniable.

KEY POINTS

- Pleural tapping or thoracocentesis is very important tool for the evaluation of pleural effusion.
- In case of undiagnosed exudative pleural effusion in endemic country for tuberculosis like India it is an important part of management.
- Preprocedural USG chest is recommended to quantify the amount of effusion and selection of site.
- Proper aseptic precautions should be followed.
- The complications of the procedure should be explained and the operator should be competent enough to deal with them.

REFERENCES

1. Wiederhold BD, Amr O, Modi P, O'Rourke MC. Thoracentesis. In: StatPearls [Internet]. Treasure Island (FL): StatPearls Publishing; 2023.
2. Havelock T, Teoh R, Laws D, Gleeson F, on behalf of the BTS Pleural Disease Guideline Group. Pleural procedures and thoracic ultrasound: British Thoracic Society pleural disease guideline 2010. Thorax. 2010;65(Suppl 2):ii61-76.
3. Dezube R. (2022). How to do Thoracentesis. [online] Available from https://www.msdmanuals.com/en-in/professional/pulmonary-disorders/how-to-do-pulmonary-procedures/how-to-do-thoracentesis. [Last accessed October, 2023].
4. Asciak R, Bedawi EO, Bhatnagar R, Clive AO, Hassan M, Lloyd H, et al. British Thoracic Society Clinical Statement on pleural procedures. Thorax. 2023;78(Suppl 3):s43-68.
5. Keeling D, Tait RC, Watson H; British Committee of Standards for Haematology. Peri-operative management of anticoagulation and antiplatelet therapy. Br J Haematol. 2016;175(4):602-13.
6. Light RW. Pleural Diseases, 6th edition. Philadelphia: Lippincott Williams and Wilkins; 2013. p. 524.
7. Teleflexinterventionalcatalog. Arrow Thoracentesis Kits. [online] Available from https://www.teleflexinterventionalcatalogue.com/peripheral-intervention/drainage/arrow-thoracentesis-kits. [Last accessed October, 2023].
8. Rocket Medical LLC. R51551 Rocket Thoracentesis Catheter - 6Fg. [online]. Available from https://sales.rocketmedical.com/rocket-thoracentesis-catheter-6fg. [Last accessed October, 2023].
9. Roberts ME, Rahman NM, Maskell NA, Bibby AC, Blyth KG, Corcoran JP, et al. British Thoracic Society Guideline for pleural disease. Thorax. 2023;78(Suppl 3):s1-s42.

CHAPTER

17

Intercostal Drainage Tubes and Pleural Drainage Systems

Ashish Kumar Prakash, Anand Jaiswal

INTRODUCTION

Intercostal drainage (ICD) or chest tubes or thoracostomy tubes are the most important armamentarium to deal with pleural pathologies. An ICD or intrapleural chest tube is also called a *Bülau drain* or an intercostal catheter (ICC).[1] Though the concept of ICD was first described by *Hippocrates*[2] many years ago but was used first time in a 22-month-old infant in 1918 by *Dr C Pope* to drain postpneumonic empyema.[3] The postoperative use of ICD was first done in 1922[4] and then was routinely used in Word War II in post-thoracotomy patients. They are now frequently used in the practice of pulmonary medicine while dealing with pneumothorax,[5] hemothorax, pleural effusion, or empyema. They can also be used to instill medication such as talc, doxycycline, betadine, and Picibanil (OK-432) for pleurodesis and fibrinolytic agents, such as streptokinase and tenecteplase.

As per the latest British Thoracic Society (BTS) guidelines the indication of chest tube insertion is:[6]

- Pneumothorax failing other treatments
- Simple drainage of large benign or malignant pleural effusions
- Symptomatic pleural effusions in patients on mechanical ventilation
- Talc pleurodesis
- Pleural infection
- Traumatic hemothorax and/or pneumothorax
- Post-thoracic cavity procedures (i.e., medical thoracoscopy, thoracic, esophageal, or cardiac surgery)

In the USA around 1,330,000 ICDs were estimated to be placed in the year 1995.[7] It is very important to understand the various types of ICDs and the methodology for insertion for each one. In this chapter different types of ICD and different pleural drainage systems. Management of ICD, problems related with the issues of insertion, and respective complications will be discussed in the next chapter; however, their indications have been discussed elsewhere in previous chapters of the book.

Intercostal drainage classification is enumerated in **Box 1**.

BOX 1 Intercostal drainage (ICD) classification.

Intercostal drainage classification can be based on:

- *Size of tube measured in French(F) like*:
    - 10F, 12F up to 32F size ICD are available
- *Types*:
    - First generation—ICD without trocar
    - Second generation—ICD with trocar
    - Third generation—with guidewire
        - Leader catheter
        - Thal quick
        - Malecot
        - Pigtail
    - Fourth generation—indwelling pleural catheter
        - Pleurax or rocket catheter
- *Types of insertion technique*:
    - With Seldinger technique
    - With direct insertion through a trocar
    - Without trocar insertion
    - Tube thoracoscopy through a single-port thoracoscope

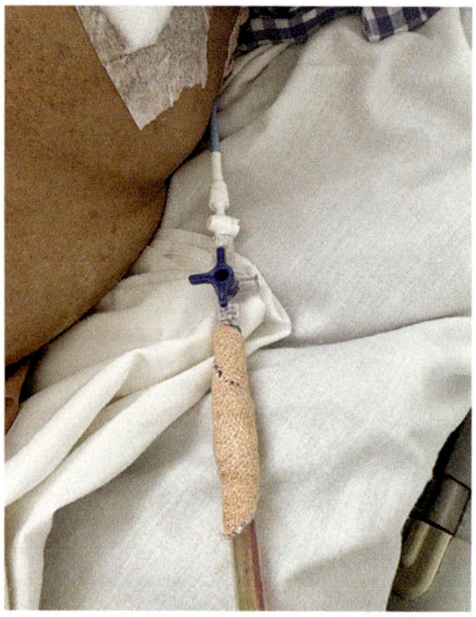

FIG. 1: Intercostal drainage (ICD) attached with three cannulas.

SIZE OF INTERCOSTAL DRAINAGE (CHEST TUBES)[8]

Though ICD are available with various sizes starting from 10 to 32F.

It is recommended to use a smaller size between 10 and 14F. Small bore tubes cause less pain and are easier to insert. However, the drawback of small-bore chest tubes is that they are very prone for blockage and often require flushing. We many times attach ICDs to the bag through a three-way cannula for ease of flushing **(Fig. 1)**.

Small-bore ICD are recommended:

- When pleurodesis is performed.
- For the treatment of pneumothorax.
- To treat a complicated parapneumonic effusion

Large bore ICD (>20F) are recommended:

- Patients of barotrauma-induced pneumothorax (mechanical ventilation)
- Patients with hemothorax
- Empyema (thick pus)

TYPES OF INTERCOSTAL DRAINAGE (CHEST TUBES)

Various tubes have been developed for the purpose of drainage of fluid or pus from the different sites of the body such as percutaneous drainage tube, pigtail catheter, leader catheter, and nephrostomy tube. Tubes that might be developed for any purpose can be used as a chest tube depending upon feasibility, availability, cost, and ease of insertion.

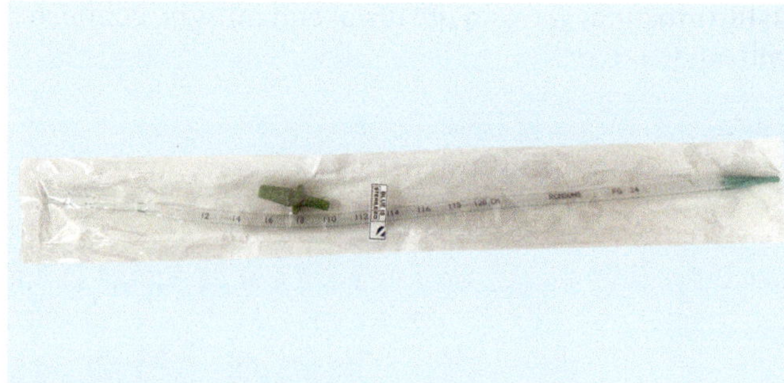

FIG. 2: Intercostal drainage (ICD) without trocar.

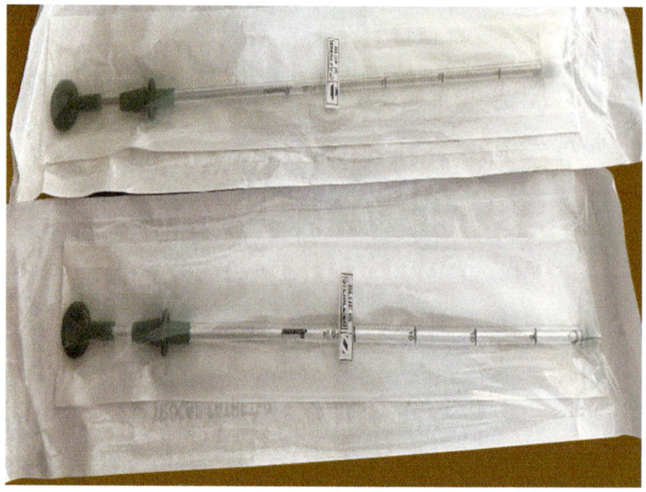

FIG. 3: Intercostal drainage (ICD) with trocar.

Intercostal Drainage without Trocar (Fig. 2)

Intercostal drainage tube without trocar is very cheap and widely available. It has a proximal end and distal end the proximal end has multiple pores to facilitate drainage and is kept inside the pleural cavity. The distal end which must be connected with the ICD bag does not have any trocar inside it. That is why the insertion of this ICD is difficult. In this case, we can say that this is the first-generation intercostal tube and now with the advancement the newer generation containing either a trocar or other various mechanisms to make the job of surgeon or interventional pulmonologist easier.

Intercostal Drainage with Trocar (Fig. 3)

The next generation ICD tube is the ICD with trocar and cannula. This has the simplest version of ICD with a trocar inside the cannula. The trocar helps while guiding the tube inside the chest wall. Like the simplest tube, it also has its proximal and distal tip with multiple fenestrations in the proximal end and the distal end must be connected with an ICD bag.

Leader Catheter or Central Venous Catheter (Fig. 4)

The use of a central venous catheter with very small gauge-like indwelling 16G is very efficacious in draining of large uncomplicated pleural effusions. It is very well tolerated by patients, very easy to insert, and is associated with minimal complications.[9] Many a times large pleural free fluid requires multiple thoracentesis in that case to avoid the use of large-bore chest tubes, it is very helpful.[10] But it requires a guidewire and the Seldinger technique is used for its insertion.[11] It has a potential for earlier blockage hence not fruitful if a long stay of ICD is anticipated (>2 days).

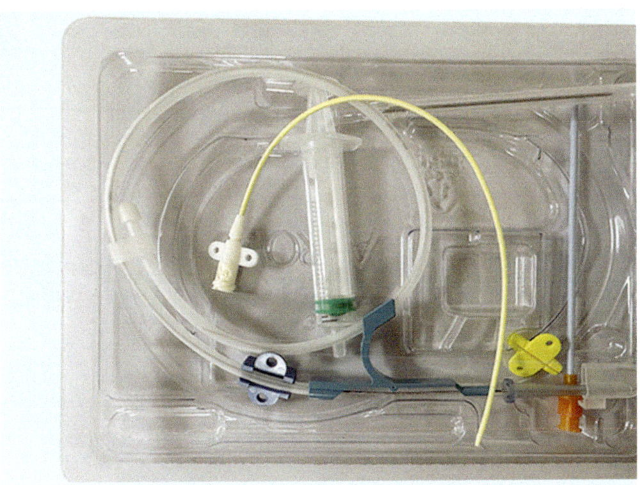

FIG. 4: Leader catheter or central venous catheter.

Pigtail (Fig. 5)

This is the more advanced version of ICD though has been derived for various purposes, it is basically made for percutaneous drainage of pus or any type of unwanted body fluid. The radiopaque catheter material enhances X-ray visualization. Pigtail catheters have a comparable efficacy to ICD in patients with pneumothorax.[12] It is now very commonly used for drainage of air or pleural fluid drainage because of its many advantages such as:

- Easy to insert with the Seldinger technique
- Non collapsibility (tough material)
- It cannot spontaneously or incidentally come out because the tip has a pigtail proximal end which is tied with thread
- Can be used for pleurodesis
- Can be kept for a long period

Thal Quick (Figs. 6A and B)

This is another type of ICD which has a tough material and not collapsible. It also comes with various sizes it is also put

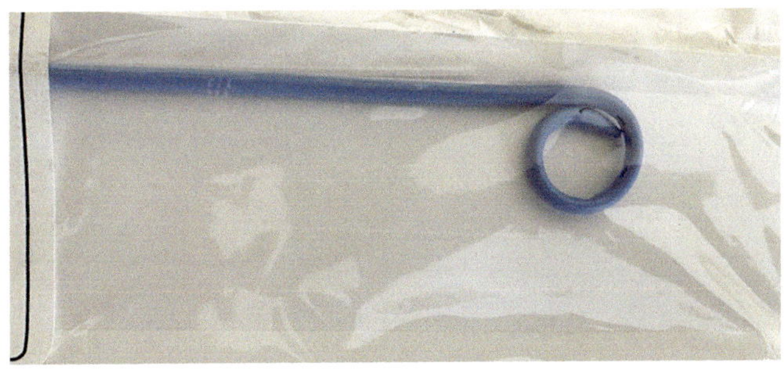

FIG. 5: Pigtail catheter.

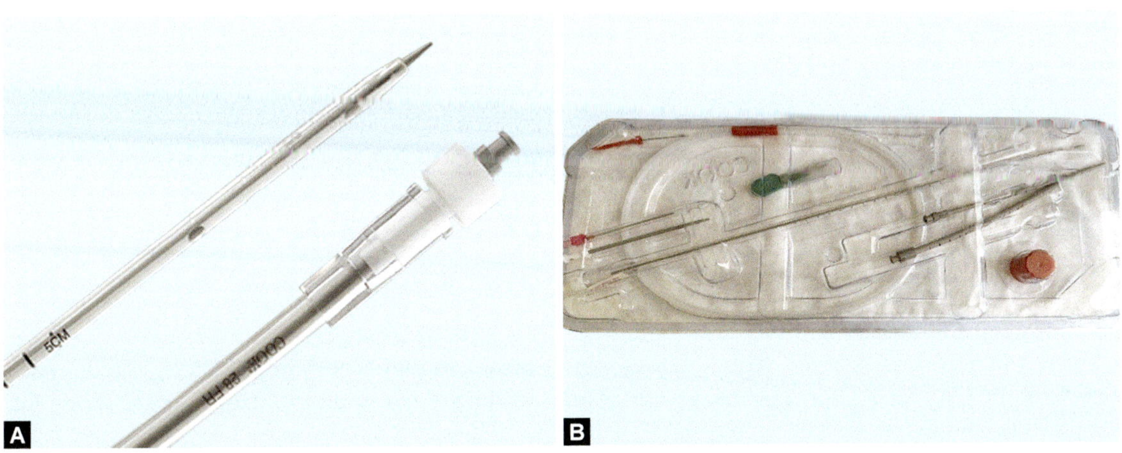

FIGS. 6A AND B: (A) Thal quick and (B) Thal quick intercostal drainage (ICD) set.

with the help of guidewire through Seldinger technique. The only drawback is that does not have a curved end like a pigtail catheter hence can have chances of spontaneous removal, but this happens less likely as all ICD are tied with sutures. It has a clear polyvinyl chloride catheter with having radiopaque stripe which allows fluid to be seen during the drainage procedure. Its proximal side hole is positioned on the radiopaque stripe to help confirming catheter positioning via X-ray. Having a double lumen set in it (additional lumen available) has an extra benefit for aspiration or infusion.

Malecot (Fig. 7)

Malecot catheter is another type of ICD with a curved and flower-shaped proximal end which helps to keep the tube inside. It was initially of rubber material, but nowadays a newer version is coming with tough material and can be put by guidewire.

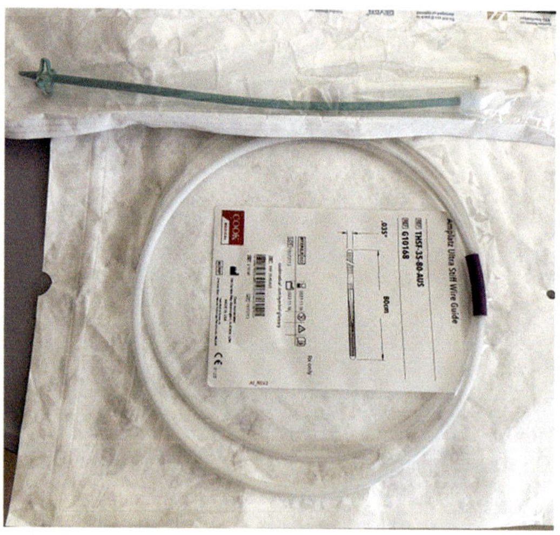

FIG. 7: Malecot catheter and guidewire.

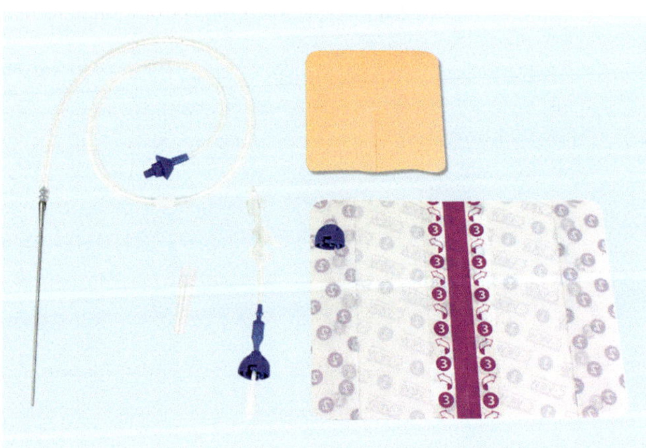

FIG. 8: Indwelling pleural catheter set.

Pleurax or Rocket (Indwelling Pleural Catheter) (Fig. 8)

This is the latest and most advanced form of ICD made to use in malignant pleural effusion. It is basically made of silicon material to be kept inside the pleural cavity for a long time. The distal end is outside the chest wall. The outer tip of the catheter is kept closed most of the time and is used off and on for pleural fluid drainage. The output bottle sometimes has negative suction or a vacuum made inside to drain the fluid automatically. To put the Pleurax inside the chest is a little bit tedious and complicated but it can be kept for a long time. The whole methodology of inserting it and maintaining it comes with manufacturer design[13] or can be seen at BTS guidelines.[14]

INSERTION OF INTERCOSTAL DRAINAGE (CHEST TUBES)

Intercostal drainage insertion is done by four basic methodologies:

1. With Seldinger technique (tube thoracostomy with a guidewire and dilators)
2. With direct insertion through trocar (tube thoracostomy with a trocar)
3. Without trocar insertion (operative tube thoracostomy)
4. Tube thoracoscopy through a single-port thoracoscope

Till date there are no controlled studies to compare among the efficacy of the different methods of chest tubes insertion.[15,16]

General Consideration and Patients' Preparation

Before ICD insertion it is very important to understand the requirements and prerequisites such as the site of insertion, training required by the performer, antibiotics prophylaxis, history and physical examination, and analgesia/sedation. Various safety issues and procedural guidance are also mentioned in many societies like BTS guidelines for Local Safety Standards for Invasive Procedures (LocSSIPs).[14]

Insertion Site

Most of the times the ICD or catheters are placed at the fourth or fifth intercostal space in the anterior or midaxillary line[16-19] while posterior approach has high chance of neurovascular damage it should be avoided.

The bundles may not be covered by the lower flange of the rib in that position.[20] Most chest tubes should be placed in the "triangle of safety" **(Fig. 9)**. This triangle is directly above a rib to avoid iatrogenic puncture of the intercostal vessels.[21] The anatomical border and landmarks are depicted in **Figure 9**.

- The lateral edge of latissimus dorsi
- The lateral border of pectoralis major
- Below the base of axilla
- Superior to the horizontal level of the fifth intercostal space

This triangle minimizes the risk to underlying neurovascular bundles and cause least damage to muscle and breast tissue. In emergency condition the landmarks should be nipple line in males and in case of female inframammarycreases. In prepubescent females more care should be given to avoid potential damage of developing breast tissue. The insertion site within the pleural cavity must be guided by the indication of ICD *(fluid gets collected in a dependent portion while the air gets collected in nondependent portion)*. If tube is placed for fluid, it would be more effective if it is placed in lowest dependent chest with the help of ultrasound guidance (signs elicited if different chapter). To drain hemopneumothorax the ICD should be directed posteriorly because the goal in this case is to drain the blood and monitor blood loss also. The better site for drainage of pneumothorax is second intercostal space in midclavicular line, as this pierces the pectoralis muscle small bore ICD around 10–14F is used. In case of uncomplicated pneumothorax this approach is least painful and can be performed at bedside in emergency condition like Tension pneumothorax.[22] In the 10th edition of ATLS (advance trauma life support) guideline in case of tension pneumothorax for needle thoracostomy lateral approach is also recommended, however other literature support decompression or ICD or catheter placement via an anterior approach.[23] In the case of anticipated transportation anterior site seems to be more stable.

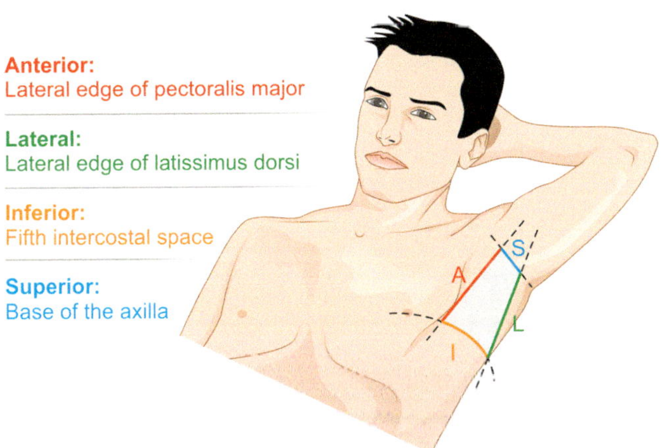

FIG. 9: Anatomical border and landmarks.

Experienced Operator

As per the ACCP recommendations minimum 10 procedures should be performed under supervision to attain basic competency. To maintain this a dedicated interventionist or pulmonologist must perform minimum five procedures per year.[24] Other safety procedural guidance is also mentioned in BTS guidelines for LocSSIPs.

Antibiotics Prophylaxis

The use of universal precautions and sterile preparation of the insertion site with a full body drape is required for all the patients. It is the clinical conditions that determines the use of prophylactic antibiotics and are explained in respective chapters of the book. Prophylaxis has a major role in the adult trauma population, rest conditions are debatable. In the case of spontaneous pneumothorax, it is not indicated.[25-27] In the case of penetrating trauma prophylactic antibiotics is warranted. One meta-analysis done of five trials found this to be significant in reducing the risk of pneumonia and empyema,[28] while in the case of elective thoracic surgery antibiotics are used as a preoperative dose only. The timing of prophylactic antibiotic administration and subsequent rates of surgical site infections (SSIs) is mentioned in **Table 1**.[29]

To continue antibiotics there is no evidence to support. In randomized controlled trial (RCT) of 245 adults the rate of surgical site infection was comparable in both arms either patient treated with extended postoperative antibiotic prophylaxis or placebo (six vs. five patients).[30,31] In case of noncardiac surgery, the antibiotics used as a

TABLE 1: Timing of prophylactic antibiotic administration and subsequent rates of surgical site infections (SSIs).

Time of administration (time-incision)	Percent with SSI	Odds ratio	95% confidence interval (CI)
Early (before 2–24 hours)	3.8	4.3	1.8–10.4
Preoperative (before 0–2 hours)	0.6	1	–
Perioperative (within 3 hours)	1.4	2.1	0.6–7.4
Postoperative (>3 hours)	3.3	5.8	2.4–13.8

prophylaxis mainly targeted to cover the organisms such as *Staphylococcus aureus, Staphylococcus epidermidis, Streptococci,* and enteric gram-negative bacilli. The selection of antibiotics should also be in concordance with the hospital antibiotic stewardship program.

History and Physical Examination

Proper history and clinical examination are very important before ICD insertion. Chest X-ray and other tests such as ultrasonography (USG) of the chest and computed tomography (CT), i.e., CT of chest play a crucial role in determining the lesion and abnormal anatomy. Few important things need to be worked up before putting an ICD such as a mediastinal tumor, cardiomegaly, situs inversus, prior thoracic surgery or thoracostomy tube or catheter placement or pleurodesis, and presence of any medical devices (such as central venous lines/port, pacemaker or defibrillator, shunt tubing, and nerve stimulator). Patients' history of coagulopathy, antithrombotic therapy obesity, any abnormality such as scoliosis and chest wall deformity. There are various factors that can elevate the diaphragm and may lead to false ICD placement also warrants attention—obesity, pregnancy, Trendelenburg position, hemoperitoneum, air in stomach/intestines from positive pressure ventilation, and bowel obstruction.

In case of pediatric population various other factors also play major role, which include:

- Congenital malformations, cysts, and pulmonary abnormalities that mimic pneumothorax on a radiograph
- Congenital or traumatic diaphragmatic defects
- Children when cries or take rapid breath or hyper-ventilate creates issues
- Any anomalies like TOF (tracheoesophageal fistula)
- In prepubescent females the developing breast tissue

Analgesia/Sedation

The ICD insertion by any means or methodology and at any site is a painful procedure. It should always be done with analgesia; however, in emergency condition, it can be performed under local anesthesia (1–2% lignocaine) with or without nerve block. The maximum dose of lignocaine to avoid toxicity is 5–7 mg/kg with epinephrine. While doing elective ICD in addition to local anesthesia oral or intravenous sedation can be administered. The author's preference is intravenous tramadol (opioid analgesia) prior to ICD along with antiemetic like ondansetron. It is important to note that operative tube thoracotomy is very painful. Hence, it is highly recommended that patients be given an anxiolytic or narcotic 10–15 minutes before the procedure and that a good dose of local anesthetic be used.[32]

- *With Seldinger technique (ICD with a guidewire and dilators)* **(Figs. 10 and 11)**: This method is the most common and probably the easiest way of ICD insertion. Nowadays, the interventional radiologist and pulmonologist are using this method quite often. It can be done based on clinical examination with chest X-ray and is many a times under ultrasound or CT guidance.[33,34] The things which are required for ICD insertion is mentioned in **Box 2**.

As described initially, there are various commercial kits available for guidewire ICD **(Box 1)**. The use of Seldinger technique with guidewires and dilators is very well known. Through thin gauge needle (24–26G) local anesthesia to the skin, periosteum and parietal pleura as done for any pleural procedure like pleural biopsy is given. It is our common practice to check air or water through the needle after piercing the parietal pleura at the end of local anesthesia. Then a cannula 16–18 is inserted after confirming the fluid or air from same. Again, fluid or air is aspirated to confirm the intrapleural position of the cannula. Plastic cannula is kept in situ and the thick metallic inner needle is withdrawn to put the guidewire through it (modified seldinger technique). While maintain zero contact with the atmosphere through thumb, the syringe is removed. The "J" wire is threaded through the needle in the anticipated direction into the pleural space. After that at the same site, a small nick is made in the skin. As skin is the toughest organ its incision should be of ample size, so that the dilator can easily pass through it. The smallest dilator is inserted, and with a rotating movement, it is advanced into the pleural space over the guidewire. The first dilator is removed, leaving the wire in place. Then the next size dilator is advanced over the guidewire into the pleural space and removed. Finally, the chest tube containing the inserter is threaded over the guidewire as shown in **Figures 10A to F**. The tube should pass readily, following the path made by the dilators and guided by the wire. It is important to make certain that all of the side holes in the tube are in the pleural space. Once the tube is in place, the inserter and the guidewire are withdrawn. The tube is then clamped until it is attached to the chest drainage system. In our practice, we attach a three-way cannula before attaching the tube. This three-way cannula helps us in operating the ICD in further management (either flushing or blocking the ICD) **(Fig. 1)**. The tube is then anchored in place by means of a long suture through the skin and around the tube and tied with the thread. The incision is sutured without tension to avoid necrosis of the skin next to the tube. The skin over the incised area is cleaned and is covered with plain 4 × 4 gauze

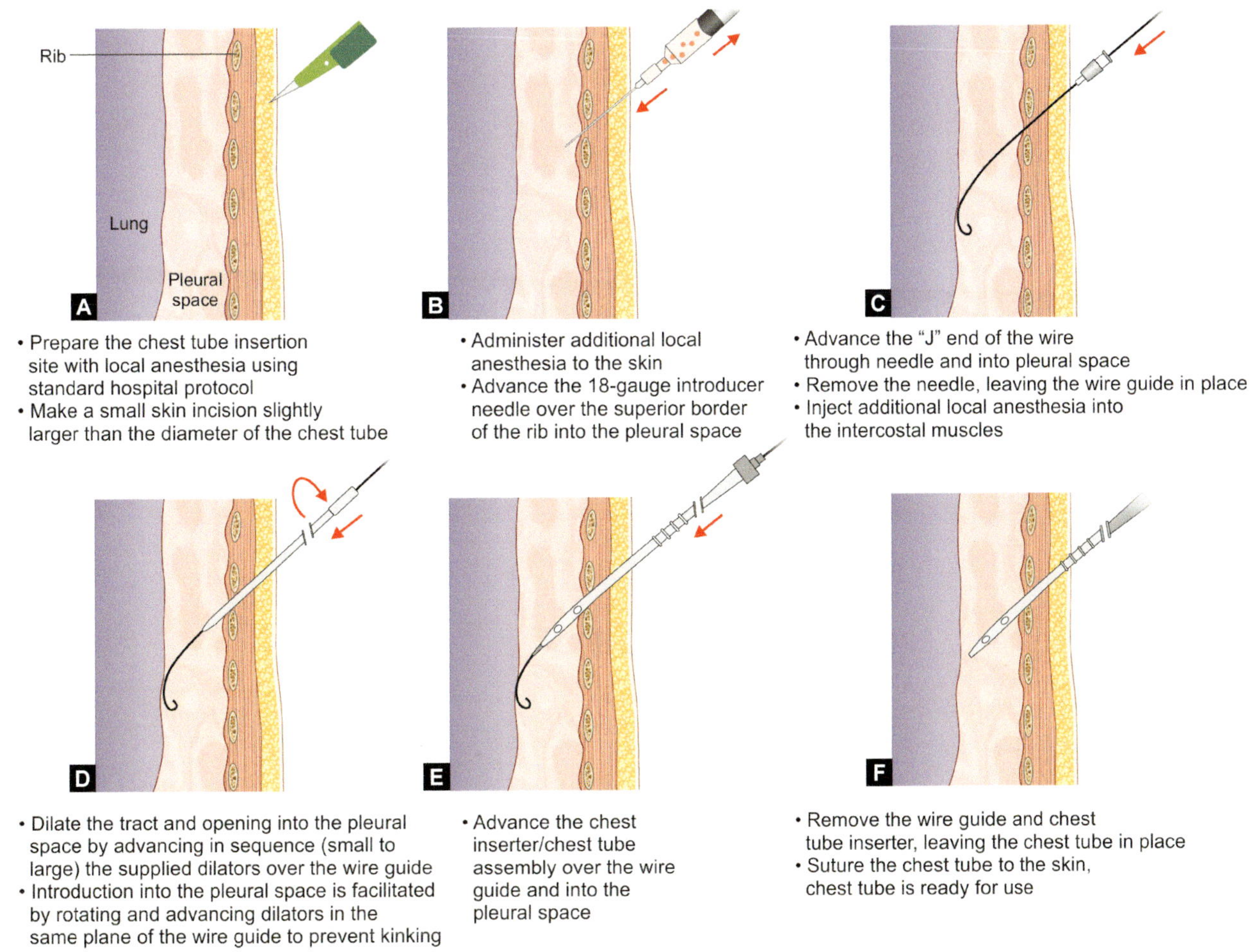

FIGS. 10A TO F: Intercostal chest drain (ICD) insertion via Seldinger technique.

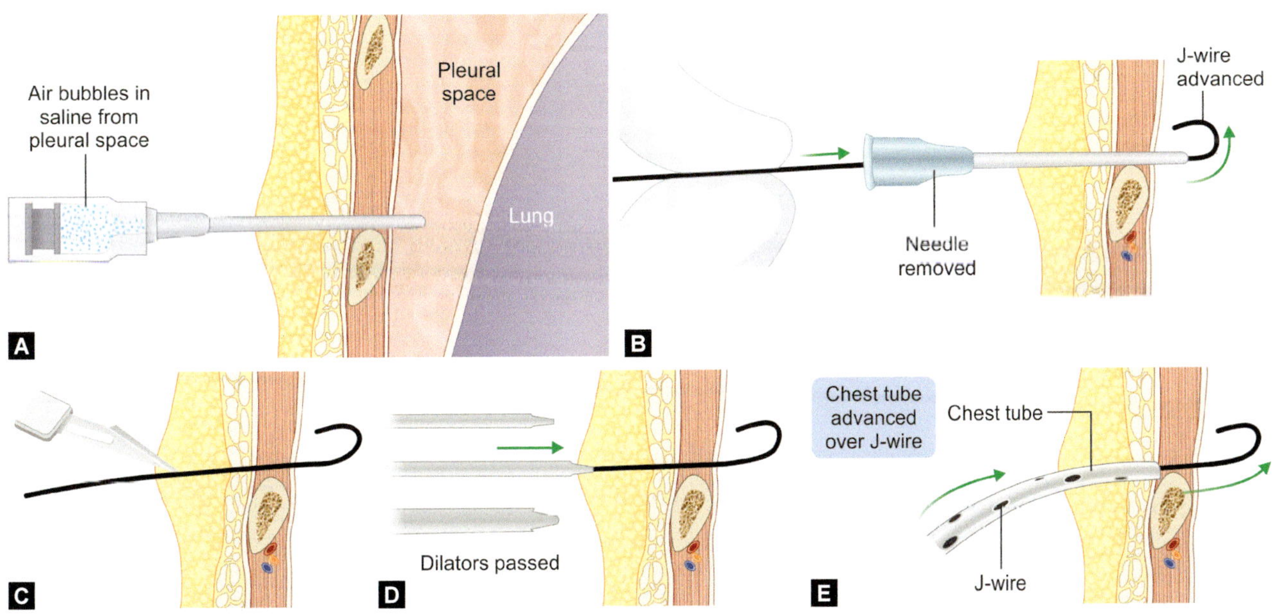

FIGS. 11A TO E: Modified Seldinger.

Note: An appropriately sized catheter (e.g., ≤14 French pigtail) can be placed immediately over a wire into the pleural space using a modified Seldinger technique.

BOX 2 Equipment list required for intercostal drainage (ICD).

- 1 or 2% lidocaine
- Needles (size 25 and size 18–21) and syringes for anesthetizing the skin
- Scalpel, with No. 10 or 11 blade
- Three Kelly clamps
- Straight scissors
- Chest tube
- Silk suture (1-0)
- Needle holder
- Petroleum gauze
- Drain sponges
- Elastic tape
- Sterile drapes, gown, and gloves
- Mask and protective eyewear
- 2% chlorhexidine or povidone–iodine
- Drainage system

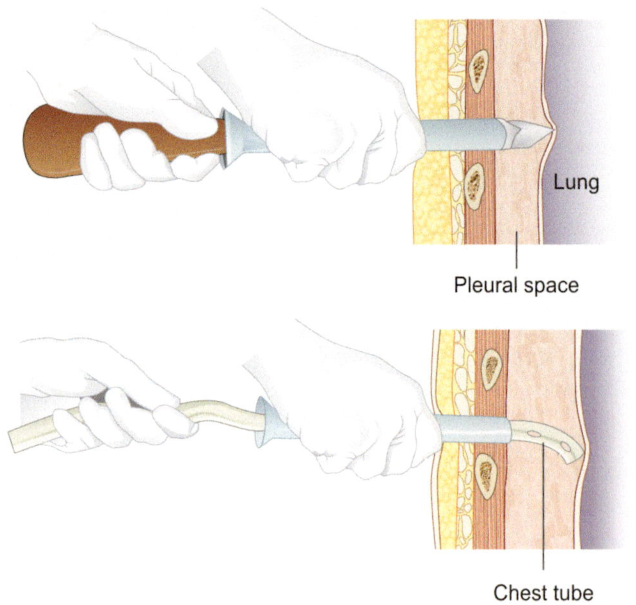

FIG. 12: Trocar tube thoracostomy.

pads and then covered with the help of Dynaplast or micropore. Commercial kits are made so that chest tubes from 8 to 36F can be put. The smaller kits of chest tubes < 12F have no dilators. The Thal-Quick chest tube sets come with chest tube sizes from 8 to 36F. The modified seldinger technique is more or less similar to seldinger technique, but here metallic needle is not used and guidewire is inserted through plastic canula. An appropriately sized catheter (e.g., ≤14 French pigtail) can be placed immediately over a wire into the pleural space **(Figs. 11A to E)**.

- *Direct insertion through a trocar (tube thoracostomy with trocar)* ***(Figs. 12 and 13)***: This methodology is like the guidewire tube thoracostomy, but there is no guidewire or dilators. In general, it is less recommended (when the first one is not available, or the performer is not familiar with the Seldinger technique) because its use appears to be associated with more complications.[35] The use of trocar catheter is discouraged by some, but its popularity depends on the operator's experience.[36,16] This methodology requires a 2–4-cm incision which is made parallel to the superior border of the rib through the skin and subcutaneous tissues once local anesthesia is obtained. After that the trocar can then be inserted between the ribs into the pleural cavity, while the flat edge of the stylet tip is kept cephalad to prevent damage to the intercostal vessels **(Fig. 12)** because it requires significant force to insert the trocar, the hand which is not applying the force should be placed next to the patient's chest wall and control the depth of penetration or sometimes another operator must keep chest wall fixed. Once the trocar is in the pleural space (a give-way feeling is appreciated

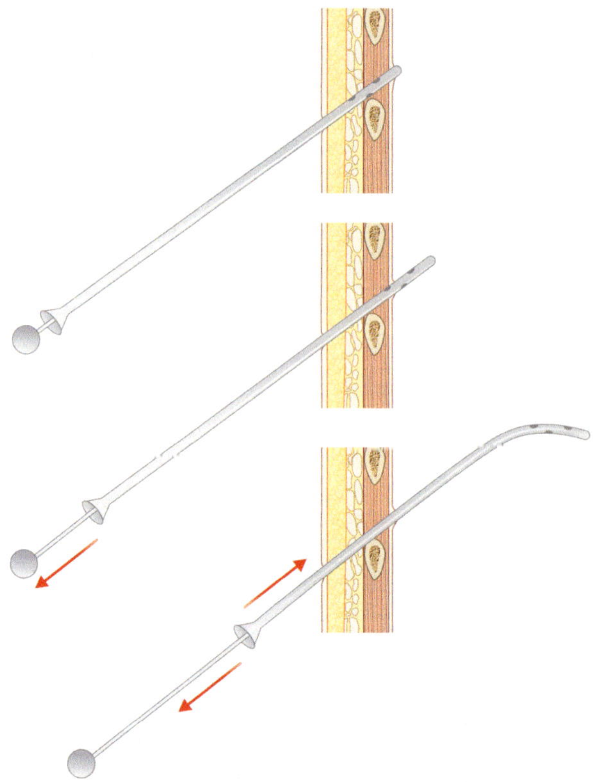

FIG. 13: Newer trocar cannula insertion.

there by the operator), the stylet is then removed. While the stylet is removed, the zero contact from the atmosphere is made by the operator immediately by covering the trocar with the thumb. This maneuver will help to prevent a pneumothorax. After that, when the operator's thumb is removed, the chest tube, with a clamped distal end, is quickly inserted into the pleural space. The trocar is removed by sliding it back over the tube. When the trocar has been removed from the chest, the ICD needs to be clamped between the trocar and the chest wall so that the clamp on the distal end of the ICD can be removed. The ICD must remain clamped until it is attached to an underwater seal (either bag or box) to prevent air from entering the pleural space.

An alternate trocar method uses an ICD with a trocar inside positioned to the pleural cavity directly **(Fig. 13)**. This ICD with a trocar inside has almost the same methodology as the previous one. This type of trocar with ICD is more commonly used nowadays as it is less complicated and easy to insert. Once the pleural cavity is entered by the trocar and cannula, the inner trocar is gradually removed from the ICD. When the proximal end containing the trocar and cannula clears the chest wall, it is clamped between the trocar and the chest wall till the trocar can be completely removed and the tube attached to a water-seal drainage system.

- *Without trocar insertion (Operative tube thoracostomy)* ***(Figs. 14A to G)***: There is a video created by Dev et al.[37] on performing operative tube thoracostomy,

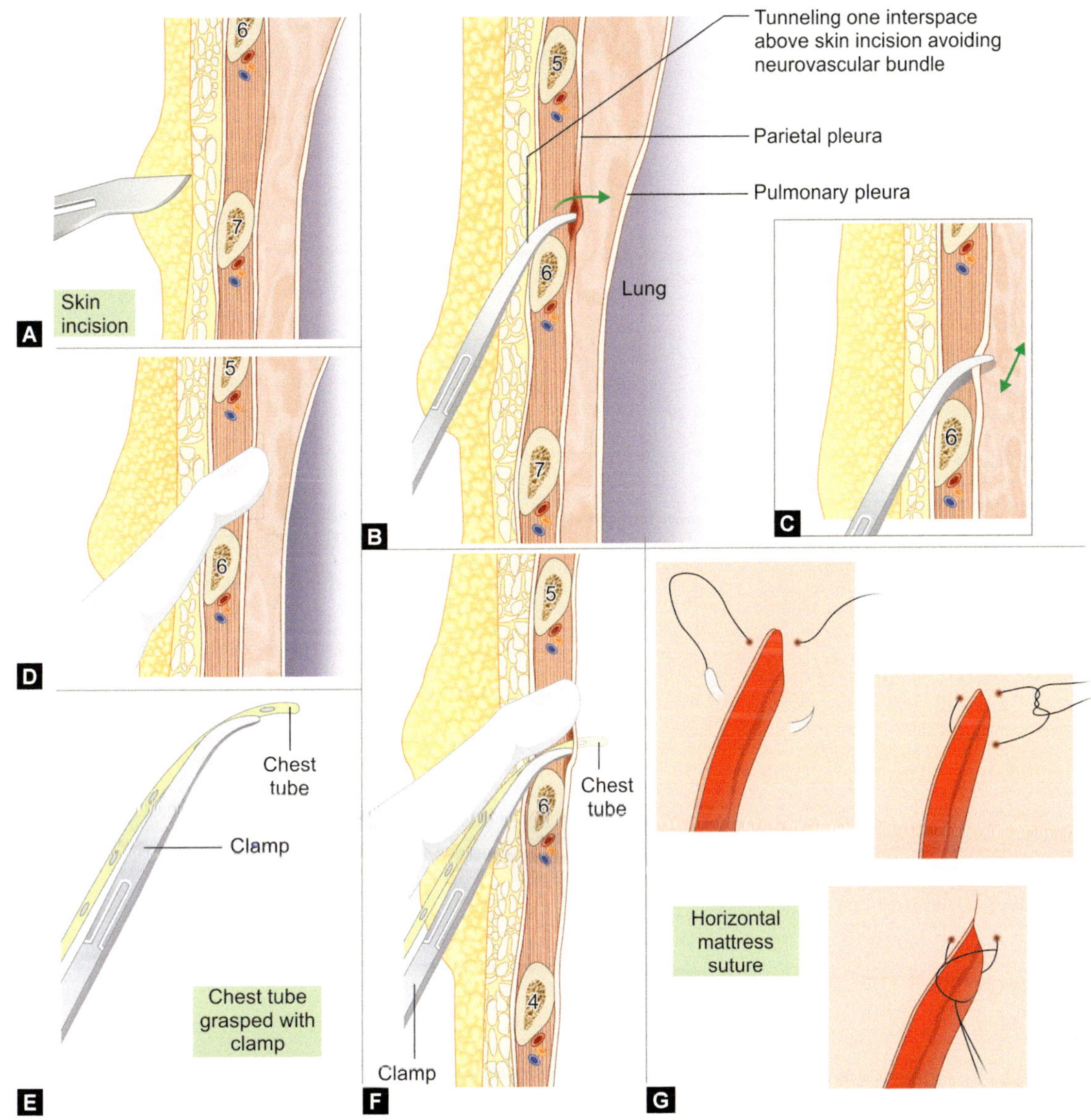

FIGS. 14A TO G: Blunt dissection (operative thoracostomy). (A) An incision is made one to two interspaces inferior to the proposed point of thoracostomy tube insertion; (B) Blunt dissection through the subcutaneous tissue is performed using a clamp; (C) The clamp is spread after entering the pleural space; (D) If patient size allows, a probing finger is inserted to confirm entry into the pleural space and to identify the diaphragm and any adhesions. In the presence of rib fractures, the operator should proceed cautiously to avoid injury; (E and F) The chest tube is gripped with a clamp and inserted (using a finger as a guide if patient size allows using caution to avoid provider injury); and (G) The chest tube is sutured securely in place.

it is recommended that operators should see the video before performing their first operative tube thoracostomy. In this method, a blunt dissection is made in the chest wall (same as done in thoracoscopy). This superficial and deep fascia is then incised throughout the length of the incision, with care must be taken not to cut the muscle. After that muscle fibers are spread with a blunt-tipped hemostat until the intercostal interspace is identified. Through the help of dissection forceps, the external and internal intercostal is split with minimum damage to the muscles. Operator then put his finger (mostly index or little finger) inside the dissected portion and split the muscles. Through to help of forceps or scapula the parietal pleura is then pierced. Though this is a more extensive procedure as compared with guidewire tube thoracostomy or trocar tube thoracostomy, but it is safer. The whole ICD process depends upon the skill and experience of the operator. Sometimes in case of thick pleural rind this method may not be successful. After piercing pleura (the give-way feeling) the gush of fluid or air is seen or appreciated. Again, the adhesions between the lungs and pleura if present are broken with the help of a finger. After that, the ICD insertion is done and is connected with the drainage system.

- *Tube thoracoscopy through a single-port thoracoscope*: This is the novel method though less commonly used by us but for discussion, it should be learned. By this method, ICD can be inserted through a single-port thoracoscopy (Zgoda et al.).[38] Here under direct visualization, the chest tube was placed into the costodiaphragmatic gutter, and after that telescope was removed. In this technique, rigid scope was used. This method will be more friendly for the operators/surgeons who are adept at thoracoscopy. The advantage of ICD placement under direct visualization is kept in mind **(Fig. 15)**.

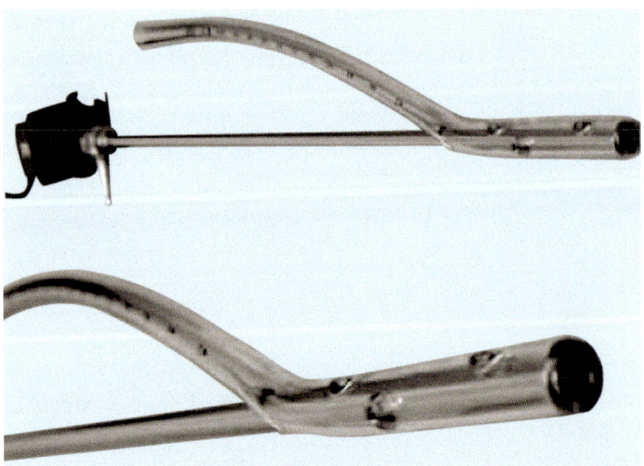

FIG. 15: Hopkins rod lens-telescope.

PLEURAL DRAINAGE AND COLLECTION SYSTEM

The ICD insertion is not the only job of the clinician, it is very important to have an in-depth knowledge of the drainage system to be attached with the tube. Which drainage system has to be applied and may require to shift to another one is the clinician's decision and is very dynamic depending upon the disease condition and severity. Once a chest tube is secured, we want the air or fluid present in the pleura to continuously drain out and at the same time there should not be any air entering into the pleural cavity from outside. We all know that pleural cavity is a negative pressure zone, and it can suck air from the atmosphere, if only tube is inserted into it without any drainage system it will cause an iatrogenic pneumothorax. To prevent this, various types of bags and bottle system have been developed. Initially, a single bottle system was used which has now been replaced by many advanced collection systems but all of them are basically based on the same principle as the one-bottle system to prevent air entry and remove unwanted pleural fluid or air. The drainage systems can be basically classified into four types, which are as follows:[39]

1. One-way Heimlich valve
2. Bottle system or analog three-container systems
3. Digital or electronically controlled devices
4. Vacuum bottles (for IPC drainage)

One-way (Heimlich) Valve (Fig. 16)

It is the simplest drainage system. This is a one-way rubber flutter valve which is attached to the chest tube. Whenever the pressure inside the tube is less than the atmospheric pressure, the valve closes, and it opens as soon as the pressure inside the tubing rises above the atmospheric pressure. Overall, it is closed while inspiration when there is negative intrapleural or intratubal pressure, preventing the atmospheric air entering the pleural cavity, and open while expiration when pleural cavity has a positive pressure allowing exit of air or fluid from pleura to outside **(Fig. 17)**. It is much more useful in a case of pneumothorax as compared to a case of pleural fusion. It is very helpful for the management of ambulatory patients and allows full mobility with ICD in situ.[40] Now, there are commercially available self-contained one-way Heimlich valve with vent in India[28] and outside also [rocket pleural Vent **(Fig. 18)**].

The cheaper version and local use of this one-way valve system can be availed simply by the urobag, which is also the one-way valve system mainly used for urine drainage. Our team has a satisfactory outcome with this system and mainly used when the patients are being discharged with ICD in situ. The drawback with this

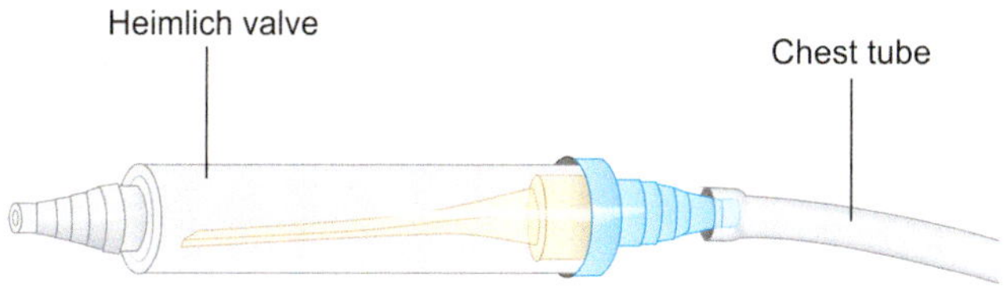

FIG. 16: Heimlich valve.

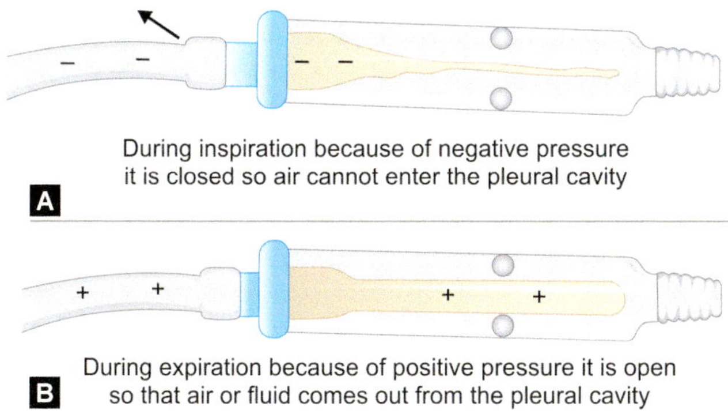

FIGS. 17A AND B: (A) During inspiration (B) during expiration.

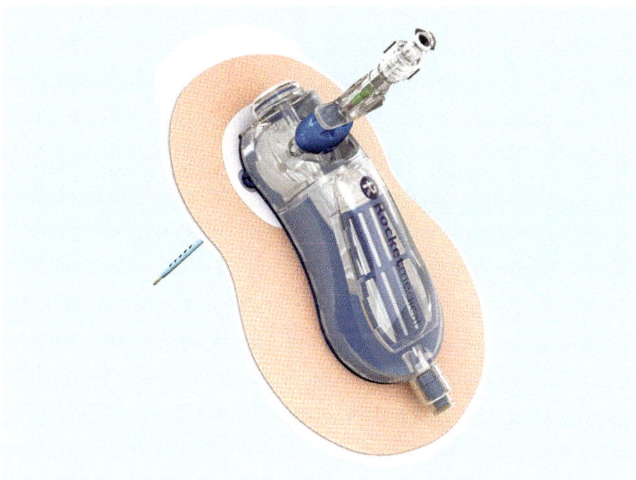

FIG. 18: Rocket pleural vent.

system is that we cannot monitor column movement with this. The urobag must be emptied at regular interval so that the pneumothorax is vented continuously. If it is not followed, then bag will fill up and prevent further removal of the pneumothorax and may cause tension pneumothorax. Because of this the outlet must be kept open (while the patient sleeping at night) so that air can escape as the bag fills up.

There are few literatures supporting the use of the urosac or urobag for this purpose. Sharma et al. had used this in 20 patients of spontaneous pneumothorax and it was found to be efficient, safe, and economical.[41] Another Indian study published in Lung India of 85 patients demonstrating use of urosac with pigtail. In that study the conventional drainage system with ICD was compared with the pigtail with urosac used as ambulatory chest drainage (ACD). The ACD was found to be simple, cheap, and effective in various clinical situations. It can avoid prolonged and expensive.[42]

Bottle System or Analog Three-container Systems

Nowadays we rarely see the bottle system because the commercially manufactured drainage systems have subsequently switched to plastic bag or box instead of the bottle system. But the basic principle behind all the drainage system is best explained by this bottle system; hence, it is required to have detail knowledge of this mechanism to understand all types of pleural drainage system **(Table 2)**.

One Bottle Collection System (Fig. 17)

This system is the combination of collection container and a water seal. ICD bag most commonly used nowadays is physiologically this system. It is a sterile bottle with a rigid straw to which the chest tube is connected. Fluid such as normal saline or sterile water is filled in this bottle to a level (around 2–3 cm water) so that the tip of the rigid straw is approximately 2 cm below the surface of the fluid. The stopper of the bottle has a vent that prevents the pressure from building up when air or fluid is drained from the pleural space and collected in the bottle. In the absence of the vent, pressure will develop inside the bottle which can result even in a tension pneumothorax. Due to the fluid or air present in pleural, the pleural pressure is positive, this makes the pressure in the rigid tube also positive. If the pressure in the rigid tube is greater than the pressure of fluid level in the collection bottle, the fluid or air present in the pleura will drain into the collection bottle. In a case of pleural effusion, the fluid level in the bottle will increase with drainage of the effusion and the pressure due to fluid will also increase. Once the pressure in the bottle rises above the pressure in the rigid straw, fluid from the bottle enters the rigid straw and acts as a barrier between the atmosphere and the pleura. This creates a water seal and does not allow any more fluid or air to enter back into the pleural cavity. In a simple pneumothorax, there is no rising fluid level in the bottle and so the simple one-bottle system works well.

Two Bottle Collection System (Fig. 18)

To overcome the limitations of one-bottle system in patients with large pleural effusions, two-bottle collection system was brought into work. The chest tube is connected to a bottle which acts as a collection system. This bottle

TABLE 2: Various ICD drainage system.

Features	One way valve	One bottle	Two bottles	Three bottles
Example	• Heimlich valve • Urosac	ICD bag	ICD box	ICD box
Figures	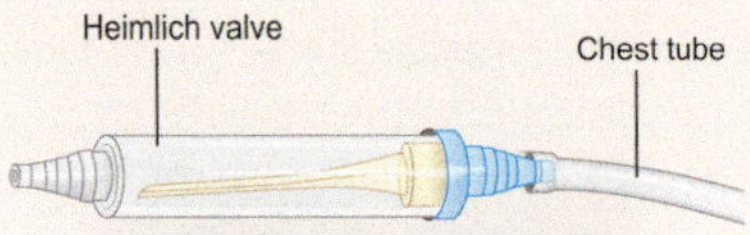 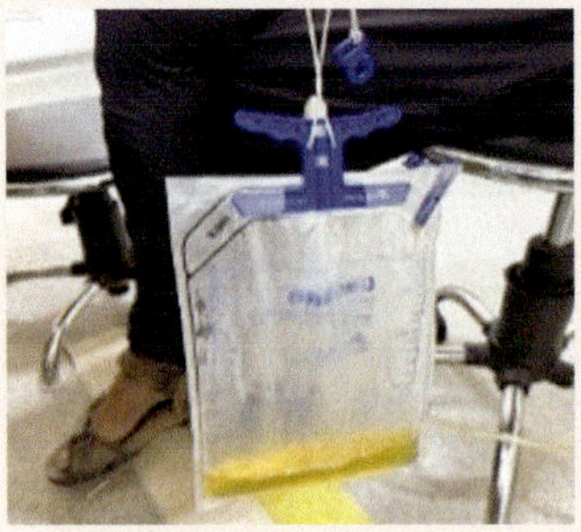	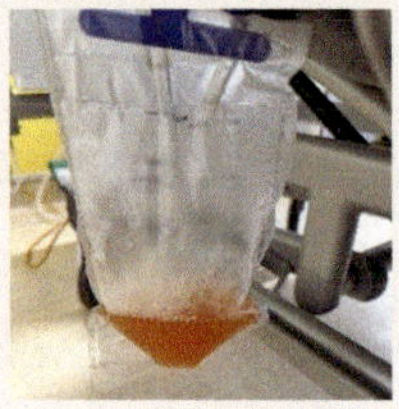	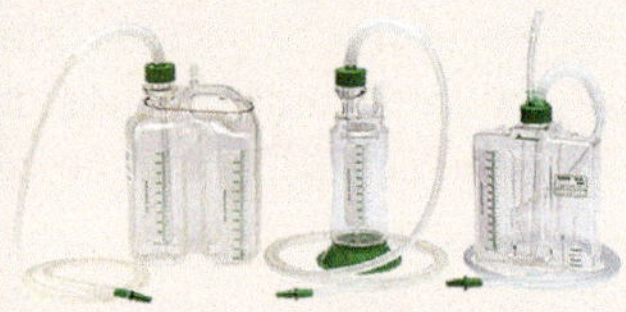	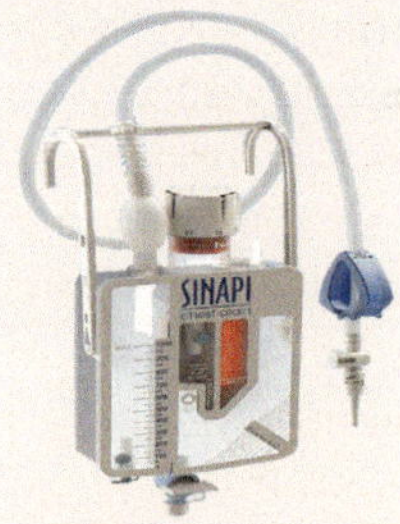
Used in	Spontaneous pneumothorax	• Pneumothorax • Pleural effusion	• Massive pleural effusion • ICD with suction	ICD with controlled suction
Advantage	• Ambulatory • Small • Cheaper	• Ambulatory • Small • Cheaper • Column movement seen	Can be used for large effusion or pneumothorax or when negative pressure is to be applied	Can be used to apply controlled negative pressure in large pneumothorax or effusion
Disadvantage	• Not useful in effusion or massive pneumothorax • Cannot be used if suction is required • Column movement not visualized	• Cumbersome • More chance of blockage and infection	• Cumbersome • Expensive • Once filled box needs to be changed • Controlled suction cannot be applied	• Nonambulatory • Expensive • Once filled, the box needs to be changed

is connected to the second bottle which acts as a water seal and vent. Since the pressure does not increase in the second bottle working as a water seal, there is no risk of developing it into a closed system leading to malfunction or pneumothorax. The first bottle directly connected to the tube must be emptied once it is filled to a level at which it starts touching the tip of the chest tube connected to this bottle. Both one and two-bottle collection system work on gravity dependence principle. In both system the water-seal functions in similar manner.

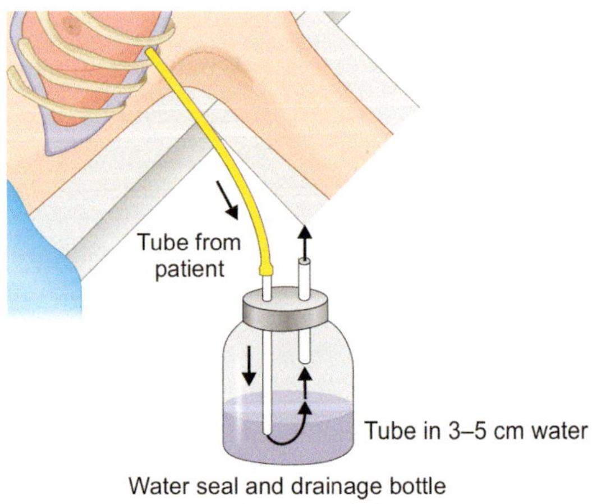

FIG. 19: One bottle system.

Three Bottle Collection System (Figs. 19 to 21)

Sometimes in cases of large effusions and pneumothorax and for re-expansion of lungs so that it is opposed with the parietal pleura, a negative suction is preferred. In 1967, for the first time a three-bottle system was brought into use. The first bottle connected to the chest tube acts as a collection bottle, which is connected to a second bottle acting as a water seal and vent, just like two-bottle collection system. Negative suction can be directly connected to the one- or two-bottle system also. Most healthcare settings have wall suction which is difficult to regulate and may cause more harm than benefit to the patient. In a three-bottle system controlled negative suction is applied with the third bottle. The second bottle acting as a vent and seal is connected to a third bottle which has a rigid pipe same as the first bottle and this is in direct contact with the outside atmosphere and inside the bottle it is submerged in fluid. Third bottle also had a vent which is connected to the negative suction. When the suction is started it sucks air in the bottle from the atmosphere through the rigid tube but only when the negative pressure in bottle is more than the depth to which the rigid tube is submerged. The suction pressure is controlled by the fluid level inside the third bottle. Amount of negative pressure depended on the depth to which the rigid tube was submerged in the fluid. Whatever, the suction pressure in the third bottle, the same pressure exists in second bottle because they are directly connected. By altering the length of the rigid tube inside the fluid in the third bottle, the amount of negative pressure applied can be changed.

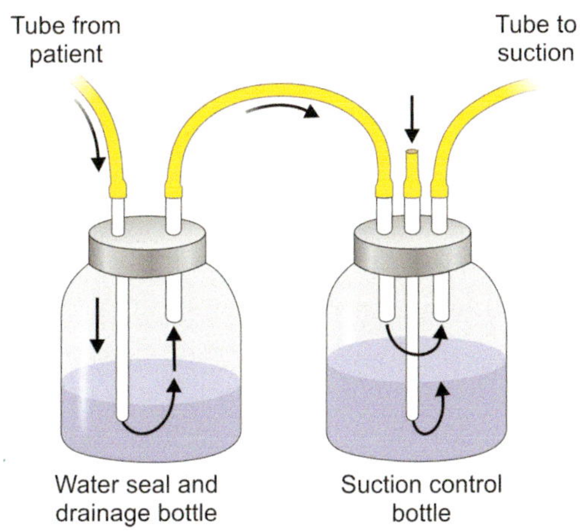

FIG. 20: Two bottle system.

Nowadays, negative suction systems are also commercially available. These are much more compact and convenient than three-bottle collection system. Patient mobilization and drain management are much simpler with these commercially available drainage systems, e.g., the Pleur-evac system, atrium system, and Sinapi Chest Drain.

The drainage system must have **(Fig. 22)**

- Visible water-seal—to easily see if the tube is patent or not and if there is any air leak
- Sufficient volume can be stored
- Markings in the collection chamber to calculate the amount of fluid drained
- Measure to control suction
- The system should still be functional in case negative suction is removed or stops working

Commercial Three Bottle System (Pleur-Evac/Sinapi) (Fig. 23)

It works on the same principle as of three-bottle collection system, in the right most we have a collection system connected to water-seal chamber, which is connected to the suction control chamber in the leftmost. The negative pressure depends on the difference of height of water in the suction control chamber, and the water-seal chamber. This drainage system also has a vent which lets air out when the pressure is >2 cm of water. It has a nob that

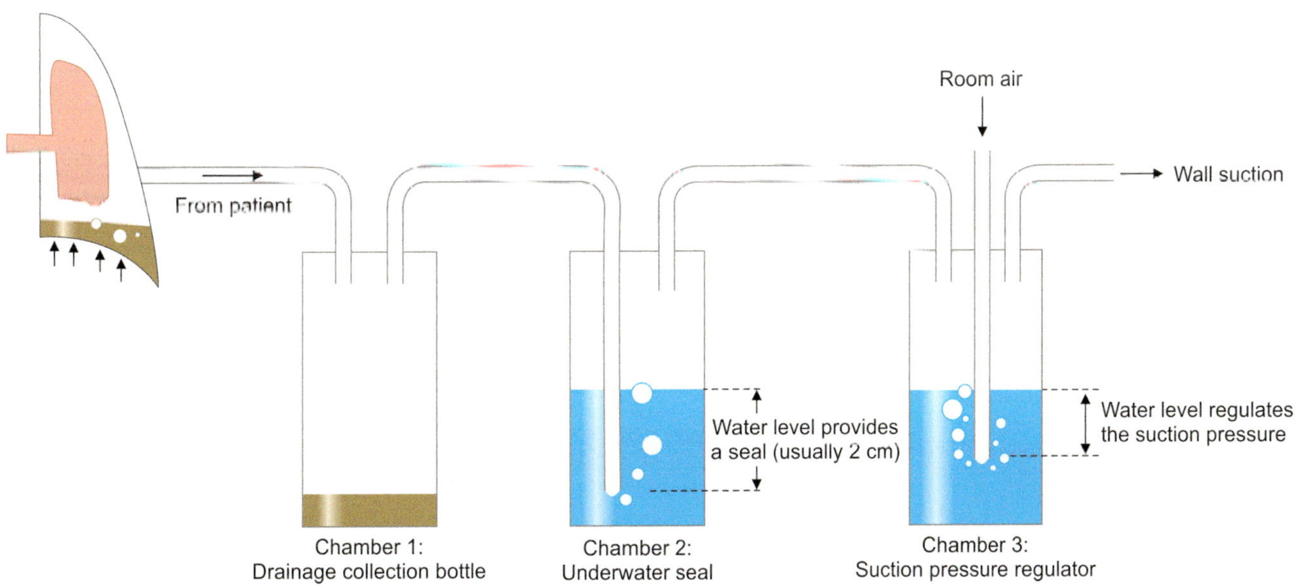

FIG. 21: Three bottle system.

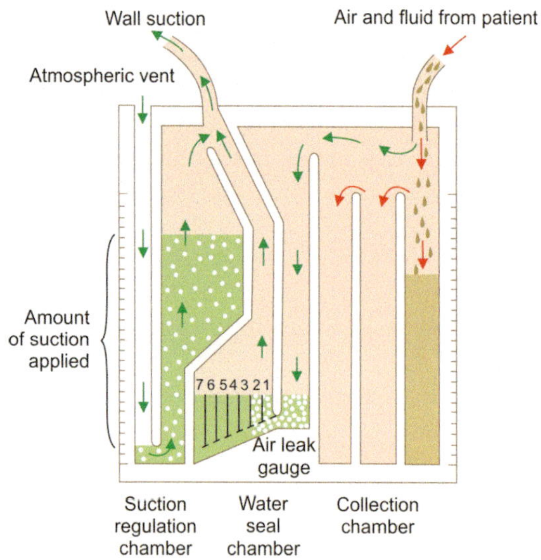

FIG. 22: Details of commercially available three bottle system.

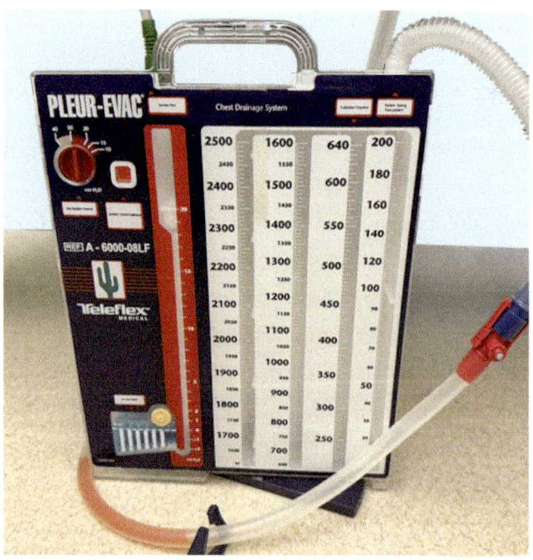

FIG. 23: Three bottle drainage system.

can be used to control the amount of negative pressure applied. The amount of negative suction applied can vary from –10 cm of water to –40 cm of water; although, negative suction has been under scrutiny in the recent times. In cases of pneumothorax application of negative suction might keep the leak patent which may have closed on its own. Surgeons prefer negative suction over physicians as they treat a pneumothorax with surgical sutures. So, the negative suction only helps by keeping the visceral pleura as opposed to the parietal pleura and helps in lung expansion.

Digital or Electronically Controlled Devices (Figs. 24A to C)

This is the latest and most advance version of the chest tube drainage system. It has a feature of all the previously mentioned drainage system and most important part of this device is that the pressure is digitally controlled. It allows the optimal desired pressure to be applied for the chest drainage management. This helps in objective and reliable monitoring of the ICD drain. It has two units one is the electronic machine **(Fig. 24A)** and other part is the canister which is disposable. The most common commercially available device is Medela-Thopaz.[43] Other commercial devices are also available such as Atmos; Dentrex and Redax. It is battery-operated with a charger, lightweight, and compact. This device is portable which makes it very convenient for carrying. This helps in early mobilization of patients even who requires negative pressure **(Fig. 24C)**. This device can reduce the interobserver variability in leak assessment as they provide a 24-hour digital recording of fluid drainage, air leak, and intrapleural pressure.[44] It can help in maintaining predetermined intrathoracic negative pressure and the system automatically intervenes as needed to achieve the optimum value The only drawback of this system is that it is very costly and not available everywhere. The electronic device is the one-time buy and is reusable but the canister

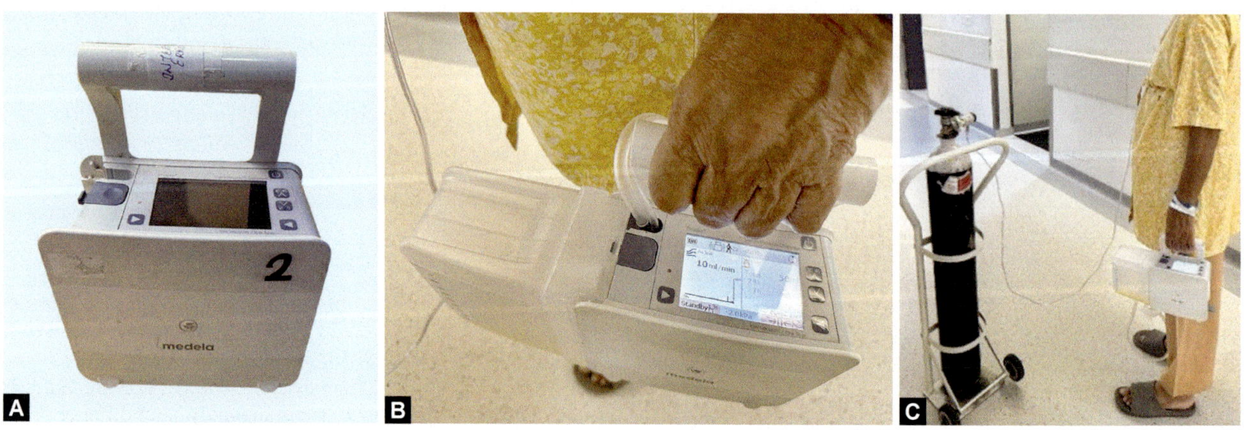

FIGS. 24A TO C: Electronic drainage system.

that is attached to it is one-time use and also costly. There are various literatures favoring use of this technically advance digital drainage system in case where controlled suction is required for ambulatory patients.[45,46]

Vacuum Bottles Used in Indwelling Pleural Catheter (Fig. 25)

This has been explained earlies in this chapter while discussing ICD. The drainage system of IPC has collection bottle which are disposable drainage vacuum bottles of different capacities depending upon the IPC manufacturer, such as 200, 400, 600, and 1,000 mL capacity. These bottles are costly and of single use. Sometimes, for cost issues different catheters are used where manual pump being attached to the collection bag in line. Here, the patients can themselves operate it by squeezing it to start the vacuum effect and draining out the fluid to the collection bag.[47] This drainage system is mostly used in malignant pleural effusion where pleurodesis fails. It is useful in early ambulation and one-time suction.

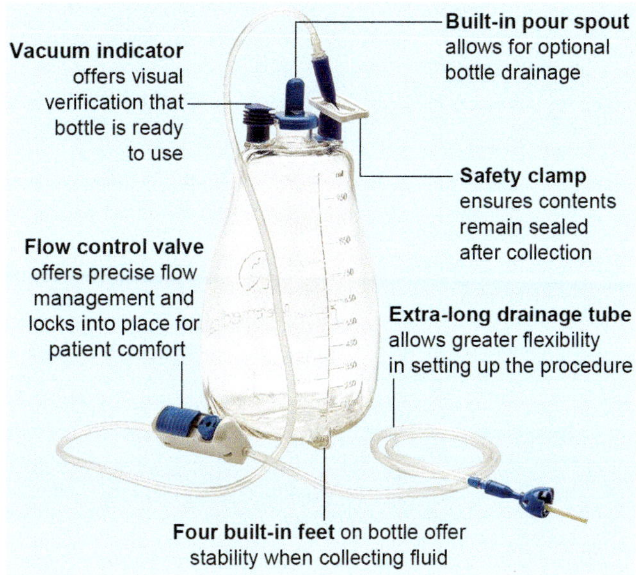

FIG. 25: Suction drainage of indwelling pleural catheter (IPC).

KEY POINTS

- ICD is the most important tool to deal with the pleural pathologies such as pneumothorax and pleural effusion of any etiology such as empyema and malignant effusion.
- It comes in various sizes and of various types like with or without trocar, pigtail, and indwelling pleural catheter. The most used ICD is the pigtail and trocar cannula.
- There are various modes of ICD insertion and among them most important is the Seldinger technique.
- Most of the time small bore ICD is recommended unless hemothorax or empyema with thick pus is suspected.
- Triangle of safety is the most convenient site for ICD insertion as it causes minimal risk to underlying neurovascular bundles and least damage to muscle and breast tissue.
- The insertion site within the pleural cavity must be guided by the indication of ICD (fluid gets collected in a dependent portion while the air gets collected in a nondependent portion).
- The insertion site within the pleural cavity must be guided by the indication of ICD (fluid gets collected in a dependent portion while the air gets collected in a nondependent portion).
- While ICD insertion good pain management is recommended, and routine use of prophylactic antibiotic is not necessary.
- Pleural drainage system is an important part of the ICD system. One bottle (urosac and Heimlich valve) is commonly used for pneumothorax with ambulatory patients, two bottle (underwater seal bag) is used for pneumothorax and pleural effusion.
- Three-bottle system Is used when a large effusion with negative pressure is required and many a times helpful in applying a controlled system.
- Recent advances in the pleural drainage system are the digital or electronically-controlled devices (Medela), which are battery-operated with a charger, lightweight, and compact. This device is portable which makes it very convenient for carrying.

REFERENCES

1. Wikipedia. org. (2023). Chest tube. [online] Available from https://en.wikipedia.org/wiki/Chest_tube [Last accessed November, 2023].
2. Adams F. Genuine Works of Hippocrates. Sydenham, London: Sydenham Society; 1849.
3. Graham ME, Bell CR. Open Pneumothorax: Its relation to the treatment of empyema. Am J Med Sci. 1918;156(6):839-71.
4. Lilienthal H. Resection of the lung for suppurative infections with a report based on 31 operative cases in which resection was done or intended. Ann Surg. 1922;75(3):257–320.
5. MacDuff A, Arnold A, Harvey J; BTS Pleural Disease Guideline Group. Management of spontaneous pneumothorax: British Thoracic Society pleural disease guideline 2010. Thorax. 2010;65:ii18-31.

6. Asciak R, Bewadi EO, Bhatnagar R, Clive AO, Hasan M, Lloyd H, et al. British Thoracic Society Clinical Statement on pleural procedures. Thorax. 2023;78(Suppl 3):1-25.
7. DeFrances CJ, Cullen KA, Kozak LJ. National Hospital Discharge Survey: 2005 annual summary with detailed diagnosis and procedure data. Vital Health Stat 13. 2007;165:1-209.
8. Baumann MH. What size chest tube? What drainage system is ideal? And other chest tube management questions. Curr Opin Pulm Med. 2003;9(4):276–81.
9. Singh K, Loo S, Bellomo R. Pleural drainage using central venous catheters. Crit Care. 2003;7(6):R191-4.
10. Grodzin CJ, Balk RA. Indwelling small pleural catheter needle thoracentesis in the management of large pleural effusions. Chest. 1997;111(4):981-8.
11. Cooper CM. Pleural aspiration with a central venous catheter. Anaesthesia. 1987;42(2):217.
12. Kulvatunyou N, Vijayasekaran A, Hansen A, Wynne JL, O'Keeffe T, Friese RS, et al. Two-year experience of using pigtail catheters to treat traumatic pneumothorax: a changing trend. J Trauma. 2011;71(5):1104-7.
13. Rocket Medical LLC. R54400-16-MT Rocket IPC Pleural & Peritoneal Catheter Insertion Set with metal tunneller. [online] Available from https://sales.rocketmedical.com/rocket-ipc-indwelling-pleural-catheter-insertion-set-with-metal-tunneller dated 08/08/2023 [Last accessed November, 2023].
14. British Thoracic Society. British Thoracic Society Guidance to support the implementation of Local Safety Standards for Invasive Procedures (LocSSIPs) - Bronchoscopy and Pleural Procedures, 2020. [online] Available from https://www.brit-thoracic.org.uk/qualityimprovement/clinical-resources/interventional-procedures/national-safetystandards-for-invasive-procedures-bronchoscopy-and-pleural-procedures/ [Last accessed November, 2023].
15. Light RW. Pleural controversy: optimal chest tube size for drainage. Respirology. 2011;16(2):244-8.
16. Symbas PN. Chest drainage tubes. Surg Clin North Am. 1989;69(1):41-6.
17. Keeling AN, Leong S, Logan PM, Lee MJ. Empyema and effusion: outcome of image-guided small-bore catheter drainage. Cardiovasc Intervent Radiol. 2008;31(1):135-41.
18. Brims FJ, Lansley SM, Waterer GW, Lee YC. Empyema thoracis: new insights into an old disease. Eur Respir Rev. 2010;19(117):220-8.
19. Dalbec DL, Krome RL. Thoracostomy. Emerg Med Clin North Am. 1986;4(3):441-57.
20. British Thoracic Society. Pleural procedures. [online] Available from https://www.brit-thoracic.org.uk/quality-improvement/clinical-statements/pleural-procedures/ [Last accessed November, 2023].
21. Salamonsen M, Dobeli K, McGrath D, Readdy C, Ware R, Steinke K, et al. Physician-performed ultrasound can accurately screen for a vulnerable intercostal artery prior to chest drainage procedures. Respirology. 2013;18(6):942-7.
22. Kulvatunyou N, Erickson L, Vijayasekaran A, Gries L, Joseph B, Friese RF, et al. Randomized clinical trial of pigtail catheter versus chest tube in injured patients with uncomplicated traumatic pneumothorax. Br J Surg. 2014;101(2):17-22.
23. Cantin L, Chartrand-Lefebvre C, Lepanto L, Gianfelice D, Rabbat A, Aubin B, et al. Chest tube drainage under radiological guidance for pleural effusion and pneumothorax in a tertiary care university teaching hospital: review of 51 cases. Can Respir J. 2005;12(1):29-33.
24. Ernst A, Silvestri GA, Johnstone D; American College of Chest Physicians. Interventional pulmonary procedures: guidelines from the American College of Chest Physicians. Chest. 2003;123(5):1693-717.
25. LeBlanc KA, Tucker WY. Prophylactic antibiotics and closed tube thoracostomy. Surg Gynecol Obstet. 1985;160(3):259-63.
26. Stone HH, Symbas PN, Hooper CA. Cefamandole for prophylaxis against infection in closed tube thoracostomy. J Trauma. 1981;21(11):975-7.
27. Olgac G, Aydogmus U, Mulazimoglu L, Kutlu CA. Antibiotics are not needed during tube thoracostomy for spontaneous pneumothorax: an observational case study. J Cardiothorac Surg. 2006;1:43.
28. Sanabria A, Valdivieso E, Gomez G, Echeverry G. Prophylactic antibiotics in chest trauma: a meta-analysis of high-quality studies. World J Surg. 2006;30(10):1843-7.
29. Huggins JT, Carr SR, Woodward GA. (2023). Thoracostomy tubes and catheters: Indications and tube selection in adults and children. [online] Available from https://www.uptodate.com/contents/thoracostomy-tubes-and-catheters-placement-techniques-and complications?search=thoracostomy%20tube&source=search_result&selectedTitle=1~150&usage_type=default&display_rank [Last accessed November, 2023].
30. Oxman DA, Issa NC, Marty FM, Patel A, Panizales CZ, Johnson NN, et al. Postoperative antibacterial prophylaxis for the prevention of infectious complications associated with tube thoracostomy in patients undergoing elective general thoracic surgery: a double-blind, placebo-controlled, randomized trial. JAMA Surg. 2013;148(5):440-6.
31. Bosman A, de Jong MB, Debeij J, van den Broek PJ, Schipper IB. Systematic review and meta-analysis of antibiotic prophylaxis to prevent infections from chest drains in blunt and penetrating thoracic injuries. Br J Surg. 2012;99(4):506-13.
32. Luketich JD, Kiss M, Hershey J, Urso GK, Wilson J, Bookbinder M, et al. Chest tube insertion: a prospective evaluation of pain management. Clin J Pain. 1998;14(2):152-4.
33. Moulton JS. Image-guided management of complicated pleural fluid collections. Radio Clin North Am. 2000;38(2):345-74.
34. Munnell ER. Thoracic drainage. Ann Thorac Surg. 1997;63(5):1497-502.
35. Fishman NH. Thoracic drainage: A manual of procedures. United States: Mosby; 1983. pp. 32-66.
36. Dev SP, Nascimiento B Jr, Simone C, Chien V. Videos in clinical medicine. Chest-tube insertion. N Engl J Med. 2007;357(15):e15.
37. Zgoda MA, Lunn W, Ashiku S, Ernst A, Feller-Kopman D. Direct visual guidance for chest tube placement through a single-port thoracoscopy: a novel technique. Chest. 2005;127(5):1805-7.
38. Porcel JM. Chest tube drainage of the pleural space: A Concise Review for Pulmonologists. Tuberc Respir Dis (Seoul). 2018;81(2):106-15.
39. Gogakos A, Barbetakis N, Lazaridis G, Papaiwannou A, Karavergou A, Lampaki S, et al. Heimlich valve and pneumothorax. Ann Transl Med 2015;3(4):54.
40. Indiamart.com. Rocket R54565 Pleural Vent. [online] Available from https://www.indiamart.com/proddetail/rocket-r54565-pleural-vent-19282453612.html [Last accessed November, 2023].
41. Sharma TN, Agnihotri SP, Jain NK, Madan A. Spontaneous pneumothorax: use of urosac as pneumosac. Indian J Tuberc. 1987;34:194-96.

42. Desai U, Joshi JM. Use of pigtail catheter and urosac: Numero uno for ambulatory chest drainage! Lung India. 2018;35(5): 395-400.
43. www.medelahealthcare.com. Thopaz Digital Chest Drainage and Monitoring System. [online] Available from https://www.medelahealthcare.com/en-IN/solutions/chest-drainage/thopaz [Last accessed November, 2023].
44. Arai H, Tajiri M, Kameda Y, Shiino K, Ando K, Okudela K, et al. Evaluation of a digital drainage system (Thopaz) in over 250 cases at a single site: a retrospective case-control study. Clin Respir J. 2018;12(4):1454-9.
45. Pompili C, Brunelli A, Salati M, Refai M, Sabbatini A. Impact of the learning curve in the use of a novel electronic chest drainage system after pulmonary lobectomy: a case-matched analysis on the duration of chest tube usage. Interact Cardiovasc Thorac Surg. 2011;13(5):490-3;discussion 493.
46. Zisis C, Tsirgogianni K, Lazaridis G, Lampaki S, Baka S, Mpoukovinas I, et al. Chest drainage systems in use. Ann Transl Med. 2015;3(3):43.
47. Gillen J, Lau C. Permanent indwelling catheters in the management of pleural effusions. Thorac Surg Clin. 2013;23(1):63-71,vi.

CHAPTER 18

Chest Tube Monitoring, Complications, and Its Management

Ashish Kumar Prakash, Anand Jaiswal, Mayank Pratap Singh

INTRODUCTION

The job of a treating clinician is not just over after putting an intercostal chest drain (ICD). Though it gives immense pleasure to the operator that a successful insertion of ICD has been done but it needs a follow-up. Monitoring the ICD, its drain, air leak, and management of the complications is far more important than the ICD insertion.

FOLLOW-UP AFTER INTERCOSTAL CHEST DRAIN INSERTION

- Confirmation of ICD placement in the pleural space
- Postprocedural complications and its management
- Monitoring of ICD drain
- Air leak
- ICD drainage systems
- ICD removal

CONFIRMATION OF INTERCOSTAL CHEST DRAIN PLACEMENT IN THE PLEURAL SPACE

Once the ICD is inserted it needs to be verified that the ICD is in pleural space. It is highly recommended by the authors and team that before confirming the ICD in pleural space, do not stop the procedure and before fixing the tube with skin it should be rechecked. There is various way to confirm the pleural position. Clinically at the bedside, inside the tube, we can see:[1]

- Fluid level inside the chest drain in internal pipe swings.
- When the patient is asked to cough the prime-level fluid bubbles
- In the case of pleural effusion pleural fluid drains from the chest
- In the case of pneumothorax, the chest drain fogs up

While inserting the local anesthesia fluid or air in the syringe can give a hint as described during the insertion procedure. Once ICD is placed and a trocar or guide wire is removed, again through a 10–20 cc syringe suction is done to check fluid or air. A three-way canula is good to be put at the distal end of ICD and then the drainage system is connected. Sometimes it is not feasible to directly connect the ICD tube (with trocar-canula) to the drainage system, in that case, various types of connectors are commercially available and should be used as required for individual systems **(Figs. 1A to C)**.

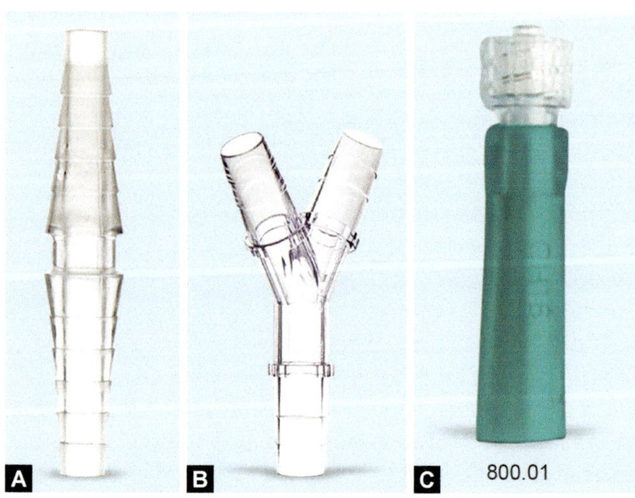

FIGS. 1A TO C: Types of connectors. (A) Universal 3/8″ straight connector; (B) 3/8″ Y-connector; and (C) Vygon Heimlich Valve Adaptor.

Radiology has a very important role in pleural pathology and the basic chest X-ray PA and lateral view most tell us about the position of ICD. Very rarely thoracic ultrasound or chest computed tomography (CT) is required for confirmation of ICD and its drainage holes whether left subcutaneously can be needed. With CT, the tube can be visualized over its entire course with the exact location of its tip. It can also tell us whether the ICD is lying near fissures or if any lung penetrations have been done.[2] In case of multiple loculated empyema of hemothorax, contrast-enhanced computed tomography (CECT) can help to differentiate between the visceral and parietal pleura also. That will help in giving the exact location of the ICD and the need for another ICD if the in-situ ICD is not communicating with the another locules.[3]

POSTPROCEDURAL INTERCOSTAL CHEST DRAIN MANAGEMENT AND COMPLICATIONS

Malpositioning

Intercostal chest drain malpositioning is the most common complication of thoracostomy tube insertion.[4,5] A study done by Curtin et al. demonstrated 58% (38 out of 66) of ICDs done in emergency for trauma were within the fissure. However, there was no any evidence of decreased functional effectiveness because of this position. It can be possible because of the repositioning of ICD in the fissure after the fluid was drained.[6] In another study of 77 thoracostomy tubes placed in emergency in trauma patients, malpositioning was detected in 20 out of 51 patients (26%) via CT.[7] Among them the tubed were placed nine in intrafissural, five in intraparenchymal, and two in subcutaneous position. So, it is mandatory to get a CT scan if a patient's chest X-ray is consistent with malpositioned ICD or ICD nonfunctional, i.e., not draining in spite of radiolucency or lesion present clinically. ICD or catheters that are not in the correct position may represent a form of penetrating trauma and managed accordingly. Multidisciplinary consultation with a pulmonary and cardiothoracic and vascular surgery (CTVS) (thoracic surgery) service should be done before making any changes in a stable patient where the tube is malpositioned. If it is an intraparenchymal ICD or catheter, it need not be removed until a second functioning ICD has been inserted into the pleural space. Every preparation should be made by the treating clinician to manage bleeding as well as an anticipated immediate massive air leak, when the malpositioned ICD removal is planned. In case of tension pneumothorax always place a second functioning tube before removing the first one. As per the guidelines when another ICD is needed because of a nonfunctioning intercostal tube, the previous track must be avoided while inserting the new drain.

Tube Blockage

The ICD blockage is a common sequalae (would not label as a complication) and is almost with every ICD if not managed properly. The lesser the diameter more is the chance of blockage.[6] As the latest guidelines are focusing more on small bore ICD, this sequalae should always be kept in mind and need to be evaluated on a daily basis in ICD-inserted patients. The author's team has a common practice to check for blockage on a daily basis. The simple clinical art to check for blockage is the column movement. With an ICD patient, the water column inside the visible tube moves and it goes toward the pleura while inspiration (because of negative pleural pressure) and moves toward the drainage tube, i.e., away from the pleura during expiration. The material with which the cannula or tube is made is one of the most important factors for blockage This art of checking column movement in an ICD water seal bag also tells us about the air leak or bronchopleural fistula (BPF). In the case of BPF the ICD bag has air bubbles inside **(Fig. 2)**. To check for column movement, one has to be aware of the drainage system. To look for the column movement ICD with underwater seal drainage system is required. It may not be appreciated many a times if the ICD is connected with a one-way valve like a urobag or Heimlich valve. Column movement is also difficult to monitor if ICD is connected with suction directly or suction control drainage system.

The next thing that has to be understood is the factors that are responsible for blockage:[8]

- Kinking or angulation of tube (pigtails and leader catheter are very prone to that) and maximum time

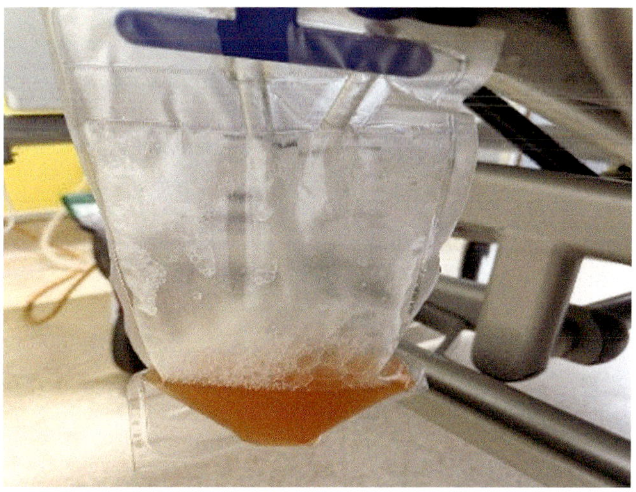

FIG. 2: Intercostal chest drainage (ICD) showing air leak.

they are kinked just at a junction in chest wall outside where the tube is fixed with the suture
- ICD filled with cast, lung tissue, or drained material that has blocked the tube
- Pleurodesis is done and chemicals are left inside the tube causing a blockage
- In hemothorax blood clots block small bore ICD almost daily
- ICD is clamped by an attendant or staff nurse while transportation
- After anticipated drainage the ICD is intentionally blocked to prevent reperfusion pulmonary edema.
- The manufacturing material of the tube is very delicate, and the tube gets blocked almost daily in case of a leader catheter or fenestrated angiocatheter used to drain pneumothorax (not recommended for long-term use or in effusion)

The simple and most convenient remedy for blockage is ICD flushing. Flushing can be done according to the ICD and its connection with the drainage system. The three-way cannula attached or the connector has an important role while flushing. If three-way is used, then the flushing becomes very easy and can be done even in ward rounds with a simple use of a 10–20 cc syringe, and normal saline is instilled with the help of stopper guidance **(Fig. 3)**. In that case both tubes can be flushed either the ICD tube inside the pleural cavity or connections to the drainage system. In the case of other tubes where the three-way connections are not possible the Toomey 50 cc syringe **(Fig. 4)** can be fitted in the ICD tube and flushing can be done. The authors also used the tip of the Ryles tube to facilitate the flushing through a normal syringe. The Ryles tube is cut from its proximal end and only 2–3 cm of the cannula is remained which can be tightly fitted to the ICD and flushing can be done **(Figs. 5A to C)**. Milking of ICD is one of the other methods to remove blockage. Nowadays, because of better newer generations of ICDs and better flushing mechanisms, this is rarely used. In case of kinking and angulation sometimes ICD proper positioning and proper fixation with the chest wall is required. Very rarely it may be required to change the ICD if recurrent blockage is creating issues.

Infection

Putting something inside the human body is always the risk of introducing of infection inside the body. Closed ICD is classified as "clean-contaminated" and hence the risk of infection of the wound is 7.7%.[9] Empyema secondary to ICD has been reported around 1–25% as a complication.[10,11] Prolonged ICD or retained hemothorax increases the risk of infection. In case of penetrating chest trauma, these risk factors for infection should be kept in mind.[12] Blood is a good culture media for bacterial growth hence in the case of hemothorax it requires extra attention. In the case of retained hemothorax early fluid drainage decreases the incidence of empyema, and contrast chest CT is more useful than plain films in further management.[13]

The skin infection at the surgical site has a wide spectrum and ranges from cellulitis to necrotizing soft tissue infection. ICD drainage for empyema thoracis as anticipated has a higher chance of giving rise to necrotizing soft tissue infection. This complication can be prevented with adequate skin preparation prior to ICD insertion. Necrotizing fasciitis after ICD has been reported as a complication of empyema thoracis,[14] in patients with Werdnig-Hoffman disease[15] and in secondary spontaneous pneumothorax for tuberculosis.[16] Skin infection at the site starts with an area of redness that later gives rise to dusky and purplish skin. Later on, signs of tissue necrosis such as putrid discharge, bullae, severe pain, and subcutaneous emphysema, and sometimes

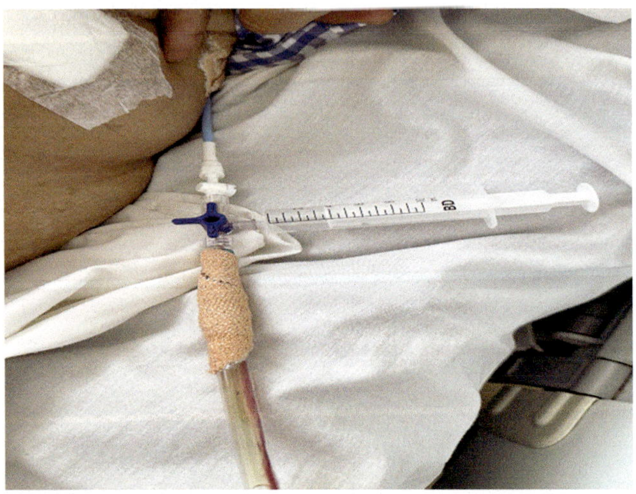

FIG. 3: Intercostal chest drainage (ICD) attached with a normal syringe through a three-way canula and flushing done.

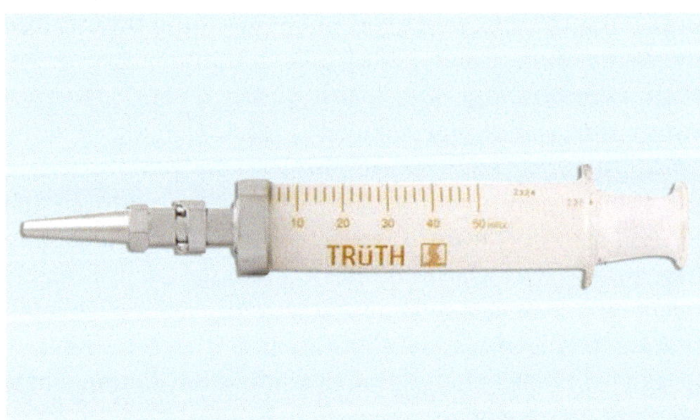

FIG. 4: Toomey syringe.

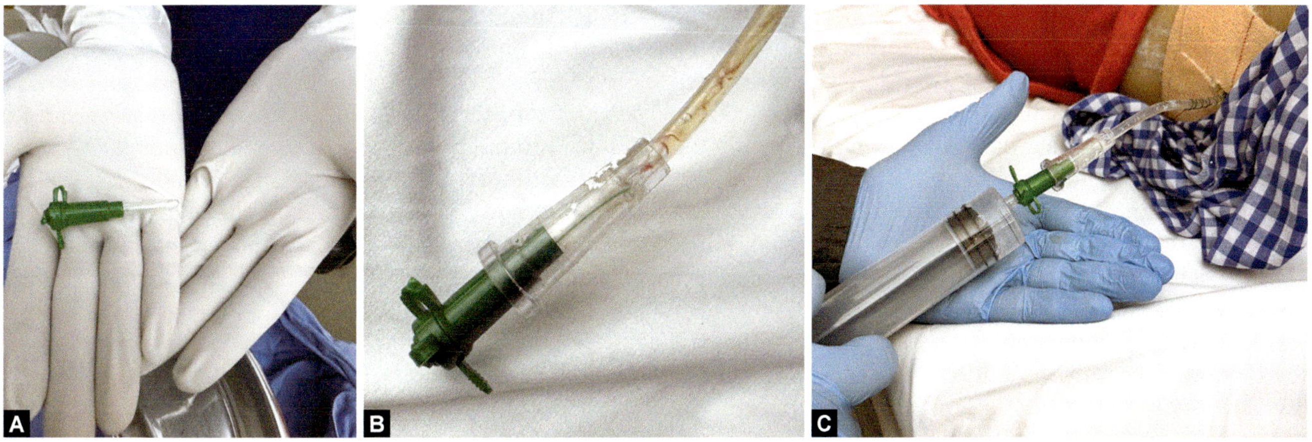

FIGS. 5A TO C: (A) Cut part of Ryles tube; (B) Cut cart of Ryles tube connected with ICD; and (C) Flushing of ICD through Ryles tube.

systemic features appear. Chest CT and X-ray will show the presence of gas in the subcutaneous plane. The skin infection usually responds well to antibiotics. Apart from antibiotics sometimes aggressive surgical debridement, and repeated debridement according to the case may be required. After infection control role of a plastic surgeon for skin grafting may be vital. A free flap sometimes may be needed. Microsurgical reconstruction had been done with a latissimus dorsi-free flap for pleural reconstruction and chest wall stabilization.[17]

Chest Drain Dislodgment

There is always a chance of accidental dislodgment of ICD if proper care is not taken. This could be partial or total. This happens mostly during the transportation of patients, mobilization, or during sleep. Sometimes in ICU settings patients are critically ill with multiple tubes in situ and is very difficult to handle all lines and tubes while mobilization out of bed is done. The dislodgment of the tube can be taken care of by proper training and instruction to the caregiver and patients. It can further be prevented with meticulous care and good anchorage of the drain. The use of a stay-in or mattress suture is therefore recommended.[18] As per the latest BTS guidelines also all ICDs have to be fixed with the holding suture.[19] Purse string suture is discouraged as it increases the chance of skin necrosis and does not prevent air leaks.[20] Even if for dislodgment the new ICD is planned with full aseptic condition, the previous track must be avoided while inserting the new drain.

Subcutaneous Emphysema

It is a well-known complication of ICD. It can be clinically detected by crepitation felt subcutaneously or by simple chest X-ray. Sometimes this becomes very massive and causes disfigurement, discomfort, anxiety, and rarely pacemaker dysfunction[21] or obstruction of upper airways.[22] It is more commonly associated with preexisting or concomitant ailments such as chest trauma, large and bilateral pneumothorax, and BPF or in mechanically- ventilated patients. In case of poor tube placements, tube blockage, prolonged tube placements, two or more ICDs in situ, and most importantly migration of one or more ports inside the chest wall the occurrence of subcutaneous emphysema is well established.[23] Overall, this complication leads to increased morbidity and mortality.

Most of the time this complication resolves on its own and is not life-threatening. In case of massive and life-threatening issues, an incision in the skin and subcutaneous fascia below the clavicle *(infraclavicular blow hole)* has been tried for air to escape.[24] To get rid of tension subcutaneous emphysema other modalities such as subcutaneous pigtail,[25] fenestrated angiocatheter in the subcutaneous planes,[26] and large bore ICD has been also used.[27]

Organ Injury

Lung as obvious is the most common organ to be injured which is ICD. Till date as per literature, it has been reported in around 0.2–1.4% of ICD insertion. Many a times abnormal lung parenchyma which is adhered with the chest wall is mistaken for pleural adhesions. In that case, it is important to anticipate the lung injury and one should be more aware and prefer to do the procedure under ultrasound guidance. Another organ damage though rarer but has been reported. The organ damage is very much dependent on the operator's skill and clinical assessment prior to the ICD insertion. An interesting survey done by Griffiths et al., on junior doctors while inserting ICD about the anatomical landmarks, revealed that 45% were placed outside the safe area. Among them 20% inserted ICD too low.[28] There is a greater probability of organ damage when the ICD is inserted low. Rarely these serious complications had been detected in autopsy, like pulmonary perforation which had been not anticipated antemortem.[29,30]

- *Nerve injuries*: Nerve injuries because of ICDs are rare but can be manifested and there are various literature. The nerve injury reported in the adult and pediatric populations as Horner's syndrome.[31,32] It is basically an oculosympathetic paresis that results from damage of second-order preganglionic neurons. The clinical manifestations are miosis, ptosis, ipsilateral hemifacial anhidrosis, and enophthalmos. Other nerves likely to be injured are phrenic nerve injury leading to diaphragmatic paralysis,[33,34] ulnar neuropathy[35] and injury to the long thoracic nerve.[36]
- *Cardiac and vascular injuries*: Cardiovascular systems is also prone for injury with interventions done with ICD insertion. There are chances of perforation to the heart. Injuries of almost all chambers of the heart have been reported because of ICD insertion. Rare case reports of perforation of either atria (left or right) and ventricle (left or right) is there.[37-41] These complications are though rare but catastrophic and life-threatening. The factors responsible for these complications were cardiomegaly, chest wall deformity, trauma, and critically ill patients. Blunt dissection with trocar, i.e., first-generation ICDs was the main cause along with the patient's background, such as postpneumonectomy condition[42] and dense pleural adhesions.[43,44] Rare cardiovascular complications like subclavian artery occlusion have been also reported by Flower in a premature baby whose ICD was done after surgical repair of tracheoesophageal fistula with esophageal atresia.[45]

  Sometimes during dissection during chest tube insertion intercostal arteries may get damaged and bleed profusely. There is variability of intercostal artery (ICA) in the elderly, it is more tortuosity near the vertebral body. Hence where the ICA enters the costal groove it is a risk zone to puncture. The juxta-vertebral zone is less risky in the upper half as compared with the lower half and it extends more laterally in males than females. To avoid the damage of variably positioned superior neurovascular bundle and inferior collateral artery in the intercostal space, ICD should be inserted in between 50 and 70% of the way down in the interspace.[46] Rarely after ICD can intercostal artery and subcutaneous vein cause systemic A–V malformation.[47]
- *Cardiac dysrhythmia*: ICD insertion can complicate to arrhythmias rarely. This could be because of irritation of the vagus nerve or because of mechanical irritation to the heart or pericardium. A sudden death has been reported because of hemorrhage and vagus nerve irritation after ICD insertion.[48]
- *Esophageal perforation:* This can happen either in the normal esophagus or at the site of anastomosis/myotomy following repair of esophageal atresia.[49,50]

  Herniation of a lung bulla through the insertion site. Chylothorax is also one of the complications and it has been discussed separately in different chapters of this textbook.

Tumor Recurrence at Insertion Sites

Sometimes there could be a local spread or metastasis from the different sites. This is found more with surgical or postprocedure ICD insertion and is less common with newer-generation percutaneous procedure. Two cases of tumor recurrence were reported by Hayes-Jordan et al. after intraoperative thoracostomy at the insertion site because of a huge spillage of malignant epithelial thymoma and pleuropulmonary blastoma.[51]

Re-expansion Pulmonary Edema

This complication is though rare but serious. Re-expansion pulmonary edema (RPE) occurs because of rapid re-expansion of a lung that had been collapsed for at least the last 3 days either due to pneumothorax or effusion. Initially, it was reported more after the drainage of pneumothorax;[52] but in later literatures, it has been reported more with pleural effusions drainage.[53] When a retrospective review of the literature is done, the total incidence comes to around 0–1%. One study with 172 adult patients being treated for spontaneous pneumothorax 27 case of RPE was found and attributed to the size and duration of pneumothorax but not because of suction settings.[54]

Rarely RPE has been reported in:

- Re-expansion of lung after decortications[55]
- Re-expansion after excision of giant mediastinal tumor[56]
- Transthoracic sympathectomy is done for primary hyperhidrosis[57]
- Puncture of a giant bulla[58]

Re-expansion pulmonary edema generally happens on the ipsilateral side but there are cases where RPE occurred on the contralateral of the expanded lung[59] or rarely bilateral.[60] Clinically it presents with cough breathlessness and hypoxia. The pathophysiology of RPE is yet unknown but few hypotheses have been regarding it.

The etiopathogenesis of increased permeability and loss of integrity of capillo-endothelial membrane which leads to protein-rich exudation are as follows:[8]

- There is a mechanical stress to normal blood vessel which happens during re-expansion
- In chronically collapsed lung the surfactant level reduces. In case of rapidly lowering intrapulmonary pressure and a further decrease in perivascular pressure of pulmonary capillaries low surfactant level leads to pulmonary edema.[61]
- Collapse of the lung itself leads to the destruction of microvascular endothelium occur. Most likely mechanical or anoxic stress to the endothelium by change of lymphatics or blood cells leads to pulmonary edema.
- In collapsed or diseased lung there is aggravated leucocyte sequestration, monocyte chemoattractant protein-1 (MCP-1), and interleukin-8 (1L-8).[62] An increased xanthine oxidase activity has also been reported.[63] These chemokines not only affect the ipsilateral lungs but also the contralateral ones leading to bilateral pulmonary edema.
- Shift of mediastinum because of compression atelectasis of the contralateral lung is thought to be the main cause of bilateral involvement.[64]
- Increase in oxygen-free radical (ROS) and increase catalytic activity of its scavenger and other enzymes.[65] ROS may injure capillary endothelium. The evidence to support this hypothesis is that increase in FiO_2 (40%) prevents pulmonary edema in the re-expanded lung.[66]

The management of re-expansion pulmonary edema is first to reduce the chance of occurring it, that is where the preventive methods are applied. In that case, it is very important for the clinicians to anticipate where it is likely to happen. After understanding the etiopathogenesis discussed it becomes easier to point the potential patients to land up in RPE. Younger patients with age <40 years, large-size pneumothorax, i.e., >30% of a single lung, chronic collapse or collapse for >3 days, rapid lung expansion, and patients with large negative suction pressure applied to ICD are at risk of developing RPE. The preventive measure is avoiding negative suction to the spontaneous pneumothorax in young patients and limiting the ICD drain in case of massive pleural effusion.[67,68] Underwater seal drainage is preferred rather than negative pressure apparatus. Fluid drainage must not be done rapidly or >1 L in one go if pleural pressure is not monitored. There are studies to elaborate that pleural manometry may be helpful. If the gradient is not allowed to exceed > 17 cm of water there is low portability of RPE to develop.[69] Treatment is mainly supportive as this disease is self-limiting. Better positioning in case of unilateral pulmonary edema helps a lot. The lateral decubitus of the patients so that the affected side is up, that will reduce intrapulmonary shunting and improve oxygenation. If needed positive pressure ventilation has to be applied along with fluid restriction. There is no evidence to support the use of nonsteroidal anti-inflammatory drugs (NSAIDs) and diuretics is not avoided.

Fistula

The pathological communication between the bronchus, pleural space, and subcutaneous tissue is called bronchocutaneous fistula. It is also one of the complications of ICD. The detailed discussion regarding BPF is discussed in different chapter of the textbook.

INTERCOSTAL CHEST DRAIN REMOVAL

When and how to remove ICD is always a neglected part during discussion. Specifically, monitoring of pleural fluid drainage as a criterion for tube removal is not yet standardized. Either no fluid drainage or <500 mL/day can be used as a hint to remove ICD. Though early removal of ICD does not appear to be harmful. A noninferiority RCT done comparing removal without accounting for the drainage rate to a conservative threshold (2 mL/kg body weight/day) may better inform tube management. It is never a better decision to have unwanted foreign material inside the human body for a long time. So, to get the best result with the least infection and minimum complications the ICD should be removed as soon as possible when it is clinically indicated. There is no major study to support the right time for ICD removal. Hence following criteria have to be met before the ICD removal.

If ICD was put in for pneumothorax:

- The lung is fully expanded, both clinically and radiologically.
- There should be no visible air leak.
- If suction has been applied then air should not accumulate when suction is removed.
- Few clinicians prefer to clamp prior to removal in case of a high leak and massive column movement (as happens in loculated pneumothorax with pleural rind), and patient not fit for surgery.
- If there is suspicion of that a leak has not been completely sealed, some clinicians clamp the tube, but this is usually not necessary.[70]
- Radiological imaging (chest X-ray, ultrasound) can be obtained to identify any possible air reoccurrence that may or may not be clinically apparent.

- In the case of mechanically ventilated patients with ICD (done for pneumothorax), whether to maintain ICD is controversial. Some believe it should be kept till the patient is on positive pressure ventilation but there is a chance of infection if it is kept prolonged unnecessarily.

If the ICD was done for effusion.

- When the lung is expanded.
- In the case of empyema there are chances that still other pockets of fluid remaining. If most of them have been drained, and the patient is clinically doing well [no fever, normal white blood cells (WBC) and now has good appetite], and apposition between visceral and parietal pleura has occurred along with documented radiographic imaging, the remaining abnormality is likely to be resolved with antibiotics alone.
- When the daily drainage is <100–300 mL/day; however, there are no studies to suggest a clear-cut threshold.[71]
- The threshold of daily drainage is individualized depending upon the indication for the ICD insertion and patient demographics [e.g., weight and height (or length)]. But till date, unfortunately, there are no clear guidelines and data that address fluid output amount for a given patient size.

Removal Technique

If the removal criteria above are met, the suction is eliminated. Prior to removing the thoracostomy tube or catheter, the likelihood of developing respiratory distress due to recurrent.

KEY POINTS

- Monitoring the ICD, its drain, air leak and management of the complications is far more important than the ICD insertion.
- Most important part in ICD maintenance is the column movement and amount of daily fluid drainage.
- The three-way canula has to be attached with the tube (may require various connector) which will help in flushing the ICD or needed to instil any drug while doing pleurodesis or pleurolysis.
- Various complication can occur during the ICD journey like, tube blockage, dislodgement, malfunction, infection, re-expansion pulmonary edema. While procedure the organ injury can happen.
- Subcutaneous edema is well-known complication of ICD. It can be clinically detected by crepitation felt subcutaneously or by simple chest X-ray.
- When another ICD is needed because of a non-functioning intercostal tube, the previous track must be avoided while inserting the new drain.
- RPE occurs because of rapid re-expansion of a lung which had been collapsed for at least last 3 days either due to pneumothorax or effusion.
- The pathophysiology of RPE is yet unknown but it is mainly because of increased permeability and loss of integrity of capillo-endothelial membrane which leads to protein rich exudation.
- Once the removal criteria are met, clinician decision is most important for ICD removal.
- It can be removed at end-inspiration or at end-expiration. The procedure is invariably painful and need to explain this to patient before removing ICD.

REFERENCES

1. Kuhajda I, Zarogoulidis K, Kougioumtzi I, Huang H, Li Q, Dryllis G, et al. Tube thoracostomy; chest tube implantation and follow-up. J Thorac Dis. 2014;6(Suppl 4):S470-9.
2. Gayer G, Rozenman, Hoffmann C, Apter S, Simansky DA, Yellin A, et al. CT diagnosis of malpositioned chest tubes. Br J Radiol. 2000;73(871):786-90.
3. Webb WR, LaBerge JM. Radiographic recognition of chest tube malposition in the major fissure. Chest. 1984;85(1):81-3.
4. Stark DD, Federle MP, Goodman PC. CT and radiographic assessment of tube thoracostomy. AJR Am J Roentgenol. 1983;141(2):253-8.
5. Lim KE, Tai SC, Chan CY, Hsu YY, Hsu WC, Lin BC, et al. Diagnosis of malpositioned chest tubes after emergency tube thoracostomy: is computed tomography more accurate than chest radiograph? Clin Imaging. 2005;29(6):401-5.
6. Curtin JJ, Goodman LR, Quebbeman EJ, Haasler GB. Thoracostomy tubes after acute chest injury: Relationship between location in a pleural fissure and function. AJR Am J Roentgenol. 1994;163(6):1339-42.
7. Kesieme EB, Dongo A, Ezemba N, Irekpita E, Jebbin N, Kesieme C. Tube thoracostomy: Complications and its management. Pulm Med. 2012:2012:256878.
8. Collop NA, Kim S, Sahn SA. Analysis of tube thoracostomy performed by pulmonologists at a teaching hospital. Chest. 1997;112(3):709-13.
9. Chan L, Reilly KM, Henderson C, Kahn F, Salluzzo RF. Complication rates of tube thoracostomy. Am J Emerg Med. 1997;15(4):368-70.
10. Helling TS, Gyles NR 3rd, Eisenstein CL, Soracco CA. Complications following blunt and penetrating injuries in 216 victims of chest trauma requiring tube thoracostomy. J Trauma. 1989;29(10):1367-70.
11. Maxwell RA, Campbell DJ, Fabian TC, Croce MA, Luchette FA, Kerwin AJ, et al. Use of presumptive antibiotics following tube thoracostomy for traumatic hemopneumothorax in the prevention of empyema and pneumonia--a multi-center trial. J Trauma. 2004;57(4):742-8; discussion 748-9.

12. Ahmad T, Ahmed SW, Soomro NH, Sheikh KA. Thoracoscopic evacuation of retained post-traumatic hemothorax. J Coll Physicians Surg Pak. 2013;23(3):234-6.
13. Velmahos GC, Demetriades D, Chan L, Tatevossian R, Cornwell EE 3rd, Yassa N, et al. Predicting the need for thoracoscopic evacuation of residual traumatic hemothorax: chest radiograph is insufficient. J Trauma. 1999;46(1):65-70.
14. Kalkat MS, Rajesh PB, Hendrickse C. Hendrickse, Necrotizing fasciitis of chest wall complicating empyema thoracis. Interact Cardiovasc Thorac Surg. 2003;2(3):358-60.
15. de Castro FCR, Rodriguez P, Santana N, Freixinet J. Necrotizing fasciitis of thoracic wall complicating chest tube drainage. Asian Cardiovas Thorac Ann. 2001;9(1):76-7.
16. Hsu SP, Wang HC, Huang IT, Chu KA, Chang HC. Tube thoracostomy-related necrotizing fasciitis: a case report. Kaohsiung J Med Sci. 2006;22(12):636-40.
17. Barbosa RF, Pinho CJ, Costa-Ferreira A, Cardoso A, Reis JC, Amarante JM. Microsurgical reconstruction of chest wall defect after necrotizing fasciitis. Microsurgery. 2006;26(7):519-23.
18. Laws D, Neville E, Duffy J. BTS guidelines for the insertion of a chest drain. Thorax. 2003;58(Suppl 2):ii55-9.
19. Asciak R, Bedawi EO, Bhatnagar R, , Clive AO, Hassan M, Lloyd H, et al. British Thoracic Society Clinical Statement on pleural procedures. Thorax. 2023;78(Suppl 3):s43-68.
20. Tang AT, Velissaris TJ, Weeden DF. An evidence-based approach to drainage of the pleural cavity: evaluation of best practice. J Eval Clin Prac. 2002;8(3):333-40.
21. Giroud D, Goy JJ. Pacemaker malfunction due to subcutaneous emphysema. Intern J Cardiol. 1990;26(2):234-6.
22. Gibney RT, Finnegan B, FitzGerald MX, Lynch V. Upper airway obstruction caused by massive subcutaneous emphysema. Intensive Care Med. 1984;10(1):43-4.
23. Jones PM, Hewer RD, Wolfenden HD, Thomas PS. Subcutaneous emphysema associated with chest tube drainage. Respirology. 2001;6(2):87-9.
24. Herlan DB, Landreneau RJ, Ferson PF. Massive spontaneous subcutaneous emphysema. Acute management with infraclavicular "blow holes". Chest. 1992;102(2):503-5.
25. Crouch JD, Keagy BA, Delany DJ. "Pigtail" catheter drainage in thoracic surgery. Am Rev Respir Dis. 1987;136(1):174-5.
26. Perkins LA, Jones SF. Resolution of subcutaneous emphysema with placement of subcutaneous fenestrated angiocatheter. Respir Med Extra. 2007;3(3):102-4.
27. Kelly MC, McGuigan JA, Allen RW. Relief of tension subcutaneous emphysema using a large bore subcutaneous drain. Anaesthesia. 1995;50(12):1077-9.
28. Griffiths JR, Roberts N. Do junior doctors know where to insert chest drains safely? Postgrad Med J. 2005;81(957):456-8.
29. Fraser RS. Lung perforation complicating tube thoracostomy: pathologic description of three cases. Hum Pathol. 1988;19(5):518-23.
30. Resnick DK. Delayed pulmonary perforation. A rare complication of tube thoracostomy. Chest. 1993;103(1):311-3.
31. Ozel SK, Kazez A. Kazez, Horner's syndrome secondary to tube thoracostomy. Turk J Pediatr. 2004;46(2):189-90.
32. Kaya SO, Liman ST, Bir LS, Yuncu G, Erbay HR, Unsal S. Horner's syndrome as a complication in thoracic surgical practice. Eur J Cardiothorac Surg. 2003;24(6):1025-8.
33. Nahum E, Ben-Ari J, Schonfeld T, Horev G. Acute diaphragmatic paralysis caused by chest-tube trauma to phrenic nerve. Pediatr Radiol. 2001;31(6):444-6.
34. Hwang MS, Chu JJ, Su WJ. Diaphragmatic paralysis caused by malposition of chest tube placement after pediatric cardiac surgery. Intern J Cardiol. 2005;99(1):129-31.
35. Rosing JH, Lance S, Wong MS. Ulnar neuropathy after tube thoracostomy for pneumothorax. J Emerg Med. 2012;43(4):e223-5.
36. Hassan WU, Keaney NP. Winging of the scapula: an unusual complication of chest tube placement. Jf Accid Emerg Med. 1995;12(2):156-7.
37. Kerger H, Blaettner T, Froehlich C, Ernst J, Frietsch T, Isselhorst C, et al. Perforation of the left atrium by a chest tube in a patient with cardiomegaly: management of a rare, but life-threatening complication. Resuscitation. 2007;74(1):178-82.
38. Deshpande SP, Chow JH, Odonkor P, Griffith B, Carr SR. Misadventures of a Pigtail: Case Report of Accidental Insertion of a Chest Tube Into the Left Atrium During Interventional Radiology-Guided Placement. A A Pract. 2018;11(10):273-5.
39. Meisel S, Ram Z, Priel I, Nass D, Lieberman P. Lieberman, Another complication of thoracostomy--perforation of the right atrium. Chest. 1990;98(3):772-3.
40. Abad C, Padrón A. Accidental perforation of the left ventricle with a chest drain tube. Texas Heart Inst J. 2002;29(2):143.
41. Kopec SE, Conlan AA, Irwin RS. Perforation of the right ventricle: a complication of blind placement of a chest tube into the postpneumonectomy space. Chest. 1998;114(4):1213-5.
42. Klalingen KW, Stam J, Rauwerda J. Complications of thoracostomy. Chest. 1991;100(3):886-7.
43. Sundaramurthy SR, Moshinsky RA, Smith JA. Non-operative management of tube thoracostomy induced pulmonary artery injury. Interact Cardiovasc Thorac Surg. 2009;9(4):759-61.
44. Takanami I. Pulmonary artery perforation by a tube thoracostomy. I Interact Cardiovasc Thorac Surg. 2005;4(5):473-4.
45. Fowler CL. Subclavian artery compression from a chest tube after thoracotomy in a premature infant. Pediatr Radiol. 1995;25(6):458-9.
46. Wraight WM, Tweedie DJ, Parkin IG. Neurovascular anatomy and variation in the fourth, fifth, and sixth intercostal spaces in the mid-axillary line: a cadaveric study in respect of chest drain insertion. Clin Anat. 2005;18(5):346-9.
47. Coulter TD, Maurer JR, Miller MT, Mehta AC. Chest wall arteriovenous fistula: an unusual complication after chest tube placement. Ann Thorac Surg. 1999;67(3):849-50.
48. Ward EW, Hughes TE. Hughes, Sudden death following chest tube insertion: an unusual case of vagus nerve irritation. J Trauma. 1994;36(2):258-9.
49. Shapira OM, Aldea GS, Kupferschmid J, Shemin RJ. Delayed perforation of the esophagus by a closed thoracostomy tube. Chest. 1993;104(6):1897-8.
50. Johnson JF, Wright DR. Chest tube perforation of esophagus following repair of esophageal atresia. J Pediatr Surg. 1990;25(12):1227-30.
51. Hayes-Jordan AA, Daw NC, Furman WL, Hoffer FA, Shochat SJ. Tumor recurrence at thoracostomy tube insertion sites: a report of two pediatric cases. J Pediatr Surg. 2004;39(10):1565-7.
52. Mahfood S, Hix WR, Aaron BL, Bales P, Watson DC. Reexpansion pulmonary edema. Ann Thorac Surg. 1988;45(3):340-5.
53. Feller-Kopman D, Berkowitz D, Boiselle P, Ernst A. Large-volume thoracentesis and the risk of reexpansion pulmonary edema. Ann Thorac Surg. 2007;84(5):1656-61.
54. Morioka H, Takada K, Matsumoto S, Kojima E, Iwata S, Okachi S. Re-expansion pulmonary edema: evaluation of risk factors in 173 episodes of spontaneous pneumothorax. Respir Investig. 2013;51(1):35-9.

55. Yamanaka A, Hirai T, Ohtake Y, Watanabe M, Nakamura K, Tanabe T. Surgery for thoracic empyema concurrent with rupture of lung abscesses in a child. J Pediatr Surg. 1998;33(9):1408-10.
56. Matsumiya N, Dohi S, Kimura T, Naito H. Reexpansion pulmonary edema after mediastinal tumor removal. Anesth Analg. 1991;73(5):646-8.
57. Lin TS, Wang NP, Huang LC. Pitfalls and complication avoidance associated with transthoracic endoscopic sympathectomy for primary hyperhidrosis (analysis of 2200 cases). Int J Surg Investig. 2001;2(5):377-85.
58. Fukuda T, Okutani R, Kono K, Ishida H, Yamanaka N, Okamoto E. [A case of reexpansion pulmonary edema during fenestration of a giant hepatic cyst]. Masuiol. 1989;38(11):1509-13.
59. Steckel RJ. Unilateral pulmonary edema after pneumothorax. N Engl J Med. 1973;289(12):621-2.
60. Ragozzino MW, Greene R. Bilateral reexpansion pulmonary edema following unilateral pleurocentesis. Chest. 1991;99(2): 506-8.
61. Katz S, Knight R. Re-expansion pulmonary edema. Am Fam Physician. 1976;13(3):94-5.
62. Sakao Y, Kajikawa O, Martin TR, Nakahara Y, Hadden WA 3rd, et al. Association of IL-8 and MCP-1 with the development of reexpansion pulmonary edema in rabbits. Ann Thorac Surg. 2001;71(6):1825-32.
63. Saito S, Ogawa J, Minamiya Y. Pulmonary reexpansion causes xanthine oxidase-induced apoptosis in rat lung. Am J Physiol Lung Cell Mol Physiol. 2005;289(3):L400-6.
64. Sohara Y. Reexpansion pulmonary edema. Ann Thorac Cardiovasc Surg. 2008;14(4):205-9.
65. Jackson RM, Russell WJ, Veal CF. Endogenous and exogenous catalase in reoxygenation lung injury. J Appl Physiol (1985). 1992;72(3):858-64.
66. Pavlin DJ, Nessly ML, Cheney FW. Hemodynamic effects of rapidly evacuating prolonged pneumothorax in rabbits. J Appl Physiol (1985). 1987;62(2):477-84.
67. MacDuff A, Arnold A, Harvey J; BTS Pleural Disease Guideline Group. Management of spontaneous pneumothorax: British Thoracic Society Pleural Disease Guideline 2010. Thorax. 2010;65(Suppl 2):ii18-31.
68. Kira S. Reexpansion pulmonary edema: review of pediatric cases. Paediatr Anaesth. 2014;24(3):249-56.
69. Hassaballa AS, Mostafa A, Hikal T, Elnori A, Elsayed HH. Pleural manometry during thoracocentesis in patients with malignant pleural effusion: A randomized controlled trial. Can J Respir Ther. 2023;59:33-44.
70. Baumann MH, Strange C, Heffner JE, Light R, Kirby TJ, Klein J, et al. Management of spontaneous pneumothorax: an American College of Chest Physicians Delphi consensus statement. Chest. 2001;119(2):590-602.
71. Utter GH. The rate of pleural fluid drainage as a criterion for the timing of chest tube removal: theoretical and practical considerations. Ann Thorac Surg. 2013;96(6):2262-7.

CHAPTER

19 Pleural Effusion in Pulmonary Embolism

Hardeep Kaur Grewal, Manish Bansal

INTRODUCTION

Venous thromboembolism (VTE) is a disorder characterized by blood clot formation in the veins. It includes deep vein thrombosis and pulmonary thromboembolism (PTE). Acute PTE is the most serious presentation of VTE which could be potentially life-threatening or can lead to chronic disease and disability. Although thrombotic occlusion of pulmonary arteries is the most common cause of pulmonary embolism (PE), there are other nonthrombotic pulmonary emboli sources also, such as air, fat, tumors, and talc.

The annual incidence of PE, as reported by various epidemiological studies, varies from 30 to 115 per 100,000 people, and is increasing with the passage of time.[1] Acute PTE accounts for approximately 300,000 deaths and is included among the top causes of death from cardiovascular disease.[1] Pulmonary embolism is also known to be one of the leading causes of mortality among hospitalized patients, accounting for 5–10% of the deaths in them.[2,3] Due to advancements in the management of PE, PE-associated mortality has decreased in recent years,[4,5] and in most of the cases, poor outcomes are preventable.

Pleural effusion is one of the complications seen in PE. Although, PE is the fourth most common cause of pleural effusion after congestive heart failure, malignancy, and parapneumonic effusion,[6,7] it is also the most underdiagnosed cause.[8,9] Pleural effusion is a marker of poor prognosis in PE and is associated with disease progression and increased risk of death. Therefore, the possibility of underlying PE should always be considered in all patients with unexplained pleural effusion, and appropriate confirmatory tests to rule out PE should be performed.

INCIDENCE OF PLEURAL EFFUSION IN PULMONARY EMBOLISM

The exact incidence and prevalence of pleural effusion in PE are not clear as different studies have reported conflicting results.[10]

A recent meta-analysis of 29 prospective and retrospective studies involving 13,430 patients of PE demonstrated a 41.2% pooled incidence of pleural effusion in patients with PE. The incidence in the individual studies ranged from 16.3 to 68.9%.[11] Another review by Agarwal et al. also reported a similar (19–61%) incidence of pleural effusion in PE patients.[12]

The incidence of pleural effusion in PE varies according to the diagnostic modality used for detecting it.[13] As per the review by Agarwal et al., the incidence was high (43%) if computed tomography (CT) was used to detect pleural effusion as compared to when chest X-ray (30.5%) was used.[12] Other studies have also demonstrated that CT is more sensitive than chest radiographs in detecting pleural effusion.[14]

Most of the patients who develop pleural effusion secondary to PE tend to have a small effusion. In a study by Kiris et al.,[15] 463 patients diagnosed with acute PE were evaluated retrospectively using computed tomography pulmonary angiography (CTPA). Almost one-fourth of the acute PE patients (25.9%) had pleural effusion, and most had only small-sized pleural effusions (21.4%). Moderate pleural effusion was detected in 4.5% of the patients, whereas large pleural effusion was present in only one patient. Bilateral pleural effusions were detected in 13.8% of the patients.

Since pleural effusion associated with PE is generally small, most of the patients cannot undergo pleural tapping, which often results in diagnostic uncertainty. This observation raises the suspicion that the true prevalence might be higher.[16,17] It also implies that a more extensive diagnostic work-up is needed to establish the true etiology.

MECHANISM OF PLEURAL EFFUSION IN ACUTE PULMONARY EMBOLISM

Although the exact mechanism responsible for pleural effusion in PE is not known, increased permeability of pulmonary capillaries appears to be the dominant cause.[9,18] There are two possible events that may make the pulmonary vasculature more permeable in PE. First, and possibly the most important mechanism, is that the embolic occlusion of pulmonary vessels results in the release of inflammatory mediators and vascular endothelial growth factor (VEGF) from platelet-rich thrombi. VEGF is one of the most potent factors responsible for increasing capillary permeability.[19] As a result, there is an accumulation of fluid in the lung interstitial space. Normally, approximately 20% of the fluid that enters the lung interstitium leaves through the pleural space. However, the increased pulmonary vasculature permeability leads to an increase in the amount of fluid in the interstitial space which overwhelms the capacity of the lymphatic vessels to remove this excess fluid.[18] As a result, the fluid traverses the visceral pleura and accumulates in the pleural space resulting in exudative pleural effusion. Second, and the less likely mechanism responsible for an increased pulmonary capillary permeability is the ischemia of the distal pulmonary capillary bed caused by the proximal embolus; however, it may have limited significance as the pulmonary capillaries are predominantly supplied by the bronchial circulation. Nonetheless, the above mechanisms might explain the role of pulmonary infarction and C-reactive protein levels as independent predictors of pleural effusion due to PE.

Although the pleural effusion secondary to PE is mostly exudative in nature, rarely it may be transudative also. This is possibly due to increased right ventricular (RV) pressure overload.[9,16] Acute PE causes pulmonary hypertension and increased RV pressure, which results in an increased systemic venous pressure on the parietal pleura. This, in turn, increases the amount of fluid entering the pleural space.[16] In addition, the lymphatic clearance of the pleural fluid is also impeded because of increased pressure in the systemic veins due to increased RV pressure overload. For both these reasons, the patients of PE with pulmonary hypertension and right heart failure may rarely have transudative pleural effusions.[20] This also explains how pleural effusion in PE could be an indicator of RV failure, contributing to poorer clinical outcomes; however, transudative pleural effusion in these patients could be due to other causes as well, such as congestive heart failure.[16]

IMPACT OF PLEURAL EFFUSION ON PROGNOSIS IN PULMONARY EMBOLISM

There are not many studies that have evaluated the impact of pleural effusion on prognosis in PE patients; however, the inclusion of a relatively large number of subjects in these studies strengthens the evidence-base. A meta-analysis of such studies by Zuin et al. showed that pleural effusion in patients with PE was associated with a higher short-term risk of death.[21] Similarly, another meta-analysis by Li et al., which included seven studies with 4,707 patients, also showed increased 30-day mortality and in-hospital mortality in patients with PE who also had pleural effusion.[11] Pleural effusion is also associated with longer hospital stays.[22]

Pleural effusion in PE is also associated with increased mid- and long-term mortality. A Chinese study showed that all-cause mortality at 3-month and 1-year follow-up was significantly higher in patients of PE who had pleural effusion.[22] Kiris et al. also demonstrated a significantly higher (55%) long-term total mortality in patients with pleural effusion than those without it (23%). The mortality was higher in those who had bilateral pleural effusion.[15] The association between pleural effusion and 30-day and long-term mortality was independent of other relevant risk markers. In contrast, a study by Choi et al. did not find pleural effusion to be a predictor of short-term outcomes or length of hospital stay.[23] However, in this study, pleural effusion was associated with a higher incidence of tachycardia, hypotension, and a greater proportion of patients having high-risk Simplified PE Severity Index.

The exact cause of increased mortality risk in patients of PE with pleural effusion is not known. Patients with more severe PE are more likely to develop pleural effusion.[23] The RV failure resulting from PE could be responsible for an increased mortality risk in these patients.[22,24] Right ventricular dilatation is also considered to be a poor prognostic marker with an increased risk of PE-related in-hospital shock, the need for cardiopulmonary resuscitation, and PE-related mortality.[25,26] Central PE and RV dilatation were significantly more common in PE patients with pleural effusion than those without pleural effusion.[23] N-terminal pro-B-type natriuretic peptide levels were also found to be high in the effusion group.

Overall, the available evidence points toward a poorer prognosis of PE patients with pleural effusion. Therefore, it is important that in patients with undiagnosed pleural effusion, a thorough clinical history and appropriate tests are performed to rule out PE.

CLINICAL PRESENTATION OF PULMONARY EMBOLISM PATIENTS WITH PLEURAL EFFUSION

Patients with PE can present with a variety of symptoms that predominantly fall into three categories—(1) pleuritic chest pain and/or hemoptysis, (2) isolated dyspnea, and (3) circulatory collapse. Pleuritic chest pain is quite common and is seen in almost 75% of the patients. It is generally described by the patients as a "stabbing" or "shooting" type of pain which increases in intensity on deep inspiration, sneezing, and coughing. Since the majority of the patients with PE and pleural effusion present with pleuritic chest pain, the presence of such type of chest pain in a patient with pleural effusion should strongly suggest the possibility of underlying PE.[27] Branch and McNeil reported that 55% of the patients younger than 40 years of age who presented to the outpatient department with pleural effusion and pleuritic chest pain had underlying PE.[28]

Another common symptom in these patients is dyspnea which is usually out of proportion to the size of the pleural effusion. This symptom is seen in almost 70% of the patients. Nearly, half of the patients of PE with pleural effusion may have cough and fever, whereas hemoptysis may be seen in 15% of the patients.[9]

Pulmonary infarction syndrome and circulatory collapse are two common complications seen in patients with PE and pleural effusion, though the overall incidence has been varying.[17,29] In the Computerized Registry of Patients with Venous Thromboembolism (RIETE), which included 4,145 patients with PE, 27% of patients with pulmonary infraction syndrome, 16% with circulatory collapse, and 12% with isolated dyspnea had pleural effusion.[29] In the Prospective Investigation of Pulmonary Embolism Diagnosis (PIOPED) study, pleural effusion was present in 56% of the patients with pleuritic chest pain or hemoptysis and 26% of those with isolated dyspnea but none of those with circulatory collapse.[27] In a study by Stein et al., pleural effusion was detected in 56% of the PE patients presenting with pulmonary infarction syndrome, 26% of those with isolated dyspnea, and none with circulatory collapse.[30] In contrast, in another study by Panjwani et al., the most common presentation in PE patients with pleural effusion was isolated dyspnea followed by pulmonary infarction and circulatory collapse. Collectively, these studies show that there is no clear pattern of association between the clinical presentation of PE and the presence of pleural effusion.[17]

Diagnostic Evaluation

The possibility of PE should be considered in any patient who has pleural effusion of unknown cause, especially in the presence of predisposing factors for PE or symptoms such as dyspnea out of proportion to the size of effusion, and/or pleuritic chest pain. These patients can be empirically started on anticoagulation until the diagnosis is confirmed using CTPA. The clinical pretest probability of PE, using the Wells score or Geneva score, should be assessed in each patient before further testing.[31,32]

Pulmonary embolism can be easily missed in patients presenting with pleural effusion. Most of the pleural effusions secondary to PE are small and unilateral. However, one-third of the patients with PE may present with bilateral pleural effusion.[13] They generally increase to maximum size by the third day. Any increase in size after three days or appearance of pleural effusion on the contralateral side is usually suggestive of recurrent PE, infection in pleural space, or hemothorax.[9,12]

Chest X-ray and Computed Tomography

Chest radiographs are not very sensitive or specific for diagnosing PE. They are usually done to exclude alternate causes of symptoms such as pneumonia and pneumothorax, rather than for diagnosing PE per se. Various radiographic signs and symptoms of PE have been described. These include Hampton hump (a peripheral wedge of airspace opacity implying pulmonary infarction), Westermark sign (regional oligemia), Fleischner sign (enlarged pulmonary artery), knuckle sign (abrupt tapering or cut off of pulmonary artery due to pulmonary embolus), Palla sign (enlarged right descending pulmonary artery), and Chang sign (dilated right descending pulmonary artery with a sudden cut-off).

Two multicenter studies enrolled 6,352 patients of PE and demonstrated that the incidence of pleural effusion, using chest radiograph, was 23 and 21%, respectively.[33,34] The incidence was much higher when CT was used. Porcel et al. found a 32% incidence of pleural effusion in patients of PE when only a chest radiograph was considered, which increased to 47% by using a CT scan.[14] In another study by

Findik et al.,[35] CT demonstrated pleural effusions in more than one-third of the patients with massive PE.

Pleural effusion in PE is generally small and unilateral with mean size equal to almost 15% of the hemithorax. The PIOPED study showed that 86% of the pleural effusions manifested only as costophrenic angle blunting and none of the patients presented with effusion exceeding one-third of the hemithorax.[27] Porcel et al. also showed that 85% of the pleural effusions were unilateral and 90% of the effusions were small with the involvement of less than one-third of the hemithorax.[14]

While most of the studies have shown that pleural effusions in PE are mostly unilateral, other studies have shown that bilateral pleural effusions are not uncommon. In a study by Agarwal et al., bilateral pleural effusions were seen in 6.5–15% of PE patients on chest radiographs and in 25–43% on CT scan.[12] In the study by Panjwani et al., almost two-thirds of the patients had bilateral pleural effusion.[20] Coche et al. also demonstrated that almost half of the patients with PE had bilateral pleural effusions detected on CT chest.[36]

The pleural effusions with PE are mostly free-flowing. However, at times, they can be loculated as well, especially if the diagnosis is delayed by >2 weeks after the onset of symptoms.[14,37] In the study by Porcel et al., CT showed loculations of the pleural fluid in 21% of the patients.[14] In another study by Reissig et al., 12 out of 39 patients with PE had loculated pleural effusions.[38] Interestingly, majority of the loculations resolve with effective anticoagulant therapy.[37]

Although PE increases the incidence of pleural effusion, it does not seem to affect the size of the effusions. Whether the location of the emboli has any relevance to the development of pleural effusion is not clear with various studies showing conflicting results. In the study by Panjwani et al., peripheral emboli were more commonly associated with pleural effusion, whereas Yap et al. found that most of the PE patients with pleural effusion had concomitant central and peripheral emboli.[39] In contrast, Liu et al. showed that the location of PE had no relation to the occurrence of pleural effusions.[13]

CTPA is considered to be the best modality to evaluate the possibility of PE in patients with undiagnosed pleural effusion.[38,40,41] This is because patients with pleural effusion often have emboli in the central, lobar, segmental, or subsegmental pulmonary arteries and CTPA can accurately detect emboli in these locations.[9]

Many other findings can be seen on CT in patients with PE with pleural effusion. Various types of pulmonary parenchymal opacities, including wedge-shaped opacities, consolidation, atelectasis, linear opacities, and ground glass attenuation can be seen. In one series, pulmonary infiltrates were present in 5–45% of these patients.[9] These infiltrates are pleural-based with convexity toward the hilum and are more commonly seen in the lower lobes of the lungs. Liu et al.[13] demonstrated that parenchymal opacities were more commonly seen in PE associated with pleural effusion than without it. A significant association was seen between the presence of pleural effusion and atelectasis, consolidation, and wedge-shaped opacities. In contrast, Panjwani et al.[17] found that consolidation had the strongest association with pleural effusion in PE patients.

Electrocardiography

The diagnostic usefulness of electrocardiogram (ECG) is limited as many ECG abnormalities that are seen in patients with PE are also common in patients without PE.[3,14] Most of the patients usually show only nonspecific ST-T wave changes. Electrocardiogram abnormalities suggestive of PE such as S wave in lead I, Q wave in lead III, and an inverted T wave in lead III (S1Q3T3) pattern or right bundle branch block can be seen in only 15% of the patients.[42]

Arterial Blood Gas Analysis

Acute respiratory alkalosis, hypocapnia, and hypoxemia are the most common arterial blood gas abnormalities in PE. However, almost one-fourth of the patients with PE have normal arterial oxygen pressure and saturation.[42] Hypoxemia in PE occurs due to ventilation–perfusion mismatch and the shunt resulting from hypoxemic vasoconstriction, atelectasis, and other associated abnormalities.

Pleural Fluid Findings

Diagnostic pleural tapping is generally not performed in patients with pleural effusion when the diagnosis of PE is already established; however, it may be needed in two scenarios: (1) To exclude pleural infection in a febrile patient, and (2) to exclude hemothorax when the size of effusion is increasing.

A few studies have described the composition of pleural fluid in PE patients with pleural effusion.[14,43,44] Most of the pleural effusions in PE are exudative in nature.[14,16,43] The pleural fluid may be clear, blood-tinged, or bloody in appearance.[14,16,43,44] The bloody appearance of pleural fluid is one of the characteristic features, and in the absence of trauma or malignancy, a workup to confirm or rule out the diagnosis of PE must be initiated.

The pleural fluid red blood cell (RBC) count in these patients is highly variable. In a study by Candeira et al., pleural fluid examination was performed in 60 patients with underlying PE. The RBC count was <10,000/mm^3 in 33% of patients, between 10,000 and 100,000/mm^3 in 48% of patients, and >100,000/mm^3 in the remaining patients.[43] Half of the patients in this study were receiving heparin therapy when pleural tapping was performed and the effect of the heparin therapy on the RBC count in the effusion could not be clearly ascertained.

The pleural fluid pH in these patients is usually > 7.3 and the glucose level is almost the same as serum glucose. The differential white blood cell count may show predominantly polymorphonuclear leukocytes or lymphocytes. In one series, the pleural fluid showed a large numbers of mesothelial cells or eosinophils.[9] However, pleural fluid eosinophilia due to PE is not a consistent finding and the frequency varies between 0 and 33%. A mesothelial reaction is seen more frequently in pleural fluids due to PE.[43] Indeed, the presence of mesothelial cells may help in identifying PE as the underlying etiology of pleural effusion.[43]

In summary, pleural effusions in PE patients are almost always exudative in nature and most of the cases show increased RBC count. High leukocyte count with predominant neutrophilia may be present. Marked mesothelial hyperplasia is a frequent feature. Eosinophilia can also be seen in a few patients. In the absence of trauma or malignancy, these findings should raise the possibility of PE.

MANAGEMENT OF PLEURAL EFFUSION IN PULMONARY EMBOLISM

The treatment protocol for PE with or without pleural effusion is not different and depends on the overall risk category of the PE. The mainstay of therapy is anticoagulation, and the hemorrhagic effusion is generally not a contraindication for anticoagulation or thrombolysis.[12]

Pleural effusion in PE gradually resolves with treatment, especially when there are no infiltrates. In the absence of radiographically proven pulmonary infarction, pleural effusion generally peaks in volume by day 3 and then resolves over a period of 7–10 days. In contrast, large pleural effusions or effusions in patients with radiographic pulmonary infarction take a longer time to resolve and usually clear in 2–3 weeks.[14,45] In one of the series, pleural effusion resolved completely with treatment in 64% of the patients without pulmonary infiltrates but in none of those with pulmonary infiltrates.[9]

An increase in the size of pleural effusion in a patient on anticoagulant therapy, or the development of effusion on the contralateral side, should suggest the possibility of recurrent PE, or another complication such as parapneumonic effusion or hemothorax.[9,12] Therefore, in such situations when pleural effusion increases in size, a diagnostic pleural tap should be performed to rule out infection and hemothorax. If there is a bloody tap, the hematocrit of the pleural fluid should be assessed, and a hematocrit >50% of that of peripheral blood means hemothorax. A massive hemothorax involves blood loss of >1.5 L. In these cases, anticoagulation should be stopped immediately, and a chest tube should be inserted.

The most common cause of spontaneous hemothorax in patients of PE with pleural effusion is anticoagulation therapy. Rarely, a spontaneous hemothorax may occur in association with pulmonary infarction or spontaneous pneumothorax. Rostand et al. reported eleven cases of hemothorax in patients with PE, as a complication of anticoagulant therapy.[46] Out of these 11 cases, five were receiving only heparin, four were receiving both heparin and warfarin, and two were receiving only warfarin. It was observed that the hemothorax usually became obvious about 4–7 days after the initiation of anticoagulant therapy. The coagulation parameters in those who developed hemothorax were mostly within the therapeutic range. The hemothorax almost always develops on the side of the original pulmonary embolus, raising the possibility of rupture of the intrapleural hemorrhagic pulmonary infarct.[46] Spontaneous hemothorax in PE is not limited only to anticoagulation therapy with unfractionated heparin or vitamin K antagonists but has also been reported with low molecular weight heparins and the novel, nonvitamin K oral anticoagulants.[47-49] Nearly half of the enoxaparin-related major bleeding complications are seen after the third day of therapy.[50,51]

Rarely, hemothorax can also occur spontaneously, in the absence of anticoagulation therapy, due to pulmonary infarct rupture. Pulmonary infarct rupture is a rare and fatal complication and may occur spontaneously or iatrogenically due to overaggressive anticoagulation.[52] It should be suspected in every patient of PE who suddenly develops circulatory and respiratory failure, especially after 7–10 days of anticoagulant therapy.[52] It is very difficult to distinguish secondary hemothorax in pulmonary infarction cases from overt rupture of the infarcted area. The increase in the vascular hydrostatic pressure due to reperfusion of the necrotic tissue in the zone of pulmonary infarct increases the possibility of pleural rupture.

CONCLUSION

Pleural effusion is not uncommon in patients with PE and has prognostic implications. Most of the pleural effusions in PE are generally small and unilateral, although bilateral pleural effusions are also not uncommon. The presence of pleural effusion in a patient with PE generally does not change the management approach but is a warning sign of increased mortality risk. Hence, it is recommended that PE should be considered as an important possibility in patients with pleural effusion presenting with pleuritic chest pain or those who have undiagnosed exudative pleural effusion. These patients may require more aggressive treatment and closer monitoring because of their worse short-term prognosis.

KEY POINTS

- Pulmonary embolism (PE) is common yet one of the most underdiagnosed causes of pleural effusion.
- Pleural effusion in a patient of PE is a marker of poor prognosis.
- PE-associated pleural effusions are mostly small and unilateral, although bilateral pleural effusions are also not uncommon.
- Pleural effusions in PE patients are almost always exudative in nature with increased red blood cell count. Marked mesothelial hyperplasia is also a common feature.
- Pleural effusion in PE gradually resolves with treatment, especially when there are no infiltrates.
- An increase in the size of pleural effusion in a patient on anticoagulant therapy, or the development of effusion on the contralateral side, should suggest the possibility of recurrent PE, or another complication such as parapneumonic effusion or hemothorax.
- The possibility of underlying PE should always be considered in all patients with unexplained pleural effusion.

REFERENCES

1. Konstantinides SV, Meyer G, Becattini C, Bueno H, Geersing GJ, Harjola VP, et al. 2019 ESC Guidelines for the diagnosis and management of acute pulmonary embolism developed in collaboration with the European Respiratory Society (ERS). Eur Heart J. 2020;41(4):543-603.
2. Alikhan R, Peters F, Wilmott R, Cohen AT. Fatal pulmonary embolism in hospitalised patients: a necropsy review. J Clin Pathol. 2004;57(12):1254-7.
3. Bikdeli B, Wang Y, Jimenez D, Parikh SA, Monreal M, Goldhaber SZ, et al. Pulmonary Embolism Hospitalization, Readmission, and Mortality Rates in US Older Adults, 1999–2015. JAMA. 2019;322(6):574-6.
4. Furfaro D, Stephens RS, Streiff MB, Brower R. Catheter-directed Thrombolysis for Intermediate-Risk Pulmonary Embolism. Ann Am Thorac Soc. 2018;15(2):134-44.
5. Lee T, Itagaki S, Chiang YP, Egorova NN, Adams DH, Chikwe J. Survival and recurrence after acute pulmonary embolism treated with pulmonary embolectomy or thrombolysis in New York State, 1999 to 2013. J Thorac Cardiovasc Surg. 2018;155(3):1084-90.e12.
6. Jany B, Welte T. Pleural Effusion in Adults—Etiology, Diagnosis, and Treatment. Dtsch Arztebl Int. 2019;116(21):377-86.
7. Light RW. Clinical practice. Pleural effusion. N Engl J Med. 2002;346(25):1971-7.
8. Light RW. The undiagnosed pleural effusion. Clin Chest Med. 2006;27(2):309-19.
9. Light RW. Pleural effusion in pulmonary embolism. Semin Respir Crit Care Med. 2010;31(6):716-22.
10. Porcel JM, Light RW. Pleural effusions due to pulmonary embolism. Current opinion in pulmonary medicine. 2008;14(4): 337-42.
11. Li P, An J, Wang S, Hu X, Zeng T, Wan C, et al. Incidence and Prognostic Role of Pleural Effusion in Patients with Pulmonary Embolism: A Systematic Review and Meta-Analysis. J Clin Med. 2023;12(6):2315.
12. Agarwal R, Singh N, Gupta D. Pleural Effusions Associated with Pulmonary Thromboembolism: A Systematic Review. Indian J Chest Dis Allied Sci. 2009;51:159-64.
13. Liu M, Cui A, Zhai ZG, Guo XJ, Li M, Teng LL, et al. Incidence of pleural effusion in patients with pulmonary embolism. Chin Med J. 2015;128(8):1032-6.
14. Porcel JM, Madronero AB, Pardina M, Vives M, Esquerda A, Light RW. Analysis of pleural effusions in acute pulmonary embolism: radiological and pleural fluid data from 230 patients. Respirology. 2007;12(2):234-9.
15. Kiris T, Yazici S, Koc A, Köprülü C, Ilke Akyildiz Z, Karaca M, et al. Prognostic impact of pleural effusion in acute pulmonary embolism. Acta Radiol. 2017;58(7):816-24.
16. Findik S. Pleural effusion in pulmonary embolism. Curr Opin Pulm Med. 2012;18(4):347-54.
17. Panjwani A, Zaid T, Alawi S, Al Shehabi D, Abdulkarim ES. Pleural effusion in acute pulmonary embolism in Bahrain: Radiological and pleural fluid characteristics. Lung India. 2019;36(2):112-7.
18. Wiener-Kronish JP, Broaddus VC, Albertine KH, Gropper MA, Matthay MA, et al. Relationship of pleural effusions to increased permeability pulmonary edema in anesthetized sheep. J Clin Invest. 1988;82(4):1422-9.
19. Cheng D, Rodriguez RM, Perkett EA, Rogers J, Bienvenu G, Lappalainen U, et al. Vascular endothelial growth factor in pleural fluid. Chest. 1999;116(3):760-5.
20. Wiener-Kronish JP, Matthay MA, Callen PW, Filly RA, Gamsu G, et al. Relationship of pleural effusions to pulmonary

hemodynamics in patients with congestive heart failure. Am Rev Respir Dis. 1985;132(6):1253-6.
21. Zuin M, Rigatelli G, Turchetta S, Pasquetto G, Roncon L, Bilato C. Mortality risk in patients with pulmonary embolism with pleural effusion. Am J Cardiol. 2022;179:122-3.
22. Zhou X, Zhang Z, Zhai Z, Zhang Y, Miao R, Yang Y, et al. Pleural effusions as a predictive parameter for poor prognosis for patients with acute pulmonary thromboembolism. J Thromb Thrombolysis. 2016;42(3):432-40.
23. Choi SH, Cha SI, Shin KM, Lim JK, Yoo SS, Lee SY, et al. Clinical Relevance of Pleural Effusion in Patients with Pulmonary Embolism. Respiration. 2017;93(4):271-8.
24. Olgun Yildizeli Ş, Kasapoglu US, Arikan H, Çimşit C, Çimşit NÇ, Süzer Aslan M, et al. Pleural effusion as an indicator of short term mortality in acute pulmonary embolism. Tuberk Toraks. 2018;66(3):185-96.
25. Alerhand S, Sundaram T, Gottlieb M. What are the echocardiographic findings of acute right ventricular strain that suggest pulmonary embolism? Anaesth Crit Care Pain Med. 2021;40(2):100852.
26. Brixey AG, Light RW. Pleural effusions occurring with right heart failure. Curr Opin Pulm Med. 2011;17(4):226-31.
27. Stein PD, Terrin ML, Hales CA, Palevsky HI, Saltzman HA, Thompson BT, et al. Clinical, laboratory, roentgenographic, and electrocardiographic findings in patients with acute pulmonary embolism and no pre-existing cardiac or pulmonary disease. Chest 1991;100(3):598-603.
28. Branch WT Jr, McNeil BJ. Analysis of the differential diagnosis and assessment of pleuritic chest pain in young adults. Am J Med. 1983;75(4):671-9.
29. Lobo JL, Zorrilla V, Aizpuru F, Uresandi F, Garcia-Bragado F, Conget F, et al. Clinical syndromes and clinical outcome in patients with pulmonary embolism: findings from the RIETE registry. Chest. 2006;130(6):1817-22.
30. Stein PD, Henry JW. Clinical characteristics of patients with acute pulmonary embolism stratified according to their presenting syndromes. Chest. 1997;112(4):974-9.
31. Wells PS, Anderson DR, Rodger M, Stiell I, Dreyer JF, Barnes D, et al. Excluding pulmonary embolism at the bedside without diagnostic imaging: management of patients with suspected pulmonary embolism presenting to the emergency department by using a simple clinical model and d-dimer. Ann Intern Med. 2001;135(2):98-107.
32. Le Gal G, Righini M, Roy PM, Sanchez O, Aujesky D, Bounameaux H, et al. Prediction of pulmonary embolism in the emergency department: the revised Geneva score. Ann Intern Med. 2006;144(3):165-71.
33. Elliott CG, Goldhaber SZ, Visani L, DeRosa M. Chest radiographs in acute pulmonary embolism. Results from the International Cooperative Pulmonary Embolism Registry. Chest. 2000;118(1):33-8.
34. Monreal M, Munoz-Torrero JF, Naraine VS, Jiménez D, Soler S, Rabuñal R, et al. Pulmonary embolism in patients with chronic obstructive pulmonary disease or congestive heart failure. Am J Med. 2006;119(10):851-8.
35. Findik S, Erkan L, Light RW, Uzun O, Atici AG, Akan H. Massive pulmonary emboli and CT pulmonary angiography. Respiration. 2008;76(4):403-12.
36. Coche EE, Muller NL, Kim KI, Wiggs BR, Mayo JR. Acute pulmonary embolism: ancillary findings at spiral CT. Radiology. 1998;207(3):753-8.
37. Erkan L, Fyndyk S, Uzun O, Atycy AG, Light RW. A new radiologic appearance of pulmonary thromboembolism: multiloculated pleural effusions. Chest. 2004;126(1):298-302.
38. Reissig A, Heyne JP, Kroegel C. Ancillary lung parenchymal findings at spiral CT scanning in pulmonary embolism. Relationship to chest sonography. Eur J Radiol. 2004;49(3):250-7.
39. Yap E, Anderson G, Donald J, Wong CA, Lee YC, Sivakumaran P. Pleural effusion in patients with pulmonary embolism. Respirology. 2008;13(6):832-6.
40. Enden T, Klow NE. CT pulmonary angiography and suspected acute pulmonary embolism. Acta Radiol. 2003;44(3):310-5.
41. Coche E, Verschuren F, Hainaut P, Goncette L. Pulmonary embolism findings on chest radiographs and multislice spiral CT. Eur Radiol. 2004;14(7):1241-8.
42. Currier PF, Hales CA. Pulmonary embolism and deep vein thrombosis. In: Yuan JXJ, Garcia JGN, Hales CA, Rich S, Archer SL, West JB, (Eds). Textbook of pulmonary vascular disease, 1st edition. New York: Springer; 2011. pp. 1231-8.
43. Romero Candeira S, Hernandez Blasco L, Soler MJ, Munoz A, Aranda I. Biochemical and cytologic characteristics of pleural effusions secondary to pulmonary embolism. Chest. 2002;121(2):465-9.
44. Bynum LJ, Wilson JE 3rd. Characteristics of pleural effusions associated with pulmonary embolism. Arch Intern Med. 1976;136(2):159-62.
45. Stein PD, Fowler SE, Goodman LR, Gottschalk A, Hales CA, Hull RD, et al. Multidetector computed tomography for acute pulmonary embolism. N Engl J Med. 2006;354(22):2317-27.
46. Rostand RA, Feldman RL, Block ER. Massive hemothorax complicating heparin anticoagulation for pulmonary embolus. South Med J. 1977;70(9):1128-30.
47. Mrug M, Mishra PV, Lusane HC, Cunningham JM, Alpert MA. Hemothorax and retroperitoneal hematoma after anticoagulation with enoxaparin. South Med J. 2002;95(8):936-8.
48. Huang J, Lin W, Lv D, Wu L, Jin H, Deng Z, et al. Dabigatran-Induced Massive Spontaneous Hemothorax. Drug Saf Case Rep. 2017;4:12.
49. Hariri BA, Alharafsheh A, Nashwan AJ, Mohamedali MG, Abusriwil HM. Spontaneous Hemothorax caused by Rivaroxaban treatment for pulmonary embolism. [online] Available from https://www.researchsquare.com/article/rs-2926991/v1 [Last accessed November, 2023].
50. Noble S, Peters DH, Goa KL. Enoxaparin. A reappraisal of its pharmacology and clinical applications in the prevention and treatment of thromboembolic disease. Drugs. 1995;49(3):388-410.
51. Antman EM, McCabe CH, Gurfinkel EP, Turpie AG, Bernink PJ, Salein D, et al. Enoxaparin prevents death and cardiac ischemic events in unstable angina/non-Q-wave myocardial infarction. Results of the thrombolysis in myocardial infarction (TIMI) 11B trial. Circulation. 1999;100(15):1593-601.
52. Wick MR, Ritter JH, Schuller D. Ruptured pulmonary infarction: a rare, fatal complication of thromboembolic disease. Mayo Clin Proc. 2000;75(6):639-42.

CHAPTER

20 Pleural Effusion due to Heart Diseases

Avi Kumar, Bhavana Mastebhakti

INTRODUCTION

Cardiovascular diseases have consistently been on top of the list of leading causes of death worldwide. Increasing cardiovascular disease means increasing heart failure with accompanying pleural effusions, which are the accumulation of fluid in one or both pleural spaces. Congestive cardiac failure from left-sided heart disease is the most common cause of cardiogenic pleural effusions and less commonly, diseases of pericardium and different types of cardiac injury, including heart surgery, may lead to pleural effusion. Diagnosing cardiac-related pleural effusions is usually unambiguous and treatment is mainly focused on managing underlying heart disease.

EPIDEMIOLOGY

In the last 50 years, the three most common causes of pleural effusions have been cardiac diseases, tuberculosis, and/or malignancy, with the prevalence order varying according to the location where the surveys have been conducted. In industrialized countries, cardiovascular disease usually tops the list of etiologies of pleural effusion. Congestive cardiac failure accounts for 500,000 of the 1,337,000 estimated annual cases of pleural effusion in the United States, according to Light.[1]

ETIOLOGY (TABLE 1)

- Congestive cardiac failure
- Pericarditis
- Postcardiac injury syndrome
- Coronary artery revascularization
- Other causes—pulmonary embolism (PE), pneumonia, and antiarrhythmic agents

PATHOGENESIS

The small volume of pleural fluid which is normally present in healthy humans originates from microvessels which are branches of the systemic circulation that perfuse the parietal pleura. This low-protein ultrafiltrate traverses the parietal surface of the pleural membrane into the pleural space. Physiologically, none of the liquid enters the pleural spaces through the visceral pleura from the lungs. In contrast, some portion of the liquid is removed via the visceral pleura.[2] Other pathways for the removal of cells, protein, particles, and excess liquid (if present) are lymphatics that drain the pleural space through stomata which are microscopic openings that are found only on the parietal surface of the pleura.[3]

The collection of fluid in the pleural spaces of patients with congestive cardiac failure comes from the lungs via the visceral pleura and its formation is regulated by the hydrostatic and oncotic forces that affect filtration across the microvessels of the pulmonary circulation. Once left ventricular (LV) end-diastolic pressure increases, pulmonary capillary wedge pressure rises correspondingly, and filtration of fluid increases in the lungs. However, pleural effusion becomes evident later in the course of the underlying heart disease, well after the onset of congestive cardiac failure as various protective mechanisms work to prevent the development of pulmonary edema, in order to preserve gas exchange across the alveoli. But when these mechanisms exhaust, fluid begins to accumulate, first in the peribronchovascular interstitial space and then inside the alveoli.[4] The peribronchovascular interstitium has to be at least partially filled with fluid before it percolates from the subpleural interstitium into the pleural space due to the pressure gradient across the visceral pleura.[5,6] This fluid leakage across the visceral

TABLE 1: Common causes and characteristics of cardiogenic pleural effusion.[8-33]

	CCF	Pericarditis	Postcardiac injury syndrome	P/CABG	Other
Causes	• Hypertension • Ischemic heart disease • Cardiomyopathy • Valvular heart disease	• Acute pericarditis • Chronic constrictive pericarditis	• Postpericardiotomy syndrome • Dressler's syndrome • Blunt trauma • Implantation of a pacemaker	• Immediate • Early • Late	Pulmonary embolism, pneumonia, and antiarrhythmic agents
Pleural fluid	Mostly transudative and bilateral	Small, left-sided or bilateral	Usually exudative	Small, left-sided	Usually exudative and occupies less than one third of the hemithorax
NT-proBNP	≥4,000 ng/L	–	–	–	–
Clinical features	• PND • Orthopnea	• Fever • Sharp retro-sternal pain • Pericardial friction rub • ECG changes	• Fever • Signs of pleural, pericardial, and pulmonary inflammation	• *Immediate*: Pain, impaired movement of left hemidiaphragm, and rapid and shallow breathing • *Late*: Dyspnea and pleura thickening	• Dyspnea out of proportion to the size of the pleural effusion • Pleuritic chest pain
Management	Diuretics	• Symptomatic treatment with anti-inflammatory agents such as aspirin • Colchicine	Symptomatic treatment with anti-inflammatory agents	• *Immediate*: Pain management and deep breathing exercises • *Late*: Anti-inflammatory agents, multiple thoracenteses, tube thoracostomy, pleural sclerosis, and pleurectomy	• Treatment of underlying etiology • Therapeutic thoracentesis is rarely necessary

(CABG: coronary artery bypass grafting; CCF: congestive cardiac failure; ECG: electrocardiography; NT-proBNP: N-terminal prohormone of brain natriuretic peptide; PND: paroxysmal nocturnal dyspnea)

pleura acts as a mechanism for the lungs to get rid of the excess liquid that would otherwise accumulate within the alveoli, thus slowing down the onset of alveolar flooding in order to preserve gas exchange.

The protein concentration of cardiogenic pleural effusion is usually low, but not as low as in healthy humans, and studies have showed that the protein concentrations within the lungs, pleural fluid, and in the lymphatics that drain the lungs were similar.[5] These results show that the pleural effusion in patients with congestive cardiac failure is formed by movement of fluid from the lungs into the pleural space and also explains the reason behind the low protein concentration found in the pleural fluid to that of the plasma.[7] Although the mechanism of pleural fluid formation in normal individuals and in patients with congestive cardiac failure differ, the routes of spontaneous clearance are similar, largely, via lymphatic channels draining the parietal pleura. Therefore, any increase in systemic venous pressure (as seen commonly in congestive cardiac failure) into which these lymphatics drain leads to a decrease in lymph flow which would retard the rate of pleural clearance.

Congestive Cardiac Failure

The most common causes of cardiogenic pleural effusion are ischemic heart diseases from coronary artery disease or hypertension, cardiomyopathies, and valvular heart diseases.

Patients with congestive cardiac failure and pleural effusion present with orthopnea, paroxysmal nocturnal dyspnea, and on the examination have fine crackles. Pleural effusions unless large enough may not be detected on physical examination. Chest X-ray [lateral and postero-anterior (PA) views] and high-resolution computed tomography (HRCT) chest may show cardiomegaly, Kerley B lines, and bilateral pleural effusions, generally the right effusion being larger than the left **(Figs. 1 to 3)**. Pleural effusions unless larger than 300 mL can be missed even on high-quality films. However, lateral decubitus X-rays can detect a collection of 100 mL or more.[8] Serum and pleural fluid NT-proBNP (N-terminal prohormone of brain natriuretic peptide) levels are significantly elevated in patients with pleural effusion, owing to congestive cardiac failure. NT-proBNP cutoff value of 4,000 ng/L

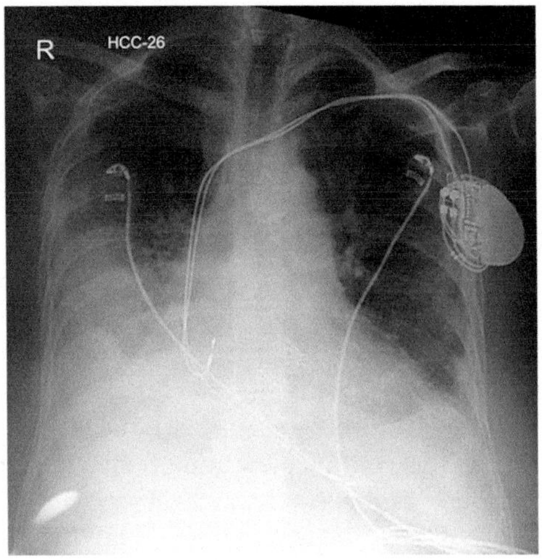

FIG. 1: Bilateral pleural effusion due to congestive cardiac failure in a patient with permanent pacemaker.

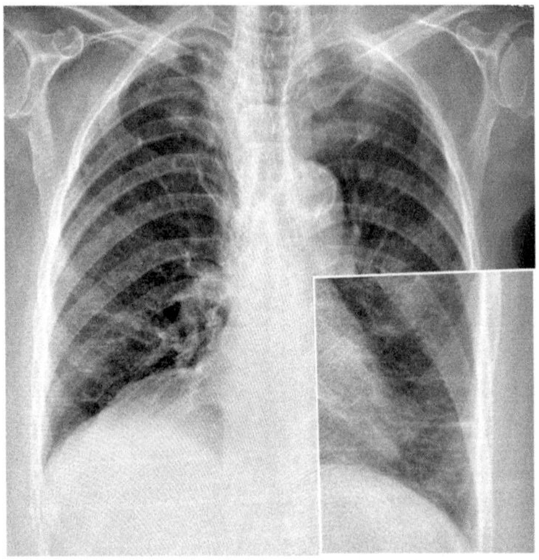

FIG. 2: Kerley B lines—thickened subpleural interlobular septa due to pulmonary edema.

in pleural fluid and serum showed comparably high diagnostic accuracies of 92% and 91%, respectively, in the diagnosis of heart failure-related pleural effusion.[9]

Cardiogenic pleural effusions are typically transudative in nature.[10] However in patients on diuretic therapy, protein and lactate dehydrogenase (LDH) levels may increase to levels found in exudative pleural effusion. This happens because in patients treated with diuretics, water is removed at a faster rate than protein, which causes the pleural-serum protein concentration ratio to increase.[11] LDH levels may also increase as a result of cell lysis and trauma from multiple thoracocentesis. There is also a subsequent reduction in serum LDH due to the relief of hepatic congestion from diuretic therapy. These mechanisms contribute to the increased pleural-serum LDH ratio to levels consistent with an exudate.

The increased pleural-serum protein and LDH ratios in patients with heart failure on diuretic therapy can misclassify the per se transudative nature of these pleural effusions into psudoexudative ones. To overcome this, the difference between pleural and serum albumin should be considered, which if >1.2 g/dL, is likely to be a transudative pleural effusion.[12] Another surrogate marker for the presence of a cardiac hydrothorax is high level of NT-proBNP in serum or in pleural fluid.[9] It has been validated that the measurements of NT-proBNP is better than the pleural-serum albumin gradient to identify patients with cardiogenic pleural effusions misclassified as exudates according to Light's criteria.[13]

Pleural effusions due to congestive cardiac failure often worsen and remit due to the waxing and waning nature of the underlying cardiac disease. However majority of the time, these effusions improve rapidly once diuretic therapy is commenced. Thoracocentesis is usually not indicated, except for in cases with respiratory distress

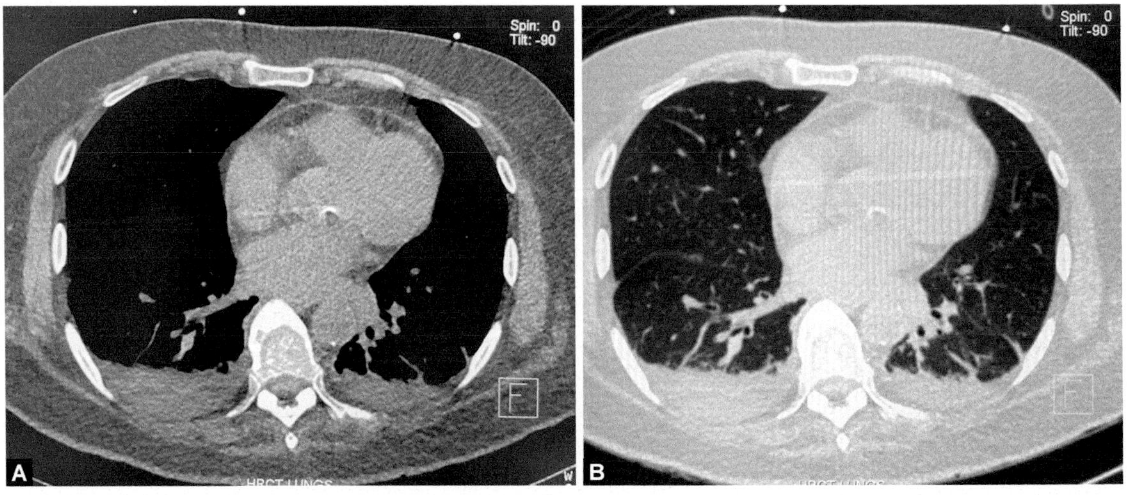

FIGS. 3A AND B: Bilateral pleural effusion due to congestive cardiac failure.

due to massive pleural effusion or unilateral left-sided pleural effusion with suspicion of a superadded infection. In patients with persistent or recurrent symptomatic pleural effusion refractory to medical therapy, the role of sclerotherapy has been controversial. According to a study, 10 out of 12 patients treated with pleurodesis had successful outcomes.[14] As mentioned earlier, the development of pleural effusions in congestive heart failure serves to reduce pulmonary edema; pleurodesis may worsen pulmonary edema in the ipsilateral lung but will not have any effect on the opposite side.

Pericarditis

Symptoms include fever and sharp retrosternal pain, which typically is worse when supine and gets relieved by sitting and leaning forward. Signs include a pericardial friction rub and/or characteristic electrocardiographic changes. Pleural effusions are usually small and are left-sided or bilateral. Thoracocentesis is usually not indicated unless there is large pleural effusion which does not subside as the pericardial disease resolves. Treatment is directed at underlying pericardial disease. A 3-month therapy with colchicine and symptomatic treatment with anti-inflammatory agents such as aspirin is generally effective and improves the outcome.[15]

There is limited data with respect to pleural effusion in patients with chronic constrictive pericarditis, although it is a common occurrence. A large series of 35 surgically proven cases of chronic constrictive pericarditis were reported by Plumb and coworkers,[16] out of which 21 (60%) had pleural effusion(s). Out of these 21 patients, pleural effusion was bilateral in 12 patients and right-sided in 9 patients. Unilateral left-sided effusion was not observed. Tomaselli and colleagues[17] also found that 18 out of 30 patients (60%) with chronic constrictive pericarditis had hydrothorax. Out of these 18 patients, 12 patients had bilaterally symmetrical pleural effusion, 3 had right-sided involvement, and the remaining 3 had left-sided pleural effusions. Thus, the left-sided predominance seen in acute pericarditis does not happen in chronic constrictive pericarditis.

Postcardiac Injury Syndrome

The postcardiac injury syndrome (PCIS) occurs following various myocardial or pericardial injuries and has been described after cardiac surgery (postpericardiotomy syndrome), myocardial infarction (Dressler's syndrome), blunt trauma to the chest, percutaneous puncture of the left ventricle, and implantation of a pacemaker (postpericardial trauma syndrome). It affects about 15% of those undergoing cardiac surgery,[18] of whom 56–92% have evidence of pleural involvement.[19] PCIS is characterized by the appearance of fever and signs of pericardial, pleural, and pulmonary parenchymal inflammation days or weeks after the initial injury. The most important differentials for PCIS are congestive heart failure, pneumonia, and pulmonary emboli.[20] Lack of a specific diagnostic test makes the diagnosis of PCIS even more challenging. One of the common manifestations of PCIS is pleuropulmonary involvement in which the resulting pleural effusions are exudative in nature with a protein level usually ≥3.0 g/100 mL and a pH usually >7.40.[21-24] Considerable overlap exists in all of the clinical conditions except complicated parapneumonic effusions in which the pH is invariably <7.30. Therefore, finding a normal pH of the pleural fluid will eliminate the diagnosis of complicated parapneumonic effusions. The presence of a serosanguineous or bloody effusion favors either PCIS or rarely PE, but it is highly uncommon in either parapneumonic effusions or effusions due to congestive heart failure.[21-23] Treatment is generally symptomatic and includes anti-inflammatory agents and recurrences may occur.

Coronary Artery Revascularization

The temporal classification of pleural effusions after coronary artery bypass grafting (CABG) surgery by Heidecker and Sahn[25] is as follows:

1. *Immediate (during the first week following CABG)*: The prevalence of pleural effusion in the first week after CABG ranges from 41 to 87%.[25] They are usually small and unilateral, left-sided. Etiologies include impaired movement of the left hemidiaphragm due to pain from the median sternotomy, chest tube placement, and intraoperative injury to the left phrenic nerve, which in turn, make the patients breathe rapidly and shallowly. This leads to bibasilar atelectasis and small, bilateral or unilateral (left-sided) pleural effusions. Therapies directed at controlling pain and encouraging deep breathing may prevent or minimize atelectasis. These effusions resolve spontaneously within 2 weeks.

   Another reason for pleural effusion in the immediate postoperative period following CABG is injury to the adjacent parietal pleura caused at the time of internal mammary artery grafting. These effusions are generally small and occur on the same side from which the artery has been harvested.

   Other causes include congestive cardiac failure due to sustained myocardial damage (stunned myocardium), vigorous intraoperative fluid administration, or the development of perioperative myocardial ischemia. Such pleural effusions are mostly small and respond to diuretics.

2. *Early (during the first 2 months following CABG)*: These effusions can result from CABG surgery per se and can be large bloody effusions or nonbloody due to PCIS.
3. *Late (2–12 months later)*: Effusions in this period can be a manifestation of evolving cardiac injury, leading to PCIS and lymphocytic effusions. Patients are usually symptomatic with dyspnea as the predominant symptom. Complications include persistence and/or recurrences and pleural thickening with entrapment of the lung. Treatment modalities include anti-inflammatory agents, multiple thoracentesis, tube thoracostomy, pleural sclerosis, and pleurectomy.

Constrictive pericarditis is an uncommon late manifestation of CABG surgery with a reported incidence ranging from 0.2 to 2.3%.[26,27]

Also underlying myocardial damage in patients with coronary artery disease, severe enough to warrant CABG, may worsen in the months following surgery and cause congestive cardiac failure with pleural effusions in case of which measurement of NT-proBNP would help in the diagnosis.

Other Causes

Common etiologies of cardiogenic pleural effusions have been discussed earlier, but patients with heart disease are also susceptible to other noncardiogenic causes of pleural effusion as follows:

Pulmonary Embolism

Venous thromboembolism (VTE), which encompasses deep vein thrombosis and PE, is a common and challenging complication of heart failure. The relative risk of PE is at least double that of patients without heart failure and increases as LV systolic function declines.[28] PE patients with heart failure have a higher overall mortality rate than those without (17% vs. 10%).[29] In addition, PE is an independent predictor of death or rehospitalization among patients with heart failure.[30] PE is the fourth leading cause of pleural effusion. All patients with undiagnosed pleural effusion should be evaluated for PE. Pulmonary emboli-related pleural effusion is due to ischemia and the release of vasoactive cytokines. Some studies indicate accumulation of fluid in PE due to increased systemic venous pressure at the parietal pleural surface, pulmonary ischemia/infarction, vascular damage, and increased pulmonary arterial pressures. Pleuritic chest pain and dyspnea out of proportion to the size of the pleural effusion are predominant symptoms. Pulmonary emboli-related pleural effusion usually occupies less than one third of the hemithorax. Pleural fluid caused by pulmonary emboli is exudative and is rarely transudative. D-dimer testing serves as a good screening test for pulmonary emboli and if positive, a computed tomography pulmonary angiogram (CTPA) should be done to confirm the diagnosis. A therapeutic pleural tap is rarely needed because effusions are small. The presence of bloody pleural fluid is not a contraindication for anticoagulation of pulmonary emboli. One should suspect recurrent emboli or other complications (e.g., hemothorax or an empyema) if the size of the pleural effusion increases or if a new contralateral pleural effusion develops after the initiation of anticoagulant therapy. Discontinuation of anticoagulation and insertion of a chest tube is indicated if the patient has a hemothorax (pleural fluid hematocrit greater than 50% of peripheral hematocrit).[31]

Antiarrhythmic Agents

Pleural effusions are known to be induced by two antiarrhythmic drugs—amiodarone and procainamide. Amiodarone causes fibrosing interstitial pneumonitis which is an uncommon but serious and sometimes fatal manifestation in which parenchymal involvement along with pleural effusion can occur.[32] Procainamide can also cause pleural effusions as a component of drug-induced lupus reaction.[33]

KEY POINTS

- Cardiac diseases are the leading cause of pleural effusions in developed countries.
- Congestive cardiac failure is the most common cause of cardiogenic pleural effusion.
- Other causes include pericarditis, PCIS, CABG, pulmonary embolism, pneumonia, and antiarrhythmic agents.
- Detailed history, clinical symptoms, signs, chest X-ray, echo, and diagnostic pleural tap (when indicated) help to establish an etiological diagnosis.
- Treatment depends on underlying etiology.

REFERENCES

1. Light RW. Pleural Diseases, 5th edition. Philadelphia, PA: Lippincott Williams & Wilkins; 2007. p. 111.
2. Zoochi L. Physiology and pathophysiology of pleural fluid turnover. Eur Respir J. 2002;20:1545-58.
3. Staub NC, Wiener-Kronish JP, Albertine KH. Transport through the pleura. In: Chretien J, Bignon J, Hirsh A (Eds). Physiology of normal liquid and solute exchange in the pleural space. The Pleura in Health and Disease. New York, NY: Marcel Dekker Inc.; 1985. pp. 169-93.

4. Staub NC. Pathophysiology of pulmonary edema. In: Staub NC, Taylor AE (Eds). Edema. New York, NY: Raven Press; 1984: 719-46.
5. Broaddus VC, Wiener-Kronish JP, Staub NC. Clearance of lung edema into the pleural space of volume-loaded, anesthetized sheep. J Appl Physiol. 1990;68:2623-30.
6. Bhattacharya J, Gropper MA, Staub NC. Interstitial fluid pressure gradient measured by micropuncture in excised dog lung. J Appl Physiol. 1984;56:271-7.
7. Light RW, MacGregor MI, Luchsinger PC, Ball WC Jr. Pleural effusions: The diagnostic separation of transudates and exudates. Ann Intern Med. 1972;77:507-13.
8. Pare JA, Fraser RG. Synopsis of Diseases of the Chest. Philadelphia, PA: WB Saunders; 1983. p. 104.
9. Kolditz M, Halank M, Schiemanck CS, Schmeisser AS, Höffken G. High diagnostic accuracy of NT-proBNP for cardiac origin of pleural effusions. Eur Respir J. 2006;28:144-50.
10. Kalomendidis I, Rodriguez M, Barnette R, Gupta R, Hawthorne M, Parkes KB, et al. Patient with bilateral pleural effusion. Are the findings the same in each fluid? Chest. 2003;124:167-76.
11. Broaddus VC. Diuresis and transudative effusions—Changing the rules of the game. Am J Med. 2001;110:732-5.
12. Burgess LJ, Maritz FJ, Taljaard JJF. Comparative analysis of the biochemical parameters used to distinguish between pleural transudates and exudates. Chest. 1995;1604-9.
13. Porcel JM, Chorda J, Cao G, Esquerda A, Ruiz-González A, Vives M. Comparing serum and pleural fluid pro-brain natriuretic peptide (NT-proBNP) levels with pleural-to-serum albumin gradient for the identification of cardiac effusions misclassified by Light's criteria. Respirology. 2007;12:654-9.
14. Glazer M, Berkman N, Lafair JS, Kramer MR. Successful talc slurry pleurodesis in patients with nonmalignant pleural effusion. Report of 16 cases and review of the literature. Chest. 2000;117:1404-9.
15. Little WC, Freeman GL. Pericardial disease. Circulation. 2006;113:1622-32.
16. Plumb GE, Bruwer AJ, Clagett OT. Chronic constrictive pericarditis: Roentgenologic findings in 35 surgically proven cases. Mayo Clin Proc. 1957;32:555-66.
17. Tomaselli G, Gamsu G, Stulbarg JS. Constrictive pericarditis presenting as pleural effusion of unknown origin. Arch Intern Med. 1989;149:201-3.
18. Imazio M. Post-pericardiotomy syndrome. Curr Opin Pulm Med. 2012;18:366-74.
19. Alraies MC, AlJaroudi W, Shabrang C, Yarmohammadi H, Klein AL, Tamarappoo BK. Clinical features associated with adverse events in patients with post-pericardiotomy syndrome following cardiac surgery. Am J Cardiol. 2014;114:1426-30.
20. Engle MA, Zabriskie JB, Senterfit LB, Ebert PA. Postpericardiotomy syndrome: a new look at an old condition. Mod Concepts Cardiovasc Dis. 1975;44:59-64.
21. Bynum LJ, Wilson JE. Characteristics of pleural effusions associated with pulmonary embolism. Arch Intern Med. 1976;136:159-62.
22. Griner PF. Bloody pleural Ruid following pulmonary infarction. JAMA. 1967;202:947-9.
23. Potts DE, Levin DC, Sahn SA. Pleural Ruid pH in parapneumonic effusions. Chest. 1976;70:328-31.
24. Good JT Jr, Taryle DA, Maulitz RM, Kaplan RL, Sahn SA. The diagnostic value of pleural Ruid pH. Chest. 1980;78:55-9.
25. Heidecker J, Sahn SA. The spectrum of pleural effusions after coronary artery bypass grafting surgery. Clin Chest Med. 2006;27:267-83.
26. Fowler NO. Constrictive pericarditis: Its history and current status. Clin Cardiol. 1995;18:341-50.
27. Matsuyama K, Matsumoto M, Sugita T, Nishizawa J, Yoshioka T, Tokuda Y, et al. Clinical characteristics of patients with constrictive pericarditis after coronary bypass surgery. Jpn Circ J. 2001;65:480-2.
28. Beemath A, Stein PD, Skaf E, Al Sibae MR, Alesh I. Risk of venous thromboembolism in patients hospitalized with heart failure. Am J Cardiol. 2006;98:793-5.
29. Monreal M, Munoz-Torrero JF, Naraine VS, Jimenez D, Soler S, Rabunal R, et al. Pulmonary embolism in patients with chronic obstructive pulmonary disease or congestive heart failure. Am J Med. 2006;119:851-8.
30. Darze ES, Latado AL, Guimaraes AG, Guedes RA, Santos AB, de Moura SS, et al. Acute pulmonary embolism is an independent predictor of adverse events in severe decompensated heart failure patients. Chest. 2007;131:1838-43.
31. Light RW. Pleural Diseases, 4th edition. Baltimore: Lippincott, Williams & Wilkins; 2001.
32. Mittal SR, Maheshwari M. Amiodarone-induced exudative pleural effusions—A case report and review of the literature. Indian Heart J. 2006;58:352-5.
33. Smith PR, Nacht RI. Drug-induced lupus pleuritis mimicking pleural space infection. Chest. 1992;101:268-9.

CHAPTER

21

Hepatic Hydrothorax

Narendra S Choudhary, Abhishek Saini

INTRODUCTION

Hepatic hydrothorax (HH) is a complication of cirrhosis and portal hypertension and is characterized by a transudative pleural effusion (typically >500 mL) without other coexisting causes of pleural effusion such as cardiac, renal, or pulmonary etiologies. Generally, HH happens in the setting of ascites, but ascites may be absent in some cases.[1-3]

Retrospective observational studies have estimated the frequency in cirrhosis patients to be between 5 and 10%. HH was found in 15.3% of cirrhotic patients in the largest documented series; however, only 6.5% of these patients needed thoracentesis.[4,5] HH is the most common cause of pleural effusions in cirrhosis and typically affects the right side (85%); isolated left side (13%) is uncommonly involved, and sometimes both sides (2%) may be involved.[6]

Hepatic hydrothorax worsens the prognosis of a patient. O'Leary et al. compared 121 patients with HH to 736 patients with refractory ascites (RA) (and no HH) and to 1,639 patients without these. The authors noted that secondary infections, hospital stays, and intensive care unit (ICU) transfer were the highest in patients with HH. Multivariable modeling showed that patients with HH had an increased risk of acute-on-chronic liver failure (ACLF) [hazard ratio (HR) 2.37 vs. RA, HR 2.56 vs. other; $p = 0.01$] after controlling against other potential factors. The risk of inpatient mortality was the highest in the HH group (HR 2.22 vs. RA alone, HR 2.31 vs. other; $p = 0.04$).[7] Pippard et al. also showed poor prognosis in patients with cirrhosis and pleural effusion. Liver transplantation dramatically improved survival.[8]

CLINICAL FEATURES

When a patient with advanced cirrhosis presents with a unilateral pleural effusion, most frequently on the right side, the diagnosis of HH is typically considered. Ascites is detectable in over 80% of those with HH but is not required for diagnosis. Rarely, HH could be the initial sign of decompensated cirrhosis.[9] The pulmonary symptoms in HH patients vary, primarily based on the amount of fluid (effusion), how quickly it built up, and the presence or absence of an underlying cardiac condition. Patients may have significant pleural effusions and be asymptomatic or may have symptoms such as breathlessness, cough, hypoxia, or respiratory failure.[10,11] In the study by Badillo et al., the most common symptoms were dyspnea at rest (in 34%) and cough (in 22%).[6] It should be noted that while ascitic tap can be done as a large volume, a large-volume thoracentesis cannot be done due to the risk of re-expansion edema.[12]

Diagnostic Thoracentesis

To confirm a diagnosis of HH and to rule out other etiologies of pleural effusion, a thoracentesis should be carried out. In prospective research, it was discovered that 30% of the pleural effusions in 60 cirrhotic patients who had diagnostic thoracentesis were caused by diseases other than HH that included spontaneous bacterial empyema (SBE; in 15%), tuberculosis, malignancy, parapneumonic effusions, and unidentified reasons. Eighty percent of right-sided pleural effusions were uncomplicated HH; this figure dropped to just 35% in cases with isolated left-sided pleural effusions.[13]

The following diagnostic procedures should be routinely performed on the pleural fluid: Cell count (total and differential), culture in blood culture bottles, serum and fluid albumin (to calculate serum pleural albumin gradient), total protein, adenosine deaminase, and sugar. In addition to these investigations, lactate dehydrogenase (LDH), polymerase chain reaction for tuberculosis, pleural fluid pH, amylase, Gram stain and cytology for malignant cells, and triglycerides are tests that can be ordered if there is clinical suspicion for empyema, tuberculosis, pancreatitis, cancer, and chylothorax.[14-16]

Because the pleural surface is more effective at absorbing water, the analysis of ascitic and pleural fluid is slightly different. In general, pleural fluid may have slightly greater quantities of total protein, albumin, and lipids. The biochemical characteristics of pleural fluid in a case of HH are shown in **Table 1**. An uncomplicated HH has a neutrophil count of fewer than 500 cells/mm^3, serum pleural albumin gradient > 1.2, and a total protein concentration < 2.5 g/dL. However, when a patient is on diuretics, the serum/pleural fluid albumin ratio < 0.6 should be considered as transudate.[15,16]

In addition to pleural fluid analysis, other procedures, such as a chest computed tomography (CT) scan and echocardiography, can be done to rule out malignant causes and cardiac failure. Thoracoscopy and pleural biopsy may be necessary when the malignant cause is highly suspected and cytologic evaluation is negative for malignant cells.

The diagnostic algorithm is shown in **Flowchart 1**.

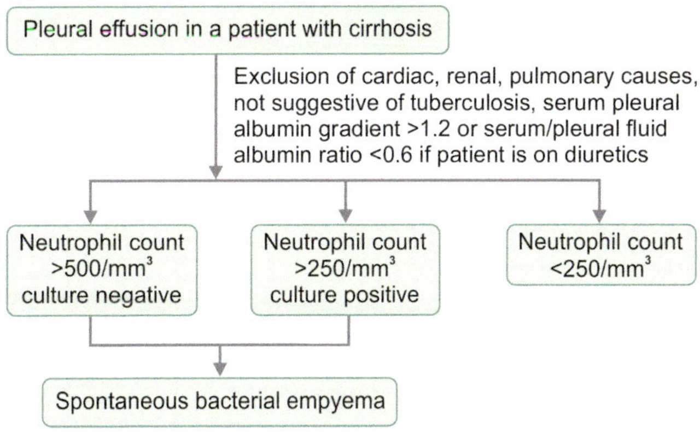

FLOWCHART 1: Diagnostic algorithm for hepatic hydrothorax.

Diaphragmatic Evaluation

Generally, diaphragmatic evaluation is not required in a typical case with cirrhosis, ascites, and transudative pleural effusion. An intraperitoneal injection of [Technetium-99]-sulfur colloid or [Technetium-99] human serum albumin may be useful when ascites cannot be seen or when the hydrothorax is on the left side. The ascites is the source of the effusion, which is confirmed by this test because radioisotopes that migrate from the peritoneal cavity into the pleural space establish communication between the two regions. The absence of the marker in the pleural space suggests a different diagnosis for the pleural effusion.[17]

TABLE 1: Management of hepatic hydrothorax (HH): Commonly used modalities.

Modality	Pros	Cons	Comments	Recommendation
Diuretics, sodium restriction, albumin	First-line measures	Difficult to use sometimes due to adverse events, diuretics-related adverse events, albumin is costly	Not tolerated in the presence of diuretic refractory ascites, may not prevent refilling of hydrothorax if not effective	C1
Drainage catheters	Rapid symptomatic relief	Not suitable for long use	Risk of bleed, infection	C1
TIPSS	Cures ascites and portal hypertension also (decreases the risk of variceal bleed)	Post TIPSS hepatic encephalopathy, liver failure (sometimes)	Provides time for liver transplant (acts as a bridge to LT, does not cure cirrhosis)	B1
Liver transplantation	Cures cirrhosis also	Graft availability takes time in the cadaveric system	The best available option, associated with good long-term outcomes, improves quality of life also	A1
Tunneled catheters, chemical pleurodesis, VATS or pleurovenous shunt	Early relief from symptoms	Adverse events, less data available as rarely used/needed, no effect on underlying cirrhosis	Case-to-case basis to patients who are not candidates for TIPSS or LT	C2

(LT: liver transplantation; TIPSS: transjugular intrahepatic portosystemic shunt; VATS: video-assisted thoracoscopic surgery)

Source: Adapted from Singh V, et al.[26]

PATHOPHYSIOLOGY

Figure 1 shows the proposed pathophysiological mechanisms leading to the development of HH. A patient will develop pleural effusion when the amount of fluid accumulation in the pleural cavity is more than the absorptive capacity of the pleural membrane. The following mechanisms have been proposed as a cause of HH in patients with decompensated cirrhosis: Decreased colloid osmotic pressure because of hypoalbuminemia, increased azygos system pressure because of portal hypertension leading to diversion of blood flow into azygous system, which causes leakage of plasma in the pleural cavity, transdiaphragmatic migration of peritoneal fluid into the pleural space, and movement of ascitic fluid in the pleural cavity through lymphatic channels.[3,10,11,18] The most widely considered mechanism is the direct movement of ascites from the peritoneal cavity to the pleural cavity through multiple diaphragmatic defects. Huang et al. suggested four different types of diaphragmatic morphology, which were associated with HH: Type 1—no visible diaphragmatic defect, type 2—blebs in the diaphragm, type 3—presence of fenestrations in the diaphragm (ruptured blebs), and type 4—multiple gaps in the diaphragm.[19]

The fact that HH happens mostly on the right side could be related to more muscular nature of the diaphragm on the left side; the right side is more tendinous because of a relationship with bare areas of the liver.[20]

Spontaneous Bacterial Empyema

Spontaneous bacterial empyema is defined as a spontaneous infection of preexisting HH. SBE happens in 13–16% of HH patients and 2.0–2.4% of cirrhotic individuals.[21-23] The pathophysiology, clinical course, and management approach of SBE are distinct from those of empyema (secondary to chest infection) since there is typically no sign of pus in the pleural cavity in SBE. SBE can be caused by spontaneous bacteremia, as in spontaneous bacterial peritonitis, or can be caused by movement of infected ascites to the pleural cavity via defects in the diaphragm. Although the movement of infected ascites across diaphragmatic defects is the likely cause in the majority of SBE cases, up to 40% patients with SBE may not be associated with ascitic fluid infection. Enterobacteriaceae are common causal pathogens causing SBE, which is intuitive given the association with SBP.[24,25]

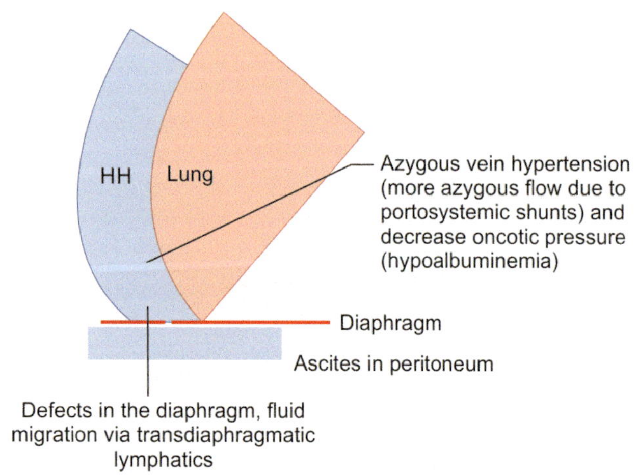

FIG. 1: Proposed mechanisms for the development of hepatic hydrothorax (HH).

A positive pleural fluid culture and a neutrophil count of >250 cells/mm^3 are required for the diagnosis of SBE to be made. When cultures are negative, the diagnosis is made by ruling out a parapneumonic infection and using a neutrophil count of >500 cells/mm^3 to confirm the diagnosis.[26] The cornerstone of the therapy is an initial course of appropriate antibiotic therapy. Given the connection to spontaneous bacterial peritonitis, the choice of antibiotics is identical, and an intravenous third-generation cephalosporin given for a duration of 7–10 days is the advised course of treatment.[27]

The placement of a drainage tube is typically not advised in SBE, even in situations where the culture is positive, as it can result in fluid depletion, protein loss, and electrolyte imbalance. Only pus in the pleural area is a sign that SBE requires chest tube drainage.[27-29]

MANAGEMENT

Medical Management[26,30,31]

The medical management of HH is discussed in **Table 1**.

The initial management is like that of abdominal ascites.

- Abstinence if alcoholic, treatment of viral hepatitis (B or C), or etiology of liver disease
- Dietary sodium should be <2 g daily.
- Diuretics—a combination of furosemide (maximum dose 160 mg) and spironolactone (maximum dose 400 mg). Doses are increased gradually as per response, as used for ascites.
- Splanchnic and peripheral vasoconstrictors (terlipressin, midodrine, octreotide) may be helpful by increasing sodium excretion in urine. Midodrine is available as an oral tablet.
- The role of intermittent albumin infusion has been studied in cases of RA, with variable results.[26] However, there are no good data available regarding the role of albumin infusions in the management of HH, but it should help.

Refractory Hepatic Hydrothorax

Many patients continue to have intractable dyspnea and respiratory impairment because of recurrent hydrothorax after receiving medical treatment with diuretics and sodium restriction. Diuretic-induced electrolyte imbalances (hyponatremia, hypo- or hyperkalemia), renal dysfunction, or precipitation of hepatic encephalopathy may also make it difficult to successfully treat pleural effusion symptoms in many patients. HH in these patients is regarded as being refractory. The only definitive treatment for refractory HH is liver transplantation.[26,32]

The goals of treatment for refractory HH include symptomatic treatment and averting pulmonary consequences in both transplant candidates and patients awaiting liver transplantation. Placement of transjugular intrahepatic portosystemic shunt (TIPSS), chest tube insertion, indwelling pleural catheter, therapeutic thoracentesis, and surgical treatments are the potential treatment options when liver transplantation is not possible.

Therapeutic Thoracentesis

- Simple and effective procedure for relief of symptoms
- Although it is said that 2 L can be removed, the authors have seen re-expansion edema at lower volumes also, and caution should be kept.
- Coagulopathy in patients with cirrhosis is not a contraindication to therapeutic thoracentesis unless it is because of disseminated intravascular coagulation. Preprocedure empirical use of platelets and fresh frozen plasma should be avoided, and a thromboelastography-guided approach is better.[33]

Chest Tube Placement and Indwelling Tunneled Pleural Catheter

In patients with HH, a chest tube should not be inserted routinely since it may result in adverse events such as protein loss, infection, pneumo- or hemothorax, hepatorenal syndrome, and electrolyte abnormalities.[illegible]

The indwelling tunneled pleural catheter (also known as PleurX or Denver catheter) was originally intended in patients with recurrent malignant pleural and ascitic effusions. It can be used in patients with HH. A recent meta-analysis on the use of this catheter for nonmalignant pleural effusions by Patil et al. showed a spontaneous pleurodesis rate of 51%; however, experience is limited, and further studies are necessary. Thirteen studies (n = 325) were included in the analysis. Congestive cardiac failure was a cause of effusion in approximately half of the patients. The following were the major complications: Empyema (2.3%), loculation (2.0%), dislodgement (1.3%), leakage (1.3%), and pneumothorax (1.2%). The following minor complications were noted: Skin infection in 2.7%, blockage/drainage failure in 1.1%, and subcutaneous emphysema in 1.1%. One mortality was related to indwelling pleural catheter use.[35]

Transjugular Intrahepatic Portosystemic Shunt

A Transjugular Intrahepatic Portosystemic Shunt is an artificial metallic shunt that connects some of the hepatic inflow (portal system) to outflow (one of hepatic veins), thus sending some of the portal flow directly to a hepatic vein (without need to cross hepatic sinusoids) and decreasing portal hypertension **(Fig. 2)**. Given the role of portal hypertension in the formation of HH, portal decompression is useful in alleviating HH also. In addition to the control of HH, TIPSS also decreases the risk of variceal bleeding. Several studies have shown that TIPSS is an effective tool to control HH.[36,37] A meta-analysis of six studies on TIPSS for HH involved 198 patients. A complete response was present in 55.8%, and a partial response was present in 17.6%.[36]

The rate of shunt dysfunction was high with bare stents; however, with the use of polytetrafluoroethylene (PTFE)-covered stents, shunt patency is improved significantly, which is also applicable to the benefit of TIPSS for HH. TIPSS can hasten liver failure in individuals who already have severe hepatic dysfunction because it shunts blood away from the liver and lowers efficient portal perfusion to the liver. Patients with a high risk of decompensation following as TIPSS functions as a bridge to transplant treatment.[38-40]

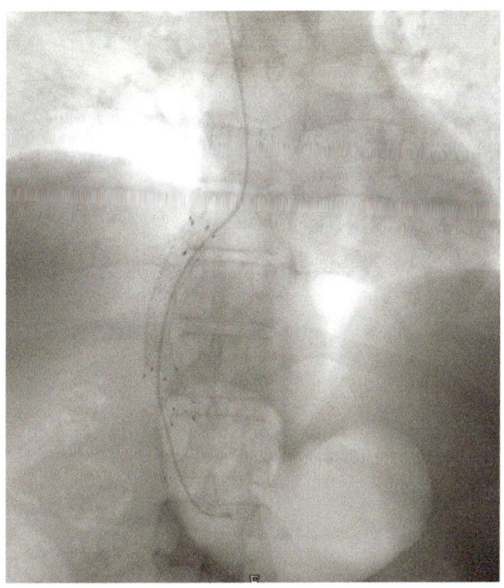

FIG. 2: A transjugular intrahepatic portosystemic shunt (TIPSS) is being placed inside liver parenchyma.

In patients with cirrhosis and RA, a higher bilirubin, a higher model for end-stage liver disease (MELD) score, and Child-Turcotte-Pugh (CTP) class C cirrhosis are associated with increased post-TIPSS complications, although there is insufficient evidence to recommend a cutoff value above which any of these parameters should be considered as a contraindication to TIPSS placement. The absolute contraindications to TIPSS creation include the American College of Cardiology/American Heart Association stage C or D heart failure, stage C or D untreated valvular heart disease, moderate-to-severe pulmonary hypertension, uncontrolled systemic infection, refractory overt hepatic encephalopathy, and anatomic barriers to TIPSS placement (multiple hepatic cysts or lesions). A MELD score > 18, age > 60 years, serum sodium < 130 meq/L, and bilirubin > 3 mg/dL are associated with poor prognosis after TIPSS. It should be noted that studies have excluded patients with a high creatinine (>1.5 or >3 in the majority of studies).[38-40]

Surgical Interventions

The following surgical approaches have been used for the management of HH:

- Pleurodesis
- Surgical repair of diaphragm defects
- Peritoneovenous shunts or pleurovenous shunting

Pleurodesis

Pleurodesis leads to ablation of pleural cavity (space between parietal and visceral pleura). It is done with a sclerosing agent or irritant (talc, tetracycline), which is administered by a chest tube or by thoracoscopy [video-assisted thoracoscopic surgery (VATS)]. A meta-analysis by Hou et al. included 180 patients with HH who underwent pleurodesis in 13 trials. The authors showed a mean success rate of 72% and symptomatic recurrences of HH occurred in 25% of cases. The rate of complete response was 72% with chest tube method and 84% with video thoracoscopic approach. The complete response rate with talc alone was 71% and with OK-432 (± minocycline) was 93%.[41]

Surgical Repair of Diaphragm Defects

In patients with refractory HH, the use of thoracoscopic mesh onlay reinforcement to prevent ascites leak has been introduced. The procedure can be performed via VATS or open thoracotomy with or without mesh, although open thoracotomy is rarely performed given the associated morbidity and mortality in patients with decompensated cirrhosis. An abdominal approach via laparoscopic repair can also be considered. The type of diaphragmatic defect may influence the repair strategy. In a recent retrospective study, patients with type I defect were treated with mesh covering only, while those with type II, III, or IV defects were treated with mesh with or without suturing. Huang et al. reported 63 patients with refractory HH who received thoracoscopic mesh onlay reinforcement to correct diaphragmatic abnormalities (mesh in 47 patients and mesh with suturing in 16 patients) in a recent surgical series. Four individuals had recurrences after a median of 20.5 months of follow-up examinations. The main reasons of mortality were sepsis, acute renal injury, bleeding (gastrointestinal), hepatic encephalopathy, and ischemic bowels.[42]

Although the results of minimally invasive approaches are encouraging, further experience is needed as patients with decompensated cirrhosis remain at a significant surgical risk.

Peritoneovenous Shunts or Pleurovenous Shunting

Peritoneovenous shunts were used at the time of no-good alternative options.[43] These are not used nowadays as better options exist, and there were technical issues, complications, and frequent failure.

Liver Transplantation

Liver transplantation is the best available option in patients with refractory HH. It is otherwise also indicated generally in these patients (presence of decompensated cirrhosis, RA, sometimes hepatocellular carcinoma). Patients with diuretic-resistant or diuretic-intractable HH, or high MELD (>15), should be referred for evaluation at a liver transplant center. The results of HH (whether refractory or not) after transplantation are highly favorable.[44]

KEY POINTS

- Hepatic hydrothorax in the setting of decompensated cirrhosis presents a challenge to management.
- It worsens the prognosis of a patient with decompensated cirrhosis.
- Liver transplantation is the best available option as it cures the underlying cause (cirrhosis).
- Medical management (diuretics, sodium restriction, intravenous albumin) is difficult to implement and is poorly tolerated.
- If liver transplantation is not possible, then TIPSS remains the next line of management if feasible (provided no contraindications).
- TIPSS is often not feasible in sick patients with liver failure.
- There is no benefit of drainage catheters in the long-term.

REFERENCES

1. Machicao VI, Balakrishnan M, Fallon MB. Pulmonary complications in chronic liver disease. Hepatology. 2014;59(4):1627-37.
2. Singh A, Bajwa A, Shujaat A. Evidence-based review of the management of hepatic hydrothorax. Respiration. 2013;86:155-73.
3. Garbuzenko DV, Arefyev NO. Hepatic hydrothorax: an update and review of the literature. World J Hepatol. 2017;9(31):1197-204.
4. Cardenas A, Kelleher T, Chopra S. Review article: hepatic hydrothorax. Aliment Pharmacol Ther. 2004;20:271-9.
5. Chen TA, Lo GH, Lai KH. Risk factors for spontaneous bacterial empyema in cirrhotic patients with hydrothorax. J Chin Med Assoc. 2003;66:579-86.
6. Badillo R, Rockey DC. Hepatic hydrothorax: clinical features, management, and outcomes in 77 patients and review of the literature. Medicine (Baltimore). 2014;93(3):135-42.
7. O'Leary J, Reddy K, Tandon P, Biggins S, Wong F, Kamath P, et al. Increased risk of ACLF and inpatient mortality in hospitalized patients with cirrhosis and hepatic hydrothorax. Dig Dis Sci. 2020;66:3612.
8. Pippard B, Bhatnagar M, McNeill L, Donnelly M, Frew K, Aujayeb A. Hepatic hydrothorax: a narrative review. Pulm Ther. 2022;8(3):241-54.
9. Kim JS, Kim CW, Nam HS, Cho JH, Ryu JS, Lee HL. Hepatic hydrothorax without ascites as the first sign of liver cirrhosis. Respirol Case Rep. 2016;4:16-8.
10. Norvell JP, Spivey JR. Hepatic hydrothorax. Clin Liver Dis. 2014;18:439-49.
11. Gur C, Ilan Y, Shibolet O. Hepatic hydrothorax—pathophysiology, diagnosis and treatment—review of the literature. Liver Int. 2004;24:281-4.
12. Thomas R, Jenkins S, Eastwood PR, Lee YCG, Singh B. Physiology of breathlessness associated with pleural effusions. Curr Opin Pulm Med. 2015;21(4):338-45.
13. Xiol X, Castellote J, Cortes-Beut R, Delgado M, Guardiola J, Sese E. Usefulness and complications of thoracentesis in cirrhotic patients. Am J Med. 2001;111:67-9.
14. Roussos A, Philippou N, Mantzaris GJ, Gourgouliannis KI. Hepatic hydrothorax: pathophysiology diagnosis and management. J Gastroenterol Hepatol. 2007;22:1388-93.
15. Porcel JM. Identifying transudates misclassified by Light's criteria. Curr Opin Pulm Med. 2013;19:362-7.
16. Light RW. The undiagnosed pleural effusion. Clin Chest Med. 2006; 27:309-19.
17. Benet A, Vidal F, Toda R, Siurana R, De Virgala CM, Richart C. Diagnosis of hepatic hydrothorax in the absence of ascites by intraperitoneal injection of 99m-Tc-Fluor colloid. Postgrad Med J. 1992;68:153.
18. Kiafar C, Gilani N. Hepatic hydrothorax: current concepts of pathophysiology and treatment options. Ann Hepatol. 2008;7:313-20.
19. Huang PM, Chang YL, Yang CY, Lee YC. The morphology of diaphragmatic defects in hepatic hydrothorax: thoracoscopic finding. J Thorac Cardiovasc Surg. 2005;130(1):141-5.
20. Holt KA, Oliviera E, Rohatgi PK. Hepatic hydrothorax demonstration by Tc-99m sulfur colloid ascites scan. Clin Nucl Med. 1999;24(8):609.
21. Xiol X, Castellote J, Baliellas C, Ariza J, Gimenez Roca A, Guardiola J, et al. Spontaneous bacterial empyema in cirrhotic patients: analysis of eleven cases. Hepatology. 1990;11:365-70.
22. Xiol X, Castellvi JM, Guardiola J, Sese E, Castellote J, Perello A, et al. Spontaneous bacterial empyema in cirrhotic patients: a prospective study. Hepatology. 1996;23:719-23.
23. Murray HW, Marks SJ. Spontaneous bacterial empyema, pericarditis, and peritonitis in cirrhosis. Gastroenterology. 1977;72:772-3.
24. Castellote J, Lopez C, Gornals J, Domingo A, Xiol X. Use of reagent strips for the rapid diagnosis of spontaneous bacterial empyema. J Clin Gastroenterol. 2005;39:278-81.
25. Reiche W, Deliwala S, Chandan S, Mohan BP, Dhindsa B, Ramai D, et al. Spontaneous bacterial empyema in cirrhosis: a systematic review and meta-analysis. World J Hepatol. 2022;14(6):1258-68.
26. Singh V, De A, Mehtani R, Angeli P, Maiwall R, Satapathy S, et al. Asia-Pacific association for study of liver guidelines on management of ascites in liver disease. Hepatol Int. 2023;17(4):792-826.
27. Tu CY, Chen CH. Spontaneous bacterial empyema. Curr Opin Pulm Med. 2012;18:355-8.
28. Orman ES, Lok AS. Outcomes of patients with chest tube insertion for hepatic hydrothorax. Hepatol Int. 2009;3(4):582-6.
29. Liu LU, Haddadin HA, Bodian CA, Sigal SH, Korman JD, Bodenheimer HJ, et al. Outcome analysis of cirrhotic patients undergoing chest tube placement. Chest. 2004;126:142-8.
30. European Association for the Study of the Liver. EASL Clinical Practice Guidelines for the management of patients with decompensated cirrhosis. J Hepatol. 2018;69(2):406-60.
31. Singh V, Dhungana SP, Singh B. Midodrine in patients with cirrhosis and refractory or recurrent ascites: a randomized pilot study. J Hepatol. 2012;56(2):348-54.
32. Baikati K, Le DL, Jabbour II, Singhal S, Anand S. Hepatic hydrothorax. Am J Ther. 2014;21:43-51.
33. European Association for the Study of the Liver. EASL Clinical Practice Guidelines on prevention and management of bleeding and thrombosis in patients with cirrhosis. J Hepatol. 2022;76(5):1151-84.
34. Runyon BA, Greenblatt M, Ming RH. Hepatic hydrothorax is a relative contraindication to chest tube insertion. Am J Gastroenterol. 1986;81:566-7.
35. Patil M, Dhillon SS, Attwood K, Saoud M, Alraiyes AH, Harris K. Management of benign pleural effusions using indwelling pleural catheters: a systematic review and meta-analysis. Chest. 2017;151:626-35.
36. Ditah IC, Al Bawardy BF, Saberi B, Ditah C, Kamath PS. Transjugular intrahepatic portosystemic stent shunt for medically refractory hepatic hydrothorax: a systematic review and cumulative meta-analysis. World J Hepatol. 2015;7:1797-806.
37. Dhanasekaran R, West JK, Gonzales PC, Subramanian R, Parekh S, Spivey JR, et al. Transjugular intrahepatic portosystemic shunt for symptomatic refractory hepatic hydrothorax in patients with cirrhosis. Am J Gastroenterol. 2010;105(3):635-41.
38. Copelan A, Kapoor B, Sands M. Transjugular intrahepatic portosystemic shunt: indications, contraindications, and patient work-up. Semin Intervent Radiol. 2014;31(3):235-42.
39. Salerno F, Cammà C, Enea M, Rössle M, Wong F. Transjugular intrahepatic portosystemic shunt for refractory ascites: a meta-analysis of individual patient data. Gastroenterology. 2007;133(3):825-34.

40. Boike JR, Thornburg BG, Asrani SK, Fallon MB, Fortune BE, Izzy MJ, et al. North American Practice-Based Recommendations for Transjugular Intrahepatic Portosystemic Shunts in Portal Hypertension. Clin Gastroenterol Hepatol. 2022;20(8):1636-62.e36.
41. Hou F, Qi X, Guo X. Effectiveness and safety of pleurodesis for hepatic hydrothorax: a systematic review and meta-analysis. Dig Dis Sci. 2016;61:3321-34.
42. Huang PM, Kuo SW, Chen JS, Lee JM. Thoracoscopic mesh repair of diaphragmatic defects in hepatic hydrothorax: a 10-year experience. Ann Thorac Surg. 2016;101:1921-7.
43. Artemiou O, Marta GM, Klepetko W, Wolner E, Müller MR. Pleurovenous shunting in the treatment of nonmalignant pleural effusion. Ann Thorac Surg. 2003;76:231-3.
44. Serste T, Moreno C, Francoz C, Razek WA, Paugham C, Belghitti J, et al. The impact of preoperative hepatic hydrothorax on the outcome of adult liver transplantation. Eur J Gastroenterol Hepatol. 2010;22:207-12.

CHAPTER 22

Pleural Effusion in Obstetrics and Gynecology

Monika Madaan Gaur, Reena Verma Prakash

INTRODUCTION

Pleural effusion is associated with varied disorders in obstetrics and gynecology. Some of the effusions are specific to obstetrics and gynecology conditions, while others may be due to associated other disease pathologies. Pregnancy in itself causes major changes in respiratory physiology in women predisposing them to certain pleural pathologies. A multidisciplinary approach is required in managing these women consisting of obstetrician/gynecologist, chest physician, and intensivist.

The varied causes of pleural effusion in obstetrical and gynecological conditions are elaborated in **Box 1**.

BOX 1 Causes of pleural effusion in obstetrics and gynecologic conditions.

Gynecological causes:
- *TES*:
  - Pleural effusion
  - Catamenial hemothorax
  - Catamenial pneumothorax
- OHSS
- Meigs syndrome
- Pseudo-Meigs syndrome

Obstetrical causes:
- *Pertaining to specific obstetric condition*:
  - Hyperemesis gravidarum
  - Preeclampsia/HELLP syndrome
  - Tocolysis with beta-adrenergic agonists
  - Peripartum cardiomyopathy
  - Benign peripartum pleural effusion
  - Pulmonary thromboembolism

Associated with other disease pathologies:
- Tuberculosis
- HIV
- Pneumonia
- Trauma
- Lymphangiomyomatosis
- Malignant pleural effusion
- Still's disease

(HELLP: hemolysis, elevated liver enzymes, low platelet; HIV: human immunodeficiency virus; OHSS: ovarian hyperstimulation syndrome; TES: thoracic endometriosis syndrome)

PLEURAL EFFUSION IN GYNECOLOGY

Thoracic Endometriosis Syndrome

Endometriosis is defined as the presence of endometrial glands and stroma outside the uterus. Classically, it presents with pelvic pain, dysmenorrhea, infertility, and dysparcunia. It affects around 5–15% of women in reproductive age.[1] Extragenital endometriosis is found in 12% of this population.[2,3] The presence of ectopic endometrial tissue in the lung parenchyma, diaphragm, and pleural surfaces is termed thoracic endometriosis syndrome (TES). It encompasses catamenial pneumothorax, catamenial hemothorax, catamenial hemoptysis, pulmonary nodules, pleural effusion, and catamenial chest pain.[4,5]

Age of Onset

Thoracic endometriosis syndrome has an older age of onset at the mean age of 35 years as compared to mean age of occurrence of 25–30 years of pelvic endometriosis.[6] Women generally experience symptoms of TES 5–7 years after development of pelvic endometriosis. TES can occur in isolation but is commonly found in association with extensive endometriosis of reproductive system in 50–85% of women.[6]

Pathophysiology

Various theories have been postulated to explain the occurrence of endometrial tissue outside the uterus. The most common explanation is retrograde menstruation theory.[7] According to this theory, the retrograde migration of endometrial implants or the menstrual blood in the peritoneal cavity further migrates transdiaphragmatically to the pleural cavity via the flow of abdominal fluid through the right paracolic gutter.

According to the coelomic metaplasia theory, the pleural and peritoneal mesothelial cells undergo metaplasia and transform into endometrial tissue, leading to endometriosis.[8] Another possible explanation is the dissemination of endometrial cells through the lymphatic or hematogenous routes, which can explain the bilateral occurrence of lesions in some cases.[9] Additionally, the bronchoconstrictor prostaglandin F2 alpha (PGF2α) may cause alveolar rupture of superficial bullae, resulting in catamenial pneumothorax. PGF2α is detected in the plasma of females during menstruation.[10]

Clinical Features

The clinical presentation of endometriosis can vary. Many females may be asymptomatic, but those with catamenial pneumothorax may experience chest pain, shoulder pain, cough, shortness of breath, and recurrent pneumothorax within 72 hours of their periods. Right-sided lesions are found in 92% of cases.[6] Bronchopulmonary thoracic endometriosis may present with hemoptysis or lung nodules. Diagnostic tools include chest X-ray, computed tomography (CT) scan, magnetic resonance imaging (MRI), and bronchoscopy. However, the diagnostic utility of bronchoscopy along with transthoracic bronchoscopy and cytological washings is limited due to the presence of endometrial implants at peripheral locations in the lungs.[11,12] The gold standard for diagnosing diaphragmatic endometriosis is video laparoscopy (VL) or video-assisted thoracoscopic surgery (VATS).[13] Sometimes the diagnosis is based on clinical features such as the temporal relation with menses, right-sided lesions, young age, and features of pelvic endometriosis such as infertility, dyspnea, and pelvic pain. A high index of suspicion is necessary as the clinical features can be variable and the association with menstruation is not always evident.

Management

Medical management is the primary treatment approach and may involve oral contraceptive pills (OCP), progesterone, danazol, aromatase inhibitors, gonadotropin-releasing hormone (GnRH) analogs, and GnRH antagonists. GnRH analogs are highly effective in suppressing the endogenous hormonal milieu/hypothalamic–pituitary–adrenal (HPA) axis, but long-term treatment (3–6 months) may lead to decreased bone mineral density, osteoporosis, and menopausal symptoms.[14,15] Discontinuation of hormonal treatment leads to recurrence, which is a disadvantage of medical therapy.[12]

Surgery is recommended for patients with refractory or recurrent lesions. Surgical options include pleurodesis, partial pleural biopsy, partial diaphragmatic resection, and pleurectomy. VATS is considered the gold standard for both diagnosis and treatment of TES.[6,11,16] Fulguration of superficial lesions can be done using diathermy, CO_2 laser, neodymium-doped yttrium–aluminum–garnet (Nd-YAG) laser, and argon laser. Deeper lesions require excision with sharp dissection.

A multidisciplinary approach involving gynecologists and transthoracic surgeon is required in treatment of both thoracic and pelvic diseases. Hysterectomy with bilateral salpingo-oophorectomy may be required in cases of recurrent and refractory lesions. Postoperative hormonal therapy suppression may be needed to reduce the recurrence of TES.

Ovarian Hyperstimulation Syndrome

Ovarian hyperstimulation syndrome (OHSS) is a complication that can occur during assisted reproductive techniques (ART), where pharmacological ovarian stimulation is used to increase the number of eggs and embryos. The disruption of normal physiological processes can result in increased vascular permeability and fluid accumulation, which can manifest as pleural effusion.

Ovarian hyperstimulation syndrome can occur in a mild form, affecting approximately one third of ART cycles. Mild OHSS is typically self-limiting and resolves spontaneously with supportive management. However in 3–8% of cases, OHSS can progress to a moderate-to-severe form.[17] In certain cases, OHSS can become critical and pose a life-threatening risk due to the potential development of thromboembolism, renal failure, and acute respiratory distress syndrome (ARDS).

Risk Factors

Risk factors for OHSS include a previous history of OHSS, polycystic ovary syndrome (PCOS), increased antral follicular count (AFC), high anti-Müllerian hormone (AMH) levels, high estradiol levels, and the presence of multiple ovarian follicles. The incidence of OHSS is higher in females who achieve pregnancy through ART or in cases of multiple pregnancies.

Pathophysiology

The pathophysiology of OHSS involves controlled ovarian stimulation using medications such as clomiphene or gonadotropins [follicle-stimulating hormone (FSH)] in ART. When human chorionic gonadotropin (HCG) is administered for oocyte retrieval or ovulation in hyperstimulated ovaries, it leads to the production of proinflammatory mediators, resulting in OHSS. There is an excessive production of estrogen, progesterone, and vasoactive substances such as cytokines [interleukin 6 (IL-6)], angiotensin, vascular endothelial growth factor (VEGF), and vasoactive intestinal peptide (VIP) among others.[18] These inflammatory mediators cause increased vascular permeability and a predisposition to thrombosis. Intravascular volume depletion and fluid shift into the third space lead to symptoms such as ascites, pleural effusions, and pericardial effusions. Severe OHSS can cause hypovolemia, hypoosmolality, and hyponatremia.[19] Pleural effusion in OHSS can occur due to protein-rich third space fluid, shift of ascitic fluid via diaphragm, or through the action of inflammatory mediators in the pleural cavity.[17] Right-sided pleural effusions are frequent (77%), though bilateral effusions are found in 15% of women.[20]

Clinical Features

Ovarian hyperstimulation syndrome can be categorized as early or late OHSS. Early OHSS is typically mild and presents within 7 days of HCG stimulation, while late OHSS is severe, occurs 10 days or more after HCG administration, and may also be influenced by endogenous HCG from early pregnancy.[21] Early-phase symptoms include abdominal discomfort, bloating, vomiting, and diarrhea. Severe OHSS is characterized by breathlessness, hypotension, decreased urine output, ascites, pleural effusion, ARDS, and thrombosis.

Management

The diagnosis and management of OHSS require a multidisciplinary approach involving ART specialists, chest physicians, and intensivists in severe cases. Initial assessment involves various tests such as complete blood count, serum electrolytes, liver and kidney function tests, serum osmolality, electrocardiogram (ECG), pelvic ultrasound, abdominal imaging, coagulation profile, and chest imaging (chest X-ray and CT scan in selected cases). Severe OHSS is suggested by the typical clinical features, elevated hematocrit, decreased serum osmolality, and decreased serum sodium levels. Treatment focuses on supportive care and volume replacement. Crystalloids are the first line of management for initial correction of dehydration. Colloids such as hydroxyethyl starch (HES) and albumin can also be used as plasma volume expanders. Intensive hemodynamic monitoring may be necessary in cases with persistent hemoconcentration despite volume replacement.[22]

Pleural fluid analysis should be performed to rule out other potential causes and drainage of pleural effusion may be required for symptomatic relief in certain cases.

Prognosis of pleural effusion complicating OHSS is good except where pulmonary embolism and ARDS develop.

Meigs Syndrome

Meigs syndrome was first reported in 1939 by Vincent Meigs and Cass, and later named Meigs syndrome by Rhodes and Terrell.[23,24] It is characterized by the presence of a benign ovarian tumor, such as fibroma, thecoma, granulosa cell tumor, or Brenner tumor, along with ascites and pleural effusion. The resolution of ascites and pleural effusion typically occurs after the surgical removal of the tumor.

Meigs syndrome accounts for approximately 1% of all ovarian tumors. Ovarian fibromas are the most commonly associated tumors, diagnosed in 2–5% of all excised ovarian tumors. It is more commonly observed in postmenopausal women around the age of 50 years, although the peak incidence is in the seventh decade of life.[25]

The exact cause of third-space fluid accumulation in the presence of an ovarian tumor is unclear. Proposed explanations include lymphatic obstruction caused by the tumor, leading to fluid escape and peritoneal inflammation induced by the tumor. Proinflammatory mediators such as IL-1, IL-6, IL-8, tumor necrosis factor-alpha (TNF-α), and VEGF can increase vascular permeability, resulting in the accumulation of fluid in the peritoneal and pleural cavities.[26]

Clinical Features

Clinical presentation of Meigs syndrome may include symptoms related to the primary tumor and ascites, such as abdominal distension, bloating, abdominal discomfort, weight loss, fatigue, and lower extremity edema. Pleural effusion can manifest as dyspnea, dry cough, and pleuritic pain. Pleural effusions in Meigs syndrome are usually right-sided, although in a minority of cases, they can be left-sided or bilateral.

Management

Diagnosis and management of Meigs syndrome involve differentiating it from malignant ovarian neoplasms. Imaging techniques such as pelvic ultrasound, CT scan and positron emission tomography (PET) scan can be helpful in diagnosing the primary tumor and distinguishing it from other conditions. CA-125 levels may be elevated in cases of Meigs syndrome, although the elevation is related to mesothelial expression of the antigen by peritoneum rather than the ovarian tumor.[27]

CA-125 returns to normal after surgical removal of the tumor. Pleural fluid should be aspirated and sent for analysis, i.e., biochemistry, cell count, cytology, and culture. Pleural fluid is of exudative nature in majority of cases, but there have been reports of transudative effusions in literature. After ruling out malignancy and other etiologies, surgical management with the removal of the tumor is the mainstay of treatment. In young women where fertility is desired, unilateral salpingo-oophorectomy may be done. In postmenopausal women, total abdominal hysterectomy with bilateral salpingo-oophorectomy is required. In females with large pleural effusion, thoracocentesis may be required initially for symptomatic relief before definitive surgical management is performed. The diagnosis is confirmed after histopathological report and resolution of ascites and pleural effusion.

Meigs syndrome has good prognosis overall and the chances of progression to fibrosarcomas are less than 5%.[28,29] The overall life expectancy is equivalent to general population postsurgery.

Pseudo-Meigs Syndrome

There is association of ascites, pleural effusion, and other benign ovarian malignant pelvic or abdominal tumor in pseudo-Meigs syndrome. The pathophysiology is same as that of Meigs syndrome.

Pseudo-pseudo-Meigs Syndrome

It is the presence of ascites, pleural effusion, and elevated CA-125 in patients with systemic lupus erythematosus (SLE). It is also called *Tjalma syndrome*. There is no association with gynecological tumor. Third-space fluid collection is attributed to immune complex deposition, lymph aggregation of plasma cells, and vasculitis of small vessels, leading to local inflammatory response.[30]

Management of Pseudo-pseudo-Meigs syndrome is based on treatment with steroids and in nonresponsive cases, azathioprine and cyclophosphamide **(Table 1)**.

PLEURAL EFFUSION IN OBSTETRICS

Alterations in Pulmonary Physiology during Pregnancy

There is significant alteration in normal physiology of respiratory system in pregnancy. Estrogen causes hyperemia, mucosal edema, and increased secretions of airways. Diaphragm is pushed upward by enlarging the uterus and there is progressive decrease in functional residual capacity (decreases by 10–20% by term). Pulmonary hyperventilation leads to respiratory alkalosis with compensatory renal excretion of bicarbonate. There is increase in blood volume and decrease in colloid osmotic pressure. During labor, pain and anxiety may lead to alveolar hypoventilation, atelectasis, and mild hypoxemia.

Causes of Pleural Effusion in Obstetrics

Hyperemesis gravidarum in severe cases may lead to esophageal perforation and pleural effusion. In pregnancies conceived by ART, severe OHSS may lead to pleural effusions in certain cases. Infections like HIV, pneumonias, and tuberculosis may complicate pleural effusions.

In the case of preterm labor, the use of beta-mimetic agents such as terbutaline, ritodrine, and isoxsuprine may cause pulmonary edema or pleural effusions due to myocardial dysfunction caused by maternal tachycardia,

TABLE 1: Management of Meigs', pseudo-Meigs', and pseudo-pseudo-Meigs' syndromes.

Meigs syndrome	Pseudo-Meigs syndrome	Pseudo-pseudo-Meigs syndrome (Tjalma syndrome)
• Benign ovarian tumor (fibroma, thecoma, granulosa cell tumor, and Brenner tumor) • Ascites • Pleural effusion	• Other benign ovarian tumor ascites • Pleural effusion	• Elevated CA-125 ascites • Pleural effusion • In systemic lupus erythematosus (SLE)
Surgical and supportive management	Same	Steroids azathioprine cyclophosphamide

increased capillary permeability, and intravenous (IV) fluids given to compensate for the maternal tachycardia.

Pregnancy-associated disorders such as preeclampsia and HELLP (hemolysis, elevated liver enzymes, lower platelets) syndrome may lead to pleural effusion in 3% of cases.[31]

Benign peripartum pleural effusion can develop spontaneously during labor and delivery and are caused by alterations in respiratory system physiology due to pregnancy. It is compounded by Valsalva maneuver during labor, leading to increased intrathoracic pressure and decreased pleural fluid and lymphatic drainage from the thoracic cavity. Majority of women are asymptomatic and effusions are detected incidentally by chest X-rays or ultrasound done for other reasons. The effusion is transudative in nature and occurs predominantly on right side. They resolve spontaneously within 7 days of delivery.[32]

Pregnancy being hypercoagulable state is prone to venous thrombosis in high-risk cases (OHSS, antiphospholipid antibody syndrome, thrombophilias, surgery, immobility, immunologic disorders, and preeclampsia). Pulmonary embolism in these women also leads to pleural effusion. Peripartum cardiomyopathy is a serious condition and usually presents postdelivery with symptoms of heart failure such as breathlessness, orthopnea, and peripheral edema.

Arterial blood gas (ABG) and chest X-ray are the primary investigations done in these cases. Ultrasound of chest can detect pleural effusion and underlying pathology. Pleural fluid aspirate is sent for cytology, biochemistry, gram staining, and acid-fast bacteria (AFB) culture. CT scan and MRI give better clinical information about the extent of disease and associated lung parenchyma. Ventilation perfusion scan or CT pulmonary angiography may be required in women presenting with pulmonary thromboembolism. Multidisciplinary approach involving obstetrician, chest specialist, and intensivist is required in the management of acutely ill patients.

Benign effusions resolve spontaneously over time. Effusions associated with preeclampsia respond to management of the underlying pathology. Thoracocentesis or tube thoracostomy may be required for larger symptomatic pleural effusions while awaiting definitive treatment of underlying disease. VATS may be done for empyema. In cases of maternal collapse, there is a role of peripartum cesarean section, thus delivering the live baby, and thereby also aiding in resuscitation of the mother.

KEY POINTS

- Pleural effusions in pregnancy may be benign or severe in certain cases, necessitating multidisciplinary approach.
- As symptoms of normal physiological changes in pregnancy and pathology overlap, it is imperative for physicians to be on high alert so that appropriate timely intervention can be done to prevent maternal and fetal morbidity and mortality.
- There are various gynecological cause of pleural effusion like TES: Pleural effusion, Catamenial hemothorax, Catamenial pneumothorax, OHSS, Meigs syndrome, Pseudo–Meigs syndrome.
- The obstetrical causes may be pertaining to specific obstetric condition like hyperemesis gravidarum, preeclampsia/HELLP syndrome, tocolysis with beta-adrenergic agonists, peripartum cardiomyopathy, benign peripartum pleural effusion, pulmonary thrombo-embolism.
- Pleural effusion may be associated with other disease pathologies:
  - Tuberculosis
  - HIV
  - Pneumonia
  - Trauma
  - Lymphangiomyomatosis
  - Malignant pleural effusion
  - Still's disease
- Pseudo-pseudo-Meigs syndrome is the presence of ascites, pleural effusion, and elevated CA-125 in patients with systemic lupus erythematosus (SLE) (Tjalma syndrome).

REFERENCES

1. Alifano M. Thoracic endometriosis: current knowledge. Ann Thorac Surg. 2006;81(2):761-9.
2. Giudice LC. Clinical practice. Endometriosis. N Engl J Med. 2010;362:2389-98.
3. Veeraswamy A, Lewis M, Mann A, Kotikela S, Hajhosseini B, Nezhat C. Extragenital endometriosis. Clin Obstet Gynecol. 2010;53:449-66.
4. Nezhat C, King LP, Paka C, Odegaard J, Beygui R. Bilateral thoracic endometriosis affecting the lung and diaphragm. JSLS. 2012;16:140-2.
5. Bobbio A, Canny E, Mansuet Lupo A, Lococo F, Legras A, Magdeleinat P, et al. Thoracic endometriosis syndrome other than pneumothorax: Clinical and pathological findings. Ann Thorac Surg. 2017;104:1865-71.
6. Korom S, Canyurt H, Missbach A, Schneiter D, Kurrer MO, Haller U, et al. Catamenial pneumothorax revisited: Clinical approach and systematic review of the literature. J Thorac Cardiovasc Surg. 2004;128:502-8.
7. Nezhat C, Nezhat F, Nezhat C. Endometriosis: Ancient disease, ancient treatments. Fertil Steril. 2012;98(6 Suppl):S1-62.

8. Alifano M, Roth T, Broet SC, Schussler O, Magdeleinat P, Regnard JF. Catamenial pneumothorax: A prospective study. Chest. 2003;124:1004-8.
9. Ueki M. Histologic study of endometriosis and examination of lymphatic drainage in and from the uterus. Am J Obstet Gynecol. 1991;165:201-9.
10. Bagan P, Le Pimpec Barthes F, Assouad J, Souilamas R, Riquet M. Catamenial pneumothorax: retrospective study of surgical treatment. Ann Thorac Surg. 2003;75:378-81; discussion 381.
11. Hilaris GE, Payne CK, Osias J, Cannon W, Nezhat CR. Synchronous rectovaginal, urinary bladder, and pulmonary endometriosis. JSLS. 2005;9:78-82.
12. Tripp HF, Thomas LP, Obney JA. Current therapy of catamenial pneumothorax. Heart Surg Forum. 1998;1:146-9.
13. Nezhat C, Nezhat F, Nezhat C. Nezhat's Video-assisted and Robotic-assisted Laparoscopy and Hysteroscopy with DVD, 4th edition. New York: Cambridge University Press; 2013.
14. Marshall MB, Ahmed Z, Kucharczuk JC, Kaiser LR, Shrager JB. Catamenial pneumothorax: Optimal hormonal and surgical management. Eur J Cardiothorac Surg. 2005;27:662-6.
15. Slabbynck H, Laureys M, Impens N, De Vroey P, Schandevyl W. Recurring catamenial pneumothorax treated with a Gn-RH analogue. Chest. 1991;100:851.
16. Nezhat C, Nicoll LM, Bhagan L, Huang JQ, Bosev D, Hajhosseini B, et al. Endometriosis of the diaphragm: Four cases treated with a combination of laparoscopy and thoracoscopy. J Minim Invasive Gynecol. 2009;16:573-80.
17. Delvigne A, Rozenberg S. Epidemiology and prevention of ovarian hyperstimulation syndrome (OHSS): a review. Hum Reprod Update. 2002;8:559-77.
18. Budev MM, Arroliga AC, Falcone T. Ovarian hyperstimulation syndrome. Crit Care Med. 2005;33(10):S301-6.
19. Evbuomwan I. The role of osmoregulation in the pathophysiology and management of severe ovarian hyperstimulation syndrome. Hum Fertil (Camb). 2013;16: 162-7.
20. Carter R, Petrie K, Sadighi A, Skene H. Ovarian hyperstimulation syndrome on the acute medical unit: a problem-based review. Acute Med. 2015;14(1):21-7.
21. Mathur RS, Akande AV, Keay SD, Hunt LP, Jenkins JM. Distinction between early and late ovarian hyperstimulation syndrome. Fertil Steril. 2000;73:901-7.
22. Practice Committee of the American Society for Reproductive Medicine. Ovarian hyperstimulation syndrome. Fertil Steril. 2008;90(Suppl 5):S188-93.
23. Meigs JV, Cass JW. Fibroma of the ovary with ascites and hydrothorax: with a report of seven cases. Am J Obstet Gynecol. 1937;33(2):249-67.
24. Rhoads JE, Terrell AW. Ovarian fibroma with ascites and hydrothorax (Meigs' syndrome): report of a case. JAMA. 1937;109(21):1684-7.
25. Saha S, Robertson M. Meigs' and Pseudo-Meigs' syndrome. Australas J Ultrasound Med. 2012;15(1):29-31.
26. Tjalma WAA. Ascites, pleural effusion, and CA 125 elevation in an SLE patient, either a Tjalma syndrome or due to the migrated Filshie clips, a pseudo-Meigs syndrome. Gynecol Oncol. 2005;97(1):288-91.
27. Riker D, Goba D. Ovarian mass, pleural effusion, and ascites: revisiting Meigs syndrome. J Bronchology Interv Pulmonol. 2013;20(1):48-51.
28. Nemeth AJ, Patel SK. Meigs syndrome revisited. J Thorac Imaging. 2003;18(02):100-3.
29. Light RW, Lee YCG. Textbook of Pleural Diseases. 2nd edition. London: Taylor & Francis; 2008.
30. McVorran S. Systemic lupus erythematosus presenting with massive ascites: a case of pseudo-pseudo Meigs syndrome. Case Rep Rheumatol. 2016;2016:8701763.
31. Haddad B, Barton JR, Livingston JC, Chahine R, Sibai BM. HELLP (hemolysis, elevated liver enzymes, and low platelet count) syndrome versus severe preeclampsia: onset at < or 1⁄428.0 weeks' gestation. Am J Obstet Gynecol. 2000;183(6):1475-9.
32. El-Naggar T. Peripartum pleural effusion. Respir Med. 1994;88(7): 541-2.

CHAPTER

23

Pediatric Pleural Diseases

Nishant Gupta, Sangeeta Basu

INTRODUCTION

Pleural effusion develops in the pleural space between the parietal and visceral pleura by the collection of body fluids and is caused by a primary phenomenon or is secondary to a variety of disorders such as infections, autoimmune processes, metabolic, tubercular, or malignancy.

The mechanism of the pleural fluid formation is same in pediatric age group as in the adult population, i.e., when the local hydrostatic pressure (pushes fluid out of the vascular space) is more than the colloidal oncotic pressure (draws the fluid inside vascular space). The Frank–Starling law controls this process.[1-3]

Pleural effusion can be further classified into: (1) Transudative or (2) exudative.

- *Transudative*: Intact membrane but abnormal hydrostatic and oncotic pressure
- *Exudative*: Increased permeability/integrity of the vessels due to inflammatory process or lymphatic drainage

ETIOLOGY

The etiological mechanisms of the pleural effusion are quite considerably different in childhood and adulthood. The most common cause of pleural effusion in children is infections,[4] while the most common causes in adults have been shown to be congestive heart failure and malignancies.

Recent studies have shown that majority of pleural effusion in pediatric age group is caused by pneumonia, followed by malignancies, renal disorders, trauma, and heart failure.

Amongst the infectious pleural effusions, bacterial infections are the most common causes that may lead to serious complications such as empyema (most commonly associated with *Streptococcus pneumonia*[5]); however, they can also occur due to viral infections that may be asymptomatic. In this context, among different serotypes of this pathogen, serotype 1 is dominant in children with empyema.

Other common causes are: *Staphylococcus aureus*,[6,7] *Haemophilus influenzae* type B,[8] coagulase-negative *Staphylococcus*, and other streptococcal species as viridans *Streptococcus*, Group A *Streptococcus*, alpha-hemolytic *Streptococcus*, and *Streptococcus pyogenes*.[9,10]

In India, a common infective cause of pleural effusion in children is pulmonary tuberculosis (TB).[11] Effusions are generally unilateral and may occur primarily from direct hematogenous invasion of the pleural space or secondary to a reactivation disease such as pulmonary parenchymal disease. It is to be noted that there are a few case reports on disseminated *Mycobacterium bovis* also reported with complicated pneumonia. Other bacteria as causative agents are *Klebsiella* species,[12] *Pseudomonas aeruginosa*,[13,14] *Legionella*,[15] and *Mycoplasma pneumoniae*.[16,17]

Among the noninfectious causes of pleural effusion, congestive heart failure is a less common cause secondary to elevated left atrial or pulmonary capillary wedge pressure.

In any previously healthy child, pleural effusion may usually be secondary to an infection by acute bacterial pneumonia or pulmonary TB. Generally, when associated with infections, effusions are unilateral in most of the cases, while bilateral empyemas are a bit unusual.

It is important to remember that certain anaerobic organisms such as *Peptostreptococcus*, *Bacteroides* species, and *Streptococcus milleri*[12] are rarely isolated in children and should be taken into consideration in any child with lung infections with delayed neurological development.

As per the data, the rate of parapneumonic effusion that complicates pneumonia is roughly around 1%. It is to be understood that the prevalence of any small parapneumonic effusion is very difficult to investigate due to several factors and also often goes undetected.

Notably in the current practice, the culture of pleural fluid is often sterile due to the usage of antibiotics administered prior to the aspiration of the pleural fluid sample.

Also, there are many case reports of methicillin-resistant *Staphylococcus aureus*,[6,7] causing empyema in children generally due to predisposing factors including immunodeficiencies, postsurgical aspiration, and sometimes trauma. It is important to understand that pleural effusion may not always be secondary to any infection and is sometimes sterile.

Other secondary causes of the pleural effusions are congenital heart disease, connective tissue disorders, renal disease, postcardio thoracic surgery, and trauma.

Another rare cause of pleural effusion is chylothorax in children that can occur congenitally or acquire from the leakage of chyle into the pleural space as a result of damage to the thoracic duct by rupture, laceration, tear, or compression.

Tubercular empyema can at times result from the progressive pulmonary TB and has been reported to account for almost 6% of all empyema cases worldwide.[11] The treatment in tubercular pleural effusions is same, namely rifampicin, isoniazid, ethambutol, and pyrazinamide. In some cases, the use of steroids is also warranted.

PLEURAL EFFUSIONS CAUSED DUE TO MALIGNANT TUMORS

In children, pleural effusions due to malignancy can either be unilateral or bilateral.[18] Malignancy as a cause of pleural effusions in pediatric age group can either be a primary or a metastatic malignancy.

Common Causes

- *Lymphoma*: It is the most common malignancy associated with pleural effusion. Lymphoma is also the most common cause of anterior mediastinal mass in children. Majority of lymphomas (>50%) are non-Hodgkin lymphoma, while the remaining are Hodgkin lymphoma. Patients with lymphoma shall usually present with an anterior mediastinal mass. And a very low percentage of these (around 5%) patients will develop pleural effusion.[19]

  Non-Hodgkin lymphoma is one of the most common cause of malignant pleural effusion (MPE) in the children.[20-23]
- *Neurogenic tumor*: Neuroblastoma and ganglio-neuroma make up to 90% of posterior mediastinal masses. Neurogenic tumors rarely cause pleural effusion.
- T-*leukemia*: Cell lymphoblastic leukemia is another cause of MPE. Pleural effusions develop in around 50–70% of lymphoblastic leukemias.
- *Germ cell tumors (GCT):* They account for about 6–18% of mediastinal masses. Close to 20% of GCT are malignant. These include seminomas and nonseminomatous tumor-like teratocarcinoma, embryonal carcinoma, choriocarcinoma, yolk sac tumor, and mixed types. These tumors may lead to encroachment to adjacent structures in mediastinum and cause respiratory symptoms. In some cases, there may be compression of tracheobronchial tree and the obstruction of the lymphatic flow by these tumors can sometimes result in the development of pleural effusions.[24,25]
- *Chest wall and pulmonary malignancy*: They can be primary and metastatic, but it is difficult to differentiate among them. For example, carcinoids tumors, Askin tumors,[26] and pleuropulmonary blastoma.
- *Carcinoid tumor*: It is common in older children and adolescents. It accounts for 80–85% of the primary malignant tumors in pediatric age group. They may cause compressive atelectasis and sometimes pneumonia that can cause the development of pleural effusion.
- *Pleuropulmonary blastoma*: It is a rare tumor in pediatrics. It is embryonal, a mesenchymal tumor which originates from lung and the pleural cavity. Diagnosis of this malignancy is often late. If tumor invades adjacent structures, then it may lead to pleural effusions.
- Askin *tumors*: They are a rare form of Ewing sarcoma or primitive neuroectodermal tumor that may arise from the ribcage, chest wall, or sometimes lungs. The tumor may invade adjacent structures such as muscle ribs, pleura, and lungs. They may lead to mass effects, along with the compression of the nearby organs and development of the pleural effusion.
- Other rare causes of pleural effusion in children include hemothorax, hypoalbuminemia, nephrosis, hepatic cirrhosis, and iatrogenic causes.

Hemothorax

Hemothorax is defined as the presence of blood in the pleural cavity. The main cause of hemothorax is generally a blunt or sharp trauma to chest. Iatrogenic hemothorax can occur as a complication to any cardiopulmonary surgery, placement of a subclavian or jugular catheters, or lung and pleural biopsies.

Chylothorax

In children, chylothorax is rare. As per the definition, it is the collection of chyle into the pleural space as a result of either damage to the thoracic duct by any rupture, tear, laceration, or any external compression.[27,28] Chyle is a milky colored fluid, which is enriched by emulsified fat (i.e., chylomicrons) that is absorbed by the intestinal cells and is the transported by the lymphatic channels that finally converge to become the thoracic duct.

Other causes may be the obstruction of superior vena cava, congenital malformations of pulmonary or thoracic lymphatic system, major neck surgeries, malignancies of mediastinum, or dysmorphic syndromes such as Turner's or Noonan's syndrome. Chylothorax is life-threatening condition that can lead to metabolic, immunological, and nutritional complications.

In chylothorax, the management is the same, despite any cause of the chylothorax, i.e., correction of underlying cause, somatostatin analogs,[29-31] low-fat diet, total parenteral nutrition (TPN),[32-34] pleurodesis,[29,30] and surgery (thoracic duct ligation[34-36] or embolization) in selected cases.

Tubercular Pleural Effusion

In developing countries like India, with very high-TB burden, TB is one of the leading cause of the pleural effusion in the pediatrics age group.

PATHOPHYSIOLOGY OF PLEURAL EFFUSIONS

The pleural space contains about 0.3 mL/kg body weight of the pleural fluid in the adult human body.[37] Any imbalance occurring between pleural fluid formation and pleural fluid drainage can cause a pleural effusion. Compared to serum, pleural fluid has much higher levels of electrolytes such as bicarbonate, low level of sodium, and almost similar levels of glucose.[38]

All these parameters get changed if there are any disease processes such as an infection that affects the lung parenchyma or vessels and can activate an immune response and the inflammation of the pleura.[39]

The increased vascular permeability shall lead to migration of inflammatory cells (mononeutrophils, lymphocytes, eosinophils, etc.) into pleural space. This process is mediated by the cytokines such as interleukin-(IL)-1, 6, 8, tumor necrosis factor alpha (TNF-α), and the platelet-activating factor—which are released by the mesothelial cells, lining the pleural space.[37]

This results in the exudative pleural effusion. This may further progress to a fibrinopurulent stage because of an increased accumulation of fluid and infective bacterial invasion across damaged pleural epithelium. The fibrin deposition in the pleural space further leads to septations or loculation of pleural effusion. Pleural infection is classically divided into three stages: (i) Exudative, (ii) fibrinopurulent, and (iii) organizational.[40]

PRESENTING SIGNS AND SYMPTOMS

The patient may present with dry cough, fever (high grade in empyema), breathlessness, sharp chest pain, poor feeding, fetor oris (halitosis), abdominal pain, tachypnea, tachycardia, lethargy, and malaise.

The child may try to lie down on the affected side due to pleuritic chest pain to create a physiological splint to temporarily relieve the pain and symptoms.

CLINICAL EXAMINATION

Inspection: Decreased chest expansion on the affected side can be observed. In chronic cases, scoliosis may be observed.

Palpation: Decreased chest expansion on the affected side. Decreased tactile vocal fremitus.

Percussion: Dull note on percussion.

Auscultation: Reduced or absent breath sounds.

ASSESSMENT

It is important to make a provisional diagnosis once the suspicion of pleural effusion is confirmed on a chest X-ray (CXR) or an ultrasonography (USG). Any child with a suspected sympneumonic effusion or a possible empyema should always be advised to get admitted to the hospital.

Diagnostic Imaging

X-ray: Posteroanterior radiographs are to be done first. Any obliteration of either of the costophrenic angle is the first sign of an underlying pleural effusion and there may be a rim of fluid, ascending the lateral chest wall (known as the meniscus sign) on a CXR. Shown further are the two CXR of the patient with pleural effusion **(Figs. 1 and 2)**.

Lateral CXR can help to identify any pneumothorax or lung abscess **(Figs. 3 and 4)**. If there is a differential of pleural effusion, it is advisable to confirm the CXR findings with the ultrasound.

Ultrasound: It is recommended to quantify the fluid in the pleural cavity and may also help to identify any loculations at present. USG can aid in identifying the echogenicity of the pleural fluid in addition to pleural thickening.[39]

Ultrasound-guided diagnostic thoracocentesis (or drain placement if massive effusion, leading to respiratory failure) should be done. If there is no clinical indication that this effusion is secondary to infection, it is advisable to send pleural fluid for cytological analysis.

Computed tomography (CT) scan: Not Recommended routinely; however, may be of use in detecting lung abscess, cavitary lesions, any endobronchial lesions, and mediastinal pathology. It may be warranted if an open thoracotomy and decortication for empyema is planned.

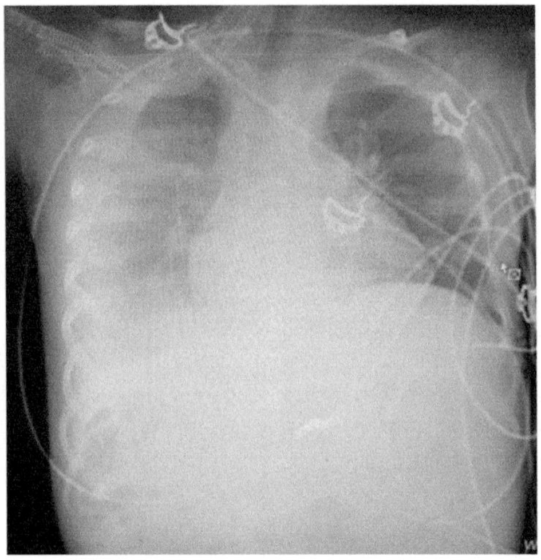

FIG. 1: Chest X-ray of a 3-year-old child who presents with fever, chest pain, and shortness of breath. Chest X-ray suggestive of right-sided pleural effusion. X-ray shows a rim of fluid ascending the lateral chest wall (known as the meniscus sign) on chest.

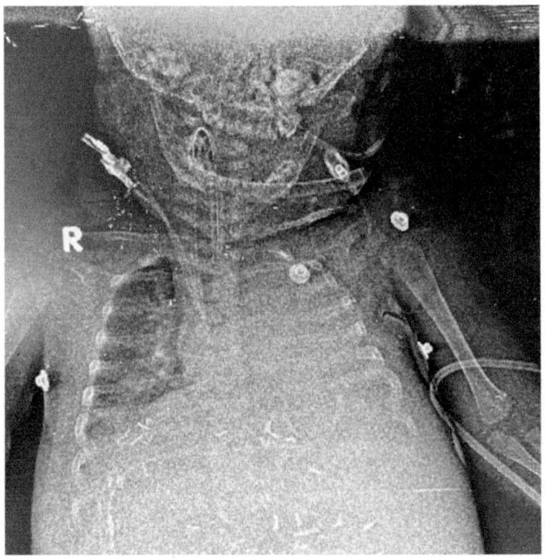

FIG. 3: Left-sided pleural effusion in a neonate. Patient presented with shortness of breath, fever, and tachypnea. X-ray shows left-sided white out lung.

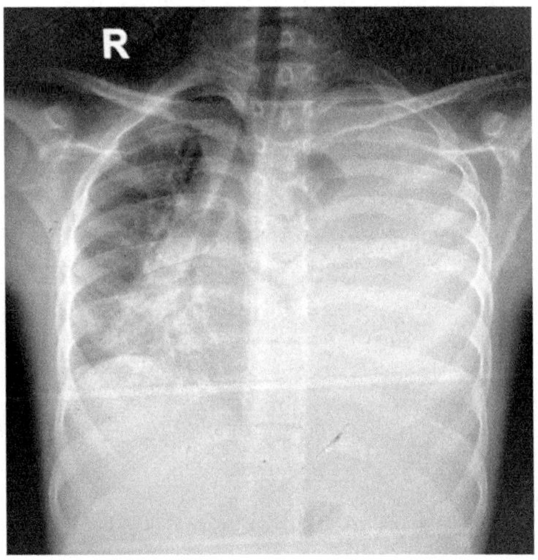

FIG. 2: Chest X-ray of a patient with massive left-sided effusion. The massive pleural effusion leads to mediastinal shift to the contralateral side.

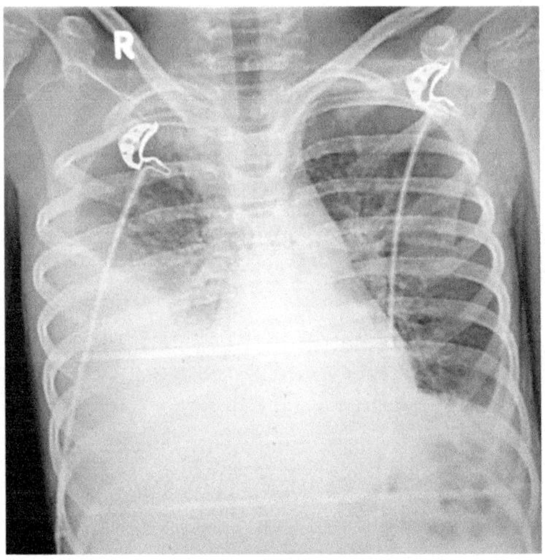

FIG. 4: Chest X-ray of a 4-year-old boy presenting with fever and shortness of breath, depicting large hazy opacity on the right side, with the obliteration of right costophrenic angle, suggestive of consolidation and possible pleural effusion on the right side.

Pleural Fluid Analysis

- Pleural fluid should be tested for microbiological tests including the Gram-stain, potassium hydroxide (KOH) stain, acid-fast bacteria (AFB) stain, GeneXpert, and routine culture.[41]
- Pleural fluid should also be evaluated for the total and differential cell count.
- In case of lymphocytosis (>70%)—a diagnosis of tubercular pleural effusion[42,43] and malignancy has to be excluded.
- For uncomplicated parapneumonic effusions/ empyema, the biochemical analysis of pleural fluid is not required. However, it is still recommended in Indian set of population due to high load of TB. Hence, it is mandatory to evaluate pleural fluid protein, glucose, lactate dehydrogenase (LDH), and adenosine deaminase (ADA) for additional work-up.
- In any patient with a milky, white colored pleural fluid and recent history of chest or abdominal surgery, we should always rule out for Chylothorax—pleural fluid triglycerides should be >110 mg/dL for the diagnosis of chylothorax.
- To rule out hemothorax—pleural fluid hematocrit of >50% of serum hematocrit

Diagnostic Analysis of Pleural Fluid Using Light's Criteria[44-48]

This helps in determination of transudate versus exudate source of pleural effusion.

Fluid is exudate if one of the following Light's criteria is present:

- Effusion protein/serum protein ratio > 0.5
- Effusion LDH/serum LDH ratio > 0.6
- Effusion LDH level greater than two-thirds the upper limit of the laboratory's reference range of serum LDH.

Other Laboratory Work-up

- A set of paired blood cultures should always be sent in children with parapneumonic effusion to rule out septicemia.[49]
- A morning sputum (fasting preferred) sample should be sent for Gramstain, KOH stain, GeneXpert, and routine culture if available.

MANAGEMENT OF PLEURAL EFFUSION

As a rule of thumb, any effusion which may be massive and/or is compromising the respiratory function will require an intercostal chest drain (ICD) to remove the fluid and cannot be managed with antibiotics alone. This will not only improve the lung function but also reduce the bacterial load. In some cases, conservative treatment may result in prolonged duration of illness and increased hospital stay.

In few cases if not properly managed, it may lead to pleural thickening, loculations, rind formation, and may further require surgical intervention.

Role of Antibiotics in Management of Pleural Effusion

- All cases of pleural effusion in pediatric age group should be managed with intravenous antibiotics and should include cover for *Streptococcus pneumonia*, group A streptococci, and *Staphylococcus aureus.*[49] In the Indian set of population, TB remains an important differential and hence always needs to be ruled out.
- Decision on antibiotics choices is recommended as per microbiology results. Local flora plays an important role in the decision regarding the antibiotics.
- Oral antibiotics are recommended on discharge for a period of 1–4 weeks and sometimes longer if there is any of the residual disease left.
- A broader spectrum of antibiotics cover is required for all the hospital-acquired infections to be guided as per indigenous flora, in addition to those that happen secondary to any surgery, trauma, or aspiration.

Chest Drains

- *Ideal chest tube/Seldinger chest drain set*:
    - Newborn: 8–12 FG
    - Infant: 12–16 FG
    - Child: 16–24 FG
    - Adolescent: 20–32 FG
- A chest drain should only be inserted under the ultrasound guidance.[50,51] The precheck includes ruling out any coagulopathy or low platelet count. It is advisable that any defect present should be corrected prior to the drain insertion.
- The ideal position for a chest drain insertion is "safe triangle."[52] It is bordered by anterior border of latissimus dorsi, lateral border of pectoralis major muscle, a line superior to the horizontal level of the nipple and apex below the axilla. It is preferred to place drains in fourth or fifth intercostal space anterior to midaxillary line—roughly at a level with the nipple or lower border of the scapula.
- Intracostal chest tube/drains/pigtail should be inserted at an optimum site, under guidance of chest ultrasound (is preferred in midaxillary line through "safe triangle") as shown in **Figure 5**.
- Intravenous sedation is preferred to general anesthesia under full monitoring equipment. Current

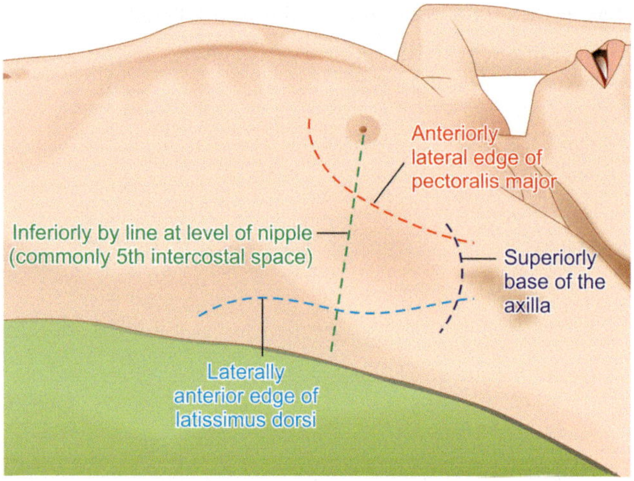

FIG. 5: Safe triangle for insertion of an intercostal chest drain (ICD) (bordered by anterior border of latissimus dorsi, lateral border of pectoralis major muscle, a line superior to the horizontal level of the nipple and apex below the axilla. It is preferred to place drains in fourth or fifth intercostal space anterior to midaxillary line—roughly at a level with the nipple or lower border of the scapula).

data suggests that there is no significant evidence that the large-bore chest drain may offer any advantage over the small drains like pigtail catheters.[53] Hence, it is preferable to use the smaller drains to minimize patient discomfort.

- Chest drains should always be attached to a unidirectional flow drainage system (like an underwater seal bottle/bag) and it should be always kept at a level below the patient's chest. In children, a negative suction at 5–10 cmH_2O can be applied but needs strict monitoring. After the tube insertion, CXR should be performed always to look for the tube placement and any complication. In case if there is any persistent air leak, chest drain should never be clamped[52] and no negative suction should be applied.
- It is advisable that the chest drain should be kept clamped for at least 1 hour after pleural fluid as per 10 mL/kg is initially removed so as to prevent re-expansile pulmonary edema in the child.
- The following criteria should be followed for the ICD removal, i.e., ICD output < 100 mL/day, clinical and radiological resolution, and no air column movement.
- However if the drain cannot be unblocked, then it should be removed immediately and be replaced if there is any significant pleural fluid left.

Intrapleural Fibrinolytics (Streptokinase, Urokinase, and Alteplase)

The use of intrapleural fibrinolytics is somewhat controversial.

- Intrapleural fibrinolytics reduce the hospital stay and hence are recommended for any case of empyema (overt pus) or a complicated parapneumonic effusion (thick fluid with loculations).
- There have been studies on urokinase[54] in randomized controlled trials in children. Urokinase should be administered through the chest tube twice daily for 3 days (6 doses in total) using 10,000 units in 10 mL (0.9% saline) for children weighing under 10 kg and 40,000 units in a 40 mL (0.9% normal saline) for children weighing 10 kg or above.

Surgery

- Any patient with an organized empyema may require an open thoracotomy or a video-assisted thoracoscopic surgery (VATS) decortication.[55]
- Any child with a persistent pleural collection/empyema which fails to resolve, despite the intracostal chest tube drainage, optimal dosage, and duration of preferable antibiotics.

PNEUMOTHORAX IN CHILDREN

Primary and Spontaneous Pneumothorax in Children

Pneumothorax is defined as air in pleural cavity. This condition occurs without an obvious etiology and can be classified as either primary or secondary.[56] Primary pneumothorax occurs in a healthy individual without any lung disease. Secondary pneumothorax occurs in patients with an underlying lung disease condition such as asthma, cystic fibrosis, foreign body aspiration, and lung or pleural infection. The term pneumothorax was coined by Itard in 1803, while Laennec described the clinical picture of pneumothorax in 1819. Though uncommon in children, but small and asymptomatic pneumothorax can be at times an incidental finding on the routine CXR in outpatient clinics.

Management of pediatric of both primary and secondary spontaneous pneumothorax (PSP and SSP, respectively) continues to be mainly extrapolated from adult-based practice and evidence till date. In the United States, pneumothorax occurs in 4 out of 100,000 male children and 1.1 out of every 100,000 female children.[57] There is a strong male predominance for PSP in adults.

Over a period of time, there is improvement in understanding of the PSP—pediatric patients and the potential role of conservative management.

Worldwide, there are mainly two guidelines which are taken into consideration: The American College of Chest Physicians (ACCP) and the British Thoracic Society (BTS). As summarized in **Table 1**, there is a significant difference

TABLE 1: Summary of the main features of the BTS and ACCP guidelines for spontaneous pneumothorax management.

	BTS	ACCP
Definition of large pneumothorax	>2 cm between lung margin and chest wall (at the level of hilum)	≥3 cm apex-to-cupola distance
First-line small PSP management	Observation if asymptomatic Aspiration is symptomatic	Observation for 3–6 hours and outpatient follow-up Aspirate or ICC if pneumothorax enlarges Presence of symptoms >24 hours does not alter treatment
First-line large PSP management	Observation if asymptomatic Aspiration is symptomatic	Insertion of ICC
First-line small SSP management	Admission and insertion of ICC Aspiration can be considered as an alternative	Admission and observation Admission of ICC if symptomatic
First-line large SSP management	Admission and insertion of ICC	Admission and insertion of ICC

(ACCP: American College of Chest Physicians; BTS: British Thoracic Society; ICC: intercostal catheter; PSP: primary spontaneous pneumothorax; SSP: secondary spontaneous pneumothorax)

in the definition and management among international clinical guidelines.

The 2003 BTS guidelines[58] recommended aspiration as a first-line intervention in large and/or clinically unstable PSP, whereas the 2001 ACCP guidelines recommend insertion of an ICD.[59]

For Small Primary Spontaneous Pneumothoraxes

As per the latest BTS guidelines, there is a recommendation of conservative management approach with observation and early discharge in the small PSP cases;[58] however, ACCP recommends only observation period, for about 3–6 hours instead.[59]

For Large Primary Spontaneous Pneumothoraxes

The ACCP recommends the insertion of a chest drain as the first-line intervention for cases of large PSP,[59] in contrast to recommendation of the BTS guidelines of aspiration.[58] It may be noted that the BTS guidelines have reserved intervention for only symptomatic cases and/or unstable cases regardless of the pneumothorax size **(Table 1)**.[60]

CLINICAL EVALUATION AND IMAGING

Common presenting symptoms: Shortness of breath and sudden-onset sharp chest pain.

Clinical examination: On auscultation, there will be reduced air entry in the affected lung, tachypnea, increased work of breathing, and reduced chest movement.

On percussion: Following findings may be noted:
- Hyper-resonant on percussion
- Decreased vocal fremitus

History: Always evaluate for:
- *Onset of symptoms*: Chest pain that may be radiating to shoulder tip, cough, and dyspnea
- Any recent lung infection
- Any history that suggests inhalation of a foreign body
- Any possible recreational drugs (especially inhaled) usage history
- *In neonates*: Birth history needs to be verified (especially, traumatic delivery)
- Expiratory CXR is not recommended for the routine diagnosis of pneumothorax.
- It is advisable to do lateral chest or a lateral decubitus X-ray in case there is a high clinical suspicion of pneumothorax, but a CXR posteroanterior view is normal. Serial inspiratory CXR should be repeated to observe the progress in pneumothorax.[61]
- Chest CT scan is recommended if we have to differentiate a pneumothorax from a complex bullous lung disease, if any ICD is misplaced, in cases of surgical emphysema or pneumomediastinum. The clinical significance of apical blebs (<2 cm) discovered on a CT scan is unclear. Apical blebs can be present in 20–45% children with PSP[62-64] and 0–15% in healthy children and young adults **(Fig. 6)**.[63,64]

Chest Tube Insertion Procedure

Site: Midclavicular line, second intercostal space, with one end positioned into the apex of lung and the other end in underwater seal.

[It is advisable to use larger chest drains (14–20F) in case of persistent leaks.]

Ideal size: 10F pigtail catheter is preferred due to less pain and does not leave any significant scar mark.

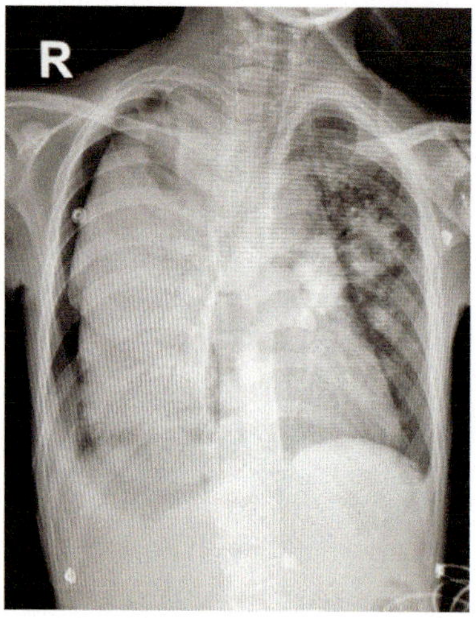

FIG. 6: Chest X-ray of a patient who presented to emergency with shortness of breath and chest pain.

Negative suction: It is required if lung fails to inflate after 24 hours and is applied at –20 cmH_2O via a controlled suction unit like a Medelar or a Pleur-evac.

When to remove the ICD: When the lung is fully expanded on CXR and there is no bubbling for 24 hours in the underwater seal

It is advisable not to clamp an ICD with active air leak. However, in case of uncertainty of air leak, we can keep it clamped for 4 hours and then unclamp it while closely observing underwater seal for any air leak or a recurrent pneumothorax.

Reexpansion pulmonary edema: It should be suspected if a patient with pneumothorax or pleural effusion develops a new-onset cough, shortness of breath, and chest tightness after an insertion of chest drain. Generally, this resolves spontaneously but may require some positive end-expiratory pressure (PEEP) if it does not.

A *tension pneumothorax* may lead to severe hypotension (obstructive shock) and can be fatal.

Signs Suggestive of Tension Pneumothorax

Tension pneumothorax is a life-threatening condition and patient may show the following signs:

- Tracheal deviation (opposite and away from side of pneumothorax)
- Cyanosis, tachypnea, hypotension, tachycardia, and decreased heart sounds
- *If tension pneumothorax is suspected, then immediately*:
    - Start high-flow oxygen via a nonrebreathable mask (NRBM)
    - Connect a syringe half filled with sterile water to large-bore cannula (14 or 16 g)
    - Insert it in second anterior intercostal space in the midclavicular line at 90° inside skin and being careful to avoid any neurovascular bundle by going over the top of the third rib.
    - Then slowly aspirate syringe until you are in pleural space (look out for air bubbles in syringe and stop going deeper as soon as you see them).
    - Remove the syringe and needle while securing the cannula. Attach the cannula to the underwater seal.
    - In the meantime, arrange for an ICD insertion on priority basis.

Recurrent pneumothoraces may occur due to blebs or bullae seen on chest high-resolution CT or CXR after an initial episode of pneumothorax were associated with ipsilateral recurrences. We suggest surgical intervention for patients with recurrent SSP and for those with underlying lung disease that is severe, progressive, or known to be associated with recurrent pneumothoraces (grade 2C). For patients with cystic fibrosis, surgical intervention is not recommended for the first occurrence of pneumothorax but is recommended for any recurrence.[65]

In such cases, there is an option to obliterate the pleural spaces using sclerosing agents such as talc or doxycycline through the chest tube or mechanically via a surgery.

An early VATS for those at high risk of recurrence like in cases with the presence of blebs or bullae is advisable.[59]

Spontaneous Pneumomediastinum

Spontaneous pneumomediastinum in children is secondary to alveolar rupture in pulmonary interstitium, followed by dissection of air toward hilum and mediastinum. Like spontaneous pneumothorax, SPM is more common in adolescent males.[66,67]

The most common known cause in children is asthma.

The clinical diagnosis consists of symptom triad, including dyspnea, chest pain, and subcutaneous emphysema. There is also evidence of Hamman's sign and the diagnosis can be confirmed by chest radiography.

The main differential diagnosis is esophageal perforation, which may require a CT scan and upper gastrointestinal endoscopy (UGIE). Spontaneous pneumomediastinum should generally resolve spontaneously in a few days.

The management consists of firstly treating an underlying cause (if diagnosed), analgesics, clinical monitoring, and rest. Any known predisposing factors should be controlled to prevent any recurrences. Spontaneous pneumomediastinum usually resolves in 2–15 days by itself. Recurrence occurs in <5% patients.[68]

In any case of an idiopathic spontaneous pneumomediastinum, it is necessary to perform a diagnostic pulmonary function test after an acute episode, as it is essential to detect whether the child has asthma.[69]

PLEURAL EFFUSION—KEY POINTS

Clinical scenario: Any child with a diagnosed or suspected para pneumonic effusion/and or empyema should be admitted to the hospital regardless of the etiology.

Diagnostic imaging: Firstly a PA view CXR should be done and if pleural fluid is suspected it is advisable to confirm the CXR findings with the USG followed by USG guided thoracentesis and ruling out any active infection, tubercular effusion, empyema and hemothorax etc.

Diagnostic analysis of the pleural fluid:

- Pleural fluid should be evaluated for the microbiological and biochemical analysis for diagnostic confirmation.
- A differential of tubercular pleural effusion should always be kept in differential in the Indian set of population.

Microbiological assessment:

- Set of paired blood cultures should be done to rule out any septicemia.
- Sputum for routine aerobic culture, gram stain and KOH stain should be sent if available.

Management:

- Massive pleural effusions or ones compromising respiratory function require an intercostal chest drainage to drain out the fluid.
- In some cases if pleural effusion is inadequately managed may require surgical intervention like open thoracotomy or a VATS decortication.

Role of antibiotics:

- All patients should be managed with the intravenous antibiotics and should always include cover for *Streptococcus pneumonia* in the pediatric age group.
- In the Indian set of population the tuberculosis remains an important differential and hence always need to be ruled out.

Chest drains:

- A chest drain should only be inserted under the ultrasound guidance in "safe triangle".
- Its advisable that drain should be kept clamped for at least 1 hour after pleural fluid as per 10 mL/kg is initially removed so as to prevent re-expansion pulmonary edema.
- Intrapleural fibrinolytics can reduce the hospital stay and hence are recommended for any case of empyema or a complicated para pneumonic effusion.
- *Surgery*: Any patient with an organized empyema may require a open thoracotomy or a VATS decortication.

PNEUMOTHORAX—KEY POINTS

- *For small primary spontaneous pneumothoraxes*: first take conservative management approach with observation and early discharge in the small PSP.
- *For large primary spontaneous pneumothoraxes*: Insertion of a chest drain is preffered.
- History of any recent lung infection, inhalation of a Foreign body, recreational drugs (especially inhaled) usage history, in neonates—traumatic delivery) should always be evaluated.

Chest tube insertion procedure:

- *Site*: Mid clavicular line, 2nd intercostal space, with one end positioned into the apex of lung and the other end in underwater seal.
- *Ideal size*: 10 F pigtail catheter is preferred.
- *Negative suction*: It is required if lung fails to inflate after 24 hours and is applied at –5 to –10 cmH_2O via a controlled suction unit like a medelar or a pleurivac.
- *When to remove the ICD*: When the lung is fully expanded on chest X-ray and there is no bubbling for 24 hours in the underwater seal.
- Re-expansion pulmonary edema should be suspected if a patient with pneumothorax or pleural effusion develops a new onset cough, shortness of breath and chest tightness after an insertion of chest drain.
- *Signs suggestive of tension pneumothorax*: It is a life-threatening condition and patient may show the following signs:
    - Tracheal deviation (opposite and away from side of pneumothorax), cyanosis, tachypnea, hypotension, tachycardia and decreased heart sounds.
    - If tension pneumothorax is suspected, then immediately start high flow oxygen via a NRBM (non rebreathable mask).
    - Large bore cannula is inserted in 2nd anterior intercostal space in the midclavicular line.
    - Attach the cannula to the underwater seal.
    - In the mean time arrange for a intercostal chest drain insertion on priority basis.
- *Spontaneous pneumomediastinum*: The most common known cause in children is asthma.
    - The clinical diagnosis consists of symptom triad including dyspnea, chest pain and subcutaneous emphysema.
    - The main differential diagnosis is esophageal perforation, which may require a CT scan and UGIE.
    - Spontaneous pneumomediastinum usually self resolves in 2–15 days by itself.
    - In any case of an idiopathic spontaneous pneumomediastinum it is necessary to perform a diagnostic pulmonary function test to rule out asthma.

REFERENCES

1. Charalampidis C, Youroukou A, Lazaridis G, Baka S, Mpoukovinas I, Karavasilis V, et al. Physiology of the pleural space. J Thorac Dis. 2015;7(Suppl 1):S33-7.
2. Charalampidis C, Youroukou A, Lazaridis G, Baka S, Mpoukovinas I, Karavasilis V, et al. Pleura space anatomy. J Thorac Dis. 2015;7(Suppl 1):S27-32.
3. Peppa VG, Solenov EI, Kalomenidis I, Tsilioni I, Gourgoulianis KI, Hatzoglou C, et al. Pleural effusion osmolality correlation with pH and glucose level of pleural fluid and its effects on the pleural membrane permeability. Respir Physiol Neurobiol. 2021;285:103581.
4. Freij BJ, Kusmiesz H, Nelson JD, McCracken GH Jr. Parapneumonic effusions and empyema in hospitalized children: a retrospective review. Pediatr Infect Dis. 1984;3:578-91.
5. Jerng JS, Hsueh PR, Teng LJ, Lee LN, Yang PC, Luh KT. Empyema and lung abscess caused by viridans streptococci. Am J Respir Crit Care Med. 1997;156:1508-14.
6. Ravitch MM, Fein R. The changing picture of pneumonia and empyema in infants and children. JAMA. 1961;175:1039-44.
7. Forbes GB. Diagnosis and management of severe infections in infants and children: a review of experiences since the introduction of sulphonamide therapy. J Pediatr. 1946;29:45-67.
8. Alkrinawi S, Chernick V. Pleural infection in children. Semin Respir Infect. 1996;11:148-54.
9. Chonmaitree T, Powell KR. Parapneumonic pleural effusion and empyema in children. Review of a 19-year experience, 1962–1980. Clin Pediatr. 1983;22:414-9.
10. Tharup J, Ellermann-Eriksen S, Stjernmholm J. Neonatal pleural empyema with group A *Streptococcus*. Acta Paediatr. 1997;86:769-71.
11. Bai KJ, Wul H, Yu MC, Chiang IH, Chiang CY, Lin TP, et al. Tuberculous empyema. Respirology. 1998;3:261-6.
12. Chang AB, Stokes K, Robinson PJ. Bilateral empyema and pneumonia due to chloramphenicol-resistant *Haemophilus influenzae*. Pediatr Pulmonol. 1996;22:207-9.
13. Mangete ED, Kombo BB, Legg-Jack TE. Thoracic empyema: a study of 56 patients. Arch Dis Child. 1993;69:587-8.
14. Mishra OP, Das BK, Jain AK, Lahiri TK, Sen PC, Bhargara V. Clinico-bacteriological study of empyema thoracis in children. J Trop Pediatr. 1993;39:380-1.
15. Bettencourt JD, Barroso A, da Mota HC. Severe pleural effusion due to *Legionella pneumophila* respiratory infection. Arch Ped Adolesc Med. 1994;148:1218-9.
16. Fine NL, Smith LR, Sheedy PF. Frequency of pleural effusions in mycoplasma and viral pneumonias. N Engl J Med. 1970;283:790-3.
17. Munglani R, Kenney IJ. Paediatric parapneumonic effusions: a review of 16 cases. Respir Med. 1991;85:117-9.
18. Asciak R, Kanellakis NI, Bibby A, Kidd A, Gerry S, Mercer R, et al. The Association Between Pleural Fluid Exposure and Survival in Pleural Mesothelioma. Chest. 2021;160(5):1925-33.
19. McCarten KM, Nadel HR, Shulkin BL, Cho SY. Imaging for diagnosis, staging and response assessment of Hodgkin lymphoma and non-Hodgkin lymphoma. Pediatr Radiol. 2019;49(11):1545-64.
20. Paradies G, Zullino F, Orofino A, Leggio S. Mediastinal teratomas in children. Case reports and review of the literature. Ann Ital Chir. 2013;84(4):395-403.
21. Viet LA, Khuyen HK, Hung DQ, Chien LH, Duc HL, Anh NM, et al. Coincidence of juvenile granulosa cell tumor and serous cystadenoma in a pediatric patient: Case report and literature review. Radiol Case Rep. 2021;16(9):2370-5.
22. Laine M, Ghorfi IA, Lambatten D, Kettani F, Abid A. Rapidly fatal Askin's tumor: a case report and literature review. Pan Afr Med J. 2014;18:104.
23. Beghetti *M, La Scala G, Belli D, Bugmann P, Kalangos A, Le Coultre C.* Etiology and management of pediatric chylothorax. J Pediatr. 2000;136(5):653-8.
24. Büttiker V, Fanconi S, Burger R. Chylothorax in children: guidelines for diagnosis and management. Chest. 1999;116(3):682-7.
25. Baniak N, Podberezin M, Kanthan SC, Kanthan R. Primary pulmonary/pleural melanoma in a 13 year-old presenting as pleural effusion. Pathol Res Pract. 2017;213(2):161-4.
26. Ahmed AA, Andraws N, Almutairi AM, Saied HM, Elbagir-Mohamed AM. Cytologic and Immunophenotypic Features of Malignant Cells in Pediatric Body Fluids. Acta Cytol. 2015;59(4):332-8.
27. Xu J, Margol AS, Shukla A, Ren X, Finlay JL, Krieger MD, et al. Disseminated Medulloblastoma in a Child with Germline BRCA2 6174delT Mutation and without Fanconi Anemia. Front Oncol. 2015;5:191.
28. Utine GE, Ozçelik U, Kiper N, Doğru D, Yalçn E, Cobanoğlu N, et al. Pediatric pleural effusions: etiological evaluation in 492 patients over 29 years. Turk J Pediatr. 2009;51(3):214-9.
29. Bender B, Murthy V, Chamberlain RS. The changing management of chylothorax in the modern era. Eur J Cardiothorac Surg. 2016;49:18-24.
30. McGrath EE, Blades Z, Anderson PB. Chylothorax: aetiology, diagnosis and therapeutic options. Respir Med. 2010;104:1-8.
31. Roehr CC, Jung A, Proquitté H, Blankenstein O, Hammer H, Lakhoo K, et al. Somatostatin or octreotide as treatment options for chylothorax in young children: a systematic review. Intensive Care Med. 2006;32:650-7.
32. Haines C, Walsh B, Fletcher M, Davis PJ. Chylothorax development in infants and children in the UK. Arch Dis Child. 2014;99:724-30.
33. Mery CM, Moffett BS, Khan MS, Zhang W, Guzmán-Pruneda FA, Fraser CD Jr, et al. Incidence and treatment of chylothorax after cardiac surgery in children: analysis of a large multi-institution database. J Thorac Cardiovasc Surg. 2014;147:678-86.
34. Shin YR, Lee H, Park YH, Park HK. Chylothorax after Surgery for Congenital Cardiac Disease: A Prevention and Management Protocol. Korean J Thorac Cardiovasc Surg. 2020;53:41-8.
35. Bazancir LA, Jensen RJ, Frevert SC, Ryom P, Achiam MP. Embolization of the thoracic duct in patients with iatrogenic chylothorax. Dis Esophagus. 2021;34:doab001.
36. Gurevich A, Hur S, Singhal S, DiBardino D, Haas AR, Hansen-Flaschen JH, et al. Nontraumatic Chylothorax and Chylopericardium: Diagnosis and Treatment Using an Algorithmic Approach Based on Novel Lymphatic Imaging. Ann Am Thorac Soc. 2022;19:756-62.
37. Quadri A, Thomson AH. Pleural fluids associated with chest infection. Paediatr Respir Rev. 2002;3:349-55.

38. Davies CH, Gleeson FV, Davies RJO. BTS guidelines on the management of pleural infection. Thorax. 2003;58(SupplII): ii18-28.
39. Chippindale AJ, Patel B, Mamtora H. A case of necro bacillosis. Thorax. 1990;45:74-5.
40. Hamm H, Light RW. Parapneumonic effusion and empyema. Eur Respir J. 1997;10:1150-6.
41. Maskell NA, Butland RJA. BTS guidelines for the investigation of a unilateral pleural effusion in adults. Thorax. 2003;58(SupplII):ii8-17.
42. Yone EW, Kenge AP, Moifo B, Kuaban C. Prevalence and determinants of extrapulmonary TB involvement in patients with pulmonary tuberculosis in a Sub-Saharan African country: a cross-sectional study. Scand J Infect Dis. 2013;45:104-11.
43. Valdes L, Alvarez D, San Jose E, Penela P, Valle JM, García-Pazos JM, et al. Tuberculous pleurisy: a study of 254 patients. Arch Intern Med. 1998;158:2017-21.
44. Porcel JM, Light RW. Diagnostic approach to pleural effusion in adults. Am Fam Physician. 2006;73:1211-20.
45. Light RW, MacGregory MI, Luchsinger PC, Ball WC Jr. Pleural effusion: the diagnostic separation of transudates and exudates. Ann Intern Med. 1972;77:507-13.
46. Burgess LJ, Martiz FJ, Talljaard JJF. Comparative analysis of the biochemical parameters used to distinguish between pleural transudates and exudates. *Chest.* 1995;107:1604-9.
47. Light RW. Diagnostic principles in pleural disease. Eur Respir J. 1997;10:476-81.
48. Vives M, Porcel JM, Vicente de Vera M, Ribelles E, Rubio M. A study of Light's criteria and possible modifications for distinguishing exudative from transudative pleural effusions. Chest. 1996;109:1503-7.
49. British Thoracic Society Standards of Care Committee. British Thoracic Society guidelines for the management of community acquired pneumonia in childhood. Thorax. 2002;57(SupplI):i1-24.
50. Stavas J, van Sonnenberg E, Casola G, Wittich GR. Percutaneous drainage of infected and non-infected thoracic fluid collections. J Thoracic Imaging. 1987;2:80-7.
51. Eibenberger KL, Dock WI, Ammann ME, Dorffner R, Hörmann MF, Grabenwöger F. Quantification of pleural effusions: sonography versus radiography. Radiology. 1994;191:681-4.
52. Laws D, Neville E, Duffy J. BTS guidelines for the insertion of a chest drain. Thorax. 2003;58(SupplII):ii53-9.
53. Clementsen P, Evald T, Grode G, Hansen M, Krag Jacobsen G, Faurschou P. Treatment of malignant pleural effusion: pleurodesis using a small bore catheter. A prospective randomized study. Respir Med. 1998;92:593-6.
54. Wells RG, Havens PL. Intrapleural fibrinolysis for parapneumonic effusion and empyema in children. Radiology. 2003;228:370-8.
55. Cohen G, Hjortdal V, Ricci M, Jaffe A, Wallis C, Dinwiddie R, et al. Primary thoracoscopic treatment of empyema in children. J Thorac Cardiovasc Surg. 2003;125:79-83.
56. Costumbrado J, Ghassemzadeh S. Spontaneous Pneumothorax. In: StatPearls [Internet]. Treasure Island (FL): StatPearls Publishing; 2023.
57. Dotson K, Johnson LH. Pediatric spontaneous pneumothorax. Pediatr Emerg Care. 2012;28:715.
58. Roberts ME, Rahman NM, Maskell NA, Bibby AC, Blyth KG, Corcoran JP, et al. British Thoracic Society Guideline for pleural disease. Thorax. 2023;78:1143-56.
59. Baumann MH, Strange C, Heffner JE, Light R, Kirby TJ, Klein J, et al. Management of Spontaneous Pneumothorax: An American College of Chest Physicians Delphi Consensus Statement. Chest. 2001;119(2):590-602.
60. Roberts ME, Rahman NM, Maskell NA; BTS Pleural Guideline Development Group. British Thoracic Society Guideline for pleural disease. Thorax. 2023;78:s1-42.
61. Robinson PD, Cooper P, Ranganathan SC. Evidence-based management of paediatric primary spontaneous pneumothorax. Paediatr Respir Rev. 2009;10:110.
62. Chiu CY, Chen TP, Wang CJ, Tsai MH, Wong KS. Factors associated with proceeding to surgical intervention and recurrence of primary spontaneous pneumothorax in adolescent patients. Eur J Pediatr. 2014;173:1483.
63. Bense L. Spontaneous pneumothorax. Chest. 1992;101:891.
64. O'Lone E, Elphick HE, Robinson PJ. Spontaneous pneumothorax in children: when is invasive treatment indicated? Pediatr Pulmonol. 2008;43:41.
65. Yellin A, Gapany-Gapanavicius M, Lieberman Y. Spontaneous pneumomediastinum: is it a rare cause of chest pain? Thorax. 1983;38:383.
66. Dekel B, Paret G, Szeinberg A, Vardi A, Barzilay Z. Spontaneous pneumomediastinum in children: clinical and natural history. Eur J Pediatr. 1996;155:695.
67. Noorbakhsh KA, Williams AE, Langham JJW, Wu L, Krafty RT, Furtado AD, et al. Management and Outcomes of Spontaneous Pneumomediastinum in Children. Pediatr Emerg Care. 2021;37:e1051.
68. Jougon JB, Ballester M, Delcambre F, Mac Bride T, Dromer CE, Velly JF. Assessment of spontaneous pneumomediastinum: experience with 12 patients. Ann Thorac Surg. 2003;75:1711.
69. Chalumeau M, Le Clainche L, Sayeg N, Sannier N, Michel JL, Marianowski R, et al. Spontaneous pneumomediastinum in children. Pediatr Pulmonol. 2001;31(1):67-75.

CHAPTER

24 Pleural Effusion due to Collagen Vascular Diseases

JN Durga Rao Yadavalli, Rajiva Gupta

INTRODUCTION

Collagen vascular diseases are a heterogeneous group of diseases that affect every part of our body. Pleural effusion is a common manifestation of some of these disorders. It can present as an asymptomatic effusion to causing respiratory compromise necessitating interventions. Some conditions characteristically present with effusion whereas in others it is a rarity. We will discuss pleural effusion in various common connective tissue diseases (CTDs) in the following sections.

SYSTEMIC LUPUS ERYTHEMATOSUS

Systemic lupus erythematosus (SLE) is a prototype autoimmune disease that presents in a heterogeneous manner with involvement in almost every organ in the body.[1] Symptoms range from asymptomatic presentation to life-threatening organ manifestations. Usually, patients present with rash, joint pains, and fever. Serositis encompassing pleural effusion, pericardial effusion and ascites is a common manifestation of SLE. About 50% of the patients have pulmonary involvement during the disease course and can present with respiratory symptoms in 4–5%.[2,3] Pleural involvement is the most common and present in about 45–60% in various studies.[3] Pleural effusion can occur at any time of diseases and it can be the presenting manifestation too. Serositis is a part of the classification criteria of SLE. Recent American College of Rheumatology (ACR)–European Alliance of Associations for Rheumatology (EULAR) classification criteria incorporated serositis with a weightage of five. A total score of ≥10 encompassing clinical and serological domains is helpful in classifying lupus.[4] Pulmonary manifestations occur more commonly in males and in adults compared to children but can be severe and life-threatening.[5,6]

Etiopathogenesis

The exact etiopathogenesis is not known. Various studies have shown the interplay of genetic, environmental, endocrine, and infective factors in the pathogenesis and origin of lupus. Serositis is due to immunological damage to the pleural lining.[7] This leads to protein and fluid leak due to altered permeability of the microvascular circulation due to pleural and peritoneal microvessel inflammation. The role of vasculitis by complement activation and immune complex deposition was described in earlier studies and noted in biopsies of the pleural and peritoneal vessel biopsy specimens.[8-10] A study by Bitran et al. showed granular immunoglobulin G (IgG) and complement deposition and along the mesothelial layer and blood vessels in SLE serositis.[11] Also reduced pleural absorptive capacity and decreased clearance cause rapid fluid accumulation. As in the case of SLE pathogenesis, the role of multiple immune cells and cytokines has been studied.

CLINICAL FEATURES

Pleural effusion can present in various ways ranging from asymptomatic incidental finding to massive effusion causing respiratory compromise.[5,6] It is bilateral in the majority of cases and in unilateral cases, there is no laterality. It occurs usually in the context of systemic disease or flare, but patients can also present with Pleural effusion as the initial or presenting manifestation. Symptoms range from dry cough, shortness of breath, and pleuritic chest pain. Patients also can have other features of SLE such as rash, joint pains, alopecia, oral ulcers, abdominal pain, frothy urine, hematuria, and proteinuria. Usually common in females and in young to middle-aged females. It can also present as a part of polyserositis such as ascites and pericarditis. It is associated with arthritis, rash, low complements, and raised double-stranded deoxyribonucleic acid (dsDNA) antibody levels. Drug-induced lupus (DIL) is a subtype of lupus that is associated with symptoms and clinical features due to some drugs. Commmon drugs causing DIL are sulfonamides, hydralazine, procainamide, and many others.[12] DIL characteristically is associated with antihistone antibodies, arthritis, rash, and serositis. Antinuclear antibodies (ANAs) positivity is seen in 100% of cases. Anti-dsDNA and Smith antigen (Sm) antibodies are rarely seen. Major organ involvement in SLE such as renal and central nervous system (CNS) involvement is almost never seen. Manifestations are usually mild and resolved by stopping offending drugs. In a few proportion of cases, treatment with steroids and other drugs may be necessary.

DIAGNOSIS

The pleural fluid typically is exudative type. Pleural fluid analysis should be done in all cases. Along with it, other tests should be done which will help in diagnosis and they may reveal anemia, leuko- or thrombocytopenia, transaminitis, active urinary sediment, proteinuria, deranged kidney function tests, low complements, and raised anti-dsDNA antibody levels. Pleural fluid is typically exudative in nature. Appearance is serosanguinous and yellowish in color. Lights criteria is used to differentiate transudative from exudative effusion. Exudative effusion has any one of the features: Pleural fluid glucose to serum glucose > 0.5, pleural fluid lactate dehydrogenase (LDH) to serum LDH ratio > 0.6, pleural fluids is more than two-thirds of the upper limit of serum LDH. In SLE patients studies have shown that the pleural fluid glucose is about 60 mg/dL, total protein > 3. 5mg/dL, and LDH < 500 IU/L.[13] Other tests to exclude infection such as adenosine deaminase (ADA) levels, Gram stain, acid-fast bacteria (AFB) stain, fungal stain, aerobic and AFB culture, and gene expert. Malignant cytology should also be done. Other differentials should be actively sought and excluded in every case of pleural effusion. The causes include infections, pulmonary embolism, heart failure, nutrition, parapneumonic effusion, empyema, tuberculosis, and others.

Antinuclear Antibody Levels

Adenosine deaminase is a highly sensitive test for lupus and is an entry criteria for SLE classification as per ACR/EULAR classification criteria.[4] Prevalence is about 99% according to newer studies. ANA-negative lupus is rare. Taking a similar analogy ANA in lupus serositis has been studied. Vinita Khare et al.[14] in their study have shown ANA positivity in 14 of 82 pleural fluid samples. About Six out of eight lupus pleuritic had ANA positivity, with high titers (>1:160, homogenous pattern) in almost all the samples. Recurrent pulmonary emboli and congestive heart failure were the diagnoses in the other two samples. The combination of pleural fluid ANA titer ≥ 1:160, with homogeneous pleural fluid ANA staining patterns and pleural fluid to serum ANA titer ratios ≥ 1 have been suggested as diagnostic tools for lupus pleuritic.[15] Pleural effusions in SLE are enriched in macrophages, neutrophils, basophils, and eosinophils followed by lymphocytes in cases of persistent effusions. Lupus erythematosus cells may be detected although they are not indicative of SLE, as they have been reported in pleural effusions not induced by SLE.[16] Immunohistological examination of pleural tissue biopsies from lupus pleuritis patients reveal deposition of IgG, immunoglobulin M (IgM), and complement (C3) immunoglobulins which show diffuse and speckled patterns within the pleural nuclei.[17,18] LE cells—initially used for lupus diagnosis were also studied in the pleural fluid of SLE patients and were specific but their routine use is not recommended.[19,20]

Pleural Fluid Biopsy

A biopsy is necessary in a few cases where the diagnosis is not found after extensive investigations. Biopsy is usually done through video-assisted thoracic surgery now. Biopsy features are nonspecific, showing lymphocytic and plasma cell infiltration, fibrinous, and fibrotic pleuritic.[20] Indicated to primarily exclude alternative etiologies. Thoracoscopy has revealed nodules on the visceral pleura and immunofluorescence of biopsy samples revealed immunoglobulin deposits.[21]

TREATMENT

It depends on the severity of effusion and other clinical manifestations. Mild effusion may resolve spontaneously or with short-course nonsteroidal anti-inflammatory drugs (NSAIDs). If not responding adequately and in case of moderate effusions steroid course is required and leads to good response.[22] Rapid and dramatic response to steroids is seen in lupus pleuritis compared to effusions in rheumatoid arthritis (RA). If recurrent, immunosuppressants should be added. Massive effusion needs Thoracentesis which can be both diagnostic and therapeutic. An intercostal chest drain (ICD) may be needed to be inserted in case of massive effusions. Pleurodesis (using tetracycline or other agents) and pleurectomy are treatment options in a few cases of refractory serositis.[23-25] Treatment of other major organ manifestations leads to resolution of serositis. There is a chance of recurrence and flares of SLE are associated with serositis. ACR-EULAR guidelines recommend low to moderated dose steroids in the range of 0.3–0.5 mg/kg daily dose for 4–6 weeks. Also, hydroxychloroquine should be used in all cases. There is no long-term data about pleural effusion in SLE.[26,27]

RHEUMATOID ARTHRITIS

Introduction

Rheumatoid arthritis is an autoimmune inflammatory disorder that mainly involves small joints though it can involve large joints too. Some patients can have systemic complications. RA can be associated with various pulmonary complications as well. Interstitial lung disease (ILD) is the most common manifestation which is clinically evident in nearly 10% of the RA population, with an additional 20–50% of participants having evidence of subclinical disease on the computed tomography (CT) scan.[28]

Bronchiectasis or bronchiolectasis is observed in up to 30% of the patients with RA studied with chest CT. Obliterative bronchiolitis can also be associated with RA but the prevalence is low and the prognosis is poor. Other forms of bronchiolar involvement may show an obstructive clinical picture and mosaicism on a CT scan similar to that seen in obliterative bronchiolitis but have a better overall prognosis and may be amenable to immunomodulatory therapy.

Rheumatoid arthritis pulmonary nodules are commonly observed as an incidental finding on chest CT or less frequently in an open lung biopsy.[29] Nodule cavitation may result in hemoptysis or pneumothorax through the rupture of subpleural nodules. Caplan syndrome consists of RA nodules associated with coal miner's pneumoconiosis. Elevated cholesterol levels resulting in sterile empyema and fibrothorax with lung restriction may rarely occur.[30]

Pleural involvement is the most frequent pulmonary manifestation of RA.[30] The incidence of pleural effusion is increasing in patients with RA. Asymptomatic pleural effusion is also common in RA. Only 5% of patients may be symptomatic and pleural disease may be identified on chest radiography in about 20% of patients. Most effusions are unilateral and associated with male gender, high levels of rheumatoid factor (RF), HLA-B8, and *Dw3* genetic subtype.[31]

Etiopathogenesis

Pleural effusion in RA is proposed to be due to dysregulation in humoral responses with high titer of cytokines mainly tumor necrosis factor-alpha levels and decreased levels of interferon-gamma.[32] Cytological examinations of pleural fluid reveal histiocytic spindle cells, multinucleated giant cells, and eosinophilic necrotic debris. The most characteristic histologic finding is the lack of a normal mesothelial cell covering.[33]

Clinical Features

The articular inflammatory activity correlates with pleural disease in most cases but not in all patients with RA. Patients may remain asymptomatic if only a small pleural effusion is present. Chest pain, shortness of breath, and/or fever may be seen in patients with large pleural effusion and pleural thickening.[34] Cough is uncommon unless parenchymal disease is present.[31]

Diagnosis

In most of cases, a chest radiograph may show pleural effusion and/or thickening. In chronic cases, contrast-enhanced computed tomography (CECT) of the chest may be needed for better information on the extent of pleural thickening and may also reveal trapped lungs.[35] A "rheumatoid effusion" is usually an exudative effusion that is sterile with a low pH (<7.3), low glucose (<60 mg/dL), and high LDH (>700 IU/L).[35] In patients with RA-associated pleural effusion, glucose levels below 20 mg/100 mL in pleural fluid and bacteria and acid-fast bacilli negative is almost diagnostic.[36] During diagnosis, usually there is a predominant neutrophil to occur consistent with empyema, and 7–11 days later, the cells in the pleural effusion are replaced by lymphocytes. The pleural effusion with predominant eosinophilia is rare.[37] The fluid can appear "pseudochylous" due to the presence of cholesterol crystals, which importantly differs from a true chylothorax by the absence of triglycerides.[30] The fluid may test positive for RF. White cell count and differential are usually variable but are more commonly lymphocytic predominant; however, neutrophil- and eosinophil-predominant cell counts are also mentioned in the literature. ADA may be high in rheumatoid effusion.[35] The "rheumatoid" nature of the pleural exudate in patients without arthritis mandates a pleural biopsy to exclude tuberculosis or malignancy.

Pleural tapping should be performed for any pleural effusion > 1 cm on decubitus imaging. Infection should always be ruled out, as low pH, low glucose, and high LDH are also typical findings of empyema. Tuberculous and malignant effusions can sometimes mimic rheumatoid effusions. Presentation with sudden onset chest pain with shortness of breath must need evaluation for pulmonary embolism. Pleural biopsy is not indicated but should be performed when the diagnosis is unclear in a rare clinical scenario.[38]

Treatment

The management of the underlying RA can cure most rheumatoid effusions. If small and asymptomatic, no therapy is needed; however, longstanding pleural inflammation can result in trapped lung physiology.[34] Pleuritic pain may be managed with NSAIDs. Glucocorticoids and other immunosuppressive drugs may be needed in chronic recurrent symptomatic effusions and intrapleural steroids efficacy is equivocal.[39,40] Some patients with recurrent large effusions may need intercostal tube drainage and pleurodesis. Decortication can be considered in a patient with trapped lung and/or pleural loculations.[41] The usefulness of cytokines in the course of rheumatoid pleural effusion and the possible role of cytokine blockade in the treatment require further evaluation.[30]

MIXED CONNECTIVE TISSUE DISEASE

Mixed connective tissue disease (MCTD) is a heterogeneous condition comprising SLE, scleroderma, RA, and idiopathic inflammatory myositis (IIM). It was first described by Sharp et al.[42] Anti-U1 ribonucleoprotein antibody (anti U1RNP Ab) and high titers of antinuclear antibody (>1:1,000). It is diagnosed based on Alarcon-Segovia criteria if more than equal to three clinical features [puffy fingers, Raynaud's phenomenon (RP), sclerodactyly, synovitis, and myositis] are present along with high titer anti-RNP Ab (>1:1,600).[43] Component diseases can present simultaneously or they can develop sequentially. RP is the most common manifestation present in 90% of cases. Patients also present with puffy fingers, shortness of breath, joint pains, and muscle weakness and are more prone to pulmonary arterial hypertension (PAH) (20–30% based on echocardiography). Renal and CNS manifestations are uncommon compared to SLE. Symptoms depend on the underlying connective tissue disease.

Pleural effusion is seen in about 50% of cases and in rare cases can be the initial manifestation of disease. It is mostly bilateral and exudative in nature with normal glucose and complement levels. Small-sized effusions are seen in the majority and they resolve spontaneously.[44,45] Treatment is in similar lines as in any CTD.

SYSTEMIC SCLEROSIS

Systemic sclerosis (SSc) or scleroderma is a rare CTD characterized by the triad of inflammation, vasculopathy, and fibrosis.[46] The hallmark feature is fibrosis which commonly manifests as skin thickening: Classified as a limited type—affecting till elbows, knees, and face and a systemic type—affecting the trunk also. ACR/EULAR classification criteria for SSc include components such as skin thickening, digital ulcers, RP, telangiectasia, and abnormal nail fold capillaroscopy, ILD, PAH, SSc-associated antibodies, and defines a score of ≥ 9 for classifying as definite SSc.[47] It is characterized by ANA positivity in 95%[48] and specific antibodies such as antitopoisomerase 1 (anti-Scl-70) with predominant lung involvement (ILD), usually in diffuse type and anticentromere Ab (anti-CENP A/B) in limited type.[49] Anti-RNA polymerase III Ab is associated with renal involvement. Raynaud's phenomenon is an important feature present in about 95%, of gastrointestinal (GI) involvement affecting the upper and lower GI tract, lung involvement in the form of ILD [most common—90% on high-resolution computed tomography (HRCT) imaging], and PAH are seen.

Pleural effusion is uncommon in SSc occurring at 7% compared to pericardial effusion in 17%.[50,51] Usually presents as mild effusion and is exudative in nature. As in other CTDS infections to be ruled out. Treatment is symptomatic with NSAIDs, colchicine, and in-resistant cases steroids are beneficial. Chronic cases necessitate immunosuppressants such as methotrexate. The majority responds to medical management, whereas in few patients surgical intervention may be necessary.[52]

SJÖGREN'S SYNDROME

Sjögren's syndrome (SjS) This is an autoimmune disease characterized by lymphocytic infiltration of exocrine glands and presents with sicca symptoms—oral, ocular, skin, and mucous membranes. It is of two types which include (1) primary—without any underlying condition and (2) secondary—with underlying autoimmune disease. Newer ACR-EULAR classification criteria for SjS gave weightage to objective features such as anti-Ro Ab,

Schirmer's test positivity, and minor salivary gland biopsy (symptoms of lymphocytic infiltration with Focus score ≥1/4 mm^2).[53] Patients present with glandular symptoms predominantly but presentation with extraglandular/systemic symptoms such as joints, heart, CNS, peripheral nervous system (PNS), and lungs is also seen in about 30–40%.[54,55] Lung involvement (clinically significant) is seen in about 9–24%.[56] Pulmonary manifestations include airway disease, ILD (lymphocytic interstitial pneumonitis—characteristic), bronchitis or bronchiolitis, pleural effusion, lymphoproliferative disorders, PAH, and pulmonary embolism. Risk factors of lung involvement are male gender, late onset of disease, smoking, and chronicity.[56-59] Lung involvement is associated with lower quality of life and higher chances of death. It is associated with high antibody levels—ANA, anti-Ro, anti-La antibodies, RF positivity, and hypergammaglobulinemia.

Pleural effusion is a rare presentation of SjS occurring in <1% of cases and described in a few case reports.[60-62] It is exudative in nature and can be both unilateral/bilateral. Levels of ANA and Anti Ro, LA Abs may be elevated in pleural fluid. It is lymphocytic and also low complements may be seen. Pleural thickening is also a rare manifestation. Diagnosis is usually made after excluding other common cases and evaluating for underlying CTDs as it is so rare in SjS. Rarely pleural biopsy may be required. No specific guidelines exist for the treatment. As it is a part of the systemic inflammatory process, controlling the inflammation leads to resolution. The treatment is done with corticosteroids.

SPONDYLOARTHRITIS

Spondyloarthritis (SpA) is a blanket term encompassing different entities such as ankylosing spondylitis (AS), psoriatic arthritis (PsA), reactive arthritis, enteropathic arthritis, and undifferentiated SpA. These present with inflammatory low backache and other seronegative features such as psoriasis, enthesitis, dactylitis, orogenital ulcers, peripheral arthritis, and good response to NSAIDs. Human leukocyte antigen B27 *(HLA-B27)* is a genetic marker associated with SpA group. The prevalence varies in different conditions from 40 to 95%. Assessment of Spondyloarthritis International Society (ASAS) proposed a classification criteria[63] in 2011 which classifies SPA with features of inflammatory low back ache with Imaging [X-ray or magnetic resonance imaging (MRI) features symptoms of sacroiliitis] or HLA-B27 positivity with other seronegative features. These conditions differ from the classical RA with respect to RF and ACPA negativity in the majority, predominant axial involvement, asymmetric peripheral involvement, HLA-B27 positivity, sacroiliitis on X-ray, and presence of seronegative features good response to NSAIDs and biologics.

Lung involvement in the form of apical fibrosis or restrictive lung disease due to chest wall involvement is common. Unlike in RA, pleural effusion is uncommon in SpA. It can be unilateral or bilateral; asymptomatic or can present with cough, pleuritic chest pain, and breathlessness. Diagnosis is in similar lines for other CTDs after excluding other diagnosis. Usually due to other causes rather than the primary disease itself. Few cases reports and case series of pleural effusion have been reported in SpA and PsA.[64,65] Majority of cases were due to drugs [methotrexate and anti-tumor necrosis factor (anti-TNF) alpha blockers] and infections. Improvement with steroids and stoppage of offending drugs is helpful.

ANTINEUTROPHIL CYTOPLASMIC ANTIBODY-ASSOCIATED VASCULITIS

Antineutrophil cytoplasmic antibody (ANCA)-associated vasculitis (AAV) is a type of small vessel vasculitis (involving arterioles, capillaries, and postcapillary venules) which consists of three different diseases—(1) granulomatosis with polyangiitis (GPA), (2) microscopic polyangiitis (MPA), (3) and eosinophilic granulomatosis with polyangiitis (EGPA). These are characterized by ANCA. They are Anti-PR3 antibodies (Anti-PR3) and Antimyeloperoxidase antibodies (Anti-MPO). Characteristic features of these diseases are lung involvement (nodules, cavities, infiltrates, and diffuse alveolar hemorrhage), renal involvement (rapidly progressive renal failure, hematuria, proteinuria, and active urinary sediments), upper respiratory tract involvement, and mononeuritis multiplex. EGPA patients have refractory asthma and atopy.

Cytoplasmic antineutrophil cytoplasmic antibody (C-ANCA) is present in 90% of GPA whereas the perinuclear antineutrophil cytoplasmic antibodies (P-ANCA) pattern is present in MPA in 80%. Either C-ANCA or P-ANCA positivity seen in about 60% in EGPA and in a small subset of GPA can have a P-ANCA pattern and MPA with a c-ANCA pattern. Anti-PR3 antibody is predominantly associated with GPA (90%), and anti-MPO antibody with MPA (90%). Biopsy of the involved organ shows necrotizing granulomatous inflammation with infiltration of small vessel walls with neutrophils and necrosis/debris (leukocytoclastic vasculitis—pathological hallmark).

Respiratory involvement is seen in about 70% at presentations and 90% during the course. Pleural effusion in the setting of ANCA vasculitis is uncommon. About 10% of GPA patients present with pleural involvement.[66] Presentation is with pleural effusion or pleural thickening.

The cause may be due to previous effusion or sequelae of inflammatory lesions extending to the pleura (e.g., nodules).[67] Other features of pulmonary involvement such as nodules, cavities, and infiltrates may be associated. Effusion is unilateral mostly, low in volume, and exudative in nature.[68,69] Biochemical analysis shows low glucose and high protein levels; neutrophilic predominant and sterile unless infected. Similar to other CTDs: Infection, malignancy, and other differentials should be ruled out first. Isolated pleural effusion is rare and it is a part of the systemic inflammatory process. Treatment is with steroids and immunosuppressive agents such as cyclophosphamide or rituximab in case of severe or life-threatening manifestations while minor organ or less severe disease is treated with methotrexate, azathioprine, or mycophenolate mofetil.[70]

MISCELLANEOUS

Sarcoidosis is a granulomatous disease affecting the lungs, lymph nodes, skin, joints, and other organs. Histopathologically characterized by granulomatous inflammation and is a close differential to tuberculosis and has anergy as a characteristic feature (Mantoux test—negative).[71,72] Lung involvement is a common manifestation seen in about 90% of cases. Pleural effusion is rare (1%). Pleural effusion is due to active granulomatous inflammation and corticosteroids are the mainstay of therapy.[73] Behçet's disease (BD) is a multisystem vasculitis of variable clinical presentation. Pulmonary involvement is uncommon, with pleural effusion being a rarer manifestation reported in few case reports.[74]

Pleurisy and pleural effusions are rarely seen with adult-onset Still's disease (AOSD). Among 28 patients with AOSD, Uppal et al.[75] reported 17.9% of patients had a pleural effusion. In patients with AOSD, the pleural fluid is exudative with an abundance of neutrophils.[76]

Familial Mediterranean fever is an autosomal recessive disease that is mostly seen in Armenians and Sephardic Jews in the Mediterranean countries.[77] It is a familial paroxysmal polyserositis which is an uncommon cause for paroxysmal attacks of fever and pleurisy, and sometimes with pleural effusion. The early attack is seen before 20 years of age and is characteristically dominated by peritoneal signs and symptoms. Chest imaging during the acute pleuritic attacks shows elevation of the ipsilateral diaphragm and occasionally minimal pleural effusion.[78] The pleural fluid analysis consists predominantly of neutrophils.[79] The attacks are recurrent within days to months, with a quiescent period between the attacks. Treatment is with colchicine; however, it is difficult to establish a diagnosis.[80]

Rarely patients with temporal arteritis,[81] Takayasu's arteritis,[82] Kawasaki disease,[83] and dermatomyositis[84] have a pleural effusion which usually results from other complications than from primary disease such as heart failure, pulmonary embolism, and pneumonia.

KEY POINTS

- Pleural effusion is a common characteristic in a few CTDs such as SLE and RA and can present as small to massive effusions.
- Diagnosis should made on a high index of clinical suspicion in case of pleural effusion as initial presentation of CTD.
- In patients with CTD, though diagnosis seems obvious, infections and other etiologies have to be ruled out before making a final decision as they are the most common underlying etiologies.
- It might suggest a flare or a part of a systemic response.
- Treatment depends on the cause and severity of presentation necessitating medical management to surgical procedures in a few cases.
- High index of suspicion and good clinical judgment should be a priority in the diagnosis.

REFERENCES

1. Tsokos GC. Systemic lupus erythematosus. N Engl J Med. 2011;365(22):2110-21.
2. Vitali C, Bencivelli W, Isenberg DA, Smolen JS, Snaith ML, Sciuto M, et al. Disease activity in systemic lupus erythematosus: Report of the Consensus Study Group of the European Workshop for Rheumatology Research. I. A descriptive analysis of 704 European lupus patients. European Consensus Study Group for Disease Activity in SLE. Clin Exp Rheumatol. 1992;10(5):527-39.
3. Crestani B. The respiratory system in connective tissue disorders. Allergy. 2005;60(6):715-34.
4. Aringer M. EULAR/ACR classification criteria for SLE. Semin Arthritis Rheum. 2019;49(3S):S14-7.
5. Ciftçi E, Yalçinkaya F, Ince E, Ekim M, Ileri M, Orgerin Z, et al. Pulmonary involvement in childhood-onset systemic lupus erythematosus: A report of five cases. Rheumatology (Oxford). 2004;43(5):587-91.
6. Rabinovich CE. Pulmonary complications of childhood rheumatic disease. Paediatr Respir Rev. 2012;13(1):29-36.
7. Bouros D, Pneumatikos I, Tzouvelekis A. Pleural involvement in systemic autoimmune disorders. Respiration. 2008;75(4):361-71.
8. Ishiguro N, Tomino Y, Fujito K, Nakayama S, Koide H. A case of massive ascites due to lupus peritonitis with a dramatic response to steroid pulse therapy. Jpn J Med. 1989;28(5):608-11.
9. Ito H, Nanamiya W, Kuroda N, Inoue M, S asaoka A, Chijiwa T, et al. Chronic lupus peritonitis with massive ascites at elderly onset: case report and review of the literature. Intern Med. 2002;41(11):1056-61.

10. Mitra B, Sengupta P, Saha K, Sarkar N, Pal J. Systemic lupus erythematosus presenting with recurrent pleural effusion without any systemic manifestation. J Assoc Physicians India. 2005;53:1073-6.
11. Bitran J, McShane D, Ellman MH. Arthritis Rounds: Ascites as the major manifestation of systemic lupus erythematosus. Arthritis Rheum. 1976;19(4):782-5.
12. Pretel M, Marquès L, España A. Drug-induced lupus erythematosus. Actas Dermosifiliogr. 2014;105(1):18-30.
13. Good JT Jr, King TE, Antony VB, Sahn SA. Lupus pleuritis. Clinical features and pleural fluid characteristics with special reference to pleural fluid antinuclear antibodies. Chest. 1983;84(6):714-8.
14. Khare V, Baethge B, Lang S, Wolf RE, Campbell Jr GD. Antinuclear antibodies in pleural fluid. Chest. 1994;106(3):866-71.
15. Porcel JM, Ordi-Ros J, Esquerda A, Vives M, Madroñero AB, Bielsa S, et al. Antinuclear antibody testing in pleural fluid for the diagnosis of lupus pleuritis. Lupus. 2007;16(1):25-7.
16. Wang DY, Yang PC, Yu WL, Shiah DC, Kuo HW, Hsu NY. Comparison of different diagnostic methods for lupus pleuritis and pericarditis: a prospective three-year study. J Formos Med Assoc. 2000;99(5):375-80.
17. Chandrasekhar AJ, Robinson J, Barr L. Antibody deposition in the pleura: a finding in drug-induced lupus. J Allergy Clin Immunol. 1978;61(6):399-402.
18. Pertschuk LP, Moccia LF, Rosen Y, Lyons H, Marino CM, Rashford AA, et al. Acute pulmonary complications in systemic lupus erythematosus. Immunofluorescence and light microscopic study. Am J Clin Pathol. 1977;68(5):553-7.
19. Naylor B. Cytological aspects of pleural, peritoneal and pericardial fluids from patients with systemic lupus erythematosus. Cytopathology. 1992;3(1):1-8.
20. Pandya MR, Agus B, Grady RF. Letter: In vivo LE phenomenon in pleural fluid. Arthritis Rheum. 1976;19(5):962-3.
21. Mathlouthi A, Ben M'rad S, Merai S, Kovitz KL, Slabbynck H, Djenayah F. Massive pleural effusion in systemic lupus erythematosus: thoracoscopic and immunohistological findings. Monaldi Arch Chest Dis. 1998;53(1):34-6.
22. Karkhanis VS, Joshi JM. Pleural effusion: Diagnosis, treatment, and management. Open Access Emerg Med. 2012;4:31-52.
23. Gilleece MH, Evans CC, Bucknall RC. Steroid resistant pleural effusion in systemic lupus erythematosus treated with tetracycline pleurodesis. Ann Rheum Dis. 1988;47(12):1031-2.
24. McKnight KM, Adair NE, Agudelo CA. Successful use of tetracycline pleurodesis to treat massive pleural effusion secondary to systemic lupus erythematosus. Arthritis Rheum. 1991;34(11):1483-4.
25. Elborn JS, Conn P, Roberts SD. Refractory massive pleural effusion in systemic lupus erythematosus treated by pleurectomy. Ann Rheum Dis. 1987;46(1):77-80.
26. Aringer M, Costenbader K, Daikh D, Brinks R, Mosca M, Ramsey-Goldman R, et al. 2019 European League Against Rheumatism/American College of Rheumatology classification criteria for systemic lupus erythematosus. Arthritis Rheumatol. 2019;71(9):1400-12.
27. Hannah JR, D'Cruz DP. Pulmonary complications of systemic lupus erythematosus. Semin Respir Crit Care Med. 2019;40(2):227-34.
28. Brown KK. Rheumatoid lung disease. Proc Am Thorac Soc. 2007;4(5):350-7.
29. Glace B, Gottenberg JE, Maretti X, Philippe R, Pereira B, Lequerré T, et al. Efficacy of rituximab in the treatment of pulmonary rheumatoid nodules: findings in 10 patients from the French autoimmunity and Rituximab/rheumatoid arthritis registry (AIR/PR registry). Ann Rheum Dis. 2012;71(8):1429-31.
30. Balbir-Gurman A, Yigla M, Nahir AM, Braun-Moscovici Y. Rheumatoid pleural effusion. Sem Arthritis Rheum. 2006;35(6):368-78.
31. Esposito AJ, Chu SG, Madan R, Doyle TJ, Dellaripa PF. Thoracic Manifestations of Rheumatoid Arthritis. Clin Chest Med. 2019;40(3):545-60.
32. Soderblom T, Nyberg P, Teppo AM, Klockars M, Riska H, Pettersson T. Pleural fluid interferon-gamma and tumour necrosis factor-alpha in tuberculosis and rheumatoid pleurisy. Eur Respir J. 1996;9(8):1652-5.
33. Faurschou P, Francis D, Faarup P. Thoracoscopic, histological, and clinical findings in nine case of rheumatoid pleural effusion. Thorax. 1985;40(5):371-5.
34. Komarla A, Yu GH, Shahane A. Pleural effusion, pneumothorax, and lung entrapment in rheumatoid arthritis. J Clin Rheumatol. 2015;21(4):211-5.
35. Yokosuka T, Suda A, Sugisaki M, Suzuki M, Narato R, Saito H, et al. Rheumatoid pleural effusion presenting as pseudochylothorax in a patient without previous diagnosis of rheumatoid arthritis. Respir Med Case Rep. 2013;10:37-9.
36. Corcoran JP, Ahmad M, Mukherjee R, Redmond KC. Pleuro-pulmonary complications of rheumatoid arthritis. Respir Care. 2014;59(4):e55-9.
37. Dodson WH, Hollingsworth JW. Pleural effusion in rheumatoid arthritis. Impaired transport of glucose. N Engl J Med. 1966;275(24):1337-42.
38. Avnon LS, Abu-Shakra M, Flusser D, Heimer D, Sion-Vardy N. Pleural effusion associated with rheumatoid arthritis: what cell predominance to anticipate? Rheumatol Int. 2007;27(10):919-25.
39. Walker WC, Wright V. Rheumatoid pleuritis. Ann Rheum Dis. 1967;26(6):467-74.
40. Chapman PT, O'Donnell JL, Moller PW. Rheumatoid pleural effusion: response to intrapleural corticosteroid. J Rheumatol. 1992;19(3):478-80.
41. Russell ML, Gladman DD, Mintz S. Rheumatoid pleural effusion: lack of response to intrapleural corticosteroid. J Rheumatol. 1986;13(2):412-5.
42. Sharp GC. Mixed connective tissue disease and antinuclear antibodies. Diagnostic criteria for classification of MCTD. Amsterdam: Elsevier; 1987. pp. 23-32.
43. Alarcon-Segovia D, Villarreal M. Classification and diagnostic criteria for mixed connective tissue disease. In: Kasukawa R, Sharp GC (Eds). Mixed connective tissue disease and antinuclear antibodies. Amsterdam: Elsevier; 1987. pp. 33-40.
44. Prakash UB. Respiratory complications in mixed connective tissue disease. Clinics Chest Med. 1998;19(4):733-46.
45. Kundi M, Assad S, Babar S, Ghani U, Hammad S, Sheikh AG, et al. Mixed connective tissue disorder complicated by polymyositis, sjogren's syndrome, pleural effusion and pericarditis. Cureus. 2016;8(12):e906.
46. Denton CP, Khanna D. Systemic sclerosis. Lancet. 2017;390(10103):1685-99.
47. van den Hoogen F, Khanna D, Fransen J, Johnson SR, Baron M, Tyndall A, et al. Classification criteria for systemic sclerosis: an ACR-EULAR collaborative initiative. Arthritis Rheum. 2013;65(11):2737-47.
48. Steen VD. Autoantibodies in systemic sclerosis. Semin Arthritis Rheum. 2005;35(1):35-42.

49. Hughes M, Allanore Y, Chung L, Pauling JD, Denton CP, Matucci-Cerinic M. Raynaud phenomenon and digital ulcers in systemic sclerosis. Nat Rev Rheumatol. 2020;16(4):208-21.
50. Thompson AE, Pope JE. A study of the frequency of pericardial and pleural effusions in scleroderma. Br J Rheumatol. 1998;37(12):1320-3.
51. Yee BL, Varada NL, Rahimi OM, Palma CF, Al-Taweel OS, Ahsan CH. Scleroderma as an Uncommon Cause of Pericardial Effusion. Kans J Med. 2022;15:257-8.
52. In: Cerinic MM, Denton CP (Eds). Practical Management of Systemic Sclerosis in Clinical Practice. Germany: Springer; 2021.
53. Shiboski CH, Shiboski SC, Seror R, Criswell LA, Labetoulle M, Lietman TM, et al. 2017. 2016 American College of Rheumatology/European League Against Rheumatism classification criteria for primary Sjögren's syndrome: a consensus and data-driven methodology involving three international patient cohorts. Arthritis Rheumatol. 2017;69(1):35-45.
54. Retamozo S, Brito-Zeron P, Zeher M, Kathy LS, Seror R, Mandl T, et al. Epidemiologic subsets drive a differentiated clinical and immunological presentation of primary Sjögren syndrome: Analysis of 9302 patients from the Big Data International Sjögren Cohort. Arthritis Rheumatol. 2017;69(Suppl 10).
55. Fox RI. Sjögren's syndrome. Lancet. 2005;366(9482):321-31.
56. Palm Ø, Garen T, Enger TB, Jensen JL, Lund MB, Aaløkken TM, et al. Clinical pulmonary involvement in primary Sjogren's syndrome: prevalence, quality of life and mortality--a retrospective study based on registry data. Rheumatology (Oxford). 2013;52(1):173-9.
57. Ramos-Casals M, Solans R, Rosas J, Camps MT, Gil A, Del Pino-Montes J, et al. Primary Sjögren syndrome in Spain: clinical and immunologic expression in 1010 patients. Medicine (Baltimore). 2008;87(4):210-9.
58. García-Carrasco M, Ramos-Casals M, Rosas J, Pallarés L, Calvo-Alen J, Cervera R, et al. Primary Sjögren syndrome: clinical and immunologic disease patterns in a cohort of 400 patients. Medicine (Baltimore). 2002;81(4):270-80.
59. Aerni MR, Vassallo R, Myers JL, Lindell RM, Ryu JH. Follicular bronchiolitis in surgical lung biopsies: clinical implications in 12 patients. Respir Med. 2008;102(2):307-12.
60. Horita Y, Miyazaki M, Kadota Ji, Watanabe T, Yamashita M, Nishiura K, et al. Type II diabetes mellitus and primary Sjögren's syndrome complicated by pleural effusion. Intern Med. 2000;39(11):979-84.
61. Tanaka A, Tohda Y, Fukuoka M, Nakajima S. A case of Sjögren's syndrome with pleural effusion. Nihon Kokyuki Gakkai Zasshi. Nihon Kokyuki Gakkai Zasshi. 2000;38(8):628-31.
62. Teshigawara K, Kakizaki S, Horiya M, Kikuchi Y, Hashida T, Tomizawa Y, et al. Primary Sjogren's syndrome complicated by bilateral pleural effusion. Respirology. 2008;13(1):155-8.
63. Rudwaleit MV, van der Heijde D, Landewé R, Akkoc N, Brandt J, Chou CT, et al. The Assessment of SpondyloArthritis International Society classification criteria for peripheral spondyloarthritis and for spondyloarthritis in general. Ann Rheum Dis. 2011;70(1):25-31.
64. Erkan L, Uzun O, Findik S, Atici AG, Ozkaya S. Isolated pleural and pericardial effusion in a patient with ankylosing spondylitis. Respir Med. 2007;101(2):356-8.
65. Venetsanopoulou AI, Markatseli TE, Iliou C, Tziortzioti Z, Argyropoulou MI, Drosos AA, et al. Pleural effusion in psoriatic arthritis patients: a case series and review of the literature. Clinical Rheumatol. 2021;40(11):4741-8.
66. Reuter M, Schnabel A, Wesner F, Tetzlaff K, Risheng Y, Gross WL, et al. Pulmonary Wegener's granulomatosis: correlation between high-resolution CT findings and clinical scoring of disease activity. Chest. 1998;114(2):500-6.
67. Kumasaka T, Mitani K, Izumi H, Miyamoto H, Takahashi K, Fukuchi Y, et al. Small vessel vasculitis limited to pleuropulmonary manifestations, possibly induced by endotoxin. Histopathology. 2003;43(2):189-93.
68. Blundell AG, Roe S. Wegener's granulomatosis presenting as a pleural effusion. BMJ. 2003;327(7406):95-6.
69. McCann JL, Morris ZQ. Wegener granulomatosis presenting as an eosinophilic pleural effusion. Chest. 2006;130:327S.
70. Diot E, Lavigne C, Renjard L, Asquier E, Valentin JF, Legras A, et al. Wegener's disease mimicking acute infectious pleurisy. Rev Pneumol Clin. 2000;56(4):265-8.
71. Hellmich B, Sanchez-Alamo B, Schirmer JH, Berti A, Blockmans D, Cid MC, et al. EULAR recommendations for the management of ANCA-associated vasculitis: 2022 update. Ann Rheum Dis. 2023;ard-2022-223764.
72. Albakri M, Ahmad M, Mohamed MFH. Rapidly recurring massive pleural effusion as the initial presentation of sarcoidosis: A case report. Medicine (Baltimore). 2021;100(6):e24027.
73. Chopra A, Foulke L, Judson MA. Sarcoidosis associated pleural effusion: Clinical aspects. Respir Med. 2022;191:106723.
74. Alkhurassi HF, Ocheltree MR, Alsomali A, Alqunfoidi RA, Saadallah A Sr. Pleural Effusion Presenting in a Young Man With Behcet's Disease. Cureus. 2020;12(9):e10273.
75. Uppal SS, Al-Mucairi M, Hayat S, Abraham M, Malaviya A. Ten years of clinical experience with adult onset Still's disease: is the outcome improving? Clin Rheumatol. 2006;26(7):1055-60.
76. Ferreiro L, Alvarez-Dobano JM, Valdes L. Systemic diseases and the pleural. Arch Bronchopneumol. 2011;47(7):361-70.
77. Sohar E, Gafni J, Pras M, Heller H. Familial Mediterranean fever. A survey of 470 cases and review of the literature. Am J Med. 1967;43(2):227-53.
78. Ehrenfeld EN, Eliakim M, Rachmilewitz M. Recurrent polyserositis (familial Mediterranean fever; periodic disease): A report of fifty-five cases. Am J Med. 1961;31(1):107-23.
79. Katsenos S, Mermigkis C, Psathakis K, Tsintiris K, Polychronopoulos V, Panagou P, et al. Unilateral lymphocytic pleuritis as a manifestation of familial Mediterranean fever. Chest. 2008;133(4):999-1001.
80. Dinarello CA, Wolff SM, Goldfinger SE, Dale DC, Alling DW. Colchicine therapy for familial Mediterranean fever. A double-blind trial. N Engl Med. 1974;291(18):934-7.
81. Marie I, Heliot P, Muir JF, Roussel F, Levesque H, Courtois H. Pleural effusion revealing giant cell arteritis. Eur Intern Med. 2004;15(2):125-7.
82. Chen L, Ma T, Wang L, Wang L, Li M, Zhu R. Unilateral pleural effusion secondary to Takayasu arteritis: a case report and literature review. J Biomed Res. 2022;36(2):141-4.
83. Hamada H, Terai M, Honda T, Kohno Y. Marked pleural and pericardial effusion with elevated vascular endothelial growth factor production: an uncommon complication of Kawasaki disease. Pediatr Int. 2005;47(1):112-4.
84. Matsuoka N, Asano T, Sato S, Sasajima T, Fujita Y, Temmoku J, et al. A case of dermatomyositis complicated with pleural effusion and massive ascites. Fukushima J Med Sci. 2020;65(3):140-5.

CHAPTER

25 Pleural Effusion due to Kidney Diseases

Amit Kumar Mahapatra, Shabd Prakash

INTRODUCTION

The prevalence of pleural effusion (PE) in kidney disease patients depends upon the type and stage of the kidney disease. The two most prominent types of kidney diseases, based on time frame, are acute and chronic. Many of times they have different etiologies and pathophysiologies and the prevalence rate of PE varies in both the cases.

In tuberculosis (TB)-endemic areas like India, tubercular PE is the most common cause of unilateral and even bilateral PE in the general population.[1] Chronic kidney disease (CKD) patients are at a 6.9–52.5-fold higher risk of developing TB than the general population.[2] Yet the incidence of transudative PE is more common than exudative PE in patients with kidney diseases.[3,4] The most common factor leading to higher incidences of transudative PE is fluid overload, followed by congestive heart failure (CHF).[5] The etiology of exudative PE in cases of CKD varies in different studies with TB being the most common cause, especially in endemic regions,[6,7] while few other studies cite uremia as the most common cause.[5] PE in patients with CKD is more prevalent in stage 5D [Kidney Disease: Improving Global Outcomes (KDIGO)[8] stage G5, dialysis dependent]. This is followed by stage 5ND (KDIGO stage G5, nondialysis dependent) and stage 4. The incidence of PE is common (as high as 21%) in long-term hemodialysis patients who are hospitalized for various reasons.[5,9]

Diagnosing and treating PE in patients with kidney disease are of utmost importance as it affects patient outcomes, with increased mortality being seen with patients on maintenance hemodialysis[10] or peritoneal dialysis[11] (PD) who have PE.

ETIOLOGY

Pleural effusion in kidney disease can be due to various etiologies as shown in **Flowchart 1**.

In this chapter, we discuss the pathophysiology of PE in patients with kidney disease and some specific situations

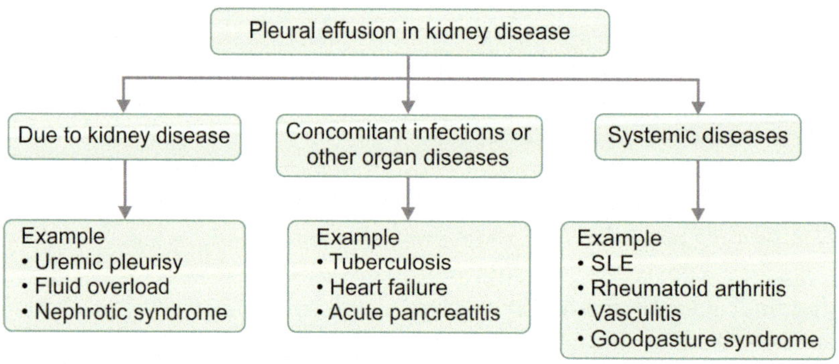

FLOWCHART 1: Pleural effusion in kidney disease.

(SLE: systemic lupus erythematosus)

of both transudative and exudative PE with underlying contributory kidney diseases.

Pleural Effusion in Acute Kidney Injury

Acute kidney injury (AKI) denotes a sudden and often reversible reduction in kidney function, as measured by glomerular filtration rate (GFR). AKI can lead to the accumulation of water, sodium, and other metabolic products along with acid–base disturbances.

The most important of these is volume overload which can lead to pulmonary edema and PE. In AKI, water retention causes increased vascular hydrostatic pressure causing fluid leakage into the interstitial space. Oliguric (<400–500 mL/day urine output in 24 h) AKI rather than nonoliguric AKI can lead more often to fluid overload. Apart from fluid overload, there is "organ crosstalk" where AKI can predispose to acute lung injury (ALI) that can lead to associated PE as well.

The proposed pathophysiology in ALI in the case of AKI is as follows:[12]

- *Inflammatory mediators*:
  - Cellular:
    - Systemic inflammation which increases CD8+ T lymphocyte trafficking to the lungs leading to apoptosis of pulmonary cells and disruption of the microvascular barrier.
    - Native macrophages in the kidney activate and increase tumor necrosis factor alpha (TNF-α) pro-inflammatory mediator which leads to an increase in neutrophil infiltration and neutrophil extracellular trap (NET) localization in the lungs.
- *Pro-inflammatory cytokines*:
  - Interleukin-6 (IL-6), IL-8, monocyte chemoattractant protein 1 (MCP-1), TNF-α, tumor necrosis factor receptor 1 (TNFR1), and caspase-3
- *Noninflammatory mediators*:
  - Uremic toxins: Indoxyl sulfate, p-cresyl sulfate, etc.
  - Indirectly increasing pro-inflammatory cytokines
  - Directly reducing pulmonary gene expressions of aquaporin 1 and 5 and epithelial Na^+ channels.
  - Reduced soluble α-klotho
  - Increased angiopoietin 2 in circulation

Concomitant cardiovascular dysfunction due to both fluid overload and organ crosstalk phenomenon can precipitate cardiogenic pulmonary edema and can lead to unilateral or bilateral PE. In most cases, both cardiogenic and noncardiogenic reasons coexist in patients who developed pulmonary edema and associated PE.[13]

Systemic diseases such as acute pancreatitis and sepsis of other organs can cause AKI and PE. The cause of PE can be both due to systemic inflammatory syndrome initiated by the primary organ and due to AKI causing fluid overload.

Pleural Effusion in Chronic Kidney Disease

Chronic kidney disease is defined as the presence of markers of kidney damage or reduced GFR < 60 mL/min/1.73 m^2 for 3 months or more. CKD is classified based on the estimated glomerular filtration rate (eGFR) and the level of proteinuria and helps to risk stratify patients. Patients are classified as G1–G5, based on the eGFR, and A1–A3, based on the albumin:creatinine ratio (ACR).[8]

Pleural effusion is caused by an imbalance in the relationship between various forces in the body, including hydrostatic pressure, osmotic pressure, and capillary permeability, as described by the Frank–Starling mechanism. The resulting effusions can be categorized as either transudate, which is caused by an increase in hydrostatic pressure or a decrease in serum oncotic pressure, or exudate, which is a protein-rich fluid caused by increased capillary permeability. Common causes of both types of pleural effusion has been described in **Table 1**.

Transudative Pleural Effusion in Chronic Kidney Disease

Alternation in the systemic factors influencing the formation and absorption of the pleural fluids leads to the accumulation of the pleural fluid and the formation of transudative PE. Pleural fluid originates from the plasma of subpleural capillaries at the rate of 0.5 mL/min or 0.4 mL/kg/h. The increased hydrostatic pressure due to hypervolemia in the case of CKD leads to an increased rate

TABLE 1: Common causes of pleural effusion in chronic kidney disease.

Types of pleural effusion	Common etiologies
Transudative pleural effusion	• Fluid overload/increased hydrostatic pressure • Reduced oncotic pressure/low albumin • Congestive heart failure (CHF) • Superior vena cava obstruction (catheter related) • Peritoneal dialysis leak • Urinothorax
Exudative pleural effusion	• Infections (TB, viral, fungal, parasitic, etc.) • Connective tissue diseases (rheumatoid, SLE, vasculitis, etc.) • Malignancy (metastatic/mesothelioma) • Uremic pleuritis

(SLE: systemic lupus erythematosus; TB: tuberculosis)

of formation of pleural fluid. This phenomenon also gets accentuated by the lower albumin, more specifically lower oncotic pressure which fails to prevent fluid flux from the capillaries.[14] In case of CHF or pulmonary embolism, the origin of PE is probably the pulmonary interstitial space which enters pleural space via visceral pleura.

In addition, pulmonary atelectasis can increase negative pressure in the pleural space leading to an increase in pleural fluid formation. When the rate of appearance of pleural fluid exceeds the rate of removal predominantly by lymphatics and subpleural venular capillaries, PE starts appearing. Lymphatic flow rates can also get reduced in cases of CHF, atelectasis, and increased abdominal pressure.

- *Fluid overload in CKD*: This is a common phenomenon, especially in advanced stages. With the decrease in GFR, renal salt handling is hampered that leads to salt retention and compensatory extracellular fluid (ECF) volume expansion. Urine output decreases in advanced kidney disease and accentuates the fluid accumulation in the body.
- *Low oncotic pressure in CKD*: In CKD patients, the higher the urine albumin excretion, the higher the risk of lower albumin. Patients who have nephrotic range proteinuria have a higher risk of developing anasarca and consequently PE. Malnutrition in cases of advanced kidney disease due to uremic decreased appetite and associated comorbidities such as chronic liver disease can also lead to hypoalbuminemia.

Congestive Heart Failure in Chronic Kidney Disease

Chronic kidney disease increases the risk of heart failure by more than one mechanism, the most common being volume overload, which is a modifiable risk factor. Associated features such as anemia, hypertension, proteinuria, arterial stiffness, and inflammation can all lead to heart failure. The precipitated heart failure, in the phenomenon of cardiorenal syndrome, can lead to further deterioration of renal function. The PE accompanying CHF is usually right sided. Jarratt and Sahn in their study found CHF to be the most common cause of PE in hospitalized CKD-5D patients.[9] Bakirci et al. had noted that transudative PE resulted from hypervolemia in 66.7% and heart failure in 22.2% of patients.[5]

Peritoneal Dialysis Leak

Patients of CKD stage 5D who are initiated on continuous ambulatory peritoneal dialysis (CAPD) have the risk of getting hydrothorax in the range of 1–10%.[15] A previously unidentified congenital or acquired defect in the diaphragmatic muscle fibers or connective tissue, which causes an abnormal communication between the peritoneum and pleural space, gets exposed after the PD fluid is put into the abdomen resulting in increased intra-abdominal pressure (IAP). This communication can lead to the translocation of dialysate into the pleural space in patients on CAPD when there is a higher pleuro-peritoneal pressure gradient due to the increased IAP. High dwell volumes, chronic cough, or straining can hasten the occurrence of hydrothorax in these patients. Diagnosis can be made by thoracentesis. "Sweet" hydrothorax is used to describe this condition due to high glucose concentration. Peritoneal scintigraphy, which involves the use of technetium-99m tagged macroaggregated albumin or Tc-99m sulfur colloid, is a noninvasive method for confirming abnormal communication between the pleural and peritoneal cavities. Treatment includes reducing PD volume or interruption of PD for 4–6 weeks which may help in healing of minor defects. For recurrent PE, pleurodesis can be attempted via videothoracoscopy or video-assisted thoracoscopic surgery (VATS). For larger diaphragmatic defects, surgical stapling by VATS can be done.

Urinothorax

Urinothorax (UT) is a rare form of PE that occurs due to the accumulation of urine in the pleural space, which is caused by a trauma or blockage of the urinary tract. The term urinothorax first coined by Friedland in 1971,[16] though its pathophysiology was explained by Corriere et al. in 1968 in an animal model.[17] A systematic review in 2017 by Toubes et al. found only 78 studies over a span of 62 years.[18]

The causes include obstructive uropathy (due to tumor, stone, stricture, prostate hypertrophy, posterior urethral valves, etc.) and trauma, both iatrogenic [nephrostomy tube, lithotripsy like percutaneous nephrolithotomy (PCNL), ureterorenoscopic lithotripsy (URSL) or shockwave lithotripsy (SWL), renal biopsy, etc.] and blunt abdominal trauma affecting kidney and urinary tract. The duration between the initial triggering incident and the onset of UT can vary from 8 hours to 2 months, with a majority of cases being identified within 2 days of the initial event.

The mechanism of urine transit to pleural space has many theories. Obstructive uropathy leading to urinoma formation can cause increased retroperitoneal or intraperitoneal pressure leading to migration of urine through diaphragmatic lymphatics. Urine can also travel through direct anatomical defects of the diaphragm. In cases of traumatic origin, the disruption of urinary excretion pathways was associated with unilateral PE. However, in the absence of trauma, unilateral ureteral or kidney obstruction does not produce UT if the contralateral kidney's function is preserved. Only obstruction of both ureters, the urethra, or the bladder can divert urine, causing ascites and subsequent UT.

The clinical scenario along with unilateral PE usually points toward the etiology. Pleural fluid analysis shows transudative character with low cell count (50–1,500) and mononuclear nature. The smell of urine may or may not be present. The diagnostic finding is pleural fluid to serum creatinine ratio > 1, low glucose level, and pH < 7.4. In fact, it is the only cause of PE which has acidic pH. Computed tomography (CT) urography or technetium-99m renal scan can point toward the origin of effusion. Early identification and understanding of the root cause are crucial in the treatment of UT, which can be reversed by addressing its primary cause.

Exudative Pleural Effusion in Chronic Kidney Disease

Uremic Pleuritis

Richard Bright in his paper in 1836 observed frequent involvement of pleura in kidney diseases (only 29 out of 100 patients with albuminous urine had normal pleura at autopsy), but fell short of mentioning pleural involvement due to uremia.[19] Hoops and Wissler in their paper in 1955 described uremic pneumonitis and accompanied fibrinous pleuritis.[20] Subsequently, uremic pleuritis was recognized as a distinct entity. As there could be multiple reasons for pleural involvement in kidney disease, uremic pleuritis always comes as a diagnosis of exclusion.

Uremia accounts for approximately 1–58% of patients with end-stage renal disease (ESRD), though the incidences are decreasing nowadays due to the timely initiation of renal replacement therapy.[21] Pleural involvement in uremia results from fibrinous inflammation leading to increased capillary permeability. The putative mechanism has not been established. It appears in patients with severe uremia, especially those who are on renal replacement therapy such as hemodialysis or PD. Nondialysis-dependent CKD (CKD-ND) have a lower chance of developing uremic PE than CKD-5D patients. Uremic PE is not related to the severity of uremia and may occur at any time during the course of kidney dysfunction, from shortly after uremia to several years later.

In uremic pleuritis, frictional rubs are usually transient and unaccompanied by pain, so they are more often missed in clinical examination and later get identified when there is significant PE. The resultant effusion is exudative, serosanguineous with a paucity of nucleated cells, predominantly lymphocytes. The uremic PE can become secondarily infected or turn hemorrhagic due to the use of heparin in case of dialysis. Pleural exudates are characterized by a high rate of fibrin formation and degradation that is reflected by high concentrations of fibrinopeptide A. PE accompanies uremic pericarditis in an average of 20% of cases and is mostly left sided.

Unlike uremic pericarditis, uremic pleuritis may not respond to dialysis. Refractory uremic PE may require repeated thoracentesis, chest tube placement, pleurodesis, and surgical pleurectomy. Corticosteroid use in refractory uremic PE has been reported in a few cases and its use is to be individualized, especially with the risk of exaggerating infection.[22]

Tuberculosis Pleural Effusion

In endemic countries like India, TB is a common cause of exudative PE in patients with CKD. Incidence of 8.7% in patients on maintenance dialysis and 12.3% in renal allograft recipients is reported.[23] Defective cell-mediated immunity and uremia are the primary reasons for high incidences of TB in CKD. The presence of diabetes and steroid therapy, especially in transplant recipients, contributes to an increased risk of reactivating TB. In kidney transplant recipients, military TB, smear-negative, and extrapulmonary TB are more frequent.[24] A definitive diagnosis of tuberculous pleurisy requires the demonstration of either *Mycobacterium tuberculosis* in pleural specimens or granulomatous inflammation in the pleura. It poses a difficulty in establishing a diagnosis most of the time. The sensitivity of acid-fast staining and culture for *M. tuberculosis* in pleural fluid is low. The activity of adenosine deaminase (ADA) is reduced in patients with CKD on dialysis, and therefore the sensitivity of this test is low in such a scenario.[25] Due to the high prevalence of TB in the general population, many times presumptive diagnosis of tubercular effusion was made and antitubercular therapy is given in exudative PE. But it sometimes leads to erroneous administration of these toxic drugs in CKD. Kumar et al.[26] have addressed this diagnostic dilemma in patients with CKD and exudative PE and found thoracoscopic pleural biopsy with histopathological examination to be 100% sensitive. Those with nonspecific pleuritis on biopsy were followed up and there was no evidence of TB in them. They also found multiplex polymerase chain reaction (PCR) employing IS6110, protein antigen b, and MPB64 to have excellent sensitivity and specificity in diagnosis.

Parapneumonic Effusion

Chronic kidney disease is an immunodeficient stage and is at a higher risk of bacterial, viral, tubercular, fungal, or parasitic pneumonia and subsequent parapneumonic effusion. The risk is even higher in patients with kidney transplant who are on maintenance immunosuppression. In a subset of patients of a kidney transplant, who have received induction agents like antithymocyte globulin (ATG) at the time of transplant or have received antirejection therapy like pulse methylprednisolone, ATG, plasma exchange, rituximab, bortezomib, etc., during episodes of cellular or antibody-mediated rejections, there can be higher episodes of subsequent infections, especially pulmonary. Apart from the standard diagnostic and treatment approach, measures to reduce the overall immunosuppression burden are vital in these patients.

KEY POINTS

- The incidence of PE in patients with kidney diseases is more common but often underappreciated.
- Fluid overload is the most common underlying reason for transudative PE in both acute and CKD patients.
- Exudative PE due to bacterial and tubercular infections happen more frequently in kidney disease patients due to lower immunity.
- Uremic pleuritis, which is specific to advanced kidney failure, is rarely seen nowadays due to improved and early initiation of renal replacement therapy.
- A low pH PE should point toward UT and the antecedent event or history of obstructive uropathy should be sought.
- PD leak leading to PE is often challenging and may require discontinuation of dialysis through the peritoneal route till a permanent treatment is done.

REFERENCES

1. Gupta R, Gupta A, Ilyas M. Spectrum of pleural effusion etiology revised in 18-70 years of age group: A tertiary care center-based study of 1000 patients. CHRISMED J Health Res. 2018;5:110-3.
2. Hussein MM, Mooji JM, Roujouleh H. Tuberculosis and chronic renal disease. Semin Dial. 2003;16(1):38-44.
3. Nitin G, Patel R, Shet T, Patil A, Mahajan S. Study of Pleural Effusion in Chronic Kidney Disease. J Med Sci Clin Res. 2019;7:383-8.
4. Venkatesh M, Arun BS, Suresh H, Sagar Reddy SL. A study of respiratory manifestations in chronic kidney disease. Int J Biomed Res. 2017;8(2):70-4.
5. Bakirci T, Sasak G, Ozturk S, Akcay S, Sezer S, Haberal M. Pleural effusion in long-term hemodialysis patients. Transplant Proc. 2007;39(4):889-91.
6. Jabbar A, Qureshi R, Nasir K, Dhrolia M, Ahmad A. Transudative and Exudative Pleural Effusion in Chronic Kidney Disease Patients: A Prospective Single-Center Study. Cureus. 2021;13(10): e18649.
7. Kumar AP, Pathrudu BM, Rani NU, Padmaja B, Naik BD, Narayana M. A study on etiology and profile of pleural effusion in chronic kidney disease. J Evol Med Dent Sci. 2015;4(68):11785-96.
8. Current Chronic Kidney Disease (CKD) Nomenclature Used by KDIGO. Transplantation. 2020;104(4S1 Suppl 1):S7.
9. Jarratt MJ, Sahn SA. Pleural effusions in hospitalized patients receiving long-term hemodialysis. Chest. 1995;108(2):470-4.
10. DeBiasi EM, Pisani MA, Murphy TE, Araujo K, Kookoolis A, Argento AC, et al. Mortality among patients with pleural effusion undergoing thoracentesis. Eur Respir J. 2015;46(2):495-502.
11. Kwan BC, Chow KM, Pang WF, Leung CB, Li PK, Szeto CC. Unexplained exudative pleural effusion in chronic peritoneal dialysis patients. Perit Dial Int. 2010;30(5):534-40.
12. Alge J, Dolan K, Angelo J, Thadani S, Virk M, Akcan Arikan A. Two to Tango: Kidney-Lung Interaction in Acute Kidney Injury and Acute Respiratory Distress Syndrome. Front Pediatr. 2021;9:744110.
13. Domenech P, Perez T, Saldarini A, Uad P, Musso CG. Kidney-lung pathophysiological crosstalk: its characteristics and importance. Int Urol Nephrol. 2017;49(7):1211-5.
14. Maher JF. Uremic pleuritis. Am J Kidney Dis. 1987;10(1):9-22.
15. Lew SQ. Hydrothorax: Pleural effusion associated with peritoneal dialysis. Perit Dial Int. 2010;30(1):13-8.
16. Friedland GW, Axman MM, Love T. Neonatal "urinothorax" associated with posterior urethral valves. Br J Radiol. 1971;44(522):471-4.
17. Corriere JN Jr, Miller WT, Murphy JJ. Hydronephrosis as a cause of pleural effusion. Radiology. 1968;90(1):79-84.
18. Toubes ME, Lama A, Ferreiro L, Golpe A, Álvarez-Dobaño JM, González-Barcala FJ, et al. Urinothorax: a systematic review. J Thorac Dis. 2017;9(5):1209-18.
19. Bright R. Tabular view of the morbid appearance in 100 cases connected with albuminous urine: with observations. Guy's Hosp Rep. 1836;1:380-400.
20. Hopps HC, Wissler RW. Uremic pneumonitis. Am J Pathol. 1955;31(2):261-73.
21. Rashid-Farokhi F, Pourdowlat G, Nikoonia MR, Behzadnia N, Kahkouee S, Nassiri AA, et al. Uremic pleuritis in chronic hemodialysis patients. Hemodial Int. 2013;17(1):94-100.
22. Park EJ, Park MA, Park SY, Lee SH. Corticosteroid therapy for refractory uremic pleurisy. Ewha Med J. 2016;39(4):125-8.
23. John GT. Infections after renal transplantation in India. Indian J Nephrol. 2003;13:14-9.
24. Taskapan H, Utas C, Oymak FS, Gulmez I, Ozesmi M. The outcome of tuberculosis in patients on chronic hemodialysis. Clin Nephrol. 2000;54(2):134-7.
25. Dussol B, Fenouillet E, Brunet P, Purgus R, Sauze N, Carrega L, et al. Kinetic study of adenosine concentrations and the expression of adenosine deaminase in mononuclear cells during hemodialysis. Kidney Int. 2004;66(4):1640-6.
26. Kumar S, Agarwal R, Bal A, Sharma K, Singh N, Aggarwal AN, et al. Utility of adenosine deaminase (ADA), PCR & thoracoscopy in differentiating tuberculous & non-tuberculous pleural effusion complicating chronic kidney disease. Indian J Med Res. 2015;141(3):308-14.

CHAPTER

26 Pleural Effusion due to Drugs and Miscellaneous Diseases

Bhawana Sharma, Mrinal Sircar

INTRODUCTION

A pleural effusion develops due to variety of causes, which are often diagnostic challenges, especially in critically ill and chronic symptomatic patients with multiple comorbidities in intensive care unit (ICU). It may be due to lung, pleura, or systemic disorder.[1] Patients with pleural effusion most commonly present with dyspnea, initially on exertion, predominantly dry cough, and pleuritic chest pain. To treat pleural effusion appropriately, it is important to determine its etiology.[2] However, the etiology of pleural effusion remains unclear in nearly 20% of cases, especially critically ill patients. During evaluation of a patient with pleural effusion, it is important to find the cause of the effusion so that appropriate and specific treatment can be instituted.[3] As we all know and as discussed in earlier chapters as well that majorities of these pleural effusions can result from a wide range of common conditions, including infections, cancer, and heart failure. Since there are numerous additional pleural effusions' causes and forms, it is very important to discuss several uncommon forms and causes of pleural effusions. In one patient, there can be more than one etiology causing pleural fluid accumulation, for example, in a chronic kidney disease (CKD) patient or postrenal transplant graft rejection case, infectious and noninfectious causes can coexist. In this chapter, an approach to the diagnosis of pleural effusions caused by various drugs and other miscellaneous disorders are discussed. Because each of these disorders has a unique etiology and mode of treatment, it is essential to recognize these entities. There are many different causes of pleural effusions (drugs and miscellaneous diseases) as listed in **Box 1**.

BOX 1 **Causes of pleural effusion due to drugs and miscellaneous diseases.**

Pleural effusion due to drugs:
- β-blockers
- Amiodarone
- Sclerotherapeutic agents
- Ergot drugs
- Minoxidil
- Methysergide
- Bromocriptine
- Chemotherapeutic agents
- Methotrexate
- Nitrofurantoin
- Dantrolene
- Interleukin 2
- Procarbazine
- Clozapine

Pleural effusion due to miscellaneous diseases:
- Asbestos exposure
- Chylothorax
- Pseudochylothorax
- Yellow nail syndrome
- Sarcoidosis
- Uremia
- Therapeutic radiation exposure
- Drowning
- Amyloidosis
- Electrical burns
- Extramedullary hematopoiesis
- Whipple disease
- Post-lung transplant
- Iatrogenic pleural effusions

DRUG-INDUCED PLEURAL EFFUSION

Drug-induced pleural disease is an uncommon entity in comparison to drug-induced pleuroparenchymal disease, but as more new drugs are developed, it is expected that an increasing number of them will be implicated in the development of pleural disease.[4] The presentation of drug-induced pleural disease may vary from an asymptomatic pleural effusion to acute pleuritis to symptomatic pleural thickening. The pathogenic mechanism for many drug-induced pleural diseases remains the same.[5] These mechanisms include:

- Hypersensitivity or allergic reaction
- Direct toxic effect
- Increased oxygen-free radical production
- Suppression of the antioxidant defenses
- Chemical-induced inflammation

Some drugs are also known to cause pleural fluid eosinophilia. Pleural fluid eosinophilia (defined as >10% of nucleated cells) may give a clinical clue to the presence of drug-induced pleural disease; however, its presence or absence is a nonspecific finding. The important causes of pleural fluid eosinophilia include pneumothorax, hemothorax, benign asbestos pleural effusion (BAPE), fungal disease, Hodgkin's lymphoma, pulmonary emboli with pulmonary infarction, and parasitic infection. These diseases are important to exclude before considering the diagnosis of drug-induced pleural disease.[6]

Cardiovascular Drugs

Minoxidil

Minoxidil acts as a peripheral vasodilator and as an antihypertensive agent. The drug has been linked with the development of fluid in the pericardial and pleural space. Drug discontinuation led to resolution of the pericardial and pleural effusions. Webb and Whale reported a case of bilateral pleural effusions in a patient who received minoxidil for 3 months.[7]

Beta-blockers

Beta-blocking agents such as practolol and oxprenolol, which were previously used in Europe, have been implicated in causing pleuropulmonary complications. With increased usage of practolol, it became evident that it was associated with complications such as pleuropulmonary fibrosis and effusions.[8] Pleuropulmonary complications with practolol occurred after doses of 300–600 mg/day were given for 12–36 months. Discontinuation of the drug did not completely prevent the development of pleuropulmonary fibrosis. Pleural fluid analysis revealed straw-colored to bloody exudates. Withdrawal of drug therapy and corticosteroid administration mitigate the pleural effusion; however, the reversal of the pleuropulmonary fibrosis is not so smooth.[9]

Amiodarone

Amiodarone, the most common antiarrhythmic used in ICU, is a class III antiarrhythmic drug, an iodinated benzofuran, approved for the treatment of supraventricular and ventricular dysrhythmias. Side effects of amiodarone are extensive and adverse pulmonary reactions occur in approximately 6% of patients, including alveolar and interstitial infiltrates, pleural thickening, and rarely, pulmonary nodules or pleural effusions.[10] Amiodarone toxicity is dose-dependent (dosage > 400 mg/day) and can develop 2–30 weeks after the start of therapy. When pleural effusions occur as a manifestation of amiodarone toxicity, concomitant parenchymal infiltrates are usually present; however, there was a single case report of amiodarone-associated pleural effusion without parenchymal involvement.[11] The amiodarone-induced pulmonary toxicity is characterized by the gradual onset of dyspnea, nonproductive cough, weight loss, and sometimes fever. Computed tomography (CT) chest shows increased parenchymal attenuation.[12] Pleural fluid analysis revealed paucicellular exudate and the presence of foamy macrophages documented as in bronchoalveolar lavage (BAL) fluid but not diagnostic for amiodarone toxicity. Therapy for amiodarone pleuropulmonary toxicity involves drug withdrawal and systemic corticosteroids for patients who have clinically important hypoxemia and marked decrease in diffusion.[13]

Serotherapeutic Agents

Sodium Morrhuate/Absolute Alcohol

Sclerotherapeutic agents are used in the management of esophageal varices, for example, sodium morrhuate and absolute alcohol, are the drugs that most commonly cause pleural effusions mostly on the right side; however, they may occur on the left or bilaterally, depending on the site of injection.[14] The incidence of pleural effusions with the use of sodium morrhuate is 40–50% and with absolute alcohol, it is 19%. The proposed mechanism for developing pleural fluid after variceal injection with these agents involves a transmediastinal spread of inflammation from the esophagus to the mediastinal pleura. Effusions can be identified radiographically within 24 hours and spontaneously resolve by 7 days.

Ergoline Drugs

Methysergide

Methysergide is used to manage migraine headaches and a serotonin antagonist.[15] It is responsible for pleuropulmonary complications in <1% of patients. During the 1960s, with increased use of methysergide, numerous literature reports of fibrosis of pleura, lung, endocardium, and pericardium were described after 1–4 years after starting the drug. The pathogenic mechanism that is responsible for methysergide-induced fibrosis is rise in serotonin levels that stimulate fibroblast activity. Serotonin was shown to stimulate fibroblast activity in vivo. Patients who have pleuropulmonary disease present with fever, dyspnea, weight loss, and pleuritic chest pain. Literature described pleural fluid as clear to bloody; pleural fluid protein was reported from 2.0–4.4 g/dL with a low-nucleated cell count.[16] Chronic pleuritis with mononuclear cell infiltrates and associated fibroblasts were found in pleural biopsies. Management of this condition consists of drug withdrawal, which causes reversal of pleural thickening in most cases but not all.

Bromocriptine

Bromocriptine ameliorates the dyskinesia that is associated with Parkinson's disease. It is an ergot derivative with strong dopamine agonist activity also used in the treatment of acromegaly. Chronic use of bromocriptine and other dopamine agents (mesulergine, lisuride, and cabergoline) is associated with pleuropulmonary changes in approximately 6% of patients. Dose-related pleural fibrosis seems to occur 12–48 months after initiation of therapy.[17] Pleural fluid typically is a lymphocyte-predominant exudate and pleural fluid eosinophilia was reported in two patients. Management includes withdrawal of drug therapy, leading to resolution of pleural effusions, but pleural fibrosis and interstitial parenchyma changes may not be reversible. Corticosteroids can be added for regression of the pleural thickening or pulmonary parenchymal lesions.[18]

Chemotherapeutic Agents

Bleomycin

Bleomycin, an antimetabolite antimicrobial agent, is used in the treatment of head and neck carcinoma, testicular carcinoma, and Hodgkin's and non-Hodgkin's lymphoma. It has been used rarely as a sclerosing agent in the management of recurrent and refractory pleural effusions. In approximately 6–10% of patients, adverse pleuropulmonary reactions are reported. The most common presentation of bleomycin-induced pulmonary reaction is the development of interstitial pneumonitis and acute respiratory distress syndrome (ARDS), which may progress into pulmonary and pleural fibrosis.[19] Pleural and pulmonary toxicity is dose- and age-related; it is common in older patients (age > 70 years) and those who receive a cumulative dose of 395 mg/m^2. Pleural effusions were reported in few patients who had bleomycin-lung toxicity. Combination of steroids and drug-therapy withdrawal may progress to resolution of the effusions and pneumonitis; however, the efficacy of treatment has not been well established.[20]

Procarbazine

Procarbazine, a methylhydrazine agent, is used in the treatment of Hodgkin's disease.[21] Pleuropulmonary effects are not common. Unilateral and bilateral pleural effusions are described in literature but may or may not be associated with parenchymal infiltrates. Pleural fluid analysis has not been reported. Symptoms and radiographic changes are resolved within a few days when the drug is discontinued.[22]

Methotrexate

Methotrexate, an antimetabolite, acts as an immune modulator and steroid-sparing agent, which is used in the treatment of malignancies, psoriasis, and autoimmune diseases. Pleuropulmonary disease occurs in 3–4% of patients who receive high-dose methotrexate. Methotrexate-induced pleuropulmonary reactions occur not only in patients who receive high-dose treatment but also with use of lower-dose methotrexate.[23] The mechanism for methotrexate-induced pneumonitis and pleural reaction is believed to be a hypersensitive reaction and can present with fever, cough, dyspnea, interstitial infiltrates, and pleural thickening or effusion.[24] The pleural manifestations are usually self-limiting and discontinuation of the drug plus corticosteroid therapy are used in a large number of patients for managing this condition.

Mitomycin

Mitomycin is an alkylating agent that is used in the treatment of lung, breast, and gastrointestinal (GI) tract malignancies. Similar to bleomycin, pleuropulmonary fibrosis has been reported with mitomycin along with its common adverse effects.[25] Ozols and coworkers reported diffuse parenchymal infiltrates in five patients who received mitomycin for ovarian cancer; two patients had bilateral pleural effusions.[26] Orwoll and colleagues reported mitomycin-induced nonspecific pleural fibrosis with lymphocytes and eosinophils aggregates in one patient.[27] Management includes withdrawal of the drug and use of systemic corticosteroids for relief in symptoms and leads to partial resolution of the radiographic findings.

Cyclophosphamide

Cyclophosphamide is an immunosuppressive-alkylating agent used in the treatment of a variety of nonmalignant and malignant conditions. Andre and coworkers first reported a case of cyclophosphamide-associated lung injury in 1967. Cyclophosphamide-induced pulmonary toxicity can be divided into early and late-onset forms. Early-onset pneumonitis is usually seen 1–6 months after drug exposure and late-onset pneumonitis occurs months to years after institution of the drug. Patients present with an insidious onset of dyspnea and cough. Typical chest radiograph features are bilateral basilar reticular or reticulonodular infiltrates and presence of pleural thickening signs of late-onset lung toxicity. Pleural effusion associated with cyclophosphamide has only been reported once.[28] Schaap and coworkers described massive pleural effusions after 2 days of high-dose cyclophosphamide infusion before bone marrow transplantation in a 37-year-old man who had chronic myelogenous leukemia.[29] Analysis of pleural fluid revealed a transudative fluid (protein 2.68 g/dL and lactate dehydrogenase 32 IU/L). Management includes drug withdrawal and corticosteroids for early-onset cyclophosphamide toxicity to relieve pulmonary symptoms and radiographic findings. Late-onset pulmonary toxicity and pneumonitis are unresponsive to corticosteroids according to literature.

Pleural Fluid Eosinophilia

Pleural fluid eosinophilia (defined as >10% of nucleated cells) is a nonspecific finding for drug-induced pleural disease. Drugs causing pleural fluid eosinophilia are discussed further.

Valproic Acid

Valproic acid is a drug used for epilepsy. Kaufman reported a single case of an eosinophilic pleural effusion in a patient who received valproic acid for 9 months.[30] Pleural fluid analysis showed an exudate with a low-nucleated cell count and differential cell count was 62% eosinophils, which increased to 84% on repeat thoracentesis. Blood eosinophils were also elevated at 26%. The effusion resolved 6 months after stopping the drug.

Propylthiouracil

Propylthiouracil is a thionamide and is used for Graves' disease. Middleton et al. described one patient who developed an eosinophilic pleural effusion after 3 weeks of starting propylthiouracil.[31] Pleural fluid analysis was exudative effusion with an initial eosinophil count of 16%, which increased to 45% on subsequent pleural fluid analysis. Chronic inflammation with an eosinophilic infiltrate is found in pleural biopsy. Pleural effusion was resolved in 3 months with drug discontinuation.

Isotretinoin

Isotretinoin is used in the treatment of severe nodulocystic acne. Milleron et al. reported a case in which the patient developed cough, fever, and pleural effusion after 1 month of isotretinoin therapy for cystic acne.[32] Pleural fluid analysis showed an exudative effusion with more than 20% eosinophils. Radiographic resolution was noted after 1 month of discontinuation of therapy. Bunker et al. described left-sided eosinophilic pleural effusion in a 49-year-old lady 7 months after starting isotretinoin for systemic sclerosis. Pleural effusion was resolved after 3 months of stopping isotretinoin.

Nitrofurantoin

Nitrofurantoin is an antimicrobial drug that is used in the treatment of urinary tract infections. Nitrofurantoin is associated with extensive adverse side effects, including dermatitis, urticaria, angioedema, GI intolerance, hepatotoxicity, neuropathy, and pulmonary reactions.[33] Acute, subacute, and chronic pleuropulmonary reactions may occur with nitrofurantoin use due to mechanism of hypersensitivity reaction in lung parenchyma and pleura. Israel and Diamond reported the first case of nitrofurantoin-induced pleuropulmonary reaction; since then, more than 2,000 cases have been reported. The acute effects may develop within 1 month of starting drug therapy.[34] Pleural effusions may be seen in up to one third of cases. Patients present with fever, dyspnea, and cough. Radiographic abnormalities include bibasilar alveolar or interstitial infiltrates. A case series of 447 patients was reported by Holmberg and Boman who had developed pulmonary reactions to nitrofurantoin; 232 (52%) had infiltrates alone, 68 (15%) had infiltrates and effusions, 14 (3%) had only an effusion, and 70 (16%) had a normal chest X-ray.[35] Nitrofurantoin-induced pleural fluid eosinophilia has been identified and are typically bilateral and treatment consists of prompt drug withdrawal. Adjunctive corticosteroids may not be very useful if they are severe at presentation. Pleural effusions rarely are associated with chronic nitrofurantoin use. Pleural thickening was seen with chronic nitrofurantoin-induced pleuropulmonary disease.

Dantrolene

Dantrolene is used as a skeletal muscle relaxant, structurally similar to nitrofurantoin and commonly seen side effects are nausea, GI atony, hepatitis, and sedation. Dantrolene-induced pleuropulmonary reaction typically presents with pleurodynia, fever, and pleural effusion.[36] Dantrolene-induced pleural effusion is usually unilateral and late sequel was described in six patients who received doses from 100–400 mg/day. Pleural effusion and fibrosis are late sequelae, with an onset of 2 months to 12 years after initiation of the drug. All reported pleural effusions were exudates with normal glucose values.[37] Pleural fluid eosinophilia is an important finding, with pleural eosinophils ranging from 33 to 66% of the total pleural fluid-nucleated cell count. Stopping the drug is associated with a dramatic reduction in symptoms and resolution of pleural effusions.

Gliclazide

Gliclazide, an oral hypoglycemic medication, was reported to cause moderate unilateral pleural effusion and parenchymal infiltrates in a male patient when given for 2 weeks. Peripheral blood eosinophilia and pleural fluid eosinophilia (80% of the total nucleated cell count in the pleural fluid) were documented.[38] After stopping gliclazide for 1 month, the patient was asymptomatic. His peripheral eosinophil count normalized and the chest roentgenogram showed complete resolution of the pleural effusion.

Other Drugs

Acyclovir

Acyclovir nucleoside analogue inhibits viral replication and is used in the treatment of herpes viral infections. Pusateri and Muder reported the case of 71-year-old man who was given acyclovir for Herpes zoster ophthalmicus and developed bilateral parenchymal infiltrates, fever, hemoptysis, and a left-sided pleural effusion 4 days into treatment.[39] Bronchoscopy revealed no infectious cause and a ventilation-perfusion scan was less probability for a pulmonary embolism. Acyclovir was discontinued on day 6 and resulted in quick resolution of the fever. Pleural effusion and parenchymal infiltrates had resolved after 10 days of drug-therapy withdrawal.

Clozapine

Clozapine is an atypical antipsychotic agent used in schizophrenia, refractory to conventional neuroleptics. Clozapine-induced pleural effusions are reported in three cases.[40] In their case report, fever with bilateral pleural effusions developed 16 days after starting clozapine. Pleural fluid analysis revealed a neutrophil-predominant exudate. Fever and pleural effusions had resolved after 9 days of discontinuation of the drug. The patient was rechallenged with clozapine and again developed pleural effusions and fever. In 1997, Chatterjee and Safferman described another case of clozapine-induced pleural effusion and pleural effusion disappeared when the clozapine was discontinued.[41] When the patient was rechallenged with clozapine at a lower dose, the left-sided pleural effusion recurred. Discontinuation of the drug resulted in resolution of the pleural effusion. In 1998, Thompson et al. described clozapine-induced bilateral pleural effusions, peripheral blood eosinophilia, hyperglycemia, hematuria, and hepatocellular dysfunction early in the course of treatment.[42] Pleural fluid analysis was not performed. All symptoms and the pleural effusion resolved promptly with clozapine discontinuation. The patient was not rechallenged.

D-penicillamine

D-penicillamine has immunosuppressive effects and is also used as a chelating agent for copper in the treatment of Wilson's disease. Because of its immunosuppressive action, it is useful in the treatment of certain autoimmune diseases. An isolated report of D-penicillamine-induced pleural effusion was described in a 35-year-old woman who had a large, left-sided pleural effusion after more than 12 years of D-penicillamine therapy for Wilson's disease.[43] Moderate straw-colored exudate was drained then cytology and extensive serologic testing (including antihistone antibody) was negative. Despite repeated thoracentesis, the effusion recurred multiple times. The patient has undergone video-assisted thoracoscopy which showed white plaques on the visceral and parietal pleura. Thoracostomy and decortication was performed. Successful reexpansion of the left lung was accomplished with the decortication. Pleura biopsy showed chronic, nonspecific inflammation without evidence of infection or malignancy. After decortication, no further sequelae were reported and D-penicillamine therapy was continued.

Granulocyte Colony-stimulating Factor

Granulocyte colony-stimulating factor (GCSF) is a hematopoietic growth factor that is used to stimulate the recovery of the bone marrow after chemotherapy-induced myelosuppression. Busmanis and coworkers reported an exudative pleural effusion 10 days after starting GCSF in a 43-year-old woman who had breast carcinoma.[44] Infection and malignancy were excluded by cytologic examination of the pleural fluid which revealed an increase of immature and mature myeloid cells. Pleural effusion resolved gradually after discontinuation of GCSF.

Interleukin-2

Recombinant human interleukin-2 (IL-2) is used in renal cell carcinoma and melanoma. Pleuropulmonary abnormalities with IL-2 occur in approximately 75% of patients.[45] The imaging patterns are nonspecific and include bilateral perihilar alveolar or interstitial infiltrates, focal infiltrates, and pleural effusions. Pleural effusion, the most common abnormality, is seen in approximately 50% of patients. Effusions usually improve following discontinuation of therapy.

Itraconazole

Itraconazole is a triazole used in systemic mycosis. Gunther et al. reported one case of itraconazole-induced pleural effusion in a 49-year-old patient who received 8 weeks of itraconazole at a dosage of 200 mg twice a day.[46] Pleural fluid analysis showed protein level of 4.3 g/dL. No signs of infection or malignancy on pleural biopsy were seen.

Mesalamine

Mesalamine is commonly used in inflammatory bowel disease. Gujral et al. described one case of pleuropericarditis that was related to the use of mesalamine. A 56-year-old man developed fever, fatigue, and chest pain after 2 weeks of oral mesalamine for ulcerative proctitis. Chest radiograph showed a small left pleural effusion without infiltrate.[47] Pleural fluid analysis was not done. Serum antinuclear antibodies (ANA) and serologic studies for viral pathogens that are known to cause pericarditis were negative. Drug-treatment withdrawal and systemic corticosteroids resulted in remission of the radiographic abnormalities over several months.

Simvastatin

Simvastatin is a 3-hydroxy-3-methylglutaryl coenzyme A reductase inhibitor that is used to treat certain forms of hypercholesterolemia. The most serious adverse effect is drug-induced hepatitis. De Groot et al. reported a case of simvastatin-induced hypersensitivity pneumonitis in an elderly male.[48] Chest radiograph demonstrated a large, right pleural effusion with pleura thickening on the left. Thoracoscopic findings revealed darkish-brown pleural fluid and pleural biopsies were negative for infection. Pleural fluid analysis was not reported. Marked symptomatic improvement within days was noted with drug-therapy withdrawal and corticosteroids.

Troglitazone

Troglitazone is used in insulin-resistant diabetes mellitus. Its most serious side effect is hepatic dysfunction. One case of troglitazone-associated pleuropulmonary reaction was described.[49] A 47-year-old man who received troglitazone for diabetes mellitus developed a productive cough, dyspnea, and night sweats after 1 week of therapy. Empiric antibiotics and antitussives did not relieve the symptoms. A chest X-ray that was obtained 1 week later showed bilateral, small pleural effusions and basilar interstitial infiltrates. After discontinuation of troglitazone, the patient's symptoms abated within 24 hours; complete resolution of the pleural effusions and parenchymal infiltrates was seen after 6 days.

Intravenous Immunoglobulin

Intravenous immunoglobulin (IVIG) is used in autoimmune diseases such as idiopathic thrombocytopenia (ITP), myasthenia gravis, and supplementation therapy for congenital immunodeficiency states because of its immunomodulating properties. A single case report of recurrent lymphocytic pleural effusion was described in a 35-year-old woman who received IVIG for ITP.[50] Pleural fluid analysis revealed a lymphocytic exudate, with glucose of 92 mg/dL, total protein of 3.3 g/dL, and lactate dehydrogenase of 274 IU/L. The pleural effusion resolved completely in 2 weeks when discontinued. Subsequent rechallenge with the same preparation of IVIG resulted in reaccumulation of pleural effusions with similar pleural fluid characteristics.

Drug-induced Lupus Pleuritis

Hoffman described lupus-like illness after treatment with sulfadiazine in 1945 and after that, more than 80 drugs have been reported to cause a lupus-like reaction or exacerbate preexisting lupus.[51] Drugs strongly linked with drug-induced lupus (DIL) include procainamide, hydralazine, chlorpromazine, isoniazid, D-penicillamine, methyldopa, and quinidine. Procainamide and hydralazine are studied well in this regard. Pleuropulmonary involvement is specifically common in DIL.[52] Approximately, 56% of patients who have procainamide-induced lupus have pleural effusions and pleuritis. Pleuropulmonary disease is reported in approximately 30% of patients who have hydralazine-induced lupus.[53] The pleural fluid characteristics of DIL are similar to idiopathic lupus; effusions are exudative with cell counts of 200–15,000 cells/mL; pleural fluid pH and glucose are usually normal but may be low on occasion; pleural fluid ANA are higher than concomitant serum values and titters frequently exceed 1:250; and cytologic examination may show the diagnostic presence of lupus erythematosus (LE) cells.[54]

Procainamide

Procainamide is the drug that is most commonly associated with DIL. More than 90% of patients will have a positive serum ANA after 1 year of therapy and of those, one third will develop a lupus-like syndrome. Procainamide-induced lupus can occur as early as 1 month, or as late as 12 years, from the initiation of therapy. Parenchymal infiltrates are noted in about 40% of patients and slightly more than 50% have pleuritis and pleural effusion.

Hydralazine

Hydralazine-induced lupus occurs in 2–21% of patients; the incidence is dependent upon the dose, duration of treatment, and acetylator phenotype. The major risk is associated with dosages > 200 mg/day or >100 g cumulative dose. Pleuropulmonary disease has been reported in approximately 30% of patients, whereas isolated parenchymal disease occurs in less than 5%. The ANA is positive in half of the patients who receive 200 mg/day; the clinical syndrome develops in 10% of these patients.

PLEURAL EFFUSION DUE TO MISCELLANEOUS DISEASES

Benign Asbestos Pleural Effusion

Asbestos-related pathological changes of the pleura include pleural plaques, malignant pleural mesothelioma (MPM), diffuse pleural thickening (DPT), and BAPE.[55] BAPE is a nonmalignant pleural disease initially described in 1964 and also termed asbestos pleuritis. Epler et al. suggested diagnostic criteria for BAPE, which consists of the follows:

- Asbestos exposure in the past
- Identification of pleural effusion by chest X-ray or pleural fluid aspiration
- Other causes of effusion should be ruled out. They also suggested that patient should be under follow-up for at least 3 years to confirm the diagnosis and also to exclude the development of malignant diseases such as MPM or lung carcinomatous pleuritis. Later Hillerdal and Ozesmi suggested only 1-year follow-up, including detailed exploration and CT scanning.[56] There is a long latency period after past asbestos exposure for development of BAPE. Before establishing the diagnosis of BAPE, pleural disease should be excluded. A detailed evaluation, including diagnostic thoracentesis cytological and bacterial analysis, thoracoscopic evaluation, and pleural biopsy should be performed to confirm a diagnosis of BAPE.

Post-lung Transplant Pleural Effusion

Judson et al. reported ipsilateral pleural effusion in nine consecutive single-lung transplant recipients and compared it with six patients who underwent other cardiothoracic operations. All lung transplant recipients developed ipsilateral pleural fluid immediately after transplantation and continued for up to 9 days. Pleural fluid output in lung transplant recipients declined steadily during the first week and was minimal by day 9, but pleural effusion due to cardiothoracic surgery declined even more rapidly.[57] Properties of pleural fluid after lung transplantation are bloody, exudative, and neutrophil predominant, similar to pleural fluid, following other cardiothoracic surgery. Judson et al. suggested to avoid analyzing pleural fluid after lung transplantation if the pleural fluid output is decreasing and the clinical course is appropriate.

Chylothorax

Chylothorax, or chylous pleural effusion, is less common form of pleural effusion with some unique features. Chylous pleural effusion is characterized by the presence of chyle (white, milky, and opalescent appearance fluid) in the pleural cavity. Chyle is a type of lymphatic fluid, predominantly with lymphocytes (particularly T-lymphocytes), immunoglobulin, and lipids that are absorbed by the digestive tract. Chylothorax suggests the presence of a chyle leak from the thoracic duct or its tributaries.[58] Causes of chylothorax are divided into traumatic and nontraumatic. Traumatic causes include invasive surgery, nonsurgical procedures, and penetrating and blunt trauma. Nontraumatic include malignancy and congenital or acquired lymphatic disorders. Traditional diagnostic criteria included pleural fluid triglyceride level (>110 mg/dL) which was less sensitive.[59] Two imaging techniques, conventional lymphangiography and lymphoscintigraphy, have been used in visualizing the lymphatic system in patients with chylothorax.[60] Due to its uncommon occurrence and diversity of potential causes, optimal management of chylothorax has not been fully defined.

Pseudochylothorax

Pseudochylothorax, also known as cholesterol pleural effusion, is a rare form of pleural effusion. It is usually a unilateral process and approximately one third of patients are asymptomatic at presentation. Similar to chylothorax, pseudochylothorax is characterized by accumulation of turbid or milky, white pleural fluid due to its high lipid content. The most common etiologies of pseudochylothorax include tuberculous pleurisy, chronic pneumothorax, chronic rheumatoid pleuritis, and chronic hemothorax.[61] Rarely, pseudochylothorax is seen with pleural paragonimiasis, echinococcosis, malignancy, or trauma. The diagnosis of pseudochylothorax is established by pleural fluid analysis. Chylomicrons are present in chylothorax but not in pseudochylothorax. In most pseudochylothorax, no specific therapy is required because effusions are associated with a benign course.

Urinothorax

Urinothorax is accumulation of urine in the pleural space. Urinothorax is a rare form of pleural effusion that often goes undiagnosed. Urinothorax needs to be considered in patients with undiagnosed pleural effusion, associated with obstructive uropathy.[62] Urinothorax causes are trauma, surgical injury, malignancy of the urinary tract, failed tube nephrostomy, lithotripsy, renal transplantation, and kidney biopsy. Proposed mechanism for the development of urinothorax is direct movement of the leaked urine in the abdomen into the pleural space via defects in the diaphragm. The appearance and odor of the pleural fluid will be consistent with urine. Early thoracentesis is essential for establishing the characteristic parameters of urinothorax. Renal scintigraphy using 99mTc-ethylene dicysteine may aid in establishing the diagnosis of urinothorax by demonstrating leakage of the tracer from the urinary tract into the pleural space. Management of urinothorax consists of treating the cause of urine leak such as relieving urinary obstruction.

Yellow Nail Syndrome

The yellow nail syndrome (YNS) is a rare disorder diagnosed by the triad of yellow and thickened nails, lymphoedema and pleural effusion, or other respiratory abnormality. Samman and White first described this condition in 1964 and after that, approximately 150 such conditions were reported in the literature.[63] The pathogenesis of YNS is not well understood. The evidence to date suggests that the lymphatic dysfunction observed in YNS is an acquired disorder rather than a heritable one. Various anatomic abnormalities of the lymphatic ducts including lymphatic hypoplasia, dilatations, and extensive collateral lymphatic network have been noted on lymphangiography in some patients with YNS.[64] Other investigators have noted functional lymphatic abnormalities based on results of lymphoscintigraphy. At present, functional lymphatic disorder rather than structural disease is favored as the shared pathogenic mechanism for the development of pleural effusions and lymphoedema. Clinical manifestations of YNS generally need supportive measures. Symptomatic and recurrent pleural effusions are controlled by therapeutic thoracenteses with pleurodesis. Persistent chylothorax is treated by thoracic duct ligation. The natural history of YNS is not well known, but the long-term prognosis of YNS is generally favorable.

SUMMARY

Drug-induced pleural disease is not so common and less commonly known to clinicians than drug-induced parenchymal lung disease. Pleural reactions from drugs manifest as pleural effusions, pleural thickening, or pleuritic chest pain, and may occur in the absence of parenchymal infiltrates. The clinician should be well aware of the possibility of a drug-induced pleural reaction. A detailed drug history, temporal relationship between symptom onset and start of therapy, and pleural fluid eosinophilia should raise the suspicion of a drug-related process. Moreover, if the cause of an exudative pleural effusion is not clinically evident after pleural fluid analysis, drug-therapy withdrawal should be a considered.

KEY POINTS

- Diagnosing the cause of pleural effusion is most important.
- Treatment is specific to each cause.
- Pleural effusion due to drugs and miscellaneous diseases.
- The etiology of pleural effusion remains unclear in nearly 20% of cases especially critically ill patients.
- In critically ill patients especially where multiorgan dysfunction with polypharmacy it is very crucial to treat pleural effusions.
- Managing the pleural effusion successfully has an important impact on patient outcome and mortality.

REFERENCES

1. Light RW. Pleural diseases, 5th edition. Baltimore (MD): Lippincott Williams & Wilkins; 2007.
2. Light RW, MacGregor MI, Luchsinger PC, Ball WC Jr. Pleural effusions: the diagnostic separation of transudates and exudates. Ann Intern Med. 1972;77:507-14.
3. Porcel JM, Light RW. Diagnostic approach to pleural effusion in adults. Am Fam Physician. 2006;73:1211-20.
4. Antony VB. Drug-induced pleural disease. Clin Chest Med. 1998;19:331-40.
5. Morelock SY, Sahn SA. Drugs and the pleura. Chest. 1999;116:212-21.
6. Porcel JM, Vives M. Etiology and pleural fluid characteristics of large and massive effusions. Chest. 2003;124:978-83.
7. Webb DB, Whale RJ. Pleuro-pericardial effusion associated with minoxidil administration. Postgrad Med J. 1982;58:319-20.
8. Fleming HA, Hickling P. Pleural effusion after Practolol. Lancet. 1974;2:120.

9. Page RL. Progressive pleural thickening during oxprenolol therapy. Br J Dis Chest. 1979;73:195-9.
10. Leech JA, Gallastegni J, Swiryn S. Pulmonary toxicity of amiodarone. Chest. 1984;85:444-5.
11. Gonzalez-Rothi RJ, Hannan SE, Hood I, Franzini DA. Amiodarone pulmonary toxicity presenting as bilateral exudative pleural effusions. Chest. 1987;92:179-82.
12. Kuhlman JE, Teigen C, Ren H, Hruban RH, Hutchins GM, Fishman EK, et al. Amiodarone pulmonary toxicity: CT findings in symptomatic patients. Radiology. 1990;177:121-5.
13. Zaher C, Hamer A, Peter T, Mandel W. Low-dose steroid therapy for prophylaxis of amiodarone-induced pulmonary infiltrates. N Engl J Med. 1983;308:779.
14. Parikh SS, Amarapurkar DN, Dhawan PS, Kalro RH, Desai HG. Development of pleural effusion after sclerotherapy with absolute alcohol. Gastrointest Endosc. 1993;39:404-5.
15. Graham JR. Cardiac and pulmonary fibrosis during methysergide therapy for headache. Am J Med Sci. 1967;254:1-12.
16. Hindle W, Posner E, Sweatnam MT, Tan RH. Pleural effusion and fibrosis during the treatment with methysergide. BMJ. 1970;1:605-6.
17. Rinne UK. Pleuropulmonary changes during long-term bromocriptine treatment for Parkinson's disease. Lancet. 1981;1:44.
18. Kinnunen E, Viljanen A. Pleuropulmonary involvement during bromocriptine treatment. Chest. 1988;94:1034-6.
19. Bauer KA, Skarin AT, Balikian JP, Garnick MB, Rosenthal DS, Canellos GP. Pulmonary complications associated with combination chemotherapy programs containing bleomycin. Am J Med. 1983;74:557-63.
20. Holoye PY, Luna MA, MacKay B, Bedrossian CM. Bleomycin hypersensitivity pneumonitis. Ann Intern Med. 1978;88:47-9.
21. Jones SE, Moore M, Blank N, Castellino RA. Hypersensitivity to procarbazine manifested by fever and pleuropulmonary reaction. Cancer. 1972;29:498-500.
22. Ecker MD, Jay B, Keohane MF. Procarbazine lung. AJR. 1978;131:527-8.
23. Abu-Shakra M, Nicol P, Urowitz MB. Accelerated nodulosis, pleural effusion, and pericardial tamponade during methotrexate therapy. J Rheumatol. 1994;21:934-7.
24. Sostman HD, Matthay RA, Putmant CE, Smith GJ. Methotrexate-induced pneumonitis. Medicine. 1976;55:371-88.
25. Gunstream SR, Seidenfeld JJ, Sobonya RE, McMahon LJ. Mitomycin-associated lung diseases. Cancer Treat Rep. 1983;67:301-4.
26. Ozols RF, Hocan WM, Ostchega Y, Young RC. MVP (mitomycin, vinblastine, and progesterone): a second-line regimen in ovarian cancer with a high incidence of pulmonary toxicity. Cancer Treat Rep. 1983;67:721-2.
27. Orwoll RS, Kiessling PJ, Patterson JR. Interstitial pneumonia from mitomycin. Ann Intern Med. 1978;89:352-5.
28. Malik SW, Myers JL, DeRemee RA, Specks U. Lung toxicity associated with cyclophosphamide use. Am J Respir Crit Care Med. 1996;154:1851-6.
29. Schaap N, Raymakers R, Schattenberg A, Ottevanger JP, DeWitte T. Massive pleural effusion attributed to high-dose cyclophosphamide during conditioning for BMT. Bone Marrow Transplant. 1996;18:247-8.
30. Kaufman J. Eosinophilic pleural effusions associated with valproic acid administration. South Med J. 1996;88:881-2.
31. Middleton KL, Santella R, Couser Jr JI. Eosinophilic pleuritis due to propylthiouracil. Chest. 1993;103:955-6.
32. Milleron BJ, Valcke J, Akoun GM, Mayaud CM. Isotretinoin-related eosinophilic pleural effusion. Chest. 1996;110:1128.
33. Larsson S, Cronberg S, Denneberg T, Ohlsson NM. Pulmonary reactions to nitrofurantoin. Scand J Respir Dis. 1973;54:103-10.
34. Israel HL, Diamond P. Recurrent pulmonary infiltration and pleural effusion due to nitrofurantoin sensitivity. N Engl J Med. 1962;266:1024-6.
35. Holmberg L, Boman G. Pulmonary reactions to nitrofurantoin: 447 cases reported to the Swedish adverse drug reaction committee. Eur J Respir Dis. 1981;62:180-9.
36. Petusevsky ML, Faling LJ, Rocklin RE, Snider GL, Merliss AD, Moses JM, et al. Pleuropericardial reaction to treatment with dantrolene. JAMA. 1979;242:2772-4.
37. Mahoney JM, Bachtel MD. Pleural effusion associated with chronic dantrolene administration. Ann Pharmacother. 1994;28:587-9.
38. Tzanakis N, Bouros D, Siarakas N. Eosinophilic pleural effusion associated due to gliclazide. Resp Med. 2000;94:94.
39. Pusateri DW, Muder RR. Fever, pulmonary infiltrates, and pleural effusion following acyclovir therapy for Herpes zoster ophthalmicus. Chest. 1990;98:754-6.
40. Daly JM, Godber RJ, Braman SS. Polyserositis associated with clozapine treatment. Am J Psychiatry. 1992;149:1274-5.
41. Chatterjee A, Safferman A. Cellulitis, eosinophilia, and unilateral pleural effusion associated with clozapine treatment. J Clin Psychopharmacol. 1997;17:232-3.
42. Thompson J, Chengappa KNR, Good CB, Baker RW, Kiese RP, Bezner J, et al. Hepatitis, hyperglycemia, pleural effusion, eosinophilia, hematuria and proteinuria occurring early in clozapine treatment. Inter Clin Psychopharmacol. 1998;13:95-8.
43. Karkos C, Moore A, Manche A, Thorpe JA. Pleural effusion associated with D-penicillamine therapy: a case report. J Clin Pharm Ther. 1996;21:15-7.
44. Busmanis IA, Beaty AE, Basser RL. Isolated pleural effusion with hematopoietic cells of mixed lineage in a patient receiving granulocyte-colony-stimulating factor after high-dose chemotherapy. Diagn Cytopathol. 1998;18:204-7.
45. Vogelzang PJ, Bloom SM, Mier JW, Atkins MB. Chest roentgenography abnormalities in IL-2 recipients: incidence in correlation with clinical parameters. Chest. 1992;101:746-52.
46. Gunther J, Lode H, Raffenberg M, Schaberg T. Development of pleural and pericardial effusions during itraconazole therapy for pulmonary aspergillosis. Eur J Clin Microbiol Infect Dis. 1993;12:723-4.
47. Gujral N, Friedenberg F, Friedenberg J, Gabriel G, Kotler M, Levine G. Pleuropericarditis related to the use of mesalamine. Dig Dis Sci. 1996;41:624-6.
48. De Groot RE, Willems LN, Dijkman JH. Interstitial lung disease with pleural effusion caused by simvastatin. J Intern Med. 1996;239:361-3.
49. Koshida H, Shibata K, Kametani T. Pleuropulmonary disease in a man with diabetes who was treated with troglitazone. N Engl J Med. 1998;339:1400-1.
50. Bolanos-Meade J, Keung YK, Cobos E. Recurrent lymphocytic pleural effusion after intravenous immunoglobulin. Am J Hematol. 1999;60:248-9.
51. Hoffman BJ. Sensitivity of sulfadiazine resembling acute disseminated lupus erythematosus. Arch Dermatol Syph. 1945;51:190-2.

52. Cush JJ, Goldings EA. Drug-induced lupus: clinical spectrum and pathogenesis. Am J Med Sci. 1985;290:36-45.
53. Yung YL, Richardson BC. Drug-induced lupus. Rheum Dis Clin North Am. 1994;20:61-85.
54. Good JT, King TE, Antony VB, Sahn SA. Lupus pleuritis: clinical features and pleural fluid characteristics with special reference to pleural fluid antinuclear antibody titers. Chest. 1983;84:714.
55. Robinson BWS, Musk AW. Benign asbestos pleural effusion: diagnosis and course. Thorax. 1981;36(12):896-900.
56. Hillerdal G, Ozesmi M. Benign asbestos pleural effusion: 73 exudates in 60 patients. Eur J Resp Dis. 1987;71(2):113-21.
57. Judson MA, Handy JR, Sahn SA. Pleural effusions following lung transplantation. Time course, characteristics, and clinical implications. Chest. 1996;109(5):1190-4.
58. McGrath EE, Blades Z, Anderson PB. Chylothorax: aetiology, diagnosis, and therapeutic options. Respir Med. 2010;104:1-8.
59. Agrawal V, Doelken P, Sahn SA. Pleural fluid analysis in chylous pleural effusion. Chest. 2008;133:1436-41.
60. Partsch H. Practical aspects of indirect lymphography and lymphoscintigraphy. Lymphat Res Biol. 2003;1:71-3.
61. Hillerdal G. Chylothorax and pseudochylothorax. Eur Respir J. 1997;10:1157-62.
62. Garcia-Pachon E, Romero S. Urinothorax: a new approach. Curr Opin Pulm Med. 2006;12:259-63.
63. Samman PD, White WF. The 'yellow nail' syndrome. Br J Dermatol. 1964;76:153-7.
64. Maldonado F, Ryu JH. Yellow nail syndrome. Curr Opin Pulm Med. 2009;15:371-5.

CHAPTER

27 Pleural Disorders in Lung Transplantation—Overview

Mohan Venkatesh Pulle, Vivek Singh, Arvind Kumar

INTRODUCTION

Pleural disease is an important aspect to consider in patients considered for lung transplantation. Pleural space disruption, temporary interruption of innate lymphatic drainage,[1] allograft rejection, and post-transplantation immunosuppression predisposes for various pleural complications after lung transplantation. In addition, if a patient already has a preexisting pleural disease, it further increases the risk of postoperative pleural complications.

PREDISPOSING FACTORS FOR PLEURAL COMPLICATIONS

The two major risk factors for postoperative pleural complications include:

1. Preexisting pleural disease
2. Size mismatch between donor and recipient lung

Preexisting Pleural Disease

The presence of preexisting pleural disease increases the intraoperative and postoperative complications of lung transplantation. To enumerate, such pleural diseases are pneumothorax, empyema thoracis, hemothorax, and chylothorax. Previous chest tube insertion and history of previous chest surgery such as lung biopsy, pleurodesis, or pleurectomy also increase the possibility of pleural adhesions. The risk factors for pleural adhesions are mentioned in **Table 1**.

All these diseases can cause dense intrathoracic vascular adhesions, which can increase the intraoperative blood loss and operative times during recipient pneumonectomy and recipient lung parenchymal injury, eventually causing pleural contamination (especially in suppurative lung diseases). This also increases the possibility of iatrogenic phrenic nerve injury, chylothorax, and reexploration rates. Excessive blood loss directly correlates with the greater number of blood transfusions, which increases the risk of primary graft dysfunction (PGD) and increased 30-day mortality.[2] In addition, intraoperative pleural contamination is a significant risk factor for the development of postoperative pleural empyema.

History of previous thoracic surgery, especially pleurodesis (mechanical/talc) should be cautiously noted by the transplant team while evaluating a patient for lung transplantation. This is because these procedures can predispose to pleural adhesions, thus more intra-

TABLE 1: Conditions predisposing for pleural adhesions.

Lung pathology	Etiology
Interstitial lung disease	Pneumothorax, history of VATS lung biopsy, and history of previous pleurodesis
Emphysema	Pneumothorax, history of previous pleurodesis, and history of lung volume reduction surgery
Suppurative lung diseases [CF **(Fig. 1)** and non-CF bronchiectasis **(Fig. 2)**]	Chronic inflammation of pleura, empyema thoracis, pneumothorax, history of previous surgery/chest tube insertion, and pleural effusion with previous history of pulmonary tuberculosis
LAM	Pneumothorax and chylothorax

(CF: cystic fibrosis; LAM: lymphangioleiomyomatosis; VATS: video-assisted thoracoscopic surgery)

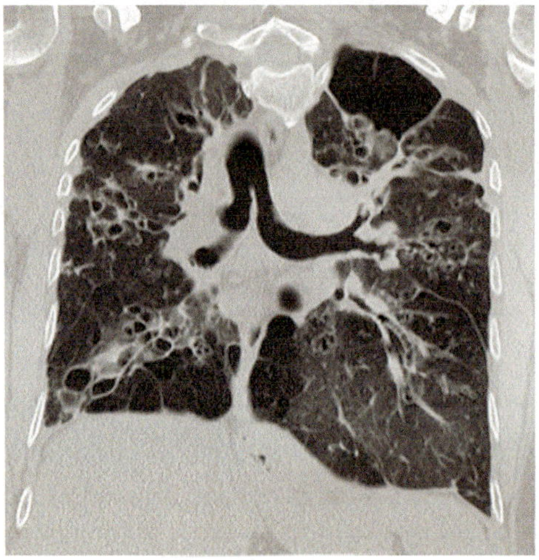

FIG. 1: Cystic fibrosis (CF)-related bilateral bronchiectasis.

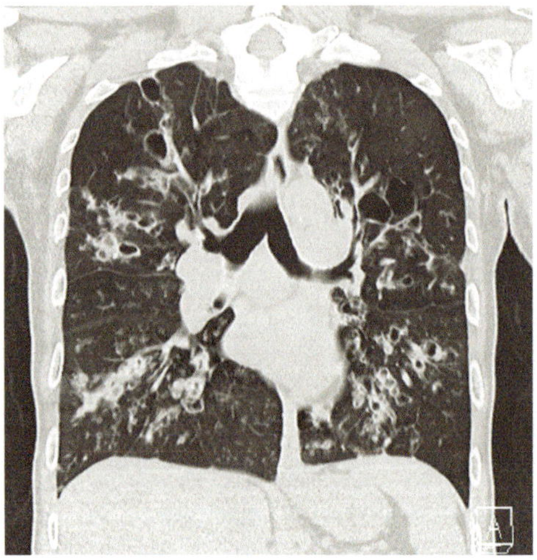

FIG. 2: Noncystic fibrosis (non-CF) bilateral bronchiectasis.

and postoperative problems. Nevertheless, previous history of pleurodesis is not a contraindication for lung transplantation. Pneumothorax in a prospective lung transplant candidate should be managed with the modality which has best, immediate outcomes.[3]

Size Mismatch between Donor and Recipient Lung

Pleural complications can be anticipated in donor–recipient size mismatch, particularly when the donor lung volume/size is smaller for the recipient. This smaller donor size can arise in three situations as follows:

1. *Lung transplantation for obstructive lung disease, i.e., emphysematous lungs*: This disease causes hyperinflation of the native recipient lungs, thus greatly increasing the chest cavity volume. In such patients, transplantation of undersized lungs can lead to persistent residual pleural space, resulting in recurrent pleural effusions.[4]
2. *Living donor lobar lung transplantation*: In this procedure, lower lobes of two donors were transplanted into the recipient. As lobar vessels and bronchus were anastomosed to main bronchus and main pulmonary vascular structures, they are prone to anastomotic complications and residual pleural space.[5]
3. *Pediatric donor lungs implanted in adult recipients*: Such situations are prone to vascular and bronchial anastomosis mismatch. This can lead to bronchial anastomotic leak, causing pneumothorax and bleeding/oozing at the site of vascular anastomosis, causing hemothorax. The undersized lungs predispose for residual pleural space, pleural effusion, and eventually empyema thoracis.[6]

PLEURAL COMPLICATIONS OF LUNG TRANSPLANTATION

Pleural complications are one of the most common problems following lung transplantation, with an incidence of 22–45%.[7] Incidence of such complications is common in the early postoperative period; however, they can occasionally occur in the late postoperative period as well. Pleural complications in the early and late postoperative period are enlisted in **Box 1**.

Pleural Effusion

Pleural effusion is the most common pleural complication that happens after lung transplantation. This can be early or late postoperative. Probable causative factors of early and late pleural effusion are mentioned in **Box 2**.

BOX 1 **Pleural complications following lung transplantation.**

Early postoperative complications:
- Pleural effusion
- Hemothorax
- Pneumothorax
- Chylothorax

Late postoperative complications:
- Chronic pleural effusion
- Empyema thoracis
- Malignant pleural effusion
- Pleural fibrosis and pleuroparenchymal fibroelastosis (PPFE)

BOX 2 Causative factors for pleural effusion after lung transplantation.

Early pleural effusion:
- Donor lung ischemia—reperfusion injury
- Pulmonary edema
- Abnormalities of pulmonary venous anastomosis

Late pleural effusion:
- Acute rejection
- Malignancy
- Infections (tuberculosis)
- Abnormalities of pulmonary venous anastomosis

Pleural Effusion in the Early Postoperative Period

- The most common cause for early pleural effusion after lung transplantation **(Fig. 3)** is increased alveolar permeability. This is due to a gross imbalance between excessive production and impaired drainage mechanisms after lung transplantation. Due to factors such as graft ischemia (warm and cold), reperfusion injury, and denervation—there is excessive pleural fluid production.[8] This situation becomes more complicated when the drainage mechanisms (lymphatic channels) are disturbed. Almost every patient who underwent lung transplantation has mild-to-moderate pleural effusion.[9] However, having a massive amount of effusion is a rarity.[10] Most of mild-to-moderate effusions resolve spontaneously with chest drains and diuretics.[11] This is the reason all of lung transplant patients are left with intercostal drains for 10–14 days after surgery. The daily decrease in the quantity of pleural fluid is directly proportional to the severity of resolution of pulmonary edema secondary to reperfusion injury.
- Pulmonary venous anastomosis abnormalities—thrombosis, kinking, and stenosis are also significant risk factors for development of either unilateral or bilateral pleural effusion. Such anatomical factors as a cause for pleural effusion are more common in the early postoperative period than in late post lung transplant.

Pleural Effusion in the Late Postoperative Period

- Pleural effusions can result from acute lymphocytic cellular rejection. The pleural fluid analysis in such patient reveals lymphocytic predominance (90%).[12] However, it is not universal that all patients with acute rejection will develop pleural effusion. If mild-to-moderate pleural effusion develops, such effusions resolve spontaneously within few days with the treatment of rejection.

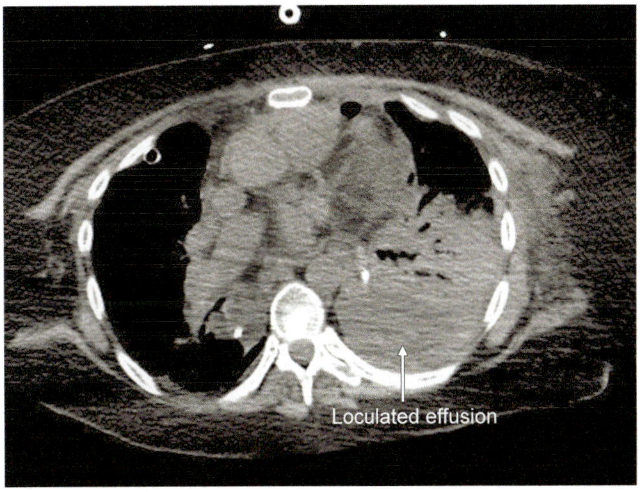

FIG. 3: Loculated pleural effusion in the early postoperative period.

- Lung transplant patients are at increased risk of developing malignancy in view of prolonged immunosuppression. The common form of such malignancy is post-transplant lymphoproliferative disorder (PTLD). However, this form of malignancy rarely causes pleural effusion.[13] However, pleural secondaries and primary malignant mesothelioma can present with hemorrhagic pleural effusion.[14]
- Pulmonary venous anastomotic issues are usually the cause of effusions in the early postoperative period. However, there are reports of pleural effusion developing due to venous anastomosis issues even after 1-year post-transplant.[15]

Management

Mild pleural effusions, if not very symptomatic, can be observed for spontaneous resolution. However, all symptomatic effusions should be treated, irrespective of the amount of fluid. The modalities commonly utilized are (1) chest drain placement with/without fibrinolytic administration, (2) indwelling pleural catheter, and (3) decortication.

- *Chest drain*: In cases of loculated pleural effusion, there is a definitive role of fibrinolytic administration into the pleural cavity. This is reported to be safe and efficacious.[4] In cases of recurrent effusions, the option of achieving pleurodesis through administration of pleurodesis agent (talc/doxycycline) through the chest drain should not be encouraged. This is because of prolonged immunosuppression; the inflammatory response will be blunted and this may predispose for development of pleural effusion into empyema thoracis.[11]

- *Indwelling pleural catheter*: This is another emerging therapeutic modality for recurrent pleural effusion with promising results of autopleurodesis.[16]
- *Decortication*: This surgical option is indicated in cases of loculated/recurrent effusions not amenable for medical management, empyema thoracis, fibrothorax, and hemothorax. If pleural effusion is left alone, it can lead to proliferation of fibroblasts within the pleura, which results in pleural fibrosis (trapped lung), thus restricting lung expansion and causing allograft dysfunction and poor survival. This procedure carries a high morbidity with about one-third of patients developing postoperative complications such as recollection, ventilator requirement, and prolonged intensive care unit (ICU) stay. The mortality rate is up to 5%.[17] Therefore, decortication as therapeutic strategy for recurrent pleural effusion with trapped lung will increase the lung volumes and improve allograft function. Early surgical intervention carries better perioperative outcomes.

Hemothorax

Hemothorax usually happens in the early postoperative period. Patients with dense intrathoracic adhesions are more prone to develop this complication, as all such adhesions should be lysed during recipient pneumonectomy, which predisposes for surface ooze and bleeding. Another source of significant bleeding is perihilar and mediastinal lymph nodes, especially subcarinal group.[18] Achieving perfect hemostasis in this region should be ensured before donor lung implantation as it becomes a very tedious and difficult task once implantation happens. Use of cardiopulmonary bypass during lung transplantation is also proven to cause higher intraoperative blood loss and requirement of blood transfusions.[11] This is because of higher anticoagulation required in comparison to central extracorporeal membrane oxygenation (ECMO). Continuous oozing of blood from the vascular anastomotic site, particularly in cases of gross size mismatch, is also a known risk factor for postoperative hemothorax **(Table 2)**.

TABLE 2: Common risk factors and source of hemothorax after lung transplantation.

Risk factors	Source
Dense pleural adhesions	Perihilar and mediastinal lymph node
Use of cardiopulmonary bypass	Ooze from vascular anastomosis
Size mismatch in vascular anastomosis	Bleeding from internal mammary artery and intercostal artery

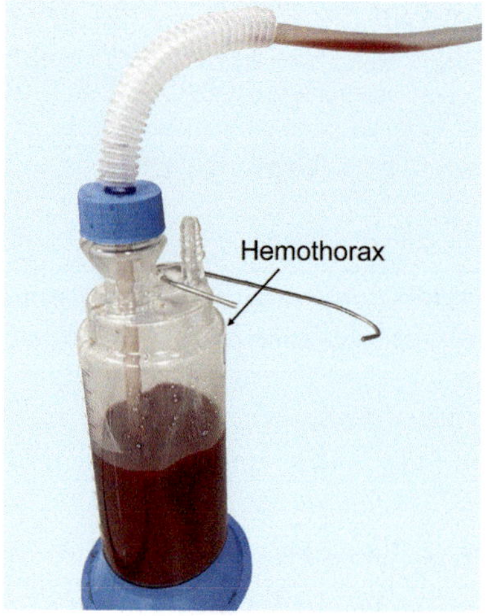

FIG. 4: Hemothorax after lung transplantation.

During the immediate postoperative period, meticulous scrutiny of discharge from thoracostomy tubes is imperative. If a substantial hemorrhagic drain output **(Fig. 4)** is noted, its cessation without intervention becomes improbable. This situation poses a great therapeutic challenge for the transplant surgeons to weigh the risks in both scenarios, i.e., the consequences of leaving a hemothorax in the pleural cavity versus the potential risks of surgical reexploration, the feasibility of pinpointing the source of bleeding, and its prompt surgical rectification. As per the literature, approximately 15% of lung transplant recipients have residual hemothorax.[8,19] The persistence of such hemothorax can potentially act as a substrate for microbial colonization, potentially precipitating further pleural complications, inclusive of lung entrapment or fibrothorax.

Pneumothorax

Pneumothorax is a known complication of lung transplantation. The etiology is multifactorial **(Box 3)**.

Size mismatch, i.e., undersized donor lung is usually the common cause of residual pleural space. Usually, such residual spaces are clinically insignificant, small,

BOX 3 Risk/Predisposing factors for pneumothorax after lung transplantation.

- Size mismatch (undersized donor lung)
- Disease in the donor lung (emphysema/bulla/blebs)
- Bronchial anastomosis leak
- Transbronchial lung biopsy to diagnose rejections
- Infection

and resolve within few weeks.[20,21] Few studies reported that ambitious negative suction application to the chest tubes may not be clinically beneficial and sometimes counterproductive.[22]

Presence of emphysematous changes/bulla/blebs in the donor lung can also be an etiology for development of secondary spontaneous pneumothorax.[23] The management includes chest tube insertion as the initial modality followed by talc pleurodesis/pleurectomy to prevent recurrences.[24]

Pneumothorax can also develop from bronchial anastomosis leak. With conservative therapy such as prolonged chest tube placement, ensuring good nutrition can alone help the air leaks to stop.[19] However if air leak persists beyond 2 weeks, anastomotic dehiscence should be suspected and be confirmed with bronchoscopic examination of anastomotic site. If anastomotic dehiscence is present, decision of tracheobronchial stenting should be considered.[11]

Bronchoscopic examination of tracheobronchial tree is very commonly done in the immediate postoperative period. In cases where rejection is suspected, transbronchial biopsy of lung should be performed for histopathological examination. Pneumothorax is a well-known complication of transbronchial lung biopsy.[25] In few cases, development of cavitary infectious lesions in the donor lung can also be a source of pneumothorax.

Chylothorax

Chylothorax is a rare complication after lung transplantation **(Fig. 5)**.[26] This can present either as early or late complication.[27] Presence of chylomicrons and triglyceride level of >110 mg/dL in the pleural fluid confirms the diagnosis of chylothorax. During lung transplantation, injury to the thoracic duct or to its tributaries causes leakage of chyle into the pleural space, leading to chylothorax. This scenario is especially common in lung transplantation for lymphangioleiomyomatosis. This can be due to spillage of chylous ascites into chest cavity transdiaphragmatically or due to excessive leakiness of lymphatic channels in the thorax.[28,29]

Treatment modalities for post-lung transplant chylothorax include somatostatin analogs, medium-chain triglyceride (MCT) diet as conservative measures and pleurodesis/pleurectomy, thoracic duct ligation, and pleuroperitoneal shunt as surgical treatment—if conservative measures fail.[30,31] Sirolimus is reported to successfully ameliorate the resistant cases of chylothorax in lymphangioleiomyomatosis with a caution that this medication should only be started 3–4 months after lung transplantation until bilateral bronchial anastomosis has completely healed.[32,33]

Empyema Thoracis

Empyema thoracis can occur in 3–7% of patients undergoing lung transplantation. Approximately, 25% of pleural effusions that develop within 3 months of lung transplantation can get converted into empyema **(Fig. 6)**.[9] The clinical symptoms may be masked compared to classical empyema presentation—in view of patient's immunosuppressive status. Therefore, a high degree of clinical suspicion is of paramount importance in diagnosing and treating this clinical entity. The etiology can be bacterial, fungal, mycobacterial, and occasionally uncommon organisms from donor lung.[34] Among all causes, fungal empyema is the most common, accounting for approximately 60% of cases. *Candida albicans* was the predominant organism.

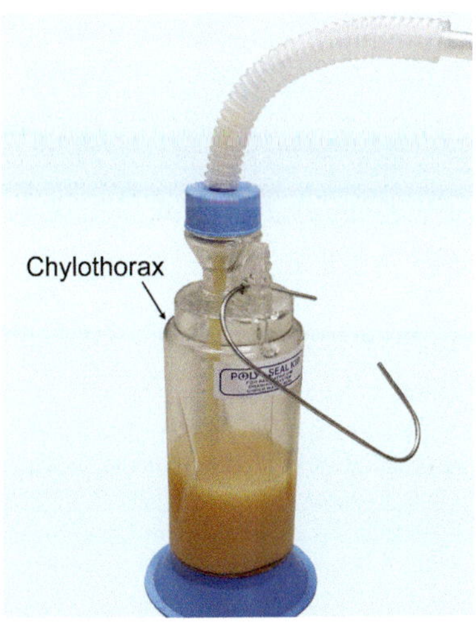

FIG. 5: Chylothorax after lung transplantation.

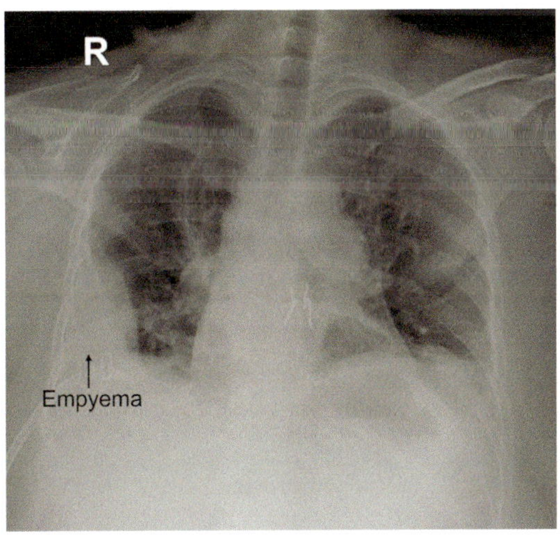

FIG. 6: Empyema thoracis (3 months post-lung transplant).

Therefore, the pleural fluid samples should be sent for bacterial cultures, acid-fast bacteria (AFB) staining, Gene-Xpert, rapid AFB cultures, potassium hydroxide (KOH) stain for fungus and fungal cultures in addition to pleural fluid adenosine deaminase (ADA) levels, and galactomannan levels.[35] Once the diagnosis is made, video-assisted thoracoscopic pleural debridement with/without decortication should be performed to control the septic source. Such pleural infections can significantly diminish 1-year survival, i.e., 67% with infection versus 87% without infection, respectively.[36]

Pleural Fibrosis and Pleuroparenchymal Fibroelastosis

This is a form of restrictive chronic lung allograft dysfunction (CLAD). This is characterized by pleural and subpleural thickening, consolidation, and fibrosis, predominantly in the upper lobes, causing volume loss in the computed tomography (CT) chest.[37,38] No treatment provides promising results for this challenging situation. Antifibrotic medications such as pirfenidone are studied as one of the treatment modalities in clinical trials.[39]

CONCLUSION

Pleura-related complications are a common entity after lung transplantation. Patients who underwent lung transplantation should be closely monitored to detect and address these complications early as they have significant impact on the allograft function and are associated with poor survival. The management of such pleural complications should involve a multidisciplinary team, involving transplant pulmonologists, lung transplant surgeons, and infectious disease specialists. Treatment should be tailored depending on the specific complication and the underlying etiology—which can range from conservative management with chest drain placement to surgical intervention will depend on the specific complication and its underlying cause, but it may include drainage procedures, medication, or surgical interventions.

KEY POINTS

- Pleura-related complications are very commonly encountered after lung transplantation.
- The two major risk factors for postoperative pleural complications are (1) preexisting pleural disease and (2) donor–recipient size mismatch.
- Commonly encountered early postoperative complications include pleural effusion, hemothorax, pneumothorax, and chylothorax.
- The late postoperative pleural complications are late pleural effusion, empyema thoracis, malignant pleural effusion, and pleuroparenchymal fibroelastosis.
- Patients who underwent lung transplantation should be closely monitored to detect and address these complications early, as they have significant impact on the allograft function and are associated with poor survival.
- High index of clinical suspicion and early intervention—key for successful long-term outcomes.

REFERENCES

1. Di Nardo M, Tikkanen J, Husain S, Singer LG, Cypel M, Ferguson ND, et al. Postoperative Management of Lung Transplant Recipients in the Intensive Care Unit. Anesthesiology. 2022;136(3): 482-99.
2. Shigemura N, Bhama J, Gries CJ, Kawamura T, Crespo M, Johnson B, et al. Lung transplantation in patients with prior cardiothoracic surgical procedures. Am J Transplant. 2012;12:1249-55.
3. Weill D. Lung transplantation: indications and contraindications. J Thorac Dis. 2018;10(7):4574-87.
4. Kao CC, Cuevas JF, Tuthill S, Parulekar AD. Pleural catheter placement and intrapleural fibrinolysis following lung transplantation. Clin Transplant. 2019;33:e13592.
5. Backhus LM, Sievers EM, Schenkel FA, Barr ML, Cohen RG, Smith MA, et al. Pleural space problems after living lobar transplantation. J Heart Lung Transplant. 2005;24:2086.
6. Keshava HB, Mason DP, Murthy SC, Brown CR, Pettersson GB. Pediatric donor lungs for adult transplant recipients: feasibility and outcomes. Thorac Cardiovasc Surg. 2012;60:275.
7. Tang A, Siddiqui HU, Thuita L, Rappaport J, Bribriesco AC, McCurry KR, et al. Natural History of Pleural Complications After Lung Transplantation. Ann Thorac Surg. 2021;111:407.
8. Siegleman SS, Sinha SB, Veith FJ. Pulmonary reimplantation response. Ann Surg. 1973;177:30.
9. Ferrer J, Roldan J, Roman A, Bravo C, Monforte V, Pallissa E, et al. Acute and chronic pleural complications in lung transplantation. J Heart Lung Transplant. 2003;22:1217.
10. Raju S, Heath BJ, Warren ET, Hardy JD. Single- and double-lung transplantation. Problems and possible solutions. Ann Surg. 1990;211:681.
11. Arndt A, Boffa DJ. Pleural space complications associated with lung transplantation. Thorac Surg Clin. 2015;25:87.
12. Judson MA, Handy JR, Sahn SA. Pleural effusion from acute lung rejection. Chest. 1997;111:1128.
13. Siegel MJ, Lee EY, Sweet SC, Hildebolt C. CT of post-transplantation lymphoproliferative disorder in pediatric recipients of lung allograft. AJR Am J Roentgenol. 2003;181:1125.

14. Chhajed PN, Bubendorf L, Hirsch H, Boehler A, Weder W, Tamm M. Mesothelioma after lung transplantation. Thorax. 2006;61:916.
15. Jing L, Chen W, Zhai Z, Pan X, Tao X, Cao L, et al. Pulmonary vein stenosis after lung transplantation: a case report and literature review. Ann Transl Med. 2021;9:181.
16. Trindade AJ, Lentz RJ, Gannon WD, Rickman OB, Shojaee S, Vandervest K, et al. Safety and utility of indwelling pleural catheters in lung transplant recipients. Clin Transplant. 2023;37:e15056.
17. Rappaport JM, Siddiqui HU, Tang A, Thuita LW, Raja S, Bribriesco A, et al. Pleural space management after lung transplant: Early and late outcomes of pleural decortication. J Heart Lung Transplant. 2021;40:623.
18. Yamamoto H, Sugimoto S, Imanishi K, Hashimoto K, Miyoshi K, Otani S, et al. Meticulous closure of collateral vessels in the perihilar mediastinal pleura to control intraoperative bleeding during lung transplantation for pulmonary hypertension. J Thorac Dis. 2021;13(10):5658-69.
19. Herridge MS, de Hoyos AL, Chaparro C, Winton TL, Kesten S, Maurer JR. Pleural complications in lung transplant recipients. J Thorac Cardiovasc Surg. 1995;110:22.
20. Griffith BP, Zenati M. The pulmonary donor. Clin Chest Med. 1990;11:217.
21. Eberlein M, Arnaoutakis GJ, Yarmus L, Feller-Kopman D, Dezube R, Chahla MF, et al. The effect of lung size mismatch on complications and resource utilization after bilateral lung transplantation. J Heart Lung Transplant. 2012;31:492.
22. Kozower BD, Meyers BF, Ciccone AM, Guthrie TJ, Patterson GA. Potential for detrimental hyperinflation after lung transplantation with application of negative pleural pressure to undersized lung grafts. J Thorac Cardiovasc Surg. 2003;125:430.
23. Spaggiari L, Rusca M, Carbognani P, Cattelani L, Rossini E, Paolucci R, et al. Contralateral spontaneous pneumothorax after single lung transplantation for fibrosis. Acta Biomed Ateneo Parmense. 1993;64:29.
24. Venuta F, Rendina EA, de Giacomo T, Ciriaco PP, Della Rocca G, Ricci C. Thoracoscopic treatment of recurrent contralateral pneumothorax after single lung transplantation. J Heart Lung Transplant. 1994;13:555.
25. McWilliams TJ, Williams TJ, Whitford HM, Snell GI. Surveillance bronchoscopy in lung transplant recipients: risk versus benefit. J Heart Lung Transplant. 2008;27:1203.
26. Jacob S, Meneses A, Landolfo K, El-Sayed Ahmed M, Makey IA, Pham SM, et al. Incidence, Management, and Outcomes of Chylothorax after Lung Transplantation: A Single-center Experience. Cureus. 2019;11:e5190.
27. Boehler A, Speich R, Russi EW, Weder W. Lung transplantation for lymphangioleiomyomatosis. N Engl J Med. 1996;335:1275.
28. Penketh AR, Higenbottam TW, Hutter J, Coutts C, Stewart S, Wallwork J. Clinical experience in the management of pulmonary opportunist infection and rejection in recipients of heart-lung transplants. Thorax. 1988;43:762.
29. Ryu JH, Doerr CH, Fisher SD, Olson EJ, Sahn SA. Chylothorax in lymphangioleiomyomatosis. Chest. 2003;123:623.
30. Fremont RD, Milstone AP, Light RW, Ninan M. Chylothoraces after lung transplantation for lymphangioleiomyomatosis: review of the literature and utilization of a pleurovenous shunt. J Heart Lung Transplant. 2007;26:953.
31. Kanou T, Nakagiri T, Minami M, Inoue M, Shintani Y, Okumura M. Peritoneovenous shunt for chylous ascites after lung transplantation for lymphangioleiomyomatosis. Transplant Proc. 2012;44:1390.
32. Ohara T, Oto T, Miyoshi K, Tao H, Yamane M, Toyooka S, et al. Sirolimus ameliorated post-lung transplant chylothorax in lymphangioleiomyomatosis. Ann Thorac Surg. 2008;86:e7.
33. Sugimoto R, Nakao A, Yamane M, Toyooka S, Okazaki M, Aoe M, et al. Sirolimus amelioration of clinical symptoms of recurrent lymphangioleiomyomatosis after living-donor lobar lung transplantation. J Heart Lung Transplant. 2008;27:921.
34. Shaver CM, Castilho JL, Cohen DN, Grogan EL, Miller GG, Dummer JS, et al. Fatal Scopulariopsis infection in a lung transplant recipient: lessons of organ procurement. Am J Transplant. 2014;14:2893.
35. Mills NL, Boyd AD, Gheranpong C. The significance of bronchial circulation in lung transplantation. J Thorac Cardiovasc Surg. 1970;60:866.
36. Wahidi MM, Willner DA, Snyder LD, Hardison JL, Chia JY, Palmer SM. Diagnosis and outcome of early pleural space infection following lung transplantation. Chest. 2009;135:484.
37. Verleden SE, Ruttens D, Vandermeulen E, Bellon H, Van Raemdonck DE, Dupont LJ, et al. Restrictive chronic lung allograft dysfunction: Where are we now? J Heart Lung Transplant. 2015;34:625.
38. Ofek E, Sato M, Saito T, Wagnetz U, Roberts HC, Chaparro C, et al. Restrictive allograft syndrome post lung transplantation is characterized by pleuroparenchymal fibroelastosis. Mod Pathol. 2013;26:350.
39. Venado A, Dewey K, Montas G, Greenland J, Leard L, Shah R, et al. Safety and tolerability of pirfenidone for restrictive chronic lung allograft dysfunction (pirclad): Interim results. Chest. 2020;158:A2389.

CHAPTER

28 Medical Thoracoscopy

Rajiv Goyal, Sandeep Katiyar

INTRODUCTION

Medical thoracoscopy or pleuroscopy is the direct telescopic visual examination of the pleural cavity with a rigid or semirigid thoracoscope, performed under conscious sedation and analgesia, through a single port in the chest wall. It is usually indicated for the diagnosis of pleural effusions, where the analysis of the pleural fluid does not provide a definite answer. The thoracoscope is used for taking biopsies from the diseased pleura under direct vision and has revolutionized the management of pleural diseases. A pleurodesis with a chemical sclerosant can be performed in the same sitting if desired.

This procedure was first performed in Ireland by *Francis Richard Cruise* in 1865,[1-3] but it was Hans Christian Jacobaeus, a Swedish internist, in 1908, who made it popular and described the procedure in detail. The word "thoracoscopy" was first used by him, which is described as *"replacing fluid with air."* He used a cystoscope to visualize the pleural cavity and later performed thoracoscopic electrocautery to lyse adhesions between the lung and chest wall as a treatment of tuberculosis (TB) and is rightfully known as the *father of thoracoscopy*. The procedure fell into disuse with the advent of chemotherapy for TB. Later, it became popular again with the availability of superior technology developed for minimally invasive surgery by pioneers such as Loddenkemper and later Philippe Astoul. It was soon realized that it could also be used for video-assisted thoracoscopic surgery (VATS). It is a tool which is now indispensable in the diagnosis of idiopathic pleural effusions and offers the highest diagnostic yield.[4] The diagnostic yield goes up to 91–95% in malignancies of the pleura.[5,6]

Video-assisted thoracoscopic surgery is in the domain of thoracic surgeons, and is performed with general anesthesia, a double-lumen endotracheal tube, and is meant for advanced surgical procedures through multiple ports. On the other hand, medical thoracoscopy or pleuroscopy is usually performed by pulmonologists, under conscious sedation and local anesthesia, mainly for diagnosis, through a single port. Traditionally, medical thoracoscopy had been done with a rigid thoracoscope; although later, a semirigid instrument for the same purpose was developed and has become very popular. We will briefly describe the instruments, methodology, indications, advantages, and complications of thoracoscopy.

INSTRUMENTS FOR THORACOSCOPY

Rigid Thoracoscopy Instruments

These consist of the following:

- *A trocar and cannula*: These are usually 5–10 mm in diameter and are needed for making the port in the chest wall, leading into the pleural cavity. This acts as a conduit for the thoracoscope to be passed inside.
- *Thoracoscope*: This instrument has within its assembly a telescope with an eyepiece and a working channel. The proximal eyepiece can be used for direct visualization or can be fitted with a camera connected to a monitor for a magnified view of the pleural cavity. The telescope can be 0° for direct end on viewing or

a 30° or 45° for lateral viewing. The working channel is used for suction, for introducing biopsy forceps, for cautery probe, and also for performing pleurodesis, all under direct vision.

- *Accessories*: These are, as mentioned earlier, a forceps used for taking biopsies, scissors for cutting through adhesions, and a probe for cauterizing bleeding tissue. Besides these, a suction cannula for sucking out pleural fluid or instilling local anesthetic, saline for irrigation, or talc for pleurodesis with the help of an insufflator (powder blower) are also used.

Instruments used for rigid medical thoracoscopy are shown in **Figures 1A to J**.

Semirigid Instruments

The semirigid thoracoscope is built like the flexible bronchoscope but with a flexible tip which is 5 cm long and a rigid proximal stem which is 22 cm in length. Like a bronchoscope, it has single-working channel for suction and biopsies, a proximal assembly with a lever for manipulating the tip, and a connection for the video processor.

Currently, two semirigid thoracoscopes by Olympus are available: LTF 160 and LTF H 290. The former one is the older version with 160/130° angulation and a 2.8-mm working channel, while the latter one is the new one, offering better angulation up to 180°. This can be helpful in taking biopsies of lesions around the port of entry. This model also has a wider channel of 3 mm for better suction. Both these models are autoclavable **(Figs. 2A and B)**.

ENDOSCOPY SUITE

Medical thoracoscopy can be performed in the bronchoscopy suite, provided strict sterility is maintained

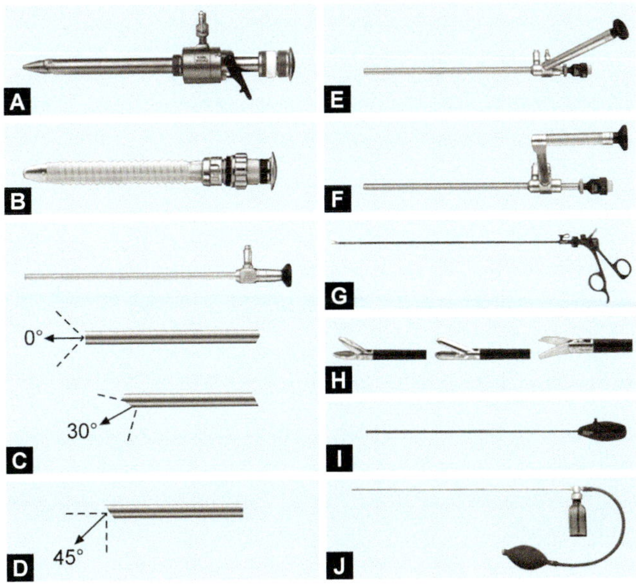

FIGS. 1A TO J: Instruments for rigid medical thoracoscopy. (A)Trocar with multifunctional valve with insufflation stopcock; (B) trocar with silicone leaflet valve; (C) telescope, particularly suited for single-incision thoracoscopy with diameter 10 mm, length 31 cm, and trocar size 11 mm; (D) various fields of view: (1) straightforward telescope 0°, (2) forward-oblique telescope 30°, and (3) 45° telescope; (E) straightforward telescope 0° with angled eyepiece, diameter 10 mm, working length 27 cm, with instrument channel 6 mm, trocar size 11 mm, single puncture. (F) Straightforward telescope 0°, with a parallel eyepiece (bayonet optic), diameter 10 mm, working length 27 cm, with instrument channel 6 mm, trocar size 11 mm, single puncture. (G) Dissecting and biopsy forceps, rotational, that can be dismantled, with connector pin for unipolar coagulation, 5 mm. (H) Single-action jaws: (1) dissecting and biopsy forceps, (2) biopsy forceps, and (3) scissors. (I) Dissecting electrodes, with connector pin for unipolar coagulation, L-shaped, size 5 mm, working length 43 cm. (J) Powder blower, with rubber bulb, size 5 mm and working length 42 cm.

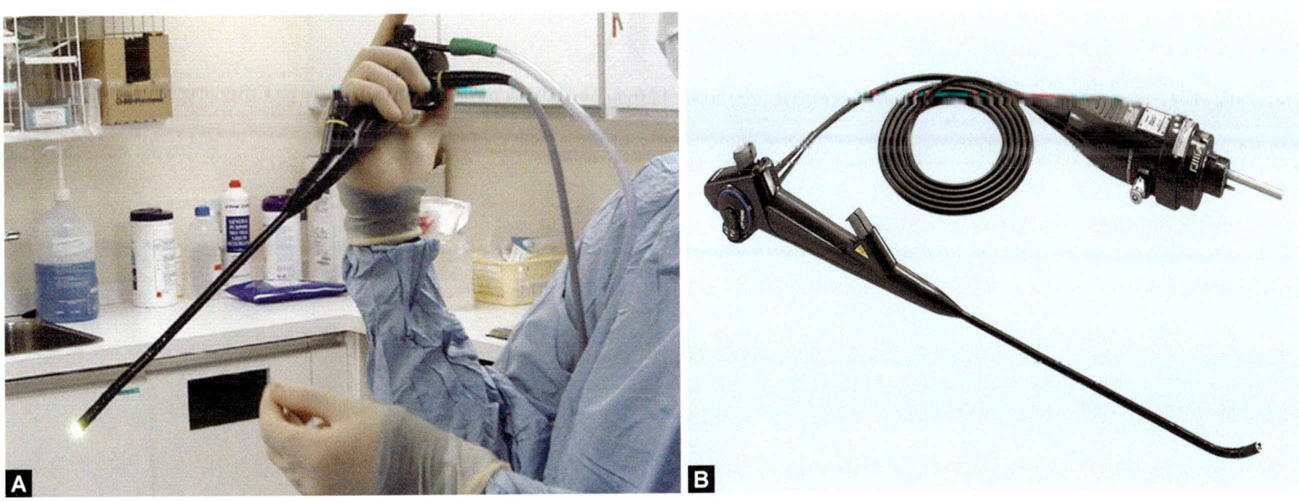

FIGS. 2A AND B: (A) Semirigid thoracoscopes; (B) LTF H-290 pleuroscope.

BOX 1 Equipment used in medical thoracoscopy.

- Thoracoscopy table
- Sterile trolley for instruments
- Sterile syringe, knife, dissecting forceps, trocar, and intercostal drainage tube
- Oxygen and suction
- Overhead light
- Resuscitation cart
- Electrocautery
- Separate mobile carts for endoscopic light sources, video equipment, and computer for recording
- Ultrasonography

during the procedure. The list of equipment is mentioned in **Box 1**.

INDICATIONS FOR MEDICAL THORACOSCOPY

Diagnostic

- Pleural effusion of indeterminate origin—this is the main indication.
- Staging of lung cancer and malignant mesothelioma
- Evaluation of cases of suspected drug-resistant TB
- For tissue acquisition in cytology-positive malignant pleural effusion

Therapeutic

- Talc poudrage in malignant and recurrent nonmalignant pleural effusion
- Parapneumonic effusions and empyema for removing adhesions and for facilitating drainage and lung reexpansion[7]
- Talc poudrage in pneumothorax[8]

Advanced procedures:
- Pleuropericardial window
- Medical sympathectomy

CONTRAINDICATIONS FOR MEDICAL THORACOSCOPY[9,10]

Absolute

- Lack of pleural space due to severe adhesions or post-pleurodesis
- Hypercapnia or severe respiratory distress
- Uncorrectable coagulopathy
- Lack of informed consent
- Inexperienced operator

Relative

- Not able to tolerate lateral decubitus position
- Refractory cough
- Poor general health and short survival expectation
- Unstable cardiovascular or hemodynamic status
- High likelihood of trapped lung
- Presence of central airway mass
- Contralateral significant lung disease
- Morbid obesity
- Severe pulmonary fibrosis
- Significant comorbid disease
- Drug hypersensitivity

Potential Complications of Medical Thoracoscopy[11-21]

Thoracoscopy is a relatively safe procedure with a few minor complications and rarely any major complication.[22]

- *Before the procedure*:
  - Air embolism, subcutaneous emphysema, and pain during pneumothorax induction
  - Shortness of breath after pneumothorax induction
  - Hypersensitivity reaction to local anesthetic
- *During the procedure*:
  - Pain
  - Hypoxemia
  - Hypoventilation
  - Hypotension
  - Cardiac arrhythmias
  - Hemorrhage
  - Injury to lung, heart, diaphragm, liver, or spleen
- *After the procedure*:
  - Reexpansion pulmonary edema
  - Pain
  - Postoperative fever
  - Wound infection
  - Hypotension
  - Empyema
  - Subcutaneous emphysema
  - Persisting pneumothorax
  - Prolonged air leakage
  - Continuing pleural fluid production
  - Seeding of chest wall by tumor cells
  - Mortality

Premedication

Medical thoracoscopy is a procedure which does not require general anesthesia and can be performed under local anesthesia with moderate sedation. The British Thoracic Society (BTS) guidelines on pleural diseases recommend 1% of lidocaine up to a maximum of 3 mg/kg[23] for infiltration of the skin and chest wall at the site selected for the initial incision and insertion of the trocar. Benzodiazepine (midazolam or lorazepam) along with narcotics (morphine or fentanyl) help in achieving further analgesia and conscious sedation. Since the procedure is performed under local anesthesia with conscious sedation, an anesthetist is not required.[24] Propofol can also be used but its use is not recommended as the drug of choice since its use is associated with higher incidence of hypoxemia, hypotension, and sudden cardiac arrest. It also requires the presence of an anesthetist.[25,26] Neither prophylactic nor routine use of antibiotics is recommended.

TECHNIQUE FOR THORACOSCOPY

An X-ray chest and electrocardiography (ECG) should be taken preferably 24 hours before the procedure. Routine blood test, coagulation profile, and viral markers are also prerequisites for the procedure.[23-28]

Any allergies should be documented and an opinion for any other comorbidity should be taken.

- Preprocedure fasting of 6 hours
- Anticoagulants to be withheld
- Warfarin 5 days
- Clopidogrel 5–7 days
- Dabigatran 2–4 days
- Rivaroxaban 2–3 days
- Apixaban 1–2 days
- Enoxaparin, fondaparinux, and aspirin 24 hours
- Heparin 4–6 hours

The technique should be well explained to the patient and a proper, informed consent should be taken.

The patient should be made to lie in a lateral decubitus position with the affected side up **(Fig. 3A)**. An ultrasound should be performed at this point to mark the point of entry. If it is not available, then an arbitrary site of 3–4th space in the midaxillary line in pneumothorax or 5–7th space (safety triangle) in case of effusion is preferred.[23,29] Patient should be cleaned from the spine up to the sternum, including the axilla and then draped. After giving proper local anesthesia, pleural fluid should be withdrawn by a syringe, thereby confirming its location. An incision of 1–2 cm parallel to the ribs is made by the surgical blade, cutting the skin and the subcutaneous tissue. If no fluid is aspirated, then an artificial pneumothorax should be created either by using a blunt Boutin needle or splitting open the parietal pleura by a blunt forceps. Further, dissection is done by a blunt "Kelly" artery forceps. On reaching the parietal pleura, the trocar is inserted perpendicular to the chest wall with a corkscrew motion while keeping the thumb on the chest wall so as not to injure the underlying lung.

Once the pleura has been breached, the cannula is pushed in by 2–3 cm and the trocar is taken out. At this point, one should be careful as in massive effusions, there can be a sudden spurt of fluid out of the cannula. It is best to cover the entry point by a gauze pad and the fluid be suctioned out gradually by a suction catheter. This should be narrower than the cannula to allow air to enter inside the pleural cavity. This replaces the fluid and thereby prevents the lung from sudden reexpansion and the subsequent pulmonary edema that can occur. Once a significant amount of fluid has been removed, the thoracoscope is inserted. Any remaining fluid is taken out by the thoracoscope and then all the pleural surfaces are inspected systematically. If adhesions prevent examination, they can be removed either by the forceps or by electrocautery. This is more easily done with the rigid thoracoscope than with the semirigid thoracoscope. Very thick or vascular adhesions are better left alone. Lower half of chest or the caudal aspect should be more than carefully inspected as 90% of malignant lesions are present there.[30,31] The biopsy should be taken from the affected area preferably over the rib as the neurovascular bundle lies inferior to it **(Figs. 3B and C)**. Pinch and peel technique offers better tissue size, especially with the semirigid thoracoscope which has a smaller forceps. Here the tissue, after closing the biopsy forceps, is lifted and then the thoracoscope is moved sideways, thereby facilitating tearing off of the tissue. At least 3–6 biopsies should be taken and be kept in different bottles, namely saline for microbiology and formalin for histopathological examination.[24,32] A chest drain is inserted through the same cannula after removing the thoracoscope, at the end of the procedure, and is usually directed to the posterior costophrenic recess. It must be anchored to the skin by tying firm sutures with it to avoid its displacement. In cases where a large amount of fluid has been removed, we prefer to intermittently clamp and reopen it at intervals of 8 hours up to a maximum of 24 hours after which it is left open to prevent reexpansion pulmonary edema. Similar experience was reported by de Campos et al. where 7 patients developed acute respiratory distress syndrome (ARDS) and 12 developed reexpansion pulmonary edema.[33] If the patient starts coughing violently on connection of the chest drain to the underwater seal, the underwater seal should be disconnected and the lung should be allowed to collapse back and then the same procedure should be followed where it is opened every hourly. The drain is removed mostly within the next 2–3 days once reexpansion has been confirmed on the chest X-ray and the drainage of fluid is <100 mL along with an absent air leak.

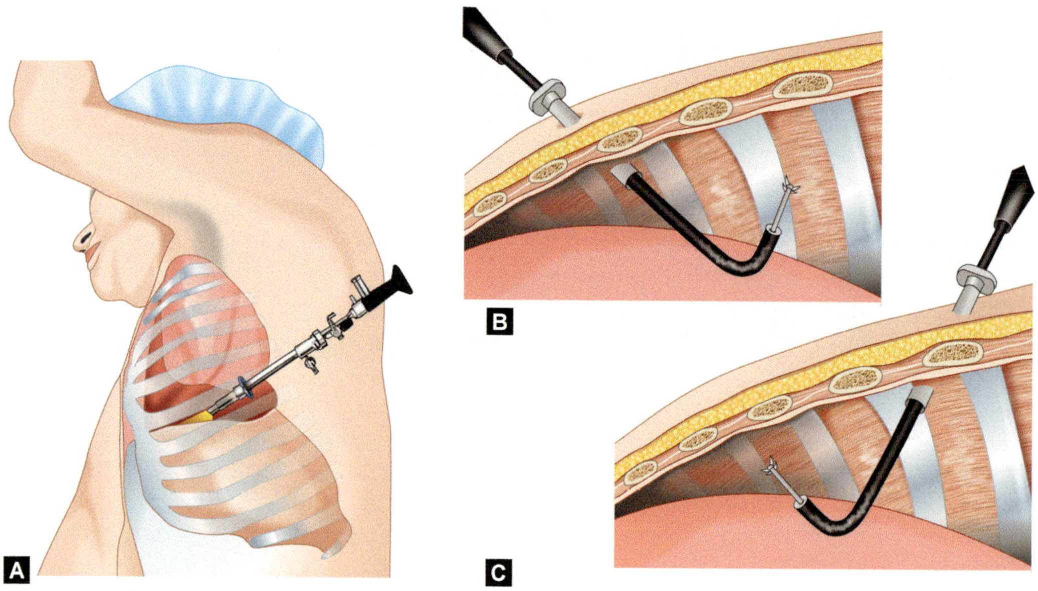

FIGS. 3A TO C: (A) Position of patient while in thoracoscopy; (B) Position of thoracoscope while visualizing posterior gutter; and (C) Position of thoracoscope while visualizing anterior gutter.

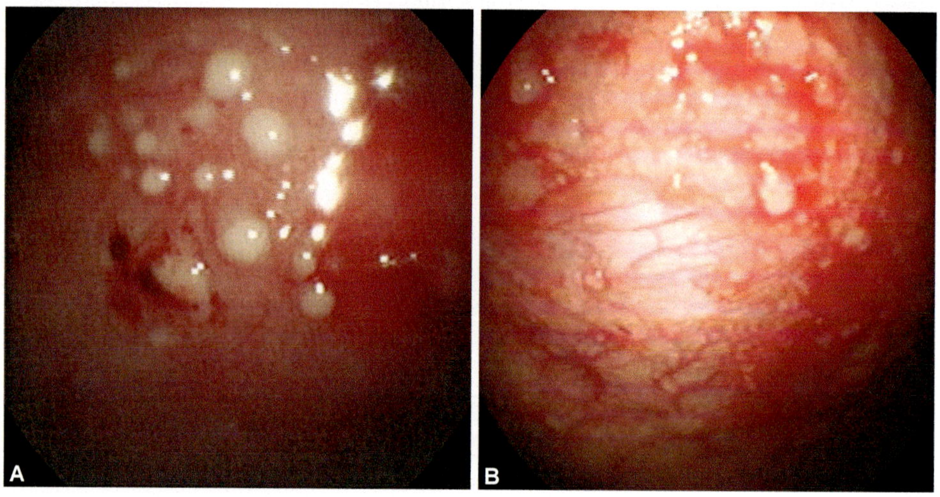

FIGS. 4A AND B: (A) Thoracoscopic image of tubercular nodules and (B) Thoracoscopic image of malignant nodules.

ENDOSCOPIC APPEARANCE OF THE PLEURA

Nodules: This is the most common presentation. These vary in size from 1 to 5 mm and may be noticed on the visceral or parietal pleural surfaces. Soft nodules are mostly associated with TB, while the harder ones are most likely malignant. The malignant nodules often have underlying neovascularization and an angry-looking pleura **(Figs. 4A and B)**.

Pleural thickening: This is the second most common presentation, where the near-transparent film is lost to a more rigid pleura, which can have an irregular and pebbly surface. In some cases, the thickening can be so severe that biopsies also become very difficult. Such appearances are called pachypleuritis **(Figs. 5A and B)**.

Masses: These are larger than nodules and can appear as large as the size of grapes. These are universally malignant. However rather than a single appearance, it is mostly a combination of the above which is present in patients **(Figs. 6A and B)**.

Adhesions: These often appear as web-like structures when flimsy and can be easily removed or band-like structures which are tougher to remove and may bleed on excision.

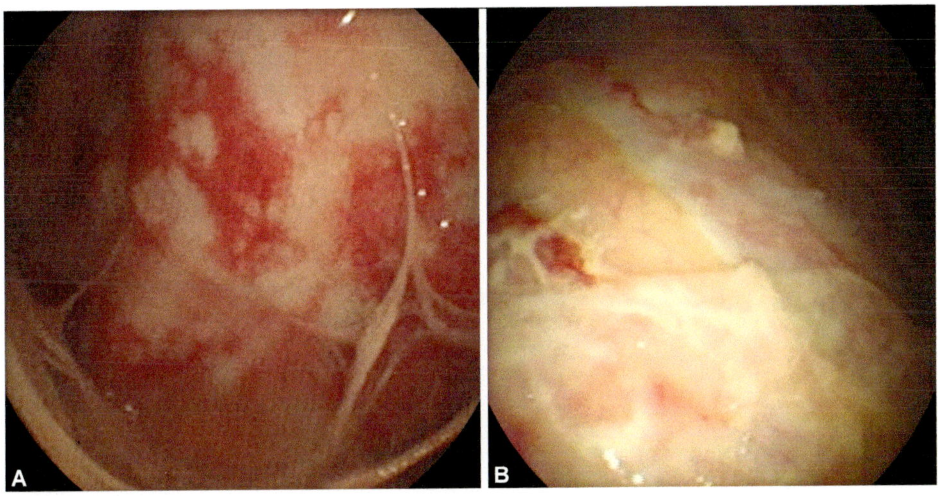

FIGS. 5A AND B: Thoracoscopic images of pleural thickening.

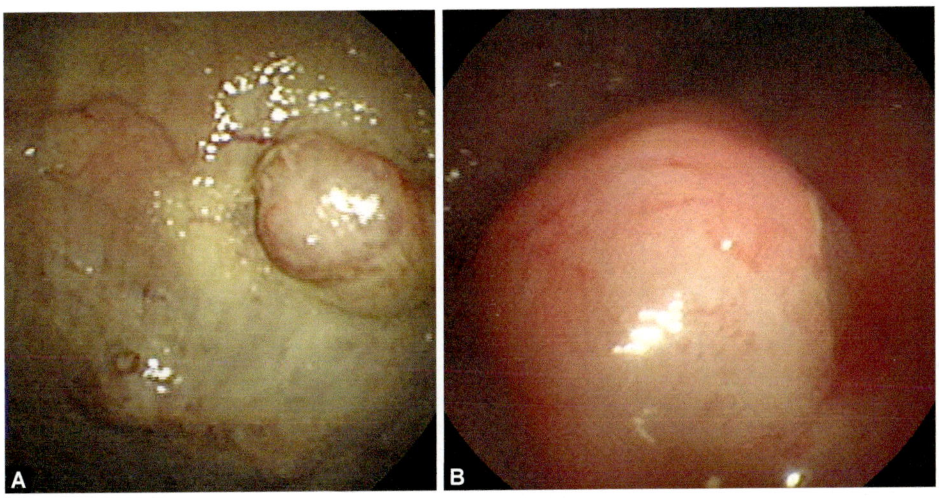

FIGS. 6A AND B: Thoracoscopic images of tumoral masses arising from the parietal pleura.

Medical Thoracoscopy in Tuberculosis

Upon its inception, medical thoracoscopy was exclusively used for TB; however nowadays, it is only a subset of cases which require exploration, namely tubercular effusions and empyemas, which either require mechanical removal of adhesions or are possible drug-resistant pleural effusion, which keep on refilling despite adequate antitubercular therapy. The diagnosis of the latter requires bacteriological confirmation of mycobacterium tubercular bacilli either by culture or GeneXpert. The cultural yield of thoracoscopic by biopsy is higher at 90–97%, while that of pleural fluid is low, anywhere between 23 and 67%.[11,34-37]

The GenXpert test can also be performed on biopsies.[29] Endoscopic appearance of TB is typical with yellowish, white soft nodules and sloughed appearance of pleura **(Figs. 7A and B)**.[36]

Medical Thoracoscopy in Pneumothorax

The incidence of pneumothorax is around 6 per 100,000 cases per year.[38] It is mostly due to rupture of blebs or bullae because of sudden violent cough or sudden changes in weather or atmospheric pressure. Pneumothorax was classified by Vanderschueren based on thoracoscopic findings.[31]

Type 1: Lung appears normal
Type 2: Adhesions are present
Type 3: Bullae or blebs < 2 cm in diameter
Type 4: Bullae or blebs > 2 cm in diameter

The role of thoracoscopy in primary spontaneous pneumothorax is limited to those patients with persistent air leak or for prevention of recurrence.[32,39] Since medical thoracoscopy interventions are generally limited to the parietal pleura, its use is restricted in pneumothorax where

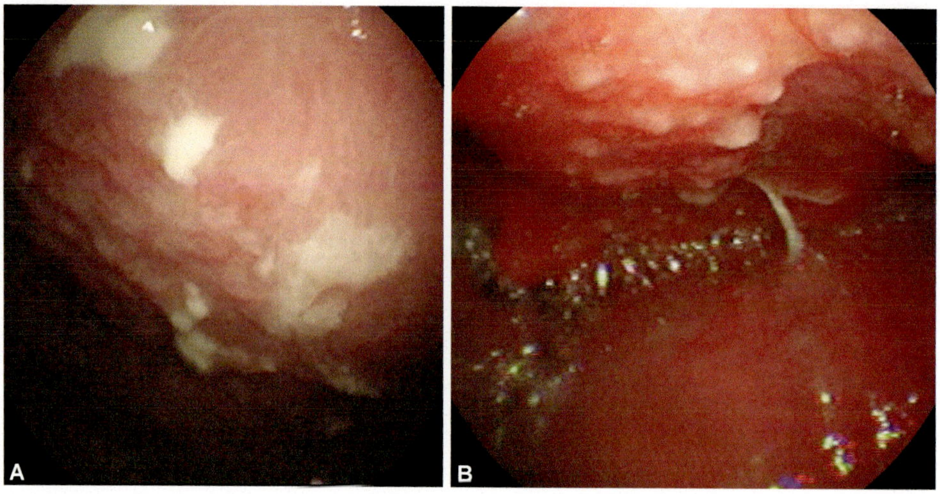

FIGS. 7A AND B: Thoracoscopic images of pleura in tuberculosis, depicting the whitish, yellowish nodules.

there is involvement of visceral pleura, to pleurodesis only.[40,41] Stapling for bullectomy, which is a standard treatment for bigger air leaks, is better performed with VATS than medical thoracoscopy.

Medical Thoracoscopy in Pleural Effusions

This forms the most common indication of medical thoracoscopy, where the origin of pleural effusion is indeterminate. Light's criteria classified pleural effusion as transudate and exudate which was later validated by Joseph et al. who stated that the absolute level of lactate dehydrogenase (LDH) in pleural fluid is the ideal marker to differentiate these two.[42,43] Thoracoscopy is indicated in exudative pleural effusions rather than transudative ones as the pleural surface is not affected by the primary pathologic process in the latter.[43] The most common cause of transudative effusion is cardiac failure followed by liver cirrhosis and nephrotic syndrome. However, a few cases of transudative pleural effusion may be caused by malignancies blocking the lymphatics.

The initial step in pleural effusion diagnosis is thoracentesis which has a yield of 50% on the first cytology and goes up to 65–70% on the second and third ones, respectively.[44] Closed pleural biopsy increases this yield by only around 7%.[14] Boutin et al. reported a positive yield of mere 36% by Abrams needle vs 87% by medical thoracoscopy in a prospective study.[11] Similar results were demonstrated by Loddenkemper et al. in Tru-cut needle biopsy and thoracoscopy.[22] The yield of medical thoracoscopy is >90% in these patients with undiagnosed pleural effusions.[45,46] Guided biopsies are recommended in cases with significant pleural thickening, leading to fusion of both the surfaces of pleura where thoracoscopy is difficult.

Often, the patients who remain undiagnosed on medical thoracoscopy are due to inadequate sampling of the pleura due to adhesions.

Malignant Pleural Effusion

Pleura is one of the most common places for malignancies to metastasize, with the most common being lung cancer followed by breast cancer.[47] Confirmation of pleural metastasis upstages a non-small cell lung cancer (NSCLC) two stage 4 (a/b), so it is recommended by the BTS to perform thoracoscopy if two samples are negative on thoracentesis.[48] Pleural malignancy is practically excluded if thoracoscopy is negative; however, autofluorescence increases the yield further by using blue light or narrowband imaging.[49] In view of the earlier, it is recommended to perform medical thoracoscopy on all patients who are cytology negative on two consecutive thoracentesis. The most common examination finding is that of nodules or masses (37%), followed by pleural thickening (26%), and a combination of the above (21%).[45]

Occasionally if the pleural fluid cytology is positive but the primary malignancy is unknown, medical thoracoscopy can be done for obtaining pleural tissue for immunohistochemistry and other diagnostic tests.

Mesothelioma

Malignant mesothelioma is a malignancy which arises from the mesothelial or submesothelial cells of either the pleura, peritoneum, or pericardium and the origin is 80% of the times from pleura.[50] It is of three major types based on history morphology—epithelioid, biphasic, and sarcomatoid. It presents as pleural effusions and cytological examination is not able to confirm the

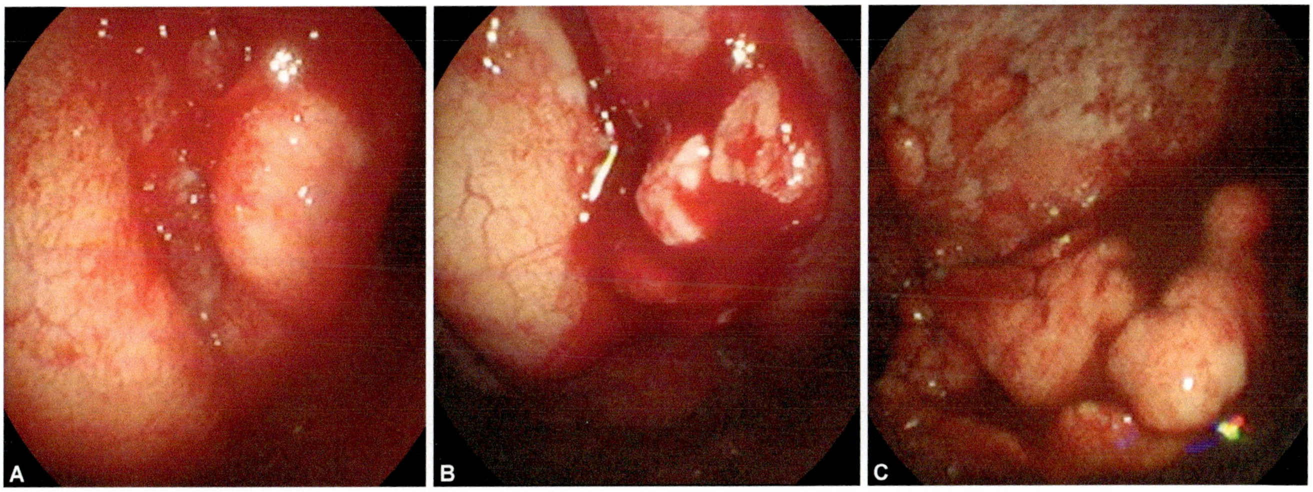

FIGS. 8A TO C: Thoracoscopic image of tumoral masses with pleural thickening in a case of malignant mesothelioma.

disease and its positivity only in 32–51.3% cases.[6,51] The diagnostic efficacy of medical thoracoscopy is around 87.5–92.6%.[52] The lower yield might be explained because in the beginning, the invasion is submesothelial which may lead to a grossly normal appearing pleura.[53] To avoid this, biopsies in these cases should be taken from different areas especially targeting plaques and nodules **(Figs. 8A to C)**.

THERAPEUTIC MEDICAL THORACOSCOPY

Pleurodesis

Talc insufflation by thoracoscopy is a safe and effective method in patients with malignant pleural effusion. A retrospective series of 327 patients had a recurrence rate of only 10% after 1 month and 80% of patients had lifelong pleural symphysis.[15] In a meta-analysis of 24 studies, talc was found to be superior to other agents such as doxycycline, povidone iodine, and bleomycin.[54] Talc slurry also has similar results and there is no statistical difference between talc insufflation and slurry.[55] About 4–8 g of sterile-graded asbestos-free talc is recommended to be used for effective pleurodesis having an average particle size of >25 μm.

Parapneumonic Effusion and Empyema

Parapneumonic effusions are a common problem, complicating pneumonias. They are present in as many as 60% of the cases of pneumonia requiring hospitalization.[56,57] Three stages are described. While the first stage, which is a simple effusion, generally responds to underlying treatment of pneumonia, the second and third one require intervention in one form or the other.

Stage 2 is the one which is most effectively managed by medical thoracoscopy, which consists of lysing the adhesions formed and drainage of all the fluid present, thereby providing for proper functioning of antibiotics and expansion of the underlying lung. The same was shown in a retrospective study of 126 patients, where 54 of the 57 patients of stage 2, i.e., 94.7% and 42 of 59 of stage 3 (71.2%) were effectively managed.[58] Other retrospective studies also had similar findings.[59]

Medical thoracoscopy is also a safe tool and can be offered to those patients who have several comorbidities and thus at high risk for VATS. The other advantages over VATS include single port, less postprocedure pain, and lesser cost.

Stage 3 involves the patients who alongside adhesions also developed pleural thickening. All these patients earlier used to be referred for VATS; however, thoracoscopy is also being used in these cases. Intercostal drain along with intrapleural fibrinolytics are also advised in stages 2 and 3, but a review of the available studies does not support their use.[60] VATS is generally required in chronic empyema where a rind is present and prevents the lung from expansion.[61]

Therefore, it is recommended that medical thoracoscopy should be used early in the course of disease where the results are better.[13,62] Apart from the debulking capabilities of medical thoracoscopy, inspection of the thoracic cavity can also help in identifying foreign bodies or esophageal fistulas and assessing the underlying lung condition.[63]

Recently, a meta-analysis on medical thoracoscopy in pleural infection demonstrated a pooled success rate of 85% when used as first-line intervention or after a failed chest tube and a complication rate of 9% only amongst 552 patients **(Figs. 9 and 10)**.[64]

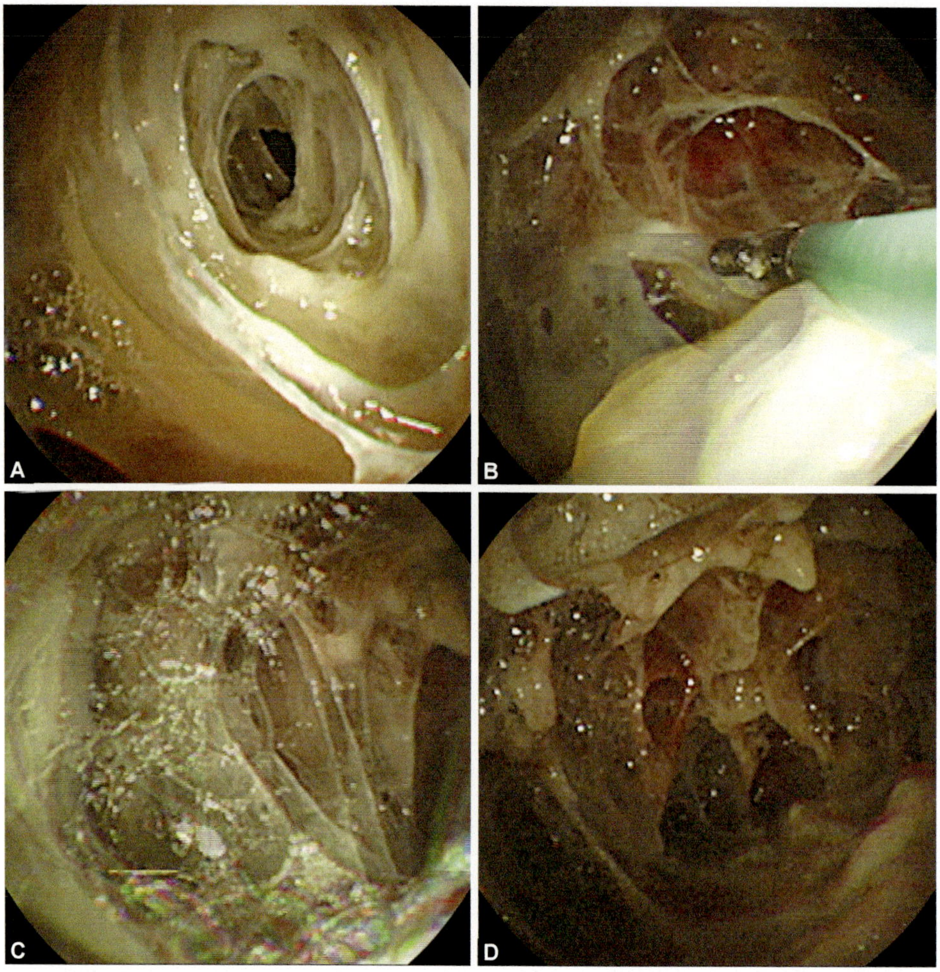

FIGS. 9A TO D: Stage 3 parapneumonic effusion (empyema) with dense adhesions.

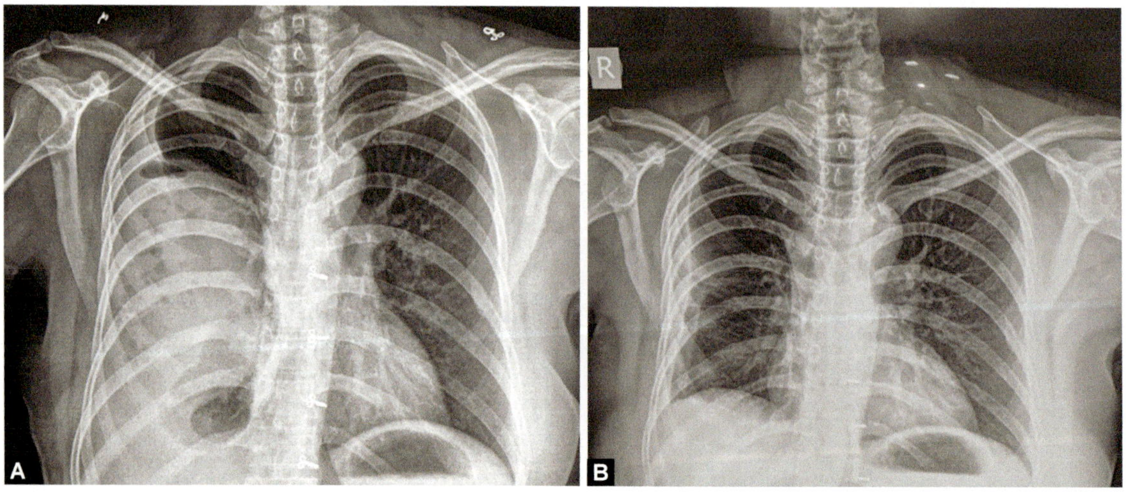

FIGS. 10A AND B: (A) Multiloculated empyema and (B) 30 days post-thoracoscopic adhesiolysis, only a small pleural rind remains.

Advanced procedures such as creation of a pleuro-pericardial window or a thoracoscopic sympathectomy to be performed by experts are beyond the scope of this chapter and will not be discussed here.

ADVANTAGES OF RIGID THORACOSCOPE OVER SEMIRIGID THORACOSCOPE

The rigid thoracoscope is cheaper, sturdier, yields larger biopsies, and can be used to break tough adhesions to free the underlying lung. The latter quality is especially useful in tackling parapneumonic effusions. In situations where the pleura is too firm and fibrous, biopsies are easier to take with the rigid instrument rather than with the semirigid one. In a randomized trial to compare the two thoracoscopes, rigid thoracoscopy was found to be superior to semirigid thoracoscopy overall, but the diagnostic yield was similar if pleural biopsy could be successfully performed.[65]

KEY POINTS

- Medical thoracoscopy is a procedure which has existed for over a century now but has undergone several changes in the last two decades.
- It is a very safe procedure in competent hands and has a simple learning curve.
- It has undisputed advantages over VATS, of being done under simple local anesthesia and conscious sedation in a bronchoscopy suite, coupled with a high diagnostic accuracy.
- It can also be used effectively for simple therapeutic procedures such as pleurodesis and adhesiolysis.
- It is an investigational tool which now has found a permanent place in the management of pleural diseases and a skill which must be taught to all aspiring pulmonologists.

REFERENCES

1. Jacobaeus HC. Über die Möglichkeit, die Zystoskopiebei Untersuchungen seröser Höhlungen anzuwenden. On the possibility, to use cystoscopy to examine serous cavities. Münch Med Wochenschr. 1910;40:2090-2.
2. Moisiuc FV, Colt HG. Thoracoscopy: origins revisited. Respiration. 2007;74:344-55.
3. Cruise FR. The endoscope as an aid to the diagnosis and treatment of disease. Br Med J. 1865;8:345-7.
4. Avasarala SK, Lentz RJ, Maldonado F. Medical Thoracoscopy. Clin Chest Med. 2021;42(4):751-66.
5. Metintas M, Ak G, Dundar E, Yildirim H, Ozkan R, Kurt E, et al. Medical thoracoscopy vs. CT scan-guided Abrams pleural needle biopsy for diagnosis of patients with pleural effusions: a randomized, controlled trial. Chest. 2010;137(6):1362-8.
6. Wang XJ, Yang Y, Wang Z, Xu LL, Wu YB, Zhang J, et al. Efficacy and safety of diagnostic thoracoscopy in undiagnosed pleural effusions. Respiration. 2015;90(3):251-5.
7. Shojaee S, Lee HJ. Thoracoscopy: medical versus surgical in the management of pleural diseases. J Thorac Dis. 2015;7(Suppl 4): S339-51.
8. Casal RF, Eapen GA, Morice RC, Jimenez CA. Medical thoracoscopy. Curr Opin Pulm Med. 2009;15(4):313-20.
9. MacDuff A, Arnold A, Harvey J; BTS Pleural Disease Guideline Group. Management of spontaneous pneumothorax: British Thoracic Society Pleural Disease Guideline 2010. Thorax. 2010;65(Suppl 2):ii18-31.
10. Jin F, Wang H, Li Q, Li S, Lai G, Huang J, et al. Expert consensus for diagnosis and treatment using medical thoracoscopy in China. J Thorac Dis. 2020;12(5):1799-810.
11. Boutin C, Viallat JR, Cargnino P, Rey F. Thoracoscopic lung biopsy. Experimental and clinical preliminary study. Chest. 1982;82:44-8.
12. Loddenkemper R, Schönfeld N. Medical thoracoscopy. Curr Opin Pulm Med. 1998;4(4):235-8.
13. Colt HG. Thoracoscopy. A prospective study of safety and outcome. Chest. 1995;108:324-9.
14. Baumgartner WA, Mark JB. The use of thoracoscopy in the diagnosis of pleural disease. Arch Surg. 1980;115:420-1.
15. Beltsios ET, Mavrovounis G, Adamou A, Panagiotopoulos N. Talc pleurodesis in malignant pleural effusion: a systematic review and meta-analysis. Gen Thorac Cardiovasc Surg. 2021;69(5):832-42.
16. Migliore M, Giuliano R, Aziz T, Saad RA, Sgalambro F. Four-step local anesthesia and sedation for thoracoscopic diagnosis and management of pleural diseases. Chest. 2002;121:2032-5.
17. Dijkman JH, van der Meer JW, Bakker W, Wever AM, van der Broek PJ. Transpleural lung biopsy by the thoracoscopic route in patients with diffuse interstitial pulmonary disease. Chest. 1982;82:76-83.
18. Mares DC, Mathur PN. Medical thoracoscopic talc pleurodesis for chylothorax due to lymphoma: a case series. Chest. 1998;114:731-5.
19. Vansteenkiste J, Verbeken E, Thomeer M, Van Haecke P, Eeckhout AV, Demedts M. Medical thoracoscopic lung biopsy in interstitial lung disease: a prospective study of biopsy quality. Eur Respir J. 1999;14:585-90.
20. Viskum K, Enk B. Complications of thoracoscopy. Poumon Coeur. 1981;37:25-8.
21. Jensen MO, Matthees DJ, Antonenko D. Laser thoracoscopy for pleural effusion. Am Surg. 1992;58:667-9.
22. Lewis RJ, Kunderman PJ, Sisler GE, Mackenzie JW. Direct diagnostic thoracoscopy. Ann Thorac Surg. 1976;21:536-9.
23. Rahman NM, Ali NJ, Brown G, Chapman SJ, Davies R, Downer NJ, et al. Local anaesthetic thoracoscopy: British Thoracic Society pleural disease guideline. Thorax. 2010;65(Suppl 2):ii54-60.
24. Loddenkemper R, Lee P, Noppen M, Mathur PN. Medical Thoracoscopy/Pleuroscopy: Step by Step. Breathe. 2011;8: 156-67.

25. Grendelmeier P, Tamm M, Jahn K, Pflimlin E, Stolz D. Propofol versus midazolam in medical thoracoscopy: a randomized, noninferiority trial. Respiration. 2014;88(2):126-36.
26. Tschopp JM, Purek L, Frey JG, Schnyder JM, Diaper J, Cartier V, et al. Titrated sedation with propofol for medical thoracoscopy: a feasibility and safety study. Respiration. 2011;82(5):451-7.
27. Murthy V, Bessich JL. Medical thoracoscopy and its evolving role in the diagnosis and treatment of pleural disease. J Thorac Dis. 2017;9(Suppl 10):S1011-21.
28. Panadero FR, Janssen JP, Astoul P. Thoracoscopy: general overview and place in the diagnosis and management of pleural effusion. Eur Respir J. 2006;28:409-21.
29. Hooper C, Lee YCG, Maskell N. Investigation of a unilateral pleural effusion in adults: British Thoracic Society pleural disease guideline 2010. Thorax. 2010;65(Suppl 2):ii4-17.
30. Canto A, Rivas J, Saumench J, Morera R, Moya J. Points to consider when choosing a biopsy method in cases of pleurisy of unknown origin. Chest. 1983;84:176-9.
31. Boutin C, Astoul P, Seitz, B. The role of thoracoscopy in the evaluation and management of pleural effusions. Lung. 1990;168(Suppl 1):1113-21.
32. Thomas M, Ibrahim WH, Raza T, Mushtaq K, Arshad A, Ahmed M, et al. Medical thoracoscopy for exudative pleural effusion: an eight-year experience from a country with a young population. BMC Pulm Med. 2017;17(1):151.
33. de Campos JR, Vargas FS, de Campos Werebe E, Cardoso P, Teixeira LR, Jatene FB, et al. Thoracoscopy talc poudrage: a 15-year experience. Chest. 2001;119(3):801-6.
34. Scerbo J, Keltz H, Stone DJ. A prospective study of closed pleural biopsies. JAMA. 1971;218:377-80.
35. Enk B, Viskum K. Diagnostic thoracoscopy. Eur J Respir Dis. 1981;62:344-51.
36. Kamholz S. Pleural tuberculosis. In: Rom W, Garay S (Eds). Tuberculosis. Boston: Little, Brown and Company; 1996. pp. 483-91.
37. Light RW. Diagnostic principles in pleural disease. Eur Respir J. 1997;10:476-81.
38. Vanderschueren RG. Thorascopie sous anesthésie local. Poumon Coeur. 1981;37:21.
39. Baumann MH, Strange C, Heffner JE, Light R, Kirby TJ, Klein J, et al.; AACP Pneumothorax Consensus Group. Management of spontaneous pneumothorax: an American College of Chest Physicians Delphi consensus statement. Chest. 2001;119:590-602.
40. Janssen JP. Thoracoscopy in the management of spontaneous pneumothorax. Int Surg. 1996;81:339-42.
41. Light RW, Macgregor MI, Luchsinger PC, Ball WC Jr. Pleural effusions: the diagnostic separation of transudates and exudates. Ann Intern Med. 1972;77:507-13.
42. Joseph J, Badrinath P, Basran GS, Sahn SA. Is the pleural fluid transudate or exudate? A revisit of the diagnostic criteria. Thorax. 2001;56:867-70.
43. Salyer WR, Eggleston JC, Erozan YS. Efficacy of pleural needle biopsy and pleural fluid cytopathology in the diagnosis of malignant neoplasm involving the pleura. Chest. 1975;67:536-9.
44. Saha K, Maji A, Bandyopadhyay A, Jash D. Diagnostic Yield of Closed Pleural Biopsy in Undiagnosed Exudative Pleural Effusions. Maedica (Bucur). 2021;16(1):34-40.
45. Boutin C, Viallat JR, Cargnino P, Farisse P. Thoracoscopy in malignant pleural effusions. Am Rev Respir Dis. 1981;124: 588-92.
46. Antony VB, Loddenkemper R, Astoul P, Boutin C, Goldstraw P, Hott J, et al. Management of malignant pleural effusions. Eur Respir J. 2001;18:402-9.
47. Pretreatment evaluation of non-small-cell lung cancer. The American Thoracic Society and The European Respiratory Society. Am J Respir Crit Care Med. 1997;156:320-32.
48. Rusch VW. A proposed new international TNM staging system for malignant pleural mesothelioma. From the International Mesothelioma Interest Group. Chest. 1995;108:1122-8.
49. Delgermaa V, Takahashi K, Park EK, Le GV, Hara T, Sorahan T. Global mesothelioma deaths reported to the World Health Organization between 1994 and 2008. Bull World Health Organ. 2011;89(10):716-24.
50. Renshaw AA, Dean BR, Antman KH, Sugarbaker DJ, Cibas ES. The role of cytologic evaluation of pleural fluid in the diagnosis of malignant mesothelioma. Chest. 1997;111(1):106-9.
51. Rakha EA, Patil S, Abdulla K, Abdulkader M, Chaudry Z, Soomro IN. The sensitivity of cytologic evaluation of pleural fluid in the diagnosis of malignant mesothelioma. Diagn Cytopathol. 2010;38(12):874-9.
52. Yang Y, Wu YB, Wang Z, Wang XJ, Xu LL, Tong ZH, et al. Long-term outcome of patients with nonspecific pleurisy at medical thoracoscopy. Respir Med. 2017;124:1-5.
53. Viallat JR, Rey F, Astoul P, Boutin C. Thoracoscopic talc poudrage pleurodesis for malignant effusions. A review of 360 cases. Chest. 1996;110:1387-93.
54. Reeder LB. Malignant pleural effusions. Curr Treat Options Oncol. 2001;2:93-6.
55. Strange C, Sahn SA. The definitions and epidemiology of pleural space infection. Semin Respir Infect. 1999;14:3-8.
56. Hamm H, Light RW. Parapneumonic effusion and empyema. Eur Respir J. 1997;10:1150-6.
57. Ghirotti C, Ravaglia C, Puglisi S, Martinello S, Gurioli C, Sultani F, et al. Medical thoracoscopy: a safe approach for treatment of pleural empyema. Eur Respir J. 2021;58:PA3788.
58. Brutsche MH, Tassi GF, Györik S, Gökcimen M, Renard C, Marchetti GP, et al. Treatment of sonographically stratified multiloculated thoracic empyema by medical thoracoscopy. Chest. 2005;128(5):3303-9.
59. Cameron R. Intra-pleural fibrinolytic therapy vs. conservative management in the treatment of parapneumonic effusions and empyema. Cochrane Database Syst Rev. 2000:CD002312.
60. Landreneau RJ, Keenan RJ, Hazelrigg SR, Mack MJ, Naunheim KS. Thoracoscopy for empyema and hemothorax. Chest. 1996;109:18-24.
61. Sendt W, Forster E, Hau T. Early thoracoscopic debridement and drainage as definite treatment for pleural empyema. Eur J Surg. 1995;161:73.
62. Weissberg D. Pleuroscopy in empyema: is it ever necessary? Poumon Coeur. 1981;37:269.
63. Mondoni M, Saderi L, Trogu F, Terraneo S, Carlucci P, Ghelma F, et al. Medical thoracoscopy treatment for pleural infections: a systematic review and meta-analysis. BMC Pulm Med. 2021;21:127.
64. Davidson AC, George RJ, Sheldon CD, Sinha G, Corrin B, Geddes DM. Thoracoscopy: assessment of a physician service and comparison of a flexible bronchoscope used as a thoracoscope with a rigid thoracoscope. Thorax. 1988;43:32732.
65. Menzies R, Charbonneau M. Thoracoscopy for the diagnosis of pleural disease. Ann Intern Med. 1991;114:271-6.

CHAPTER

29 Pleural Biopsy and Cryobiopsy

Rahul Roshan, Amit Dhamija

INTRODUCTION

Pleural biopsy is the process of obtaining tissue samples from the pleural surfaces, mainly to ascertain the specific etiology for a pathologic pleural effusion. It can be performed either without radiologic guidance for diffuse pleural involvement or with image guidance for localized pleural disease.

TYPES OF PLEURAL BIOPSY

- *Needle biopsy*: Traditionally, percutaneous pleural biopsy was done with specially designed needles. It can be either done as a closed (blinded) procedure or with image guidance. A generous local anesthetic is given at the selected site and a special needle is inserted into the pleural collection to obtain a sample of parietal pleural tissue. It gives a reasonable yield in diseases that have a diffuse pleural involvement such as tuberculous or rheumatic pleuritis. Ultrasound or computed tomography (CT) scan localization of the diseased/thickened pleura may be done beforehand to guide the needle to the correct location. Image-guided biopsy is preferable in patients with pleural masses or localized pleural diseases and gives higher yields than closed (blinded) biopsy.
- *Thoracoscopic biopsy*: Medical pleuroscopy (MP) and video-assisted thoracoscopic surgery (VATS) are two endoscopic techniques used to visualize the pleural space and obtain tissue samples.[1] Endoscopic pleural biopsy, whether through MP or VATS, has shown the highest diagnostic yield among all available sampling methods, with estimates of approximately 90% when data from multiple studies are pooled.[2] MP is performed under general anesthesia or local anesthetic with sedation. A rigid or a semirigid thoracoscope is introduced into the pleural space to visualize the abnormal areas of pleura and take targeted small pieces of tissue for examination. It is preferred in patients with patchy pleural involvement.
- *Open biopsy*: This procedure is performed under general anesthesia by a thoracotomy incision. It is used when the sample obtained from other types of biopsy is not adequate to provide a definitive diagnosis. It is a surgical procedure done under general anesthesia and a large amount of pleural tissue could be sampled, but in comparison with other procedures giving a very good yield, it is rarely required now.

Needle Biopsy

There are several methods for performing percutaneous pleural biopsy. One approach is closed pleural biopsy (CPB) which involves using special pleural biopsy needles such as the Abrams or Cope needle to obtain tissue samples. Another approach is real-time ultrasound- or CT-guided biopsy. These methods allow for the sampling of pleural tissue with minimal invasiveness.

Personnel

The guidelines from the American College of Chest Physicians recommend that personnel who perform pleural needle biopsy should be competent in thoracentesis which is the procedure to remove fluid from the pleural space. They should also be familiar with the mechanisms and techniques of the biopsy needle being used and be competent in recognizing and treating common complications associated with the procedure.

For trainees, it is recommended that they perform at least five pleural biopsies in a supervised setting to establish basic competency. To maintain competency, dedicated operators should perform at least five procedures per year.[3]

Indications for Needle Biopsy of the Pleura[4-6]

- Investigation of an accumulation of fluid in the pleural cavity with unconfirmed diagnosis on fluid analysis
  - Tubercular pleural effusion with inconclusive adenosine deaminase (ADA) or interferon-gamma levels in pleural fluid
  - Malignancy, primary or metastatic, with negative pleural fluid cytology
- Assessment of localized or widespread thickening of the pleural membrane [pleural thickening (>1 cm) or pleural nodularity on imaging]

Contraindications for Needle Biopsy of the Pleura

- Bleeding diathesis or deranged bleeding parameters
- Lack of pleural space
- Patients on anticoagulants or with uncorrected coagulopathy
- Hemodynamically unstable patients
- Platelet count below 50,000/mm^3 (platelet transfusion should be given before the procedure)
- Borderline respiratory failure (pneumothorax could worsen respiratory failure)
- Empyema (may lead to subcutaneous abscesses at the biopsy site)
- Local cutaneous lesions such as pyoderma or herpes zoster infection
- Uncooperative patient

Equipment Used for Needle Biopsy of the Pleura

- Thoracentesis kit
- Pleural biopsy needle
- Ultrasound or CT for imaging guidance
- Local anesthetic for pleural level anesthesia

Pleural Biopsy Needles

Abram's Needle[7] (Fig. 1)

- *Structure*: The Abram's needle consists of three parts—a large outer trocar, an inner cutting cannula, and an inner solid stylet. The end of the outer trocar is blunt to prevent lung laceration.
- *Incision*: A small scalpel incision is made on the anesthetized skin and subcutaneous tissue to allow insertion of the biopsy needle without excessive force. The incision should be made along the lines of cleavage to minimize scarring.
- *Locking*: The inner cutting cannula fits tightly into the outer trocar and can be locked in two positions. In the closed position, the inner cannula obstructs the notch on the outer trocar, making the needle airtight. In the open position, the inner cannula is slightly withdrawn, allowing airflow through the notch.
- *Insertion*: The stylet is placed in the inner cannula, which is then placed in the outer trocar. The inner cannula is twisted clockwise to close the distal notch of the outer trocar. The needle is inserted into the pleural space by applying firm pressure on the stylet. The large diameter and blunt tip of the needle require significant pressure for insertion.
- *Confirmation*: A popping sound may be heard as the needle enters the pleural space. If the needle cannot pass through the ribs, rotating the patient's arm and shoulder over their head can create sufficient space. Once the tip is thought to be in the pleural space, the inner stylet is removed and a syringe is attached to the inner cannula.
- *Fluid aspiration*: With the inner cannula in the closed position, pleural fluid can be aspirated through the syringe for diagnostic studies. The inner cannula is then rotated counterclockwise to lock the distal notch open, allowing fluid collection without creating a pneumothorax.
- *Biopsy and withdrawal*: A 10–20 mL syringe is attached and the inner cannula is rotated to open the distal notch. The needle is slowly withdrawn with constant aspiration until it hooks onto the pleura. When the needle hooks, it indicates that the parietal pleura is in the notch if fluid can still be aspirated.
- *Closure*: While holding the outer trocar firmly, the inner cannula is rotated into the closed position. The needle can then be safely removed.
- *The modified Abram's pleural biopsy technique*: The procedure involves drawing each tissue sample into a syringe by using suction while keeping the needle partially inserted in the chest until the entire process was finished. In contrast, both the conventional Abram's and Cope's needle techniques necessitate removing the needle from the chest after each pleural biopsy.[8]

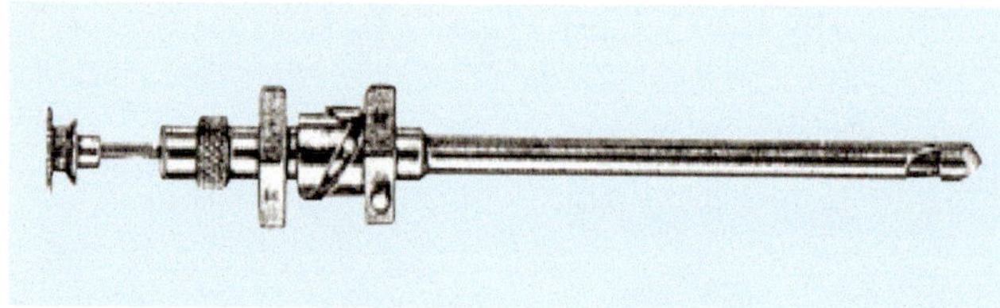

FIG. 1: Abram's needle.

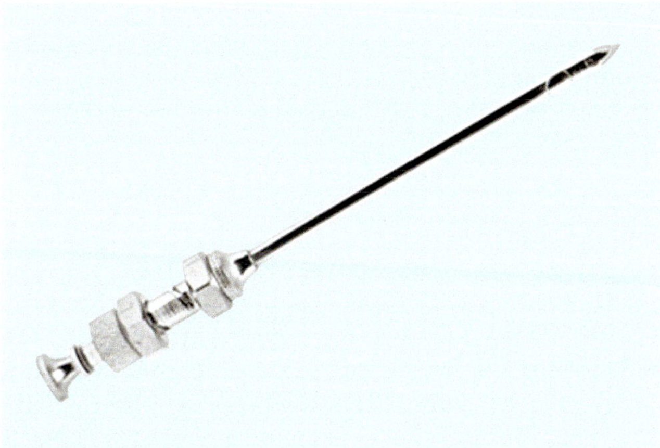

FIG. 2: Cope needle.

Cope Needle[9] (Fig. 2)

- *Structure*: The Cope needle consists of four separate parts—a large outer cannula with a square but sharp end, a hollow, blunt-tipped, hooked biopsy trocar, a hollow-beveled trocar, and a solid, thin obturator or styler.
- *Insertion*: The styler is inserted into the hollow-beveled trocar, which is then placed in the large outer cannula. The apparatus is inserted through a small skin incision into the pleural space.
- *Replacement*: The styler and hollow-beveled trocar are removed from the outer cannula and replaced by the hollow, blunt-tipped, hooked biopsy trocar. This maneuver is performed at the end of a normal expiration while the patient holds his/her breath, with the operator's thumb covering the end of the outer cannula to prevent a pneumothorax.
- *Fluid aspiration*: A syringe may be attached to the outer cannula to obtain fluid for diagnostic studies at this point.
- *Biopsy*: The hooked biopsy trocar, with a syringe attached, is inserted through the large outer cannula into the pleural space. The right-angled projection on the proximal end of the hooked biopsy trocar indicates the direction of the distal biopsy hook.
- *Tissue engagement*: The apparatus is withdrawn with the hook directed inferiorly to avoid nerve, vein, or artery entanglement until the hooked biopsy trocar engages the parietal pleura.
- *Biopsy procedure*: With one hand, the engaged hook is held steady with a continuous outward pulling motion, while the other hand advances the apparatus for biopsy.

Yield and Complications with Abram's and Cope's Needles

- *Diagnostic yield*: Blind pleural biopsies have variable diagnostic yields. The sensitivity for malignancy is reported to be <60%, while in pleural tuberculosis (TB), it ranges from 70% to 90%.[10-12] The difference is attributed to the diffuse nature of tubercular lesions and the patchy distribution of malignancy in the pleural space.
- *Safety and complications*: Closed reverse-bevel needle biopsies are associated with higher rates of complications, including pain at the biopsy site (15%), iatrogenic pneumothorax (15%), and bleeding (<2%). The overall use of blind pleural biopsies is limited and they are generally not recommended unless other methods are unavailable, there is a high prevalence of TB, and the operator is experienced.[6,13]
- *Improved yield*: Performing pleural biopsies with an Abram's needle under CT guidance has been reported to improve the diagnostic yield to around 90%, especially in cases with pleural thickening over 1 cm.[14]

Core-cutting Needle Biopsy

Core-cutting needle biopsy is a technique used to obtain percutaneous pleural biopsies and it is increasingly performed with the guidance of imaging techniques such as CT or ultrasonography (USG). Performing the biopsy under direct image guidance enhances accuracy and safety.

The procedure for core-cutting needle biopsy is like pleural aspiration in terms of asepsis and anesthesia. After preparing the patient and the site, a small incision is made in the skin. The needle is then inserted into the pleural space at a shallow angle under real-time imaging guidance. The goal is to reach the area of pleural thickening.

Once the target area is reached, the cutting part of the needle is advanced into the tissue. The aim is to include both the parietal pleura (the lining of the chest wall) and a portion of the adjacent chest wall structures in the biopsied section. This approach allows the pathologist to evaluate the involvement of subpleural structures, including the presence of fat invasion, which can be indicative of malignant diseases such as mesothelioma.

To ensure sufficient tissue for diagnosis and potential molecular profiling, it is recommended to take 8–10 core biopsies.[15] These biopsies can be obtained from one or multiple sites within the pleural space. Obtaining an adequate amount of tissue is essential for accurate diagnosis and further characterization of the disease.

Performing core-cutting needle biopsies under image guidance offers several advantages, such as improved targeting, increased diagnostic yield, and reduced risk of complications. It allows for precise sampling of the involved pleural tissue and helps guide subsequent management decisions.

Transcutaneous ultrasound (TUS) and CT guidance are both used for core-cutting needle biopsies of the pleura and studies have shown that they have similar diagnostic yields. The reported sensitivity of pleural biopsies using core-cutting needles ranges from 70% to 90%, regardless of whether CT or TUS guidance is used.[16,17]

The choice between TUS and CT guidance depends on the availability of technology. CT-guided biopsies are usually reserved for more challenging cases, such as those located in posterior regions or cases without pleural effusion. However, TUS guidance has several advantages when technically feasible. It is a safer procedure for both the patient and the operator as it does not involve radiation. TUS allows the entire procedure to be carried out in real time, enabling continuous visualization of the needle and immediate detection of any complications.[18,19] Doppler mode in TUS can be used to screen for aberrant intercostal arteries before the procedure, minimizing the risk of pleural bleeding and associated morbidity.[20]

In cases where thoracoscopy is not feasible due to patient preference, frailty, or anatomical limitations of the pleural space, image-guided biopsy becomes an alternative. TUS-guided pleural biopsies have been successful in obtaining sufficient histological diagnosis in most cases, even in patients with absent lung sliding. Combining aspiration with pleural biopsy in patients with TUS evidence of pleural thickening improves diagnostic sensitivity from 38% to 83% as compared to aspiration alone, particularly in cases of pleural malignancy.[21] Addition of TUS-guided percutaneous biopsy to thoracocentesis in patients with large pleural effusion also increases the diagnostic yield from 12.5 to 43%.[22]

Complications

Pneumothorax: It can occur during pleural biopsy due to increased communication between the pleural space and the atmosphere, particularly when using the Cope needle. Additionally, there is a risk of inadvertently incising the visceral pleura during the biopsy, leading to a small bronchopleural fistula that can result in a larger pneumothorax. Studies have shown that the incidence of pneumothorax and the need for tube thoracostomy are comparable between thoracentesis and pleural biopsy.[23]

Bleeding: It is another significant complication associated with pleural biopsy. If an intercostal artery or vein is accidentally biopsied, it can result in a hemothorax. There have been rare reports of an arteriovenous fistula developing between an intercostal artery and vein following pleural biopsy, which subsequently ruptured and caused a hemothorax.[24]

Splenic or renal injury: The pleural biopsy needle may be mistakenly inserted into the liver, spleen, or kidney. While the presence of hepatic or kidney tissue in the biopsy specimen may be demonstrated, it usually does not cause significant adverse effects in the patient. However penetration of the spleen often requires splenectomy, so caution should be exercised not to perform pleural biopsy or thoracentesis too far inferiorly on the left side to avoid spleen-related complications.[25]

Thoracoscopic Pleural Biopsy

Thoracoscopy, a procedure used for diagnostic and therapeutic purposes in the pleural cavity, utilizes an optical system. It is commonly divided into two types—surgical thoracoscopy, also known as VATS, and medical thoracoscopy (MT) or pleuroscopy. Traditionally, both VATS and MT involved the use of rigid instruments. However, the introduction of the flexi-rigid pleuroscope in the late 1990s provided an alternative, allowing proceduralists to choose between rigid or flexi-rigid instruments. Opinion on the superiority of one device over the other has been divided with limited comparative studies available to address this question. Many experienced thoracoscopists prefer the rigid scope for its ability to obtain substantial biopsies, while advocates of flexi-rigid pleuroscopy appreciate the instrument's flexibility and ease of use. The primary distinction between the two instruments lies in their ability to navigate different areas of the pleural cavity. The rigid thoracoscope is limited to a straight path and has restricted maneuverability when examining the posterior and mediastinal aspects of the thoracic cavity, particularly if the lung remains partially or fully inflated. In such cases, the operator needs to angle the scope by leveraging it against the underlying rib, potentially causing pain due to pressure on the periosteum. On the other hand, the flexi-rigid pleuroscope offers greater flexibility and enables the operator to navigate around a nondeflated lung or dense adhesions.[26]

Another major difference between the two types of scopes is the size of tissue obtained on biopsy, which is much larger with a rigid instrument but with a comparable yield between the two. Rigid instruments and accessories are considered better for adhesiolysis and clearing of septated collections.

According to an Indian study on comparison of CPB and thoracoscopy in patients with undiagnosed exudative pleural effusion (EPE), the thoracoscopy group exhibited a significantly higher procedural yield (93.2% vs. 84.5%; $p = 0.02$) compared to the closed-blind pleural biopsy (CBPB) group. The success rates were as follows: CBPB 84.5%, thoracoscopy without point-of-care ultrasonography 90.6%, and thoracoscopy with point-of-care ultrasonography 98.7%. Based on these findings, the authors concluded that MT is the preferred procedure for diagnosing undiagnosed EPE due to its higher success rate and acceptable safety profile compared to CBPB. In situations where thoracoscopy is not feasible, CBPB is recommended, particularly if image-guided procedures are available, instead of initiating empiric treatment. Both rigid thoracoscopy (RT) and semi-RT (SRT) are equally effective and the choice of thoracoscope should consider factors such as availability, the presence of pleural septations, and the necessity for additional procedures such as adhesiolysis.[27]

A meta-analysis done by Wei et al. compared the overall diagnostic effectiveness and safety between CPB and MT in patients with undiagnosed EPE based on previously published studies. The results of the analysis, which included 10 studies and a total of 1,747 patients with undiagnosed EPE, indicated that CPB is a relatively accurate tool, with a pooled sensitivity of 77% and excellent specificity of 99% in this patient population. However, the sensitivity of CPB was found to be lower compared to the pooled sensitivity of MT, which included 23 studies and 1,783 patients (93%). While the diagnostic accuracy of CPB was not superior to that of MT, the primary advantage of CPB over MT was identified as its safety profile. This meta-analysis demonstrated that CPB had lower pooled complication rates (5%) compared to MT (8%). Furthermore, in subgroup analysis, CPB showed a similar ability to diagnose nonmalignant diseases compared to MT (69% vs. 68%), while its ability to diagnose malignant diseases was lower than that of MT (72% vs. 92%). Another subgroup analysis focused on mesothelioma, revealed that the pooled diagnostic accuracy of CPB was 26% [95% confidence interval (CI) 14–38%], whereas MT had a higher pooled diagnostic accuracy of 42% (95% CI 22–62%) ($p < 0.001$).[28]

PLEURAL CRYOBIOPSY

Cryotherapy refers to the application of extreme cold to destroy tissue through rapid freeze–thaw cycles. When tissue is exposed to extremely low temperatures, cell death occurs through various mechanisms. Cryoprobe-based therapy utilizes the Joule Thomson effect in which a liquefied gas rapidly expands at a high flow rate, resulting in very low temperatures at the tip of the cryoprobe. This technique has led to significant advancements in bronchology, introducing cryobiopsy (CB) as a promising sampling method.[29]

On releasing the cryogen, a ball of ice is formed around the tip of the probe and any water-containing tissue is frozen around the probe and avulsed with a tug and pulled off the cryoprobe as a biopsy. This technique allows for the collection of larger and better-preserved tissue specimens compared to traditional forceps biopsy. Additionally, CB minimizes the occurrence of crush artifacts, enhancing the quality and interpretability of the obtained samples.[30]

Since its initial use in 1968, biopsy via cryoprobe has primarily been utilized for managing obstructive endobronchial tumors.[31] Recently, CB is now also being used in diagnosis of pleural pathologies. During MP or VATS, CB is performed by freezing a section of pleural tissue and removing it, instead of using forceps to take a small sample.

Cryobiopsy does not have any specific contraindications apart from the usual contraindications of thoracoscopy and can be performed under local anesthesia and conscious sedation in the bronchoscopy suite. A cryoprobe is inserted through a semirigid or a rigid pleuroscope. The cryoprobe, usually 1.9 or 2.4 mm, is positioned perpendicular to the parietal pleura and frozen for an average of 6–8 seconds, resulting in larger samples from parietal pleura with longer freezing times. After freezing, the pleuroscope and probe are withdrawn together, detaching the frozen parietal pleura. The sample is then thawed, detached from the cryoprobe, and the pleural biopsy site is inspected for bleeding. Intercostal drain is then inserted and connected to underwater seal system.

Pain can be a concern during cryoprobe biopsy due to forceful avulsion of the parietal pleura, but it can be overcome by infiltrating the pleural surface with lidocaine (2%) using a transbronchial needle aspiration. The cryoprobe tip should be perpendicular to the parietal pleural surface to ensure successful sample procurement, as tangential contact with the pleura often results in unsuccessful biopsies. Caution is also necessary when forcefully pulling the probe and scope, ensuring a neutral position of the scope during withdrawal to prevent damage.

The procedure is associated with a low complication rate with no major instances of bleeding or major injury being reported.

The only drawback of taking a CB is that the sample cannot be sent for cultures, both bacterial and tubercular as freezing is likely to kill the microbes. With many thoracoscopies in our country being done for undiagnosed complicated parapneumonic effusions and tubercular pleural effusions, it is advisable to always take forceps biopsies as well from a site different from the site of CB to be sent for required microbiological analysis and cultures.

During SRT, the diagnostic yield of pleural CB was found to be similar to that of flexible forceps biopsy (FFB), according to a study conducted by Dhooria et al. The study included 50 patients and the results indicated that there was no significant difference in the diagnostic yield between CB (78.0%) and FFB (76.0%; $p = 1.00$). Additionally, the study found that CB provided larger specimens compared to FFB (median size 7.0 vs. 4.0 mm; $p < 0.001$) and reached greater depths, extending up to the pleural fat or deeper (CB 65.2% vs. FFB 40.8%; $p = 0.02$). The CB procedure was also quicker than FFB, with a median duration of 10 minutes compared to 15 minutes for FFB ($p < 0.001$). There were no significant differences observed between CB and FFB in terms of the difficulty of performing the biopsy, severity of bleeding, interpretability of histology, or presence of artifacts in the specimens.[32]

In a prospective series of 80 cases with pleural effusion, Wurps et al. conducted an intrapatient comparison of parietal pleural biopsies obtained during MT using rigid forceps, flexible forceps, and cryoprobe. A total of 408 biopsies were taken, with 205 being rigid biopsies, 104 flexible biopsies, and 99 CBs. The mean surface area of rigid biopsies was measured to be 22.6 ± 20.4 mm^2, while flexible biopsies had a mean surface area of 7.1 ± 9.3 mm^2, and CBs had a mean surface area of 14.4 ± 12.8 mm^2. Rigid biopsies were significantly larger than both CBs ($p < 0.001$) and flexible biopsies ($p < 0.001$), while CBs were significantly larger than flexible biopsies ($p < 0.01$). Among rigid biopsies, 63% contained deep biopsies with fatty tissue, compared to CBs (49.5%) and flexible biopsies (39.5%). In terms of diagnostic yield, a diagnosis was obtained in 79 out of 80 cases (98.7%) through rigid biopsies. CBs achieved a diagnosis in 73 out of 80 cases (91.3%), while flexible biopsies achieved a diagnosis in 74 out of 80 cases (92.5%). The diagnostic yield of CBs was inferior to that of rigid biopsies (difference 12.7%) but noninferior to that of flexible biopsies (difference 6.5%). Authors concluded that CBs performed during MT were safe and had a high diagnostic yield. They were determined to be noninferior to flexible biopsies while providing increased tissue quantity and quality.[33]

According to a study conducted by Lee et al., which included 28 patients undergoing CB and 17 patients undergoing forceps biopsy, the diagnostic rates were 89.3% and 88.2% in the CB and forceps biopsy groups, respectively. The study concluded that pleuroscopic CB had a similar diagnostic yield to FFB and no major complications were observed in either group.[34]

Shafiq et al. evaluated seven observational studies involving a total of 586 pleural biopsies, of which 311 were CBs and 275 were flexible forceps biopsies. A meta-analysis of the data revealed a diagnostic yield of 96.5% for CB and 93.1% for forceps biopsy with no significant difference.[35]

Another systematic review and meta-analysis conducted by Giri et al. to compare pleural CB and forceps biopsy indicated that CB yielded significantly larger tissue specimens ($p < 0.01$), reached greater depths ($p < 0.01$), and exhibited better quality with fewer crush artifacts ($p < 0.01$) as compared to forceps biopsy. However, there was no significant difference observed in diagnostic yield or occurrence of mild-to-moderate bleeding events ($p = 0.57$).[36]

Most of the available data did not show superiority of CB over the thoracoscopic forceps biopsy in diagnostic yield, though deemed safe in all the studies **(Table 1)**.

TABLE 1: Characteristics of studies done on pleural cryobiopsy.

Study	Selection criteria	Cryoprobe size (in mm)	CB diagnostic rate (%)	FB diagnostic rate (%)	Significant bleeding FB	Significant bleeding FB
Dhooria et al.[32]	Randomized undiagnosed exudative pleural effusion	2.4	39/50 (78)	38/50 (76)	0/46	0/49
Wurps et al.[33]	Prospective undiagnosed exudative pleural effusion	2.4	73/80 (91.3)	74/80 (92.5)	0/80	0/80
Lee et al.[34]	Retrospective undiagnosed pleural effusion	1.9	25/28 (89.3)	15/17 (88.2)	3/28 (10.7)	1/17 (5.9)
Tousheed et al.[37]	Retrospective undiagnosed pleural effusion	2.4	86/87 (99)	50/52 (96.1)	0/87	0/52
Chen et al.[30]	Retrospective undiagnosed pleural effusion	1.9	91/92 (98.9)	84/92 (91.3)	8/92 (8.7)	6/92 (6.5)
Elsaad et al.[38]	Prospective undiagnosed exudative pleural effusion	2.4	50/50 (100)	50/50 (100)	NR	NR
Muhammad et al.[39]	Prospective undiagnosed exudative pleural effusion	2.4	30/30 (100)	30/30 (100)	NR	NR
Ahmed et al.[40]	Retrospective undiagnosed exudative pleural effusion	3	23/30 (76.7)	23/30 (76.7)	0/30	3/30

(CB: cryobiopsy; FB: forceps biopsy; NR: not recorded)

CONCLUSION

The choice of pleural biopsy method depends on various factors, such as availability of different modalities, distribution, and location of the suspected pleural condition, patient's overall health condition, expertise of the healthcare provider, cost involved, and need for hospitalization after the procedure. Each method has its advantages and considerations and the most appropriate approach must be determined based on the patient and the healthcare setting where the procedure is going to be performed. Open pleural biopsy and closed pleural needle biopsy have now been superseded by ultrasound- or CT-guided biopsy and MP techniques due to better yield. Pleural CB does give a bigger sample, but it does not translate to a better yield compared to forceps biopsy and as the sample is not fit for cultures, it is less likely to be popular in our clinical settings.

KEY POINTS

- Choice of technique of pleural biopsy should depend on yield and the procedural complications.
- Blind Abram and Cope needle biopsies have been traditionally used for pleural biopsies but gradually replaced by image-guided biopsy.
- Adequate training is must for performing pleural biopsies.
- Thoracoscopic pleural biopsies under vision have a better success rate than needle biopsies.
- Advancements in thoracoscopic technique with cryoprobe have led to larger biopsy samples, though the diagnostic yield is relatively similar to conventional forceps biopsy.

REFERENCES

1. Loddenkemper R, Lee P, Noppen M, Mathur P. Medical thoracoscopy/pleuroscopy: step by step. Breathe. 2011;8(2): 156-67.
2. Murthy V, Bessich JL. Medical thoracoscopy and its evolving role in the diagnosis and treatment of pleural disease. J Thorac Dis. 2017;9(S10):S1011-21.
3. Ernst A, Silvestri GA, Johnstone D. American College of Chest Physicians. Interventional pulmonary procedures: guidelines from the American College of Chest Physicians. Chest. 2003;123:1693-717.
4. Screaton NJ, Flower CDR. Percutaneous needle biopsy of the pleura. Radiol Clin North Am. 2000;38(2):293-301.
5. Corcoran JP, Tazi-Mezalek R, Maldonado F, Yarmus LB, Annema JT, Koegelenberg CFN, et al. State of the art thoracic ultrasound: intervention and therapeutics. Thorax. 2017;72:840-9.
6. Hooper C, Lee YCG, Maskell N. BTS Pleural Guideline Group. Investigation of a unilateral pleural effusion in adults: British Thoracic Society pleural disease guideline 2010. Thorax. 2010;65:ii4-17.
7. Abrams LD. New inventions: Pleural-biopsy punch. Lancet. 1958;1:30.
8. Kirsch CM, Kroe DM, Jensen WA, Kagawa FT, Wehner JH, Campagna AC. A modified Abrams needle biopsy technique. Chest. 1995;108(4):982-6.
9. Cope C. New pleural biopsy needle; preliminary study. J Am Med Assoc. 1958;167(9):1107-8.
10. Tomlinson J. Invasive procedures in the diagnosis of pleural disease. Semin Respir Med. 1987;9:30-60.
11. Vorster MJ, Allwood BW, Diacon AH, Koegelenberg CF. Tuberculous pleural effusions: advances and controversies. J Thorac Dis. 2015;7:981-91.
12. Bueno CE. Cytologic and bacteriologic analysis of fluid and pleural biopsy specimens with Cope's needle: study of 414 patients. Arch Intern Med. 1990;150:1190-4.
13. Bibby AC, Maskell NA. Pleural biopsies in undiagnosed pleural effusions; Abrams vs. image-guided vs. thoracoscopic biopsies. Curr Opin Pulm Med. 2016;22:392-8.
14. Metintas M, Yildirim H, Kaya T, Ak G, Dundar E, Ozkan R, et al. CT scan-guided Abrams' needle pleural biopsy versus ultrasound-assisted cutting needle pleural biopsy for diagnosis in patients with pleural effusion: a randomized, controlled trial. Respiration. 2016;91:156-63.
15. Bhatnagar R, Corcoran JP, Maldonado F, Feller-Kopman D, Janssen J, Astoul P, et al. Advanced medical interventions in pleural disease. Eur Respir Rev. 2016;25:199-213.
16. Qureshi NR, Gleeson FV. Imaging of pleural disease. Clin Chest Med. 2006;27:193-213.
17. Maskell N, Gleeson F, Davies R. Standard pleural biopsy versus CT-guided cutting-needle biopsy for diagnosis of malignant disease in pleural effusions: a randomised controlled trial. Lancet. 2003;361:1326-30.
18. Corcoran JP, Psallidas I, Ross CL, Hallifax RJ, Rahman NM. Always worth another look? Thoracic ultrasonography before, during, and after pleural intervention. Ann Am Thorac Soc. 2016;13: 118-21.
19. Hassan M, Rana M, Rahman NM. A patient with effusion undergoing pleural biopsy. Chest. 2018;154:e37-9.
20. Psallidas I, Helm EJ, Maskell NA, Yarmus L, Feller-Kopman DJ, Gleeson FV, et al. Iatrogenic injury to the intercostal artery: aetiology, diagnosis, and therapeutic intervention. Thorax. 2015;70:802-4.
21. Koegelenberg CFN, Irusen EM, von Groote-Bidlingmaier F, Bruwer JW, Batubara EM, Diacon AH. The utility of ultrasound-guided thoracentesis and pleural biopsy in undiagnosed pleural exudates. Thorax. 2015;70:995-7.
22. Botana Rial M, Briones Gómez A, Ferrando Gabarda JR, Cifuentes Ruiz JF, Guarín Corredor MJ, Manchego Frach N, et al. Tru-cut needle pleural biopsy and cytology as the initial procedure in the evaluation of pleural effusion. Arch Bronconeumol. 2014;50:313-7.
23. Poe RH, Israel RH, Utell MJ, Hall WJ, Greenblatt DW, Kallay MC. Sensitivity, specificity, and predictive values of closed pleural biopsy. Arch Intern Med. 1984;144:325-8.
24. Lai JH, Yan HC, Kao SJ, Lee SC, Shen CY. Intercostal arteriovenous fistula due to pleural biopsy. Thorax. 1990;45:976-8.

25. Mearns AJ. Iatrogenic rupture of the spleen. Br Med J. 1973; 1(5850):395-6.
26. Ernst A, Hersh CP, Herth F, Thurer R, LoCicero J 3rd, Beamis J, et al. A novel instrument for the evaluation of the pleural space: an experience in 34 patients. Chest. 2002;122(5):1530-4.
27. Maturu VN, Dhooria S, Bal A, Singh N, Aggarwal AN, Gupta D, et al. Role of medical thoracoscopy and closed-blind pleural biopsy in undiagnosed exudative pleural effusions: a single-center experience of 348 patients. J Bronchology Interv Pulmonol. 2015;22(2):121-9.
28. Wei Y, Shen K, Lv T, Liu H, Wang Z, Wu J, et al. Comparison between closed pleural biopsy and medical thoracoscopy for the diagnosis of undiagnosed exudative pleural effusions: a systematic review and meta-analysis. Transl Lung Cancer Res. 2020;9(3):446-58.
29. Schuhmann M, Bostanci K, Bugalho A, Warth A, Schnabel PA, Herth FJ, et al. Endobronchial ultrasound-guided cryobiopsies in peripheral pulmonary lesions: a feasibility study. Eur Respir J. 2014;43:233-9.
30. Chen CH, Cheng WC, Wu BR, Chen CY, Chen WC, Liao WC, et al. Feasibility and Safety of Pleuroscopic Cryobiopsy of the Pleura: A Prospective Study. Can Respir J. 2018;6746470.
31. Gage A. Cryotherapy for cancer. In: Rand R, Rinfret A, Von Leden H (Eds). Cryotherapy. Springfield, IL: John Wiley & Sons; 1968.
32. Dhooria S, Bal A, Sehgal IS, Prasad KT, Muthu V, Aggarwal AN, et al. Pleural Cryobiopsy versus Flexible Forceps Biopsy in Subjects with Undiagnosed Exudative Pleural Effusions Undergoing Semirigid Thoracoscopy: A Crossover Randomized Trial (COFFEE Trial). Respiration. 2019;98(2):133-41.
33. Wurps H, Schönfeld N, Bauer TT, Bock M, Duve C, Sauer R, et al. Intra-patient comparison of parietal pleural biopsies by rigid forceps, flexible forceps, and cryoprobe obtained during medical thoracoscopy: a prospective series of 80 cases with pleural effusion. BMC Pulm Med. 2016;16:98.
34. Lee CS, Li SH, Chang CH, Chung FT, Chiu LC, Chou CL, et al. Comparison of Diagnostic Yield and Safety between Semirigid Pleuroscopic Cryobiopsy and Forceps Biopsy for Undiagnosed Pleural Effusion. Can Respir J. 2019:5490896.
35. Shafiq M, Sethi J, Ali MS, Ghori UK, Saghaie T, Folch E. Pleural cryobiopsy: a systematic review and meta-analysis. Chest. 2020;157:223-30.
36. Giri M, Dai H, Guo S, Li Y, He L, Zhuang R. Efficacy and Safety of Pleural Cryobiopsy vs. Forceps Biopsy for Evaluation of Undiagnosed Pleural Effusion: A Systematic Review and Meta-Analysis. Front Med (Lausanne). 2022;9:847146.
37. Tousheed SZ, Manjunath PH, Chandrasekar S, Murali Mohan BV, Kumar H, Hibare KR, et al. Cryobiopsy of the Pleura: An Improved Diagnostic Tool. J Bronchology Interv Pulmonol. 2018;25:37-41.
38. Elsaad RA, Elwakil IS, Tealeb AS, Abo Sheir OM. Comparison of Parietal Pleural Biopsies by Rigid Forceps and Cryoprobe during Medical Thoracoscopy in Patients with Exudative Pleural Effusion. Med J Cairo Univ. 2020;88:367-74.
39. Muhammad R, Hussein S, Mohammad M, Ahmed M, Ali G. Thoracoscopic pleural cryobiopsy versus conventional forceps biopsy in diagnosis of exudative pleural effusion of unknown etiology. Egypt J Bronchol. 2019;13:162-9.
40. Ahmed MM, AlSharkawy SH, Shoukri AM, AbouBakr YT. Evaluation of safety and diagnostic yield of pleural cryobiopsies during thoracoscopy. Egypt J Bronchol. 2019;13:63-6.

CHAPTER

30 Surgical Management of Pleural Diseases

Harshvardhan Puri, Mohan Venkatesh Pulle, Sukhram Bishnoi

INTRODUCTION

The scope of pleural disease surgery is broad, covering diagnostic and therapeutic measures for various benign and malignant conditions. Progress in thoracoscopy has reduced the need for surgical diagnosis and palliative care. This same progress has encouraged the increased use of video-assisted thoracoscopic surgery (VATS) for managing pleural diseases. VATS has been accepted as the preferred intervention for surgically treating a pneumothorax, although when to intervene remains a topic of ongoing discussion. The application of VATS has broadened to incorporate stage II and even in stage III empyema cases, where VATS decortication is increasingly utilized for even cases with long-term, widespread pleural thickening. However, the surgical management of malignant pleural diseases is still a research topic and source of debate, with randomized controlled trials studying its role in mesothelioma, pleural metastases from thymoma, and nonsmall cell lung cancer (NSCLC).

THE ROLE OF SURGERY IN "EMPYEMA THORACIS"

A notable area where surgery assumes a pivotal role in the vast landscape of pleural diseases is in the treatment of empyema. Empyema, a condition characterized by the accumulation of pus within the pleural space **(Fig. 1)**, presents varying complexities that necessitate a thorough understanding of its types, classifications, stages, and etiology. The classification of empyema, often linked to its progression, is divided into three stages, i.e., (1) exudative, (2) fibrinopurulent, and (3) organized.[1] As per American Association of Thoracic Surgery (AATS) consensus guidelines, VATS should be considered as first-line therapy in fibrinopurulent and organized empyema.[2]

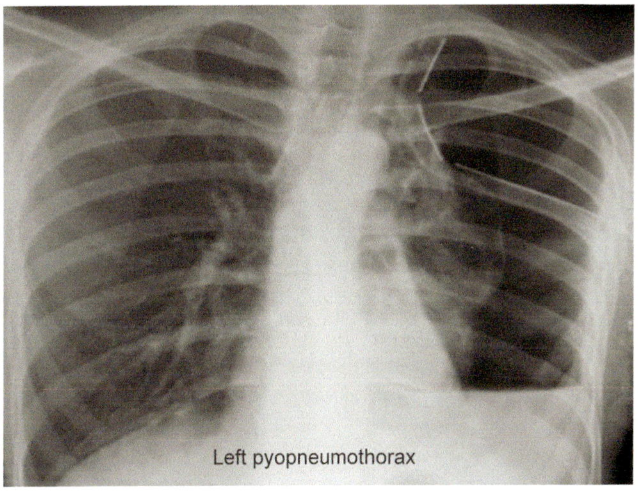

FIG. 1: Pyopneumothorax.

Indications for Surgery

- Trapped lung [thickened pleura (peel) encasing the lung parenchyma **(Fig. 2)**]
- Multiloculated pleural collection, not amenable for chest tube drainage
- Inadequate drainage of infected pleural collection despite chest tube placement
- Incomplete lung expansion despite chest tube placement
- Persistent air leak from the chest tube, suggestive of bronchopleural fistula (BPF)[3]
- Failure of resolution of sepsis within 5–7 days despite antibiotics and drainage[4]

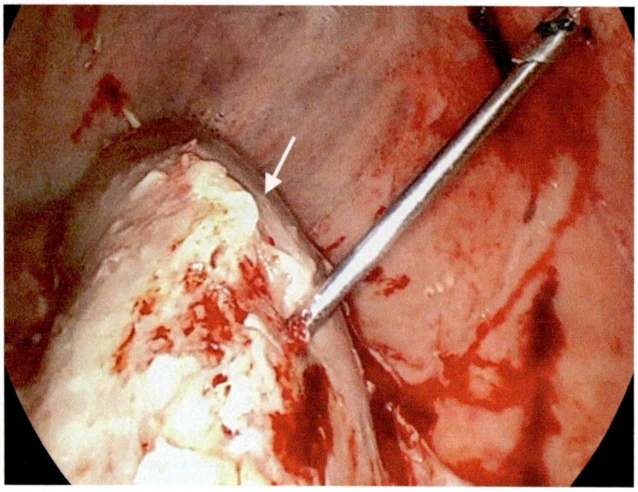

FIG. 2: Trapped lung (arrow).

Preoperative Evaluation

All the patients should undergo a comprehensive clinical examination, complemented by a posteroanterior chest roentgenogram and computed tomography (CT) of the chest, which provides a thorough overview of their disease severity. The indications of surgery were already discussed earlier in this chapter. Every patient's nutritional status is meticulously evaluated and any deficits in hemoglobin and serum albumin must be promptly addressed.

Both CT and ultrasound scanning techniques served a pivotal role in diagnosing and staging empyema.[5] While neither modality could accurately forecast the stage or predict the need for surgery, both could significantly influence the choice of procedure and facilitate intraoperative strategy. A CT scan can accurately assess the site of pleural collection, the thickness of pleural peel, and the status of underlying lung parenchyma which could potentially guide the surgeon for secure port placement and surgical decision-making. Conversely, ultrasound demonstrated superiority in identifying loculations.[6]

Special attention should be given to the CT anatomy of the hemithorax when positioning ports. Most of the patients suffering from empyema exhibit a higher diaphragm placement, which could lead to unintentional entry into the abdominal cavity if ports are created where, under normal anatomical conditions, they would overlie the chest cavity. Although an accidental penetration into the abdominal cavity may not always result in complications, it potentially endangers the underlying structures such as the liver, spleen, stomach, and bowel.

Principles of Surgery

Surgical intervention addresses two major factors and issues that should be addressed during surgery for empyema. First, the removal of the septic component, i.e., by debridement of necrotic and infective material, and second, the mechanical factor—removal of thickened pleura/peel which restricts lung expansion, i.e., by decortication. Therefore, surgery serves a dual purpose—it eliminates a persistent source of chronic infection in the chest cavity, and facilitates full pulmonary expansion, thereby circumventing the potential onset of fibrothorax and its consequential restriction of lung volumes.[7]

The four major principles of surgery in an organized stage of pleural empyema: (1) Debridement of the infected thoracic cavity, (2) visceral decortication (removal of thickened pleura/peel from lung parenchyma), (3) parietal decortication [removal of thickened parietal pleura/peel from the chest wall and diaphragm (mediastinal pleura is not excised)], and (4) reexpansion of the underlying lung. This can be achieved by either thoracotomy or thoracoscopy.

Surgical Procedure—Video-assisted Thoracoscopic Surgery Decortication

VATS decortication is performed under general anesthesia, with a double-lumen endotracheal tube inserted to achieve single lung ventilation. A preoperative CT scan guides the surgical approach. In cases where patients had a significant intrathoracic collection, the initial entry point was made where this fluid had accumulated the most. For those without significant fluid, the entry port will be through a 3 cm incision in the posterior axillary line in the sixth intercostal space. The rest of the two ports are made under vision. The two working ports are protected by using a wound protector and a camera is inserted into the chest through a trocar.

Thereafter, the first step of the procedure is debridement, where all the loculations **(Fig. 3)** were broken, and the entire necrotic and infected debris in the chest cavity was removed. Once debridement is done, the next step is visceral pleurectomy where a small area of thickened visceral peel was excised over the lung and an anesthetist is asked to expand the lung to check for the underlying lung condition and its ability to expand. Then, the whole of the visceral peel is removed to achieve complete lung mobilization from anterior to posterior hilum **(Figs. 4 to 6)**. Another important step was to separate the lung from the diaphragm. Visceral decortication is the most crucial part of the surgery. After this complete mobilization, the entire lung is examined thoroughly for any presence of BPF, which is addressed by either primary closure or lung resection.

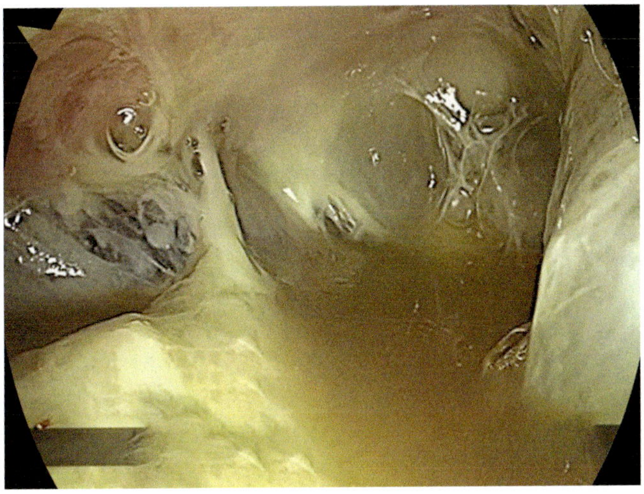

FIG. 3: Multiloculated collection.

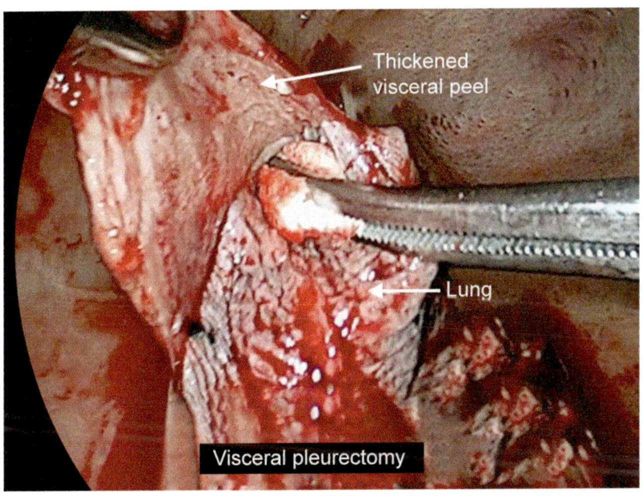

FIG. 4: Visceral pleurectomy started.

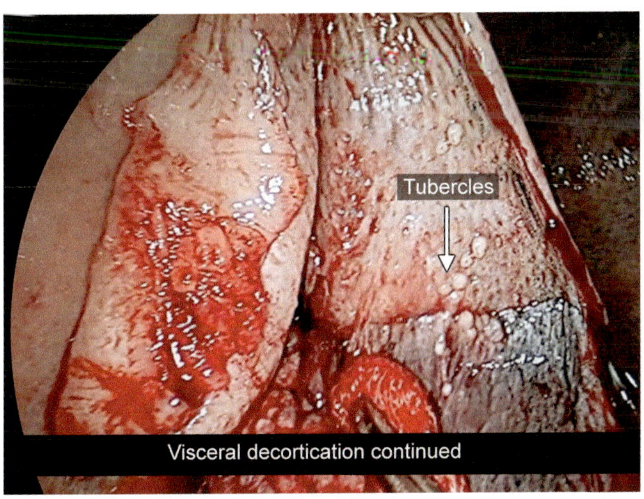

FIG. 5: Tubercles over the visceral pleura.

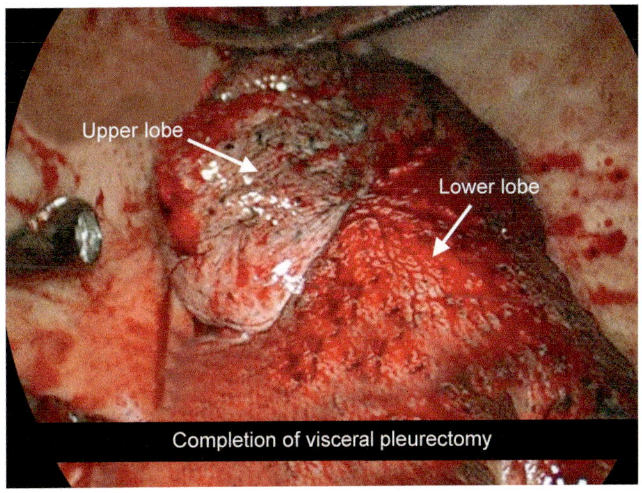

FIG. 6: Visceral pleurectomy completed—exposing normal underlying lungs.

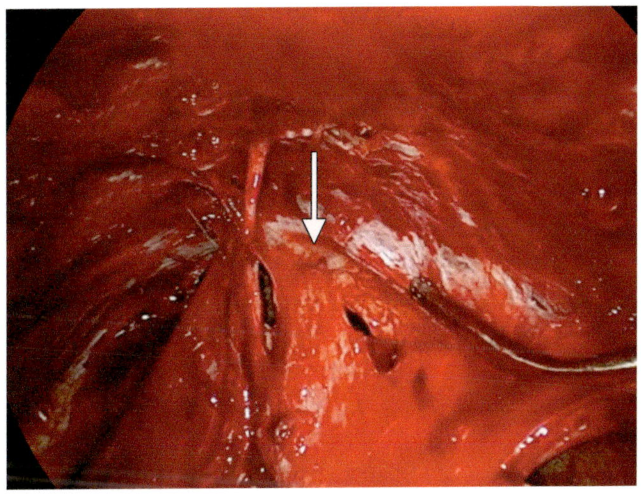

FIG. 7: Parietal pleurectomy (arrow) started.

After adequate visceral decortication, parietal pleurectomy is performed **(Figs. 7 and 8)**, where all the thickened parietal peel was mobilized from the apex of the chest to diaphragmatic attachments superoinferiorly and internal mammary vessels to the paravertebral area anteroposteriorly. Thereafter, it is vital to achieve hemostasis using either electrocautery or argon plasma coagulation spray. Finally, two chest tubes are placed (one at the base and another at the apex) **(Fig. 9)** which are connected to a negative suction device.

Role of Fibrinolytics in Empyema: Present Status

Initially, the beneficial effects of fibrinolytics were reported by various studies.[8-11] However, the latest data reveals "no benefit" when fibrinolytic agents are used alone.[12] A large randomized, double-blinded (MIST1) trial analyzed the role of streptokinase instillation in 454 patients of parapneumonic effusion/empyema, which revealed no benefit in terms of mortality, hospital stay, betterment of imaging, or referral for surgery.[13] A metanalysis by Cameron R et al., which included seven trials totaling 761 patients with parapneumonic effusion or empyema concluded that compa, red with tube thoracostomy (conservative approach), intrapleural instillation of fibrinolytics did not demonstrate any mortality benefit.[14] Therefore, the routine instillation of intrapleural fibrinolytics in parapneumonic effusions/empyema should be carefully monitored, as delay in the surgical referral would reduce the possibility of VATS surgery.[15,16]

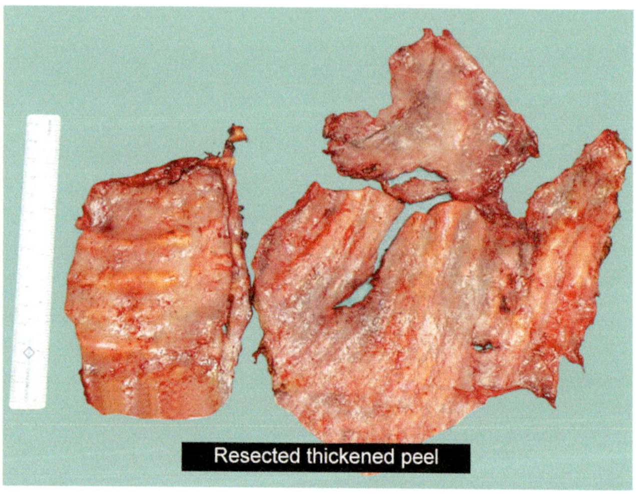

FIG. 8: Surgical specimen—excised visceral and parietal peel.

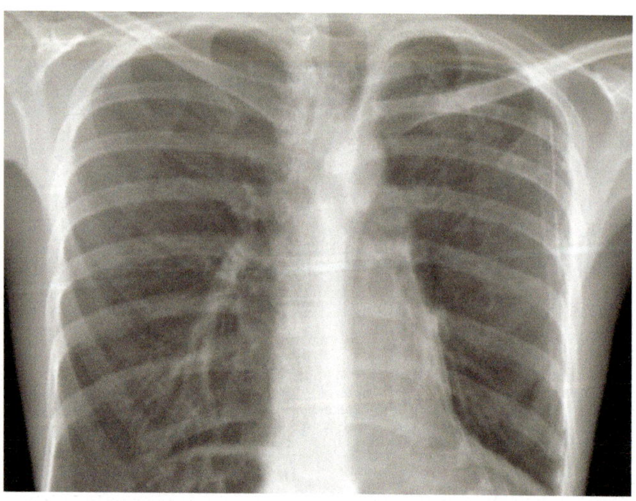

FIG. 9: Postoperative chest X-ray—completely expanded left lung.

Video-assisted Thoracoscopic Surgery versus Open Surgery: Which is Better?

The core principles of decortication surgery include debridement of the pleural cavity, visceral decortication, parietal decortication, and reexpansion of the underlying lung to prevent any residual space. With increasing experience in VATS techniques, more and more surgeons are now utilizing VATS for the management of even advanced stages of empyema thoracis. The ability of surgeons to achieve these core principles via a VATS approach has led to increased use of this technique in all stages of empyema, i.e., stage II and many cases of stage III. The role of VATS in the fibrinopurulent (stage II) stage of empyema is well established with success rates of >90%.[17,18] In addition to the stage of empyema, the state of the underlying lung parenchyma, general condition of the patient, clinical status of the patient, presence or absence of BPF, and timing of referral also should be considered as guiding factors to choose the surgical technique. Therefore, the decision of choosing VATS or an open approach based only on the stage of empyema is almost obsolete now. The indications for open approach for the management of empyema in routine clinical practice by the authors is mentioned in **Box 1**.[3]

Video-assisted thoracoscopic surgery outweighs open surgery with a shorter hospital stay,[19,20] better postoperative pain,[21] lesser duration of the chest tube and postoperative air leak,[15,22-24] fewer wound-related complications, and early return to normalcy. Surgical conversion from VATS to open thoracotomy is reported in 3–28% in stage II and 7–44% in stage III empyema.[25] The proven risk factors for conversion to open surgery included late referral (>2 weeks), stage III empyema with more pleural thickness, and proven gram-negative pleural sepsis.[26,27]

In summary, VATS is now recognized as the preferred method for treating patients with empyema, irrespective of the disease stage. If the assessment during surgery implies that a traditional open surgical approach could lead to better technical and probable clinical results, opting for this method is seen as a constructive decision, not as a setback.

BOX 1 **Indications of "open" surgery in empyema thoracis?**

- Extreme rib crowding (no space between the ribs to insert thoracoscopic ports)
- Very thich pleura (> 2 cm) as per computed tomography (CT) of the chest
- Presence of thick calcified pleura
- Presence of large volume broncho-pleural fistula (BPF)

Management of Persistent Pleural Space

Procedures to deal with a persistent space include open-window thoracostomy (OWT), (either as a permanent solution or as part of a staged procedure) and thoracoplasty. Both can be performed with or without space-filling solutions, such as the interposition of muscle and omental flaps. More recently, vacuum-assisted closure (VAC) has been described to assist in both open and closed procedures.

In carefully chosen patients, thoracoplasty is an effective treatment for the management of persistent pleural space.[28] Resection of the upper ribs reduces the space between the lung or mediastinum and the chest wall, resulting in space obliteration. Thoracoplasty can be done alone or in combination with inserting omental or muscular flaps into the cavity.[29] Based on how close they are to the residual space, pedicled muscle flaps, such as the latissimus dorsi, serratus anterior, pectoralis major, and rectus abdominis are selected.

In conclusion, patient comorbidities, postpneumonectomy status, and the presence/absence of BPF all determine the procedure of choice.

THE ROLE OF SURGERY IN "PNEUMOTHORAX"

Indications of Surgical Intervention in "Primary Spontaneous Pneumothorax"

Conventionally, surgery is indicated for recurrent pneumothorax (second ipsilateral pneumothorax or first contralateral pneumothorax).

Nevertheless, the role of definitive surgery in the first episode of pneumothorax is a matter of intense debate. Initially, all patients with the first episode of primary spontaneous pneumothorax will be managed with a conservative strategy, unless the patient is having prolonged air leak with an unexpanded lung or he/she is a high-risk professional (pilots/divers). There is a school of thought of subjecting those patients for definitive surgery even in the first episode, who had a visible bleb/bulla of size ≥ 2 cm in the CT chest since these patients had a very high chance of developing a second episode of pneumothorax.[30]

Accepted indications of surgery in the first episode of PSP:[31]

- Synchronous bilateral spontaneous pneumothorax
- Persistent air leak (despite 5–7 days of chest tube drainage) or failure of lung reexpansion
- Spontaneous hemopneumothorax
- Professions at risk (e.g., pilots and divers)
- Pregnancy

Indications of Surgical Intervention in "Secondary Spontaneous Pneumothorax"

Patients who had SSP are less likely to tolerate the symptoms, in view of underlying lung disease. Similarly, the air leak is less likely to settle spontaneously in this subset of the population. Therefore, a thoracic surgeon's opinion should be sought if (1) persistence of air leak for >48 hours of chest tube insertion, (2) persistent lung collapse. Poor performance status,[32] interstitial lung disease preoperative duration of air leak > 5 days,[33] and requirement of open surgery[34] were independent risk factors for poor postoperative outcomes.

Surgery for Pneumothorax—Principles and Procedural Details

The two major principles of surgery for pneumothorax include, first to identify the source of air leak—stop it, and second to prevent the recurrence. The success of the procedure is determined by various factors such as the type of pneumothorax (primary vs. secondary), method of surgery (open vs. VATS), method of pleurodesis (mechanical vs. chemical vs pleurectomy), and the need for lung pathology resection (blebectomy or bullectomy).

As a routine protocol, all patients will undergo computed tomography of the chest to look for any visible bleb/bulla. Underlying lung condition is also assessed to plan the surgical management.

Surgery for Primary Spontaneous Pneumothorax

All these patients will undergo surgery in general anesthesia with single lung ventilation. Three ports were created, one for the camera and the other two as working ports. A thorough pleural cavity examination will be done, and any adhesions in the chest cavity will be lysed. All the lobes will be assessed very cautiously for any abnormality, such as bleb and bulla **(Fig. 10)** and sometimes an abnormal area of telangiectasia. According to Vanderschueren's classification,[35] the pathologic lung lesions that were identified endoscopically were divided into four groups. Group I is defined as having no endoscopic abnormalities, group II as having pleuropulmonary adhesions, group III as having blebs <2 cm, and group IV as having blebs/bullae over 2 cm. Thereafter, the underwater air leak test will be done where the pleural cavity will be filled with saline and the lung will be gently ventilated to look for any air leak **(Fig. 11)** from ruptured bulla/bleb/subpleural porosity. The lung parenchyma will be immersed in the saline to check air leaks and very gentle manipulation of expanding lung parenchyma is vital to prevent any iatrogenic injury.

As per Vanderschueren's classification, the surgical procedure was as follows: Stage I: Isolated pleurectomy; stage II: Lysis of all adhesions and isolated pleurectomy; and stages III and IV: Addressing the blebs/bullae.[36] Blebs/bullous area will be stapled by using serial firing of an endoscopic linear cutter device on normal lung parenchyma **(Figs. 12 to 14)**. It is pivotal to staple over a healthy lung margin, as firing of stapler over an abnormal area can leave an abnormal area, which is a potential cause for pneumothorax recurrence even after definitive surgery. As a second part of the procedure, pleurodesis can be achieved by either mechanical pleurodesis or parietal pleurectomy **(Fig. 15)**, or talc pleurodesis **(Figs. 16 and 17)**. In mechanical pleurodesis, this will be achieved by pleural abrasion with a roll of polypropylene mesh from the apex to the costodiaphragmatic recess including the

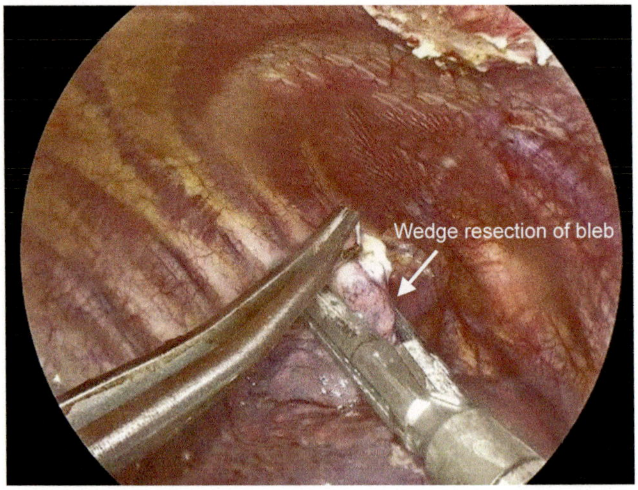

FIG. 12: Wedge resection of the lung containing bleb.

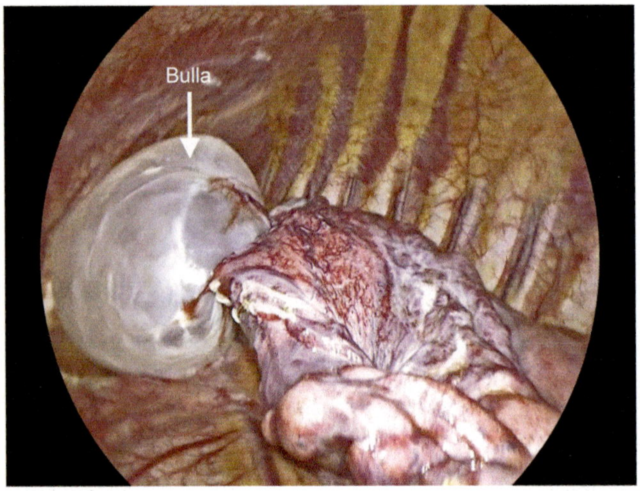

FIG. 10: Bulla arising from an apical segment of the left upper lobe.

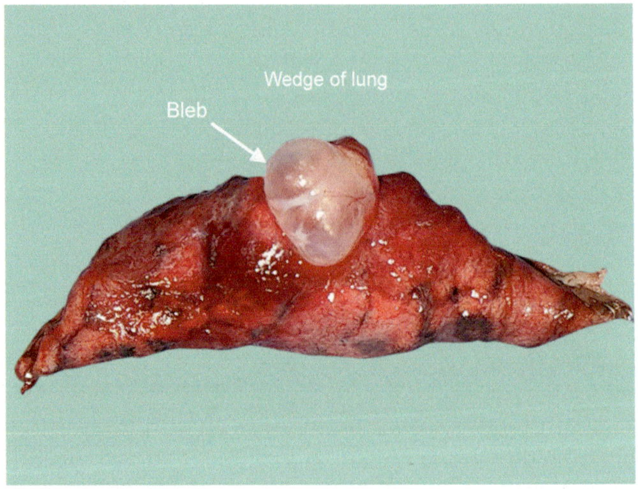

FIG. 13: Surgical specimen—a wedge of right upper lobe apical segment with bleb.

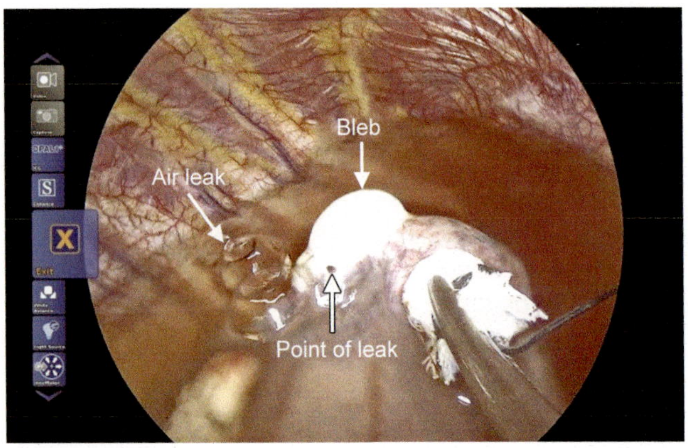

FIG. 11: Bleb in the apical segment of the right upper lobe—with active air leak.

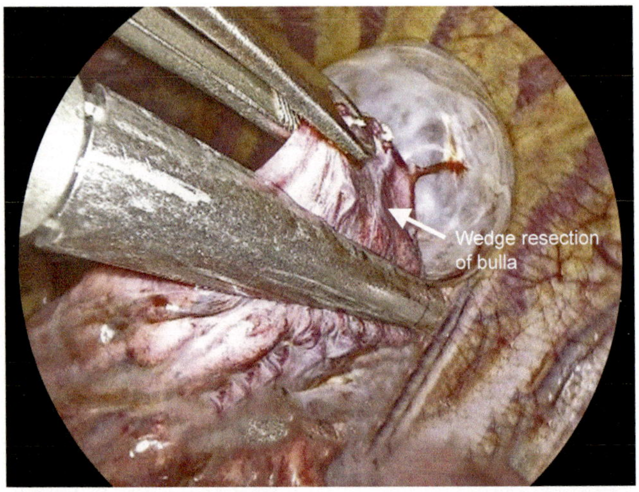

FIG. 14: Wedge resection of lung containing bulla.

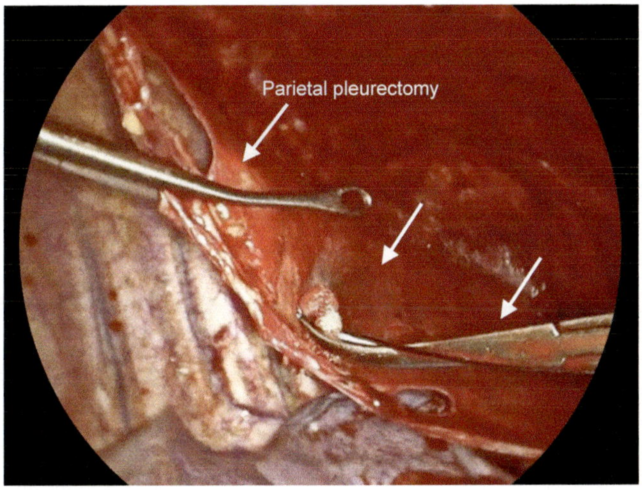

FIG. 15: Pleurectomy.

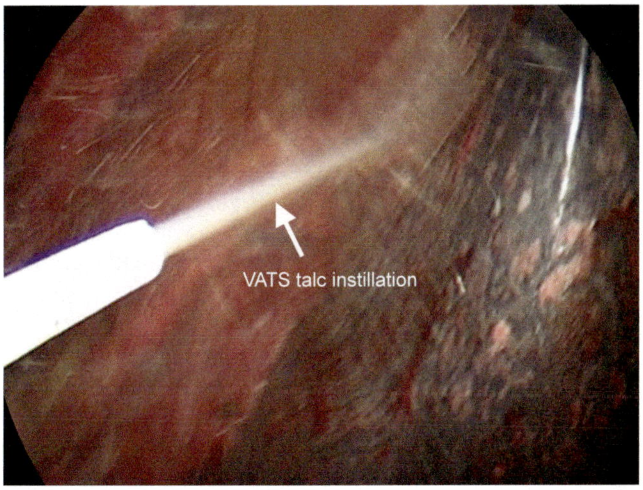

FIG. 16: Talc pleurodesis.
(VATS: video-assisted thoracoscopic surgery)

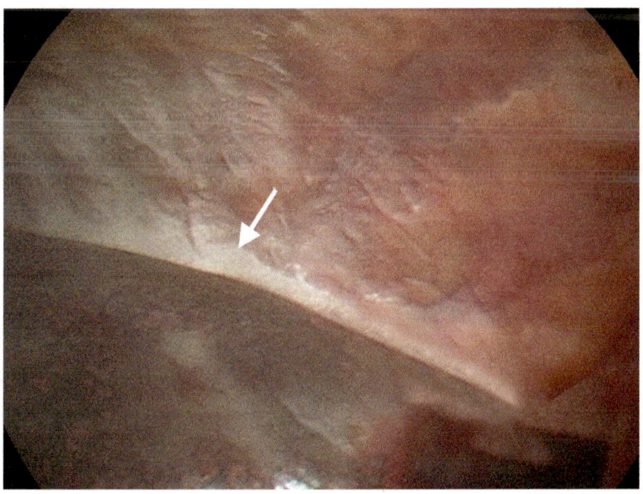

FIG. 17: Talc instilled over parietal pleura (arrow).

diaphragmatic surface to create petechial hemorrhages, which helps in pleurodesis. In parietal pleurectomy, the whole of the costal parietal pleura was removed from the internal mammary pedicle anteriorly to the paravertebral column posteriorly and the apex of the lung to diaphragmatic origin superoinferiorly. Mediastinal pleura and diaphragmatic pleura are not removed but is rubbed with a polypropylene mesh to create the raw surface. After achieving hemostasis, two chest tubes are placed (one at the base and another at the apex) which are connected to a negative suction device.

Is Wedge Resection Always Needed?

Uncertainty surrounds the role of wedge excision in preventing pneumothorax, especially in cases where morphologically no abnormality was found. Probably, this question might be answered by the WOPP (Wedge Resection plus Parietal Pleurectomy) trial[37] or (parietal pleurectomy for the treatment of recurrent primary pneumothorax) outcomes. In the contrary, there was no difference in recurrence rate was observed when comparing a wedge alone with a wedge and pleurodesis in primary spontaneous pneumothorax. However, in the subset analysis, the recurrence rate was high (7.5%) in cases where there were numerous bullae present.[38]

Surgery for Secondary Spontaneous Pneumothorax

Secondary pneumothorax arises in patients with preexisting lung disease, with the most frequent etiology being chronic obstructive pulmonary disease (COPD). Other conditions associated include interstitial lung diseases, cystic fibrosis, tuberculosis, and primary or metastatic lung malignancies. These patients experience higher morbidity and even mortality compared to primary spontaneous pneumothorax patients, in view of decreased lung reserves due to the inherent lung pathology. In cases of persistent or recurrent secondary spontaneous pneumothorax, early surgical intervention, especially VATS has gained increased acceptance. In VATS, surgeons can identify the source of air leak (ruptured bleb/bulla), which can be addressed by either resection or ligation. In addition, recurrence of pleurodesis can also be prevented by either chemical (talc) or mechanical pleurodesis. An alternative is the pleurectomy, where the parietal pleura is stripped off, achieving a similar objective of preventing recurrence. For cases, of patients who deny for VATS, bedside talc slurry installation through the chest drain is an option. The prerequisite for any kind of pleurodesis is underlying complete lung expansion. Open thoracotomy might be required in patients with very dense intrathoracic vascular adhesions. For patients with extensive underlying lung disease, perioperative pulmonary rehabilitation optimization is vital for favorable clinical outcomes.

In conclusion, the decision of surgery should be critically balanced, considering the risk-benefit ratio based on factors such as the patient's overall general condition, underlying comorbidities, and the severity of underlying lung pathology. The key to achieving the best outcomes is collaborative decision-making between thoracic surgeons, anesthesiologists, and pulmonologists.

Recurrence after Definitive Surgery and Management

Reported recurrence rates vary between 0 and 10% in multiple series.[39-43] The reasons for recurrence can be patient-related and primary surgery-related. The patient-related factors included secondary spontaneous pneumothorax, the presence of multiple blebs/bullae, and the female sex.[44] The surgery-related factors include failure to identify air leaks, no wedge resection during the surgery, and the presence of prolonged postoperative air leaks.[45] The other factor is the development of new bullae over the surgical staple line.[46]

In the case of resurgery for pneumothorax recurrence, two things should be considered (1) the surgical approach (VATS/open) and the type of pleurodesis (based on the previous method of pleurodesis). Talc pleurodesis is a superior option compared to pleurectomy and/or pleural abrasion, in view of its higher efficacy. Sometimes, recurrence can be related to the host's inflammatory response rather than to technical failure. With the emergence of VATS, redo-VATS is feasible in most of the cases of resurgery.[47]

Catamenial Pneumothorax

With a frequency of 3–6%, catamenial pneumothorax is an uncommon subset of spontaneous pneumothorax that is observed in menstruating women. Traditionally, it is described as pneumothorax occurring within 72 hours of the start of menstruation.[48] It is thought that the pathophysiology results from endometrial tissue migrating from the uterus to the pleural cavity, either by diaphragmatic porosities **(Fig. 18)**, hematogenous, or lymphatic routes.[49,50] Although thoracic endometriosis is frequently linked to catamenial pneumothorax, it is not always present. The usual clinical presentation includes chest pain and dyspnea related to menstruation.

Surgery is the definitive treatment of choice for recurrent catamenial pneumothorax when conservative therapy fails.[51] Diagnostic thoracoscopy during VATS procedure, can identify the diaphragmatic porosities and/or endometrial deposits in the thoracic cavity. The principles of surgery in this condition include wedge resection of the lung having all visible pathological lesions such as blebs or bullae and resection of endometriotic deposits.[52] This should be supplemented with chemical (talc) or mechanical pleurodesis.[53] Addressing the diaphragmatic porosities or endometrial deposits with either diaphragmatic resection or plication is of paramount importance in the surgical management of catamenial pneumothorax.[54,55] In order to decrease the recurrences, hormonal therapy with substances like gonadotropin-releasing hormone (GnRH) agonists may be used in conjunction with surgery.[56] It is important to remember that early surgical intervention in recurrent cases can result in better outcomes and lower morbidity.

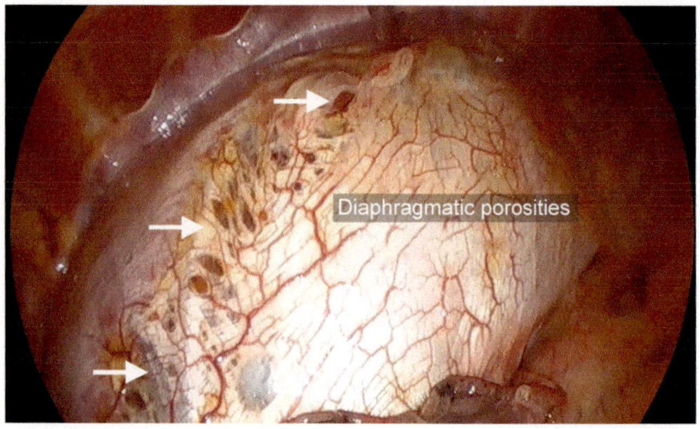

FIG. 18: Diaphragmatic fenestrations in catamenial pneumothorax.

ROLE OF SURGERY IN MALIGNANT PLEURAL MESOTHELIOMA

Only 20% of patients with mesothelioma are candidates for surgical intervention.[57] The present standard of care for surgery in malignant pleural mesothelioma (MPM) is multimodality therapy is macroscopic complete resection [macroscopic complete remission (MCR); i.e., an R0 or R1 resection] as part of a multimodality approach. Therefore, surgery is offered to patients in whom the disease is surgically resectable and is limited to one hemithorax (stage I–III as per 8th edition AJCC), without major comorbidities and having adequate cardiopulmonary reserve. Most surgeons offer surgery in only the pure epithelioid histology subtype of mesothelioma, as patients with mixed or pure sarcomatous histology subtype often have no survival benefit with surgery.[58] The poor prognostic factors or surgery include male patients, age > 50 years, male gender, platelet count > 400,000/μL, and/or white blood cell count > 15,000/μL.[59]

Spectrum of Surgical Procedures for Malignant Pleural Mesothelioma

- *Extrapleural pneumonectomy*: En bloc removal of the ipsilateral lung, pericardium, and diaphragm together with the parietal and visceral pleura. The pericardium and/or diaphragm may be left unaltered when the tumor does not affect them.
- *Extended pleurectomy/decortication (P/D)*: Parietal and visceral pleurectomy with excision of the pericardium and/or diaphragm to remove all the gross tumor.
- *P/D*: Parietal and visceral pleurectomy without diaphragm or pericardial resection to remove all the gross tumor.
- *Partial pleurectomy*: When an R0 or R1 resection is not possible, a portion of the parietal and/or visceral pleura is removed for diagnostic or palliative reasons while leaving the gross tumor alone.

Extrapleural Pneumonectomy

The morbidity and mortality related with extrapleural pneumonectomy (EPP) were decreased, and survival rates improved, with increased experience and better patient selection. The perioperative morbidity was ranging between 22 and 82% and mortality was at 0–12%.[60] The median survival after EPP (as a part of a multimodality approach) was approximately 18 months.[61] Key factors that resulted in better surgical outcomes included accurate preoperative staging, advancements in intraoperative anesthesia techniques, standardization of resection and reconstruction surgical techniques, and stringent perioperative management of procedure-related complications. The common postoperative complications included atrial fibrillation, myocardial infarction, pulmonary complications, cardiac herniation, herniation of abdominal contents into the chest cavity, BPF causing empyema, and respiratory failure.[62]

Pleurectomy/Decortication

This lung-preserving modality emerged as an alternative to EPP in carefully selected patients of MPM. This has less procedural-related morbidity and mortality in addition to the benefit of lung preservation. A large retrospective review compared EPP versus P/D, which reported that EPP was associated with higher perioperative mortality (7% vs. 4%) and worse overall survival (12 vs. 16 months).[63]

In conclusion, the choice of specific procedure (EPP vs. P/D) should be left to the judgment and expertise of the surgeon, and multimodal treatment protocols within that institution.

ROLE OF SURGERY IN NONSMALL CELL LUNG CANCER

As per AJCC 8th edition, the presence of pleural metastasis signifies stage IVB in NSCLC. The presence of ipsilateral pleural nodules is traditionally considered a systemic disease and is a contraindication for surgery in view of poor survival outcomes.[64] However, there is emerging data suggesting a potential role for aggressive local therapy, including surgical management with survival benefits in some superselected patients. Usually, these patients fall into two common clinical scenarios. First, incidentally diagnosed to have pleural metastasis intraoperatively, while the primary tumor was resectable, and second, patients were already diagnosed to have either malignant pleural effusion/pleural metastasis in the preoperative workup.

In the first scenario, i.e., patients who had incidentally diagnosed to have pleural metastasis intraoperatively, there is encouraging evidence in the literature to support the role of pleurectomy in addition to the lung resection planned.[65] Many retrospective studies have reported better survival compared to just exploratory VATS. The reported 3-year overall survival (OS) was ranging from 34.2 to 82.9%, and 5-year OS was between 16.3 and 42.7%.[66] Therefore, in patients with "unexpected" pleural metastasis during definitive lung surgery, surgeons should try to attempt/achieve complete pleurectomy (complete pathological tumor removal) in addition to lung resection. The final specimen should be sent to molecular analysis as well for the possibility of adjuvant therapy including radiotherapy.

In the second scenario, the patient was diagnosed to have pleural metastasis in a preoperative workup. Very few studies analyzed the role of surgery in this subset of patients, which reported that macroscopic clear resection and best nodal stage were independent predictive factors for survival.[67,68] The presence of pericardial effusion and having N3 disease were predictive factors for poor survival.[69] So, in selected patients with clinically metastatic disease in the preoperative workup, surgery, i.e., pathologically complete resection can still offer superior survival outcomes. Therefore, surgery can be considered an essential component in the multidisciplinary management of NSCLC in addition to systemic therapy.

In conclusion, the decision of surgery should always be considered after weighing the risk-benefit ratio. The patient's general condition, functional status, and life expectancy should be kept in mind before taking the decision.

ROLE OF SURGERY IN MALIGNANT TRAPPED LUNG

A malignant trapped lung is a manifestation of malignant pleural effusion, in which the lung is completely encased by thickened visceral peel (involved/encased with tumor), which prevents complete lung expansion.[70,71] Other causes of trapped lung included (1) pleural carcinomatosis where multiple visceral pleural metastatic tumor nodules restrict the expansion,[72] (2) chronic lung collapse/atelectasis because of proximal endobronchial obstruction, with a concomitant malignant or paramalignant pleural effusion, and sometimes (3) radiation-induced fibrosis of visceral pleura.[73] This scenario is common with extensive pleural metastasis from notably breast and lung cancers. Surgery has a definitive role in both diagnostic and therapeutic aspects for this clinical condition. In a diagnostic perspective, VATS can offer direct visualization (of visceral as well as parietal pleura) and biopsy of the nodules for the diagnosis of malignancy. with its excellent visualization offers diagnostic superiority, allowing direct visualization and biopsy of the pleura to confirm malignancy.

Beyond diagnostic purposes, surgery offers interventions that can alleviate the patient symptoms and improve the quality of life. The procedure of choice depends on the general condition of the patient, life expectancy, underlying lung condition, and the patient's severity of symptoms. VATS talc pleurodesis (poudrage) or mechanical pleurodesis is the treatment option when complete lung expansion can be achieved. For patients who are poor candidates for pleurodesis or repeatedly experience effusion recurrence, with underlying trapped lung—indwelling pleural catheters (IPCs) offer an effective solution, facilitating outpatient fluid drainage; however, this method has some potential risks such as secondary infection, catheter blockade, and possibility of tumor seedling along the catheter tract.

In selected patients, who had relatively preserved general conditions with significant symptoms—P/D can significantly improve the quality of life. The aim of this procedure is to achieve satisfactory lung expansion, not to achieve complete macroscopic tumor clearance. This surgery involves the removal of the tumor cortex from the lung parenchyma to achieve complete lung expansion. This can relieve a restrictive ventilatory deficit and helps to resolve ventilation-perfusion mismatch, decrease chest wall discomfort, and pain, and prevent recurrent pleural effusions and improve lung perfusion.[74-77] Due to its debulking nature, this surgery may also have a presumptive benefit of delaying tumor progression and thus prolonging survival.[78] The possible advantages of this surgery should always be weighed against the potential intra- and postoperative complications. The minimally invasive technique such as VATS should be the preferred surgical approach to perform this surgery as this method would reduce the surgery-related chest wall trauma, preserve chest muscle function, and therefore expedite the recovery process.[74] In conclusion, while surgery offers valuable options for patients with malignant trapped lungs, individualized assessment remains paramount to ensure optimal outcomes.

KEY POINTS

- Surgery for pleural disease encompasses both diagnostic and therapeutic measures for benign and malignant pleural conditions.
- Advancements in medical thoracoscopy techniques have minimized the need for surgery as a diagnostic and palliative modality in pleural diseases.
- Presently, VATS is the gold-standard method for managing pleural diseases.
- In pneumothorax, VATS is the preferred surgical modality, but the optimal timing for this intervention is still debated.
- The utility of VATS in empyema thoracis has expanded to treat stage II and III empyema, especially with VATS decortication for cases with significant pleural thickening.
- The diagnostic role of VATS in malignant pleural diseases (pleural metastases from NSCLC and other organs) is well established. However, the role of VATS as a definitive surgical modality is still debatable; therefore, open surgery (extrapleural pneumonectomy or P/D in malignant pleural mesothelioma and pleurectomy or pleuropneumonectomy in advanced thymoma with pleural metastasis) continues to play a major role as a definitive therapeutic strategy.

REFERENCES

1. Andrews NC, Parker EF, Shaw RP, Wilson NJ, Webb WR. Management of non-tuberculous empyema. Am Rev Respir Dis. 1962;85:935-6.
2. Shen KR, Bribriesco A, Crabtree T, Denlinger C, Eby J, Eiken P, et al. The American Association for Thoracic Surgery consensus guidelines for the management of empyema. J Thorac Cardiovasc Surg. 2017;153(6):e129-46.
3. Kumar A, Asaf BB, Lingaraju VC, Yendamuri S, Pulle MV, Sood J. Thoracoscopic Decortication of Stage III Tuberculous Empyema Is Effective and Safe in Selected Cases. Ann Thorac Surg. 2017;104(5):1688-94.
4. Davies HE, Davies RJ, Davies CW; BTS Pleural Disease Guideline Group. Management of pleural infection in adults: British Thoracic Society Pleural Disease Guideline 2010. Thorax. 2010;65(Suppl 2):ii41-53.

5. Kearney SE, Davies CW, Davies RJ, Gleeson FV. Computed tomography and ultrasound in parapneumonic effusions and empyema. Clin Radiol. 2000;55(7):542-7.
6. Medford AR, Agrawal S, Bennett JA, Free CM, Entwisle JJ. Thoracic ultrasound prior to medical thoracoscopy improves pleural access and predicts fibrous septation. Respirology. 2010;15(5):804-8.
7. Chen B, Zhang J, Ye Z, Ye M, Ma D, Wang C, et al. Outcomes of video-assisted thoracic surgical decortication in 274 patients with tuberculous empyema. Ann Thorac Cardiovasc Surg. 2015;21(3):223-8.
8. Davies RJ, Traill ZC, Gleeson FV. Randomised controlled trial of intrapleural streptokinase in community acquired pleural infection. Thorax. 1997;52(5):416-21.
9. Bouros D, Schiza S, Tzanakis N, Chalkiadakis G, Drositis J, Siafakas N. Intrapleural urokinase versus normal saline in the treatment of complicated parapneumonic effusions and empyema. A randomized, double-blind study. Am J Respir Crit Care Med. 1999;159(1):37-42.
10. Diacon AH, Theron J, Schuurmans MM, Van de Wal BW, Bolliger CT. Intrapleural streptokinase for empyema and complicated parapneumonic effusions. Am J Respir Crit Care Med. 2004;170(1):49-53.
11. Thomson AH, Hull J, Kumar MR, Wallis C, Balfour Lynn IM. Randomised trial of intrapleural urokinase in the treatment of childhood empyema. Thorax. 2002;57(4):343-7.
12. Thommi G, Nair CK, Aronow WS, Shehan C, Meyers P, McLeay M. Efficacy and safety of intrapleural instillation of alteplase in the management of complicated pleural effusion or empyema. Am J Ther. 2007;14(4):341-5.
13. Maskell NA, Davies CW, Nunn AJ, Hedley EL, Gleeson FV, Miller R, et al. U.K. Controlled trial of intrapleural streptokinase for pleural infection. N Engl J Med. 2005;352(9):865-74.
14. Cameron R, Davies HR. Intra-pleural fibrinolytic therapy versus conservative management in the treatment of adult parapneumonic effusions and empyema. Cochrane Database Syst Rev. 2008;2:CD002312.
15. Lawrence DR, Ohri SK, Moxon RE, Townsend ER, Fountain SW. Thoracoscopic debridement of empyema thoracis. Ann Thorac Surg. 1997;64(5):1448-50.
16. Striffeler H, Gugger M, Im Hof V, Cerny A, Furrer M, Ris HB. Video-assisted thoracoscopic surgery for fibrinopurulent pleural empyema in 67 patients. Ann Thorac Surg. 1998;65(2):319-23.
17. Wait MA, Sharma S, Hohn J, Dal Nogare A. A randomized trial of empyema therapy. Chest. 1997;111(6):1548-51.
18. Bilgin M, Akcali Y, Oguzkaya F. Benefits of early aggressive management of empyema thoracis. ANZ J Surg. 2006;76(3):120-2.
19. Tong BC, Hanna J, Toloza EM, Onaitis MW, D'Amico TA, Harpole DH, et al. Outcomes of video-assisted thoracoscopic decortication. Ann Thorac Surg. 2010;89(1):220-5.
20. Waller DA, Rengarajan A. Thoracoscopic decortication: a role for video-assisted surgery in chronic postpneumonic pleural empyema. Ann Thorac Surg. 2001;71(6):1813-6.
21. Chan DT, Sihoe AD, Chan S, Tsang DS, Fang B, Lee TW, et al. Surgical treatment for empyema thoracis: is video-assisted thoracic surgery "better" than thoracotomy? Ann Thorac Surg. 2007;84(1):225-31.
22. Cardillo G, Carleo F, Carbone L, Di Martino M, Salvadori L, Petrella L, et al. Chronic postpneumonic pleural empyema: comparative merits of thoracoscopic versus open decortication. Eur J Cardiothorac Surg. 2009;36(5):914-8.
23. Chung JH, Lee SH, Kim KT, Jung JS, Son HS, Sun K. Optimal timing of thoracoscopic drainage and decortication for empyema. Ann Thorac Surg. 2014;97(1):224-9.
24. Podbielski FJ, Maniar HS, Rodriguez HE, Hernan MJ, Vigneswaran WT. Surgical strategy of complex empyema thoracis. JSLS. 2000;4(4):287-90.
25. Wurnig PN, Wittmer V, Pridun NS, Hollaus PH. Video-assisted thoracic surgery for pleural empyema. Ann Thorac Surg. 2006;81(1):309-13.
26. Lardinois D, Gock M, Pezzetta E, Buchli C, Rousson V, Furrer M, et al. Delayed referral and Gram-negative organisms increase the conversion thoracotomy rate in patients undergoing video-assisted thoracoscopic surgery for empyema. Ann Thorac Surg. 2005;79(6):1851-6.
27. Stefani A, Aramini B, della Casa G, Ligabue G, Kaleci S, Casali C, et al. Preoperative predictors of successful surgical treatment in the management of parapneumonic empyema. Ann Thorac Surg. 2013;96(5):1812-9.
28. Botianu PV, Dobrica AC, Butiurca A, Botianu AM. Complex space-filling procedures for intrathoracic infections - personal experience with 76 consecutive cases. Eur J Cardiothorac Surg. 2010;37(2):478-81.
29. Garcia-Yuste M, Ramos G, Duque JL, Heras F, Castanedo M, Cerezal LJ, et al. Open-window thoracostomy and thoracomyoplasty to manage chronic pleural empyema. Ann Thorac Surg. 1998; 65(3):818-22.
30. Olesen WH, Katballe N, Sindby JE, Titlestad IL, Andersen PE, Lindahl-Jacobsen R, et al. Surgical treatment versus conventional chest tube drainage in primary spontaneous pneumothorax: a randomized controlled trial. Eur J Cardiothorac Surg. 2018;54(1):113-21.
31. MacDuff A, Arnold A, Harvey J; BTS Pleural Disease Guideline Group. Management of spontaneous pneumothorax: British Thoracic Society Pleural Disease Guideline 2010. Thorax. 2010;65(Suppl 2):ii18-31.
32. Kawai N, Kawaguchi T, Yasukawa M, Tojo T, Sawabata N, Taniguchi S. Surgical treatment for secondary spontaneous pneumothorax: a risk factor analysis. Surg Today. 2021;51(6):994-1000.
33. Jeon HW, Kim YD, Choi SY, Park JK. When Is the Optimal Timing of the Surgical Treatment for Secondary Spontaneous Pneumothorax? Thorac Cardiovasc Surg. 2017;65(1):50-5.
34. Ichinose J, Nagayama K, Hino H, Nitadori J, Anraku M, Murakawa T, et al. Results of surgical treatment for secondary spontaneous pneumothorax according to underlying diseases. Eur J Cardiothorac Surg. 2016;49(4):1132-6.
35. Vanderschueren RG. Pleural talcage in patients with spontaneous pneumothorax (author's transl). Poumon Coeur. 1981;37(4):273-6.
36. Puri HV, Asaf BB, Pulle MV, Bishnoi S, Kumar A. Video-assisted thoracoscopic surgery management of primary spontaneous pneumothorax: Results in 110 consecutive cases. Lung India. 2021;38(1):36-40.
37. Neudecker J, Malzahn U, Heuschmann P, Behrens U, Walles T. Pulmonary wedge resection plus parietal pleurectomy (WRPP) versus parietal pleurectomy (PP) for the treatment of recurrent primary pneumothorax (WOPP trial): study protocol for a randomized controlled trial. Trials. 2015;16:540.
38. Min X, Huang Y, Yang Y, Chen Y, Cui J, Wang C, et al. Mechanical pleurodesis does not reduce recurrence of spontaneous pneumothorax: a randomized trial. Ann Thorac Surg. 2014;98(5):1790-6; discussion 1796.

39. Panebianco V, Calanducci F, Poli A, Ferreri ME, Puzzo L, Pistritto A, et al. Surgical treatment of spontaneous pneumothorax: comparison of thoracotomy and thoracoscopy. G Chir. 1997;18(3):131-3.
40. Passlick B, Born C, Thetter O. Results of minimally invasive surgery in patients with recurrent or persistent primary pneumothorax. Pneumologie. 1997;51(12):1135-9.
41. Dumont P, Diemont F, Massard G, Toumieux B, Wihlm JM, Morand G. Does a thoracoscopic approach for surgical treatment of spontaneous pneumothorax represent progress? Eur J Cardiothorac Surg. 1997;11(1):27-31.
42. Ben-Nun A, Soudack M, Best LA. Video-assisted thoracoscopic surgery for recurrent spontaneous pneumothorax: the long-term benefit. World J Surg. 2006;30(3):285-90.
43. Ingolfsson I, Gyllstedt E, Lillo-Gil R, Pikwer A, Jönsson P, Gudbjartsson T. Reoperations are common following VATS for spontaneous pneumothorax: study of risk factors. Interact Cardiovasc Thorac Surg. 2006;5(5):602-7.
44. Imperatori A, Rotolo N, Spagnoletti M, Festi L, Berizzi F, Di Natale D, et al. Risk factors for postoperative recurrence of spontaneous pneumothorax treated by video-assisted thoracoscopic surgery†. Interact Cardiovasc Thorac Surg. 2015; 20(5):647-51; discussion 651-2.
45. Jeon HW, Kim YD, Kye YK, Kim KS. Air leakage on the postoperative day: powerful factor of postoperative recurrence after thoracoscopic bullectomy. J Thorac Dis. 2016;8(1):93-7.
46. Choi SY, Kim DY, Suh JH, Yoon JS, Jeong JY, Park CB. New bullae formation in the staple line increases the risk of recurrent pneumothorax following video-assisted thoracoscopic surgery bullectomy for primary spontaneous pneumothorax. J Thorac Dis. 2018;10(7):4287-92.
47. Cardillo G, Facciolo F, Regal M, Carbone L, Corzani F, Ricci A, et al. Recurrences following videothoracoscopic treatment of primary spontaneous pneumothorax: the role of redo-videothoracoscopy. Eur J Cardiothorac Surg. 2001;19(4):396-9.
48. Visouli AN, Zarogoulidis K, Kougioumtzi I, Huang H, Li Q, Dryllis G, et al. Catamenial pneumothorax. J Thorac Dis. 2014;6(Suppl 4):S448-60.
49. Van Schil PE, Vercauteren SR, Vermeire PA, Nackaerts YH, Van Marck EA. Catamenial pneumothorax caused by thoracic endometriosis. Ann Thorac Surg. 1996;62(2):585-6.
50. Bagan P, Le Pimpec Barthes F, Assouad J, Souilamas R, Riquet M. Catamenial pneumothorax: retrospective study of surgical treatment. Ann Thorac Surg. 2003;75(2):378-81; discusssion 381.
51. Joseph J, Sahn SA. Thoracic endometriosis syndrome: new observations from an analysis of 110 cases. Am J Med. 1996;100(2):164-70.
52. Marshall MB, Ahmed Z, Kucharczuk JC, Kaiser LR, Shrager JB. Catamenial pneumothorax: optimal hormonal and surgical management. Eur J Cardiothorac Surg. 2005;27(4):662-6.
53. Korom S, Canyurt H, Missbach A, Schneiter D, Kurrer MO, Haller U, et al. Catamenial pneumothorax revisited: clinical approach and systematic review of the literature. J Thorac Cardiovasc Surg. 2004;128(4):502-8.
54. Alifano M, Trisolini R, Cancellieri A, Regnard JF. Thoracic Endometriosis: current Knowledge. Ann Thorac Surg. 2006;81(12):761-9.
55. Alifano M, Jablonski C, Kadiri H, Falcoz P, Gompel A, Camilleri-Broet S, et al. Catamenial and noncatamenial, endometriosis-related or nonendometriosis-related pneumothorax referred for surgery. Am J Respir Crit Care Med. 2007;176(10):1048-53.
56. Alifano M, Magdeleinat P, Regnard JF. Catamenial pneumothorax: some commentaries. J Thorac Cardiovasc Surg. 2005;129(5):1199; author reply 1199-200.
57. Kindler HL, Ismaila N, Armato SG 3rd, Bueno R, Hesdorffer M, Jahan T, et al. Treatment of Malignant Pleural Mesothelioma: American Society of Clinical Oncology Clinical Practice Guideline. J Clin Oncol. 2018;36(13):1343-73.
58. Rusch VW, Giroux D, Kennedy C, Ruffini E, Cangir AK, Rice D, et al. Initial analysis of the international association for the study of lung cancer mesothelioma database. J Thorac Oncol. 2012;7(11):1631-9.
59. Pass HI, Giroux D, Kennedy C, Ruffini E, Cangir AK, Rice D, et al. Supplementary prognostic variables for pleural mesothelioma: a report from the IASLC staging committee. J Thorac Oncol. 2014;9(6):856-64.
60. Sugarbaker DJ, Wolf AS. Surgery for malignant pleural mesothelioma. Expert Rev Respir Med. 2010;4(3):363-72.
61. Sugarbaker DJ, Richards WG, Bueno R. Extrapleural pneumonectomy in the treatment of epithelioid malignant pleural mesothelioma: novel prognostic implications of combined N1 and N2 nodal involvement based on experience in 529 patients. Ann Surg. 2014;260(4):577-80; discussion 580-2.
62. Sugarbaker DJ, Jaklitsch MT, Bueno R, Richards W, Lukanich J, Mentzer SJ, et al. Prevention, early detection, and management of complications after 328 consecutive extrapleural pneumonectomies. J Thorac Cardiovasc Surg. 2004;128(1):138-46.
63. Flores RM, Pass HI, Seshan VE, Dycoco J, Zakowski M, Carbone M, et al. Extrapleural pneumonectomy versus pleurectomy/decortication in the surgical management of malignant pleural mesothelioma: results in 663 patients. J Thorac Cardiovasc Surg. 2008;135(3):620-6, 626.e1-3.
64. Planchard D, Popat S, Kerr K, Novello S, Smit EF, Faivre-Finn C, et al. Metastatic non-small cell lung cancer: ESMO Clinical Practice Guidelines for diagnosis, treatment and follow-up. Ann Oncol. 2018;29(Suppl 4):iv192-237.
65. Ichinose Y, Tsuchiya R, Koike T, Kuwahara O, Nakagawa K, Yamato Y, et al. The prognosis of patients with non-small cell lung cancer found to have carcinomatous pleuritis at thoracotomy. Surg Today. 2000;30(12):1062-6.
66. Ichinose Y, Tsuchiya R, Koike T, Kuwahara O, Nakagawa K, Yamato Y, et al. Prognosis of resected non-small cell lung cancer patients with carcinomatous pleuritis of minimal disease. Lung Cancer. 2001;32(1):55-60.
67. Iida T, Shiba M, Yoshino I, Miyaoka E, Asamura H, Date H, et al. Surgical intervention for non-small-cell lung cancer patients with pleural carcinomatosis: results from the Japanese Lung Cancer Registry in 2004. J Thorac Oncol. 2015;10(7):1076-82.
68. Liu T, Liu H, Wang G, Zhang C, Liu B. Survival of M1a non-small cell lung cancer treated surgically: a retrospective single-center study. Thorac Cardiovasc Surg. 2015;63(7):577-82.
69. Li H, Sun Z, Yang F, Sui X, Liu T, Wang J. Primary tumour resection in non-small-cell lung cancer patients with ipsilateral pleural dissemination (M1a): a population-based study. Eur J Cardiothorac Surg. 2019;55(6):1121-9.
70. Bonev P. Video-assisted thoracoscopic diagnosis of trapped lung in malignant pleural effusions. Trakia J Sci. 2018;3:212-7.
71. Bibby AC, Dorn P, Psallidas I, Porcel JM, Janssen J, Froudarakis M, et al. ERS/EACTS statement on the management of malignant pleural effusions. Eur Respir J. 2018;52(1):1800349.
72. Doelken P, Sahn SA. Trapped lung. Semin Respir Crit Care Med. 2001;22(6):631-6.

73. Shields TW. General Thoracic Surgery, 6th edition. Philadelphia: Lippincot Williams & Wilkins; 2005.
74. Luciano G, Waller DA. Video-assisted thoracoscopic surgery in the management of malignant pleural disease. Video-assist Thorac Surg. 2018;3:37.
75. Soysal O, Karaoğlanoğlu N, Demiracan S, Topçu S, Taştepe I, Kaya S, et al. Pleurectomy/decortication for palliation in malignant pleural mesothelioma: results of surgery. Eur J Cardiothorac Surg. 1997;11(2):210-3.
76. Ilic N. Functional effects of decortication after penetrating war injuries to the chest. J Thorac Cardiovasc Surg. 1996;111(5):967-70.
77. Swoboda L, Laule K, Blattmann HK, Hasse J. Decortication in chronic pleural empyema. Investigation of lung function based on perfusion scintigraphy. Thorac Cardiovasc Surg. 1990;38(6):359-61.
78. Rathinam S, Waller DA. Pleurectomy decortication in the treatment of the "trapped lung" in benign and malignant pleural effusions. Thorac Surg Clin. 2013;23(1):51-61.

CHAPTER

31

Pleural Diseases in COVID

Ashish Kumar Prakash, Saurabh Mandilwar, Yatin Mehta

INTRODUCTION

Coronavirus disease, which started from Wuhan, China, in November 2019, also called COVID-19, was the worst pandemic the world has seen among the people living in the current era. It has caused a spectrum of disease. Majority of those affected are asymptomatic or have febrile mild upper respiratory symptoms. Pulmonary involvement leads to moderate and severe disease. The clinical symptoms range from mild cough and breathlessness to florid acute respiratory distress syndrome (ARDS). Early inflammatory pulmonary phase is characterized by alveolitis [ground glass opacity (GGO)] and acinar shadows (consolidation and organizing pneumonia) on computed tomography (CT). This is precipitated by inflammatory cytokines and cellular infiltrates. ARDS is an exaggeration of these processes. The inflammatory phase is followed by a fibrotic phase, presenting radiologically as traction bronchiectasis, architectural lung distortion, crazy paving, or thickened interlobular septa. Pulmonary involvement was the most fatal involvement of this virus. Compared to the pulmonary manifestation, pleural disease was less reported but was very fatal. The pleural pathologies that happened because of COVID-19 disease were:[1]

- Pleural effusion and thickening
- Pneumothorax
- Pneumomediastinum (PTM)
- Empyema

PLEURAL EFFUSION AND THICKENING

Pleural effusion, its various types, etiopathology, and management have all been discussed in the previous chapters of this textbook. Although pleural effusion was less reported in the worst pandemic, it has something to discuss in terms of COVID-related illness. The topics to be discussed are:

- Incidence
- Risk factors
- Onset
- Pleural fluid characteristics
- Outcomes

Incidence of Pleural Effusion in COVID Illness

In a state-of-the-art review study done by Woon H. Chong et al., comprising 47 observational studies, the overall incidence of pleural effusions was found to be around 7.3%. It was more common in critically ill patients and those with multisystem inflammatory syndrome (MIS). On an average, it was seen in between 7 and 11 days of symptomatic patients who were hospitalized.[2] A narrative review done by Biplab K. Saha et al.,[1] on the basis of several studies and meta-analysis, showed that the pleural involvement in COVID was rare but had significant lesions, such as pleural thickening (27–52%), pleural retraction (around 56%), and pleural effusion (around

TABLE 1: Pleural involvement in COVID, a meta-analysis of several studies.

Study	No. of studies	No. of patients	+ CT scans (%) defined by studies	Pleural thickening (%)	Pleural retraction (%)	PE (%)
Bao et al.[3]	13	2,738	89.76	52.46	NS	5.88
Zhu et al.[4]	34	4,124	91.6	27.1	NS	5.3
Ojha et al.[5]	45	4,410	NS	41.7	56.5	5
Adams et al.[6]	28	3,466	89.4	34.7	NS	5.2
Xie et al.[7]	90	16,526	95.9	29.8	NS	4.2

(CT: computed tomography; NS: not specified; PE: pleural effusion)

4–6%) **(Table 1)**. One study done by Saha et al. to compare pleural lesions among various viral illnesses, mainly among those that had caused pandemics (coronavirus and influenza), elicited that compared with other viral illnesses, the incidence of pneumothorax was only 1% in COVID as compared to 11% in severe acute respiratory syndrome (SARS).[1]

Risk Factors

Among the risk factors of COVID, age was found to be very important. According to a study done by Majid et al., which was a large observational study, the frequency of pleural effusion varied with age.[8] Pleural effusion was around 7.3%, and it was found to be higher among the elderly people (age > 50 years) and was statistically significant (10% vs 5.2% with $p = 0.037$). However, few smaller studies could not elicit the same.[9,10] Although the lung involvement in COVID was found more among adults as compared to children, the same was not found in case of pleural effusion.[11] Initially, it was found that COVID pandemic was doing very little or no harm to children,[12] but later with the involvement of multiple systems called multisystem inflammatory syndrome in children (MIS-C), children were affected with severity too. MIS-C or that in adults (MIS-A) is basically the postinfective hyperinflammatory response or the complication of COVID infection because of cytokine storm.[13] Because of multisystem involvement in this condition, they are likely to develop effusions (pleural, pericardial) or ascites. Various studies have shown that they have variable presentations of MIS-C, such as pericardial effusion was present in 12.5–47.6%, while ascites was present in 19.0–37.5%. The incidence of overall pleural effusion in case of children with MIS-C was 13.9–62.5%.[12,14,15] In another case series documented by Rostad et al., the incidence of pleural effusion in children with MIS-C was statistically significant ($p < 0.01$), which was 81.8% for MIS-C as compared to 6.3% during COVID-19 infections.[16]

The next important discussion with respect to pleural lesions in COVID is pregnancy. After various reviews, it can be concluded that it had no clear-cut correlation. One reason for that is we do not have enough literature and meta-analysis to confirm correlation of pleural effusion and pregnancy with COVID. One study, though did not have enough sample size to detect statistical significance, showed incidence of pleural effusion up to 29% (12/41) in pregnancy compared to 7% (1/41) in nonpregnant women.[9] Among pregnant COVID patients, the pleural effusion developed in later stages of pregnancy (35–41 weeks) or postpartum phase. There are few explanations for this[17-19] such as transudative movement of fluid to the pleural cavity after release of pregnancy-induced systemic hypertension (HTN) in the postpartum phase. Within 24 hours of normal delivery, the gradient of pressure (increased systemic pressure and low oncotic pressure due to hypoalbuminemia) causes the movement of fluid to the pleural space. Another explanation is that because of repeated Valsalva during normal delivery, the elevated abdominal pressure due to already gravid uterus tends to further raise intrathoracic pressure and impair lymphatic drainage, leading to pleural effusion. Other risk factors for pleural effusion in case of COVID are as the same as discussed in normal patients described elsewhere in this textbook. COVID patients with sepsis, aggressive fluid supplement, hypoproteinemia, chronic kidney disease (CKD), and heart failure are at the same risk of developing pleural effusion as other patients but are mostly bilateral. Overall increased systemic inflammatory response and third space fluid retention are the possible explanations for pleural fluid in COVID. Just like other infective exacerbations, around 15% of COVID patients during their clinical course and 50% of critically ill COVID patients developed heart and kidney failure.[20,21]

Onset

The role of radiological tests such as chest X-ray and CT was extensively explored during the COVID period. These tests were done during the course of hospital admission and also follow-up. As per few observational studies done,[22-24] overall COVID-related pleural effusion had onset within 5–7 days of hospitalization and around 11 days of onset of COVID symptoms. One observational study done by Ding et al. documented that the incidence of pleural effusion increased from 9.2 to 27% from 5–7 to 15–21 days from the day of onset of COVID symptoms.[25] In another single-center retrospective cohort study, which compared chest CT findings in early versus advance phase, it was found that there was no statistically significant difference in pleural thickening (42% vs. 59%) and pleural retraction (57% vs. 54%). Pleural effusion was seen in 2.5% in early disease and 22.7% in advance disease, and it was statistically significant ($p = 0.01$).[26] One cross-sectional study on CT findings showed that pleural effusion incidence increased from 12 to 38% when done from 5th to 12th day of onset of symptoms of COVID ($p = 0.01$).[27]

Pleural Fluid Characteristics

The biochemical analysis of the pleural effusion showed exudative, lymphocytic, or neutrophilic-predominant pleural fluid, and significantly increased lactate dehydrogenase (LDH) levels and pleural fluid to serum LDH ratio. A study done by Cappelli et al. compared pleural effusion in 150 patients with nonpleural effusion (550) in COVID patients. This was a single-center retrospective study done in Pisa, Italy, between March 2020 and January 2021. This showed unilateral pleural effusion in 35 patients and bilateral in 115 patients. While quantifying the effusion among unilateral effusions, 18 patients had ≥1 cm and 17 patients had < 1 cm. Among bilateral effusion, 115 patients had <1 cm and 53 patients had ≥1 cm.[28] Few case reports and series documented that according to Light's criteria, almost all cases of COVID-related pleural effusion had exudative effusion, and pleural fluid to serum LDH ratio was 0.7 or more.[29-33]

Outcomes of COVID-19-related Pleural Effusion

To discuss the GGO and consolidation during COVID pneumonia is beyond the scope of this book. Till date, we have several meta-analyses regarding the outcome in terms of parenchymal and other residual post-COVID sequalae, and we have mixed results.[34-37] The parenchymal lesions, though were very severe, had good prognosis in terms of fibrosis among the patients who survived with severe COVID.[38,39] We have very limited data in terms of outcome with post-COVID pleural lesions. One study done by Saha et al.[1] related to outcome in case of COVID-related pleural effusion. This study was basically designed to compare the outcome as well as clinical and prognostic implications among the COVID patients with or without pleural effusion. It was found that the mortality of hospitalized patients was 36.7% among patients of COVID who had pleural effusion versus 13.8% among patients of COVID who did not have pleural effusion, and it was statistically significant ($p < 0.001$). In this study, it was found that presence of pleural effusion was associated with poor clinical outcomes. Patients of COVID who had pleural effusion had impaired gas exchange along with increased morbidity (hospital stay) and required ventilatory support, either invasive or noninvasive. Overall, the survival of the patient having pleural effusion was lower as compared with a COVID patient who did not have pleural effusion. The multivariate analysis done in the same study found pleural effusion as an independent predictor of mortality.[40] Sometimes, pleura can become thickened because of inflammation or scarring caused by COVID-19. Pleural thickening can restrict the expansion of lung, leading to respiratory distress and dyspnea on exertion, which could be mild, moderate, or severe as per the extent of pleural involvement. Overall, the summary regarding the pleural effusion in COVID is summarized in **Box 1**.

BOX 1 Pleural effusion in COVID summary.

- *Incidence*: Low, around –7.3% (number varies among several studies)
- *Comorbidities*:
  - Higher incidence was found in critically ill patients and those with MIS
  - Age = More likely in elder people
  - Pregnancy = No clear association
- Same incidence with SARS-related pleural effusions
- *Onset*:
  - 11 days from symptoms onset and 5–7 days from admission
  - Frequency increases as the course of disease advances to severe pneumonia
- *Pleural fluid nature*:
  - Exudative, lymphocytic, or neutrophilic-predominant
  - Marked increases in LDH
  - Increased pleural fluid: Serum LDH (PF:S) ratio
  - PF:S LDH ratio 1.3 < suggestive of COVID-19-related pleural effusion

(LDH: lactate dehydrogenase; MIS: multisystem inflammatory syndrome; PF:S: pleural fluid to serum; SARS: severe acute respiratory syndrome)

PNEUMOTHORAX

Although rare, a potential complication of COVID-19 was pneumothorax, a condition where air enters the pleural space, causing the lung to collapse partially or completely. Pneumothorax can result from severe lung inflammation and damage, leading to formation of air-filled pockets in the lung tissue, which can eventually rupture and cause pneumothorax. It can also be associated with PTM. Spontaneous pneumothorax (SP) is a rare complication of COVID-19 pneumonia and may occur in the absence of mechanical ventilation (MV). Pneumothorax, PTM, and subcutaneous emphysema were the most devastating outcomes of COVID pneumonia and led to the highest mortality among COVID patients **(Figs. 1 to 5)**.

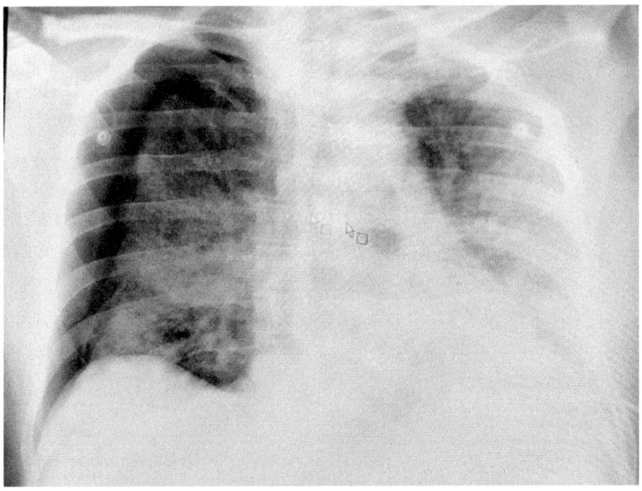

FIG. 1: Patient with bilateral lung lesion and right-sided pneumothorax.

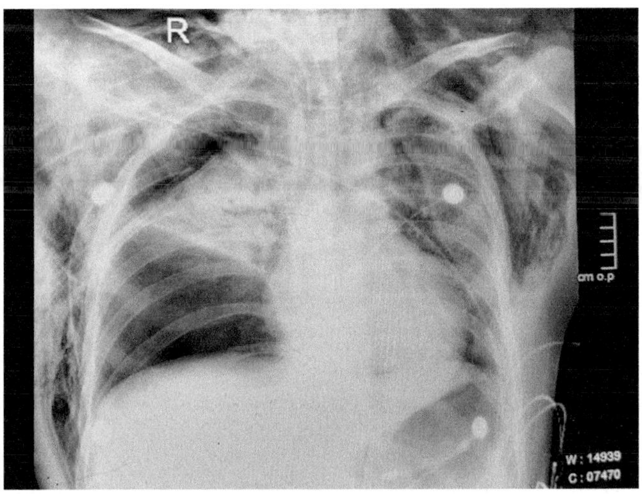

FIG. 2: COVID patient on mechanical ventilator with right pneumothorax, pneumomediastinum, and subcutaneous emphysema.

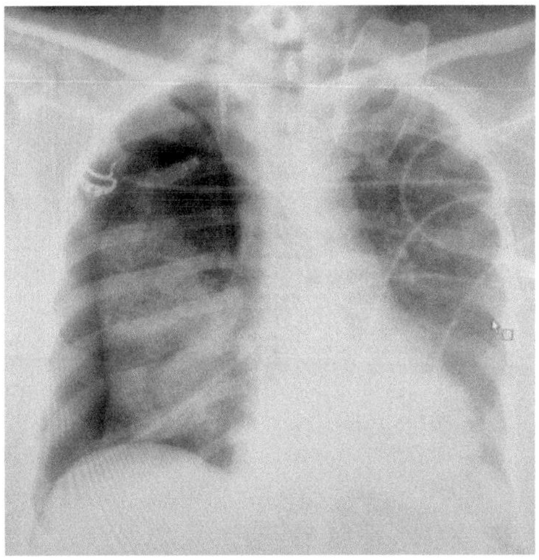

FIG. 3: COVID pneumonia with right pneumothorax.

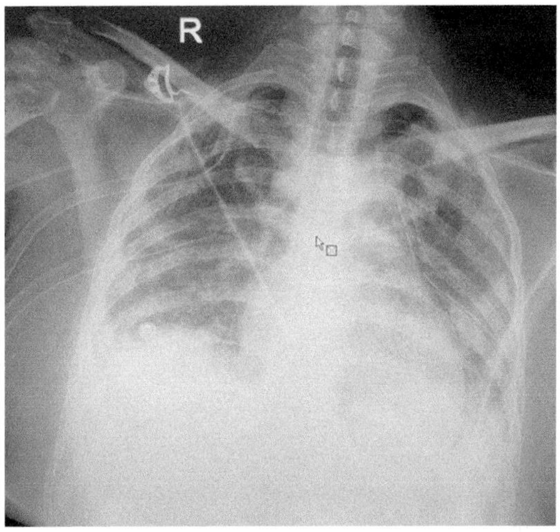

FIG. 4: Severe COVID pneumonia patient with bilateral pneumothorax (right side two and left side one intercostal chest drain in situ).

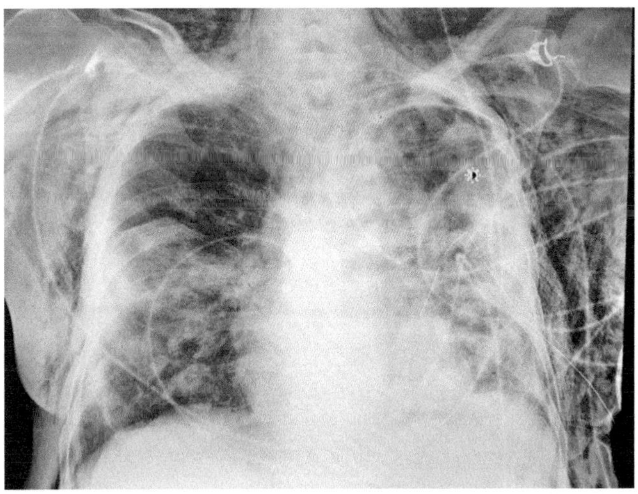

FIG. 5: COVID patient with left-sided pneumothorax (resolved) with left intercostal chest drain in situ along with subcutaneous emphysema.

Incidence of Pneumothorax in COVID Illness

Though the incidence was very low in COVID, as compared with other viral pandemics/epidemics, the mortality was substantially high. The incidence of pneumothorax was 11% in SARS, very rare in influenza, rare in Middle East respiratory syndrome (MERS), and only 1% in COVID. The viral illness versus COVID and their pleural involvement is depicted in **Table 2**.

The incidence of this complication is not yet exactly known. In a report by Chen et al., 1% (one patient) had a pneumothorax among other radiographic features[41] among all COVID-19 patients. Another study published by Yang and colleagues of 92 deceased COVID-19 patients, one (1.1%) had a pneumothorax and died as a result of it 5 days after the initial presentation.[42] While the incidence of pneumothorax in mechanically ventilated patients is high, it is believed to be even higher in those with ARDS, ranging between 14 and 87%.[43] The incidence of pneumothorax was around 10% in a study done on 334 critically ill COVID patients. It was associated with long intubation and MV with prolonged morbidity and hospital stay.[44] Previous studies have shown that the incidence of pneumothorax in patients with COVID-19 is about 1% in hospitalized patients and 2% in those needing intensive care.[41,42,45] According to Udwadia et al., the incidence of air leaks in patients with severe COVID-19 was 3.2%, which is higher than in previously reported studies. Air leaks in those patients correlate with poor outcomes and carry a mortality rate of 74%.[46]

Risk Factors and Pathophysiology of Pneumothorax in COVID Illness

The mechanism of SP in COVID-19 is due to the structural changes in the lung parenchyma. These include cystic and fibrotic changes in lung parenchyma, leading to alveolar tears, in addition to the increase in intrathoracic pressure resulting from prolonged coughing and/or MV. A systemic review was done by Shahsavarinia et al.[47] of COVID patients who had serious lesions like pneumothorax or pneumomediastinum. This included 99 studies and 139 patients, of which 96.8% of the patients developed pulmonary lesions during their hospital admission, and among them, 67.4% had pneumothorax. In the review, they found that 28.8% of the patients had developed pneumothorax after intubation or continuous positive airway pressure (CPAP). The odds of developing pneumothorax were 40–100 times higher among COVID patients compared to those without COVID, and patients on MV definitely had a high chance of pneumothorax in COVID-19 patients.[48,49] Pneumothorax was more likely in patients with neutrophilia, severe lung injury, and a prolonged clinical course. The timely diagnosis and management helped to reduce COVID-19-associated morbidity and mortality. Neutrophilia and lymphopenia can cause acute lung injury, leading to pneumothorax. Neutrophilia and lymphopenia were detected in almost all cases of COVID pneumonia who had pneumothorax. These prognostic factors exacerbated pneumothorax due to COVID-19 and may increase the length of hospital stay, thus escalating the progression of infection parameters and related morbidity-mortality. The risk of pneumothorax was increased in COVID-19 patients treated with noninvasive mechanical ventilation (NIMV) and MV. Smoking is a poor prognostic factor in COVID-19 infection and pneumothorax. One study on smoking and its outcome in COVID found that a poor clinical course was observed, and the patient died. In the study, MV/NIMV was applied in 66.6% of the smoker/ex-smoker cases, and mortality was observed in 50%. Although the clinical course of COVID-19 patients with SP in smokers was worse, and mortality was observed in three cases, there was no statistically significant difference in terms of smoking and MV/NIMV relationship and mortality and smoking. The major risk factors of developing pneumothorax were similar to the risk factors of severe COVID such as male patients, hypertension, diabetes mellitus (DM), and critically ill patients who were on endotracheal intubation and MV.[50] In one study, it was found that patients who received tocilizumab had an increased risk of developing pneumothorax.[45]

TABLE 2: Pleural involvement with outcome in various viral pandemics.

Virus	Pleural effusion	Pneumothorax	Mediastinal lymphadenopathy	Overall mortality (%)
Influenza	20–36%, early	Very rare	Approximately 20%	0.1
SARS (2003)	26% (typically later in the disease)	11%	Not reported	9
MERS (2012)	Approximately 50% (develops early, often in the first week)	Rare but associated with fatal outcome	Not reported	34
COVID-19 (2019)	4.2–5.8% (typically later in the disease)	Approximately 1%	2.9–5.4%	1–3

(MERS: Middle East respiratory syndrome; SARS: severe acute respiratory syndrome)

Outcome of Pneumothorax in COVID Illness

As discussed earlier, the occurrence of pneumothorax was mainly in severe or critically ill COVID patients and was most common in mechanically ventilated seriously ill patients. There is no doubt that the outcome will be poor among these cohorts of patients. In the systemic review by Shahsavarinia et al.,[47] the mortality of the patients was significantly related to the positive pressure ventilation (PPV) ($p = 0.0001$), but there was no statistically significant relationship between the patients' death and intercostal chest drain (ICD) insertion ($p = 0.2$). The relationship between the diagnosis of pneumothorax and the interval of time from the onset of symptoms was also not significantly related ($p = 0.7$). In that study, there was significant correlation between age and mortality [(mean age was higher in the deceased cases) ($p = 0.001$)]. A very interesting multicentric study published by Udwadia et al. in 2021,[46] who compared almost all major studies done so far on pneumothorax in COVID and their outcome, found that the outcome was very poor. Among the COVID patients who had pneumothorax, the mortality was 74% as compared with patients of COVID without pneumothorax, where the mortality was only 17% ($p < 0.001$). The various studies done so far regarding COVID pneumothorax are depicted in **Table 3**.

In one case series, delay in admission to hospital and severe pneumonia progression were detected in three patients who died due to sepsis, ARDS, and multiorgan failure. Chest tube thoracostomy was sufficient in the treatment of pneumothorax in nine cases, whereas high-dose oxygen therapy was sufficient in two cases. The lungs were expanded in all the cases, and surgery was not required. The risk of pneumothorax was increased in COVID-19 patients treated with NIMV and MV. The main cause for hospitalization in 7 out of 11 cases was pneumothorax. In the same period over the 3 years prior to the COVID-19 pandemic, a total of 40 patients were hospitalized with a diagnosis of secondary spontaneous pneumothorax (SSP). The annual number of SSP cases was found to have increased, although the difference was not statistically significant. No statistically significant difference was found between the tube thoracostomy treatment duration in the pre-COVID-19 period and that during the pandemic. In this study, compared to the previous years, the coexistence of COVID-19 infection with pneumothorax increased the number of SP cases and the rate of hospitalization and length of stay. Pneumothorax can, therefore, be considered as a poor prognostic factor in COVID-19 infection. Inflammation is common in COVID-19 pneumonia. It is possible that the developing inflammation poses a risk for SP and increases the incidence of pneumothorax. In such cases,

TABLE 3: Incidence, interventions, and outcomes in COVID-19 patients with pneumothorax.

Study	Number of patients	Patient population	Number of PTX	Pneumo-mediastinum	Tension PTX	Days post MV	Intervention	Outcomes
Chopra et al.[56]	842; 594 on MV	Critically ill patients	83 (10%); 80/83 (96%) in patients on MV	In 30% of patients concomitantly	32%	10 ± 12	Tube; thoracostomy 89%	Significantly higher in-hospital mortality 63% *versus* 49%
Rajdev et al.[55]	353; 121 on MV	Critically ill patients	23 (6.5%); barotrauma (21/121, 17% with MV and 11/232, 5% without MV)	21/353 (6%)	NS	11 (6–19) (hospital admission to barotrauma)	38% of patients received thoracostomy tubes	NS
McGuinness et al.[57]	601 on MV	Critically ill patients	77 (12.8%); 54/601 (9%) of patients suffered from PTX	59/601 (10%) of patients	NS	5.4 (0–41)	NS	No difference in survival
Miró et al.[58]	71,904	ED	40/71,904 (0.56%)	6/71,904 (0.08%)	NS	NA	73% of patients needed tube thoracostomy	Increased odds for in-hospital mortality

Continued

Continued

Study	Number of patients	Patient population	Number of PTX	Pneumo-mediastinum	Tension PTX	Days post MV	Intervention	Outcomes
Wang et al.[59]	248	Inpatient	5/248 (2.01%); 5/49 (10%) patients with ARDS. All 5 patients were mechanically ventilated	NR	NS	6–25 days	NS	4/5 (80%) died
Ekanem et al.[60]	1,619	Inpatient	22/1,619 (1.4%); 11/22 (50%) of patients on MV	NR	NR	NS	73% required tube thoracostomy	36% of patients with PTX died
Udwadia et al.[46]	1,324	Critically ill patients	18/42 (43%)	16/42 (38%)			Observation 14/42 (33%) Pleural drain 28/42 (66%) VATS 1/42 (2%) Palliative 3/71 (4.2%)	Death 31/42 (73%)
Martinelli et al.[61]	Case series of 71 patients		54/71 (76%)	11/71 (15.5%)			Observation 26/71 (36%) Pleural drain 43/71 (60%) Surgery 1/71 (1.4%)	

(ED: emergency department; IQR: interquartile range; MV: mechanical ventilation; NA: not applicable; NR: not reported; NS: not specified; PTX: pneumothorax; SD: standard deviation; VATS: video-assisted thoracoscopic surgery)

early anti-inflammatory treatment, such as corticosteroid therapy, might decrease the frequency. In addition, during the follow-up of patients with COVID-19, new symptoms and findings such as novel chest pain, onset of shortness of breath, increase in shortness of breath, or deepening of hypoxemia should be considered as warning signs for pneumothorax.[51]

PNEUMOMEDIASTINUM

Pneumomediastinum can be primary (spontaneous) or secondary to iatrogenic, traumatic, and nontraumatic causes. The incidence of spontaneous and secondary PTM is higher in patients with COVID-19 compared to the general population. So, PTM should be considered in the differential diagnosis of any patient with COVID-19 presenting with chest pain and breathlessness. A high level of suspicion is required to diagnose this condition promptly. Unlike in other disease conditions, PTM in COVID-19 has a complicated course with higher mortality in intubated patients.[52]

Incidence of Pneumomediastinum in COVID Illness

A big study of total 377 cases of PTM in COVID-19 were done among 58,484 inpatients with COVID-19 from 53 hospitals.[53] In that study period, the overall incidence of PTM was 0.64% [95% confidence interval (CI) 0.58–0.71%]. According to this study, the incidence of spontaneous PTM in COVID patients is around 0.13%, which is around 6,000 times more than the normal population, where the incidence is just 0.00002%.[54] The 120-day mortality of COVID-19 PTM patients was very high, around 52% (195/377). PTM in COVID-19 was associated with higher rates of MV. At the point of diagnosis, around 47% patients (172/377) were on MV. Till now, we have learned that MV was a very important predictor of mortality in COVID-19 PTM, and in this study also it was proven to be significant ($p < 0.001$). Just like pneumothorax, in PTM also, increasing age ($p < 0.01$) and diabetes ($p = 0.08$) were important predictors of mortality. It was also found that high flow nasal cannula (HFNC) is as good as CPAP for those patients. Switching patients from CPAP support to oxygen or HFNC after the diagnosis of PTM was not associated with significant difference in mortality.[55]

Risk Factors and Pathogenesis

Similar to pneumothorax, the risk factors for PTM in COVID were male, DM, and HTN. In the study done by James Melhorn (UK POETIC survey), the median age was 60 years. There was male preponderance (73.5% in males and 26.5% in females). The comorbidities in the demographics of that survey depicted HTN among 32.4%, DM among 21.5%, asthma among 19.4%, obesity among 10.6%, heart disease among 8.8%, and CKD among 4.5% of patients. The median symptomatic duration prior to admission was 5–10 days, while the median duration of identification of PTM since admission was 5–12.3 days. PTM appears to be a marker of severe COVID-19 pneumonitis. The majority of patients in whom PTM was identified had not been mechanically ventilated at the point of diagnosis. The pathogenesis of PTM in COVID can be very well explained by the *Macklin effect*[52] **(Fig. 6)**.

This effect demonstrates a three-step pathophysiologic process **(Figs. 7 and 8)**:

1. Blunt traumatic alveolar ruptures
2. Air dissection along bronchovascular sheaths
3. Spreading of this blunt pulmonary interstitial emphysema into the mediastinum

The presence of the Macklin effect affected neither the clinical profile nor the result of pulmonary gas analysis on hospital admission but was associated with a significant ($p < 0.001$) lengthening of the intensive care stay. The Macklin effect is present in 39% of severe blunt traumatic PTM detected by CT. Its identification does not rule out a tracheobronchial injury.[62] Overall, it is the lung parenchymal lesion that is responsible for the such devastating picture of PTM, but the incidence is very low.

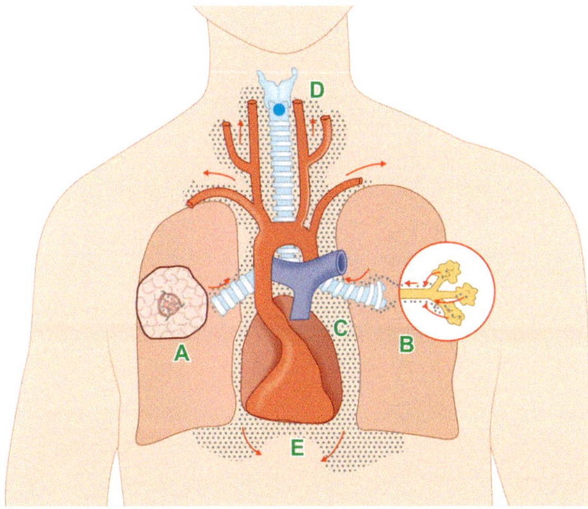

FIG. 6: Schematic representation of spread of pneumomediastinum (*Macklin effect*). It starts from (A) alveolar rupture and dissection of air into the bronchovascular sheath. (B) Spread of air as it passes along the bronchovascular sheath toward the pulmonary hilum; then air reaches the mediastinum (C), further to the subcutaneous space (D), and to the retroperitoneum (E).

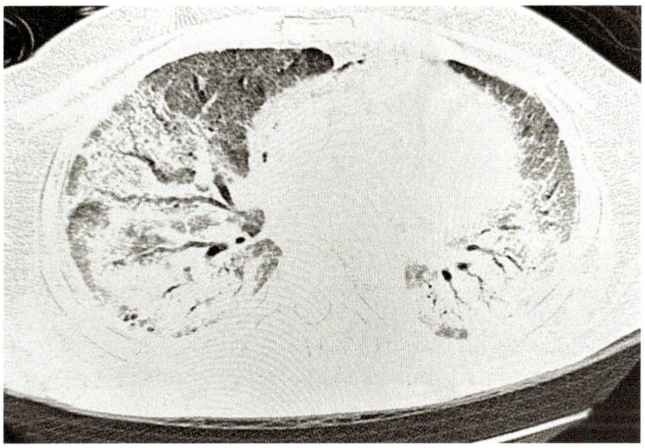

FIG. 7: Computed tomography of severe COVID patient with diffuse parenchymal lung disease.

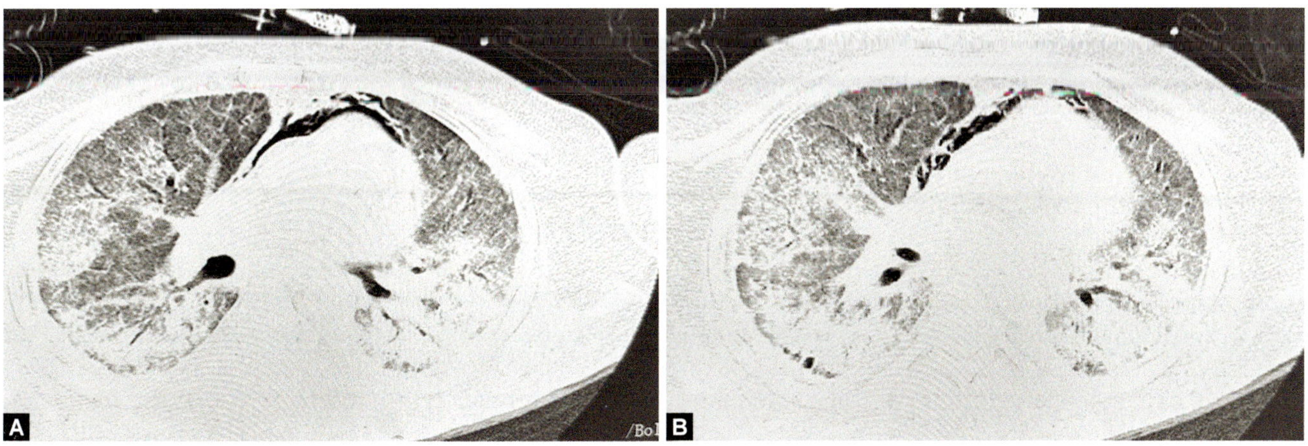

FIGS. 8A TO C: *Continued*

Continued

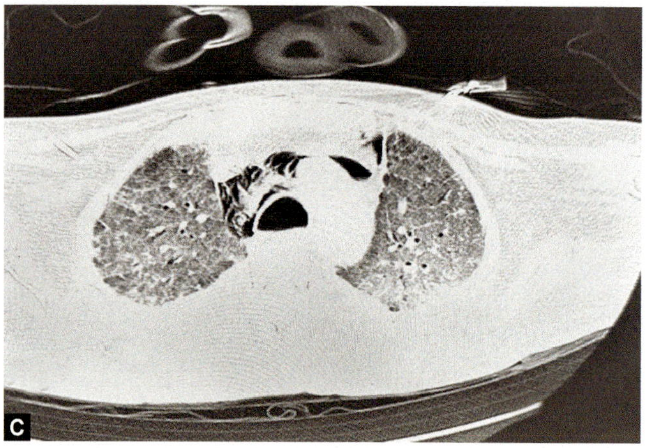

FIGS. 8A TO C: (A) Parenchymal lesion leading to pneumomediastinum. (B) Spread of pneumomediastinum. (C) Spread of pneumomediastinum.

BOX 2 Pneumothorax and pneumomediastinum (PTM) in COVID summary.

- *Incidence*: Low, around: –1 to 4% (number varies among several studies)
  - In critically ill and ventilated patients: 10–84% (number varies among several studies)
- *Risk factors*:
  - Higher incidence was found in critically ill patients
  - Age = more likely in elder people
  - Male > female
  - DM and hypertensive
  - Smokers
  - Neutrophilia and lymphopenia
  - Patients who received tocilizumab
  - Patients who were on positive-pressure ventilation
- Less incidence with SARS
- *Onset*
  - Timing of pneumothorax: 9 (0–30 days)
  - Duration of air-leak: 6–60 days
  - Duration of Invasive ventilation: 14 days (2 hours–70 days)
- *Outcome*: High mortality
  - For pneumothorax: 57–74%
  - For PTM: 34–71%

(DM: diabetes mellitus; SARS: severe acute respiratory syndrome)

Now several studies are coming depicting very low or residual lesion after follow-up of COVID;[38] hence, there is less chance of such abnormality in future. Overall, the summary regarding the summary of pneumothorax and PTM in COVID is depicted in **Box 2**.

EMPYEMA

Empyema is a condition where pus accumulates in the pleural space. It can occur as a complication of pneumonia, including pneumonia caused by COVID-19. It is very important to note that these pleural complications are relatively uncommon in COVID-19 cases. Most individuals with COVID-19 experience mild-to-moderate respiratory symptoms and do not develop these severe pleural issues. If someone has COVID-19 and experiences severe or significant breathing difficulties or chest pain, they should be evaluated for pneumonia as well as pleural complications on an urgent basis as these complications can be serious and require specialized treatment. Empyema definitely developed in long-standing cases of COVID with ICD for pleural effusion, pneumothorax, and PTM. Although empyema is rare in COVID, it has a high mortality rate, it is basically the superadded infection and is a complication of any pleural pathology with ICD. Management again is targeted antibiotics, ICD sometimes requiring video-assisted thoracoscopic surgery (VATS) (discussed in detail in empyema chapter).

KEY POINTS

- People with lung parenchymal lesions in COVID-19 are at an increased risk for complications such as pleural effusion, pneumothorax, and PTM as well as increased mortality.
- The incidence of pleural effusion is low, around 7%.
- Higher incidence was found in critically ill patients and in patients with MIS and elderly age group.
- It has the same incidence as SARS-related pleural effusions.
- Its onset is 11 days from symptoms onset and 5–7 days from admission.
- Pleural fluid nature is exudative, lymphocytic, or neutrophilic-predominant.
- Incidence of pneumothorax was very low in COVID (around 1–4%). Though it was high in critically ill and ventilated patients, ranged 10–84% in various studies.
- The risk factors were increased age, male sex, DM, HTN, and smoking.
- Higher incidence of pneumothorax and PTM was found in critically ill, neutrophilic, and lymphopenic patients, those who received tocilizumab, and those who were given positive pressure.
- Macklin effect explains well why the patients with parenchymal lesion developed pneumothorax.
- The timing of onset of pneumothorax was 9 days (0–30 days), duration of air leak was 6 days.
- It had high mortality, for pneumothorax: 57–74%, for PTM: 34–71%.
- Management is as per the protocol for specified pleural diseases, such as thoracocentesis, ICD, or VATS.
- Adherence to COVID-19 therapy as per guidelines at right time with right intervention is necessary to prevent complications related to COVID-19.

REFERENCES

1. Saha BK, Chong WH, Austin A, Kathuria R, Datar P, Shkolnik B, et al. Pleural abnormalities in COVID-19: a narrative review. J Thorac Dis. 2021;13(7):4484-99.
2. Chong WH, Saha BK, Conuel E, Chopra A. The incidence of pleural effusion in COVID-19 pneumonia: state-of-the-art review. Heart Lung. 2021;50(4):481-90.
3. Bao C, Liu X, Zhang H, Li Y, Liu J. Coronavirus disease 2019 (COVID-19) CT findings: a systematic review and meta-analysis. J Am Coll Radiol. 2020;17:701-9.
4. Zhu J, Zhong Z, Li H, Ji P, Pang J, Li B, et al. CT imaging features of 4121 patients with COVID-19: a meta-analysis. J Med Virol. 2020;92:891-902.
5. Ojha V, Mani A, Pandey NN, Sharma S, Kumar S. CT in coronavirus disease 2019 (COVID-19): a systematic review of chest CT findings in 4410 adult patients. Eur Radiol. 2020;30:6129-38.
6. Adams HJA, Kwee TC, Yakar D, Hope MD, Kwee RM. Chest CT imaging signature of coronavirus disease 2019 infection: in pursuit of the scientific evidence. Chest. 2020;158:1885-95.
7. Xie J, Wang Q, Xu Y, Zhang T, Chen L, Zuo X, et al. Clinical characteristics, laboratory abnormalities and CT findings of COVID-19 patients and risk factors of severe disease: a systematic review and meta-analysis. Ann Palliat Med. 2021;10:1928-49.
8. Majidi H, Bani-Mostafavi E-S, Mardanshahi Z, Godazandeh F, Ghasemian R, Heydari K, et al. High-resolution computed tomography finding in 552 patients with symptomatic COVID-19: first report from north of Iran. Emerg Radiol. 2020;27(6):633-9.
9. Liu H, Liu F, Li J, Zhang T, Wang D, Lan W. Clinical and CT imaging features of the COVID-19 pneumonia: focus on pregnant women and children. J Infect. 2020;80(5):e7-13.
10. Zhu T, Wang Y, Zhou S, Zhang N, Xia L. A comparative study of chest computed tomography features in young and older adults with corona virus disease (COVID-19) J Thorac Imaging. 2020;35(4):W97-101.
11. Chen A, Huang JX, Liao Y, Liu Z, Chen D, Yang C, et al. Differences in clinical and imaging presentation of pediatric patients with COVID-19 in comparison with adults. Radiol Cardiothorac Imaging. 2020;2(2):e200117.
12. Blumfield E, Levin TL, Kurian J, Lee EY, Liszewski MC. Imaging findings in multisystem inflammatory syndrome in children (MIS-C) associated with coronavirus disease (COVID-19). Am J Roentgenol. 2021;216(2):507-17.
13. Shaigany S, Gnirke M, Guttmann A, Chong H, Meehan S, Raabe V, et al. An adult with Kawasaki-like multisystem inflammatory syndrome associated with COVID-19. Lancet. 2020;396(10246):e8-10.
14. Toubiana J, Poirault C, Corsia A, Bajolle F, Fourgeaud J, Angoulvant F, et al. Kawasaki-like multisystem inflammatory syndrome in children during the COVID-19 pandemic in Paris, France: prospective observational study. BMJ. 2020;369:m2094.
15. Valverde I, Singh Y, Sanchez-de-Toledo J, Theocharis P, Chikermane A, Filippo SD, et al. Acute cardiovascular manifestations in 286 children with multisystem inflammatory syndrome associated with COVID-19 infection in Europe. Circulation. 2021;143(1):21-32.
16. Rostad BS, Shah JH, Rostad CA, Jaggi P, Richer EJ, Linam LE, et al. Chest radiograph features of multisystem inflammatory syndrome in children (MIS-C) compared to pediatric COVID-19. Pediatr Radiol. 2021;51(2):231-8.
17. Gong X, Song L, Li H, Li L, Jin W, Yu K, et al. CT characteristics and diagnostic value of COVID-19 in pregnancy. PLoS One. 2020;15(7):e0235134.
18. Zhang L, Dong L, Ming L, Wei M, Li J, Hu R, et al. Severe acute respiratory syndrome coronavirus 2 (SARS-CoV-2) infection

during late pregnancy: a report of 18 patients from Wuhan, China. BMC Pregnancy Childbirth. 2020;20(1):394.
19. Gourgoulianis KI, Karantanas AH, Diminikou G, Molyvdas PA. Benign postpartum pleural effusion. Eur Respir J. 1995;8(10):1748-50.
20. Zhou F, Yu T, Du R, Fan G, Liu Y, Liu Z, et al. Clinical course and risk factors for mortality of adult inpatients with COVID-19 in Wuhan, China: a retrospective cohort study. Lancet. 2020;395(10229):1054-62.
21. Chong WH, Saha BK. Relationship between severe acute respiratory syndrome coronavirus 2 (SARS-CoV-2) and the etiology of acute kidney injury (AKI). Am J Med Sci. 2021;361(3):287-96.
22. Han R, Huang L, Jiang H, Dong J, Peng H, Zhang D. Early clinical and CT manifestations of coronavirus disease 2019 (COVID-19) pneumonia. Am J Roentgenol. 2020;215(2):338-43.
23. Wang Y, Dong C, Hu Y, Li C, Ren Q, Zhang X, et al. Temporal changes of CT findings in 90 patients with COVID-19 pneumonia: a longitudinal study. Radiology. 2020;296(2):E55-64.
24. Song F, Shi N, Shan F, Zhang Z, Shen J, Lu H, et al. Emerging 2019 novel coronavirus (2019-nCoV). Radiology. 2020;295(1):210-7.
25. Ding X, Xu J, Zhou J, Long Q. Chest CT findings of COVID-19 pneumonia by duration of symptoms. Eur J Radiol. 2020;127:109009.
26. Zhou S, Wang Y, Zhu T, Xia L. CT features of coronavirus disease 2019 (COVID-19) pneumonia in 62 patients in Wuhan, China. Am J Roentgenol. 2020:214(6):1287-94
27. Xiong Y, Sun D, Liu Y, Fan Y, Zhao L, Li X, et al. Clinical and high-resolution CT features of the COVID-19 infection: comparison of the initial and follow-up changes. Investig Radiol. 2020:55(6):332-9.
28. Cappelli S, Casto E, Lomi M, Pagano A, Gabbrielli L, Pancani R, et al. Pleural effusion in COVID-19 pneumonia: clinical and prognostic implications—an observational, retrospective study. J Clin Med. 2023;12(3):1049.
29. Chong WH, Huggins JT, Chopra A. Characteristics of pleural effusion in severe acute respiratory syndrome coronavirus 2 (SARS-CoV-2) pneumonia. Am J Med Sci. 2021;361(2):281-4.
30. Chen H-R, Zou H, Xue M, Chen Z-B, Chen W-X. A case of childhood COVID-19 infection with pleural effusion complicated by possible secondary mycoplasma pneumoniae infection. Pediatr Infect Dis J. 2020;39(7):e135-7.
31. Mei F, Bonifazi M, Menzo S, Di Marco Berardino A, Sediari M, Paolini L, et al. First detection of SARS-CoV-2 by real-time reverse transcriptase-polymerase chain reaction assay in pleural fluid. Chest. 2020;158(4):e143-6.
32. Hussein M, Haq IU, Hameed M, Thomas M, Elarabi A, Allingawi M, et al. Pleural effusion as an isolated finding in COVID-19 infection. Respir Med Case Rep. 2020;31:101269.
33. Light RW, Macgregor MI, Luchsinger PC, Ball WC. Pleural effusions: the diagnostic separation of transudates and exudates. Ann Intern Med. 1972;77(4):507-13.
34. Hama Amin BJ, Kakamad FH, Ahmed GS, Ahmed SF, Abdulla BA, Mohammed SH, et al. Post COVID-19 pulmonary fibrosis; a meta-analysis study. Ann Med Surg (Lond). 2022;77:103590.
35. Watanabe A, So M, Iwagami M, Fukunaga K, Takagi H, Kabata H, et al. One-year follow-up CT findings in COVID-19 patients: a systematic review and meta-analysis. Respirology. 2022;27(8):605-16.
36. Sanchez-Ramirez DC, Normand K, Zhaoyun Y, Torres-Castro R. Long-term impact of COVID-19: a systematic review of the literature and meta-analysis. Biomedicines. 2021;9(8):900.
37. Zubairi ABS, Shaikh A, Zubair SM, Ali AS, Awan S, Irfan M. Persistence of post-COVID lung parenchymal abnormalities during the three-month follow-up. Adv Respir Med. 2021;89(5):477-83.
38. Datta B, Prakash AK, Yaddanapudi K, Ahlawat K, Tripathy JP, Goyal P, et al. Lung parenchymal abnormalities and outcomes in hospitalized patients with COVID 19 pneumonia: a positive message from a prospective hospital-based longitudinal study for future considerations. Respir Med. 2023;213:107261.
39. Guinto E, Gerayeli FV, Eddy RL, Lee H, Milne S, Sin DD. Post-COVID-19 dyspnoea and pulmonary imaging: a systematic review and meta-analysis. Eur Respir Rev. 2023;32(169):220253.
40. Lan C-C, Hsu H-H, Wu C-P, Lee S-C, Peng C-K, Chang H. Influences of pleural effusion on respiratory mechanics, gas exchange, hemodynamics, and recruitment effects in acute respiratory distress syndrome. J Surg Res. 2014;186(1):346-53.
41. Chen N, Zhou M, Dong X, Qu J, Gong F, Han Y, et al. Epidemiological and clinical characteristics of 99 cases of 2019 novel coronavirus pneumonia in Wuhan, China: a descriptive study. Lancet. 2020;395:507-13.
42. Yang F, Shi S, Zhu J, Shi J, Dai K, Chen X. Analysis of 92 deceased patients with COVID-19. J Med Virol. 2020;92(11):2511-5.
43. Zantah M, Dominguez Castillo E, Townsend R, Dikengil F, Criner GJ. Pneumothorax in COVID-19 disease- incidence and clinical characteristics. Respir Res. 2020;21(1):236.
44. Taha M, Elahi M, Wahby K, Samavati L. Incidence and risk factors of COVID-19 associated pneumothorax. PLoS One. 2022;17(8):e0271964.
45. Yang X, Yu Y, Xu J, Shu H, Xia J, Liu H, et al. Clinical course and outcomes of critically ill patients with SARS-CoV-2 pneumonia in Wuhan, China: a single-centered, retrospective, observational study. Lancet Respir Med. 2020;8:475-81.
46. Udwadia ZF, Toraskar KK, Pinto L, Mullerpatan J, Wagh HD, Mascarenhas JM, et al. Increased frequency of pneumothorax and pneumomediastinum in COVID-19 patients admitted in the ICU: a multicentre study from Mumbai, India. Clin Med (Lond). 2021;21(6):e615-9.
47. Shahsavarinia K, Rahvar G, Soleimanpour H, Saadati M, Vahedi L, Mahmoodpoor A. Spontaneous pneumomediastinum, pneumothorax and subcutaneous emphysema in critically ill COVID-19 patients: a systematic review. Pak J Med Sci. 2022;38(3):730-5.
48. Reddy R, Chen K, Dewaswala N, Tuarez FR, Pino J, Martinez AC, et al. High incidence of spontaneous pneumothorax in critically ill patients with SARS-COV-2. Chest. 2020;158(4):A1191.
49. Li W, Xu S, Li P, Wang G, Wang Z. Pneumothorax in 2019 novel coronavirus pneumonia needs to be recognized. Infection. 2021;49(2):367-8.
50. AlGhamdi Z, Alqahtani SY, AlDajani K, Alsaedi A, Al-Rubaish O, Alharbi A, et al. Pneumothorax in critically ill COVID-19 patients: prevalence, analysis of risk factors and clinical outcomes. Int J Gen Med. 2022;15:8249-56.
51. Ulutas H, Celik MR, Gulcek I, Kalkan M, Agar M, Kilic T, et al. Management of spontaneous pneumothorax in patients with COVID-19. Interact Cardiovasc Thorac Surg. 2022;34(6): 1002-10.

52. Ganessane E, Devendiran A, Ramesh S, Uthayakumar A, Chandrasekar V, Sadasivam AS, et al. Pneumomediastinum in COVID-19 disease: clinical review with emphasis on emergency management. J Am Coll Emerg Physicians Open. 2023;4(2):e12935.
53. Melhorn J, Achaiah A, Conway FM, Thompson EMF, Skyllberg EW, Durrant J, et al. Pneumomediastinum in COVID-19: a phenotype of severe COVID-19 pneumonitis? The results of the United Kingdom (POETIC) survey. Eur Respir J. 2022;60(3):2102522.
54. Macia I, Moya J, Ramos R, Morera R, Escobar I, Saumench J, et al. Spontaneous pneumomediastinum: 41 cases. Eur J Cardiothorac Surg. 2007;31:1110-4.
55. Rajdev K, Spanel AJ, McMillan S, Lahan S, Boer B, Birge J, et al. Pulmonary barotrauma in COVID-19 patients with ARDS on invasive and non-invasive positive pressure ventilation. J Intensive Care Med. 2021;36(9):1013-7.
56. Chopra A, Al-Tarbsheh AH, Shah NJ, Yaqoob H, Hu K, Feustel PJ, et al. Pneumothorax in critically ill patients with COVID-19 infection: incidence, clinical characteristics and outcomes in a case control multicenter study. Respir Med. 2021;184:106464.
57. McGuinness G, Zhan C, Rosenberg N, Azour L, Wickstrom M, Mason DM, et al. Increased incidence of barotrauma in patients with COVID-19 on invasive mechanical ventilation. Radiology. 2020;297:E252-62.
58. Miró Ò, Llorens P, Jiménez S, Piñera P, Burillo-Putze G, Martín A, et al. Frequency, risk factors, clinical characteristics, and outcomes of spontaneous pneumothorax in patients with coronavirus disease 2019: a case-control, emergency medicine-based multicenter study. Chest. 2021;159:1241-55.
59. Wang XH, Duan J, Han X, Liu X, Zhou J, Wang X, et al. High incidence and mortality of pneumothorax in critically Ill patients with COVID-19. Heart Lung. 2021;50:37-43.
60. Ekanem E, Podder S, Donthi N, Bakhshi H, Stodghill J, Khandhar S, et al. Spontaneous pneumothorax: an emerging complication of COVID-19 pneumonia. Heart Lung. 2021;50:437-40.
61. Martinelli AW, Ingle T, Newman J, Nadeem I, Jackson K, Lane ND, et al. COVID-19 and pneumothorax: a multicentre retrospective case series. Eur Respir J. 2020;56:2002697.
62. Wintermark M, Schnyder P. The Macklin effect: a frequent etiology for pneumomediastinum in severe blunt chest trauma. Chest. 2001;120(2):543-7.

INDEX

Page numbers followed by *b* refer to box, *f* refer to figure, *fc* refer to flowchart, and *t* refer to table.

A

B